Cardio-Oncology

Cardio-Oncology
Principles, Prevention and Management

Roberta A. Gottlieb, MD, FACC, FAHA
Professor of Medicine, Director of Molecular Cardiobiology, and
Dorothy and E. Phillip Lyon Chair in Molecular Cardiology
Barbra Streisand Women's Heart Center, Cedars-Sinai Heart Institute
Los Angeles, CA, United States

Puja K. Mehta, MD, FACC
Director of Vascular Function Research Lab, and
Co-Director of Cardio-Oncology Program
Barbra Streisand Women's Heart Center,
Cedars-Sinai Heart Institute
Los Angeles, CA, United States

AMSTERDAM • BOSTON • HEIDELBERG • LONDON • NEW YORK • OXFORD • PARIS
SAN DIEGO • SAN FRANCISCO • SINGAPORE • SYDNEY • TOKYO

Academic Press is an imprint of Elsevier

Academic Press is an imprint of Elsevier
125 London Wall, London EC2Y 5AS, United Kingdom
525 B Street, Suite 1800, San Diego, CA 92101-4495, United States
50 Hampshire Street, 5th Floor, Cambridge, MA 02139, United States
The Boulevard, Langford Lane, Kidlington, Oxford OX5 1GB, United Kingdom

Notices

Knowledge and best practice in this field are constantly changing. As new research and experience broaden our understanding, changes in research methods, professional practices, or medical treatment may become necessary.

Practitioners and researchers must always rely on their own experience and knowledge in evaluating and using any information, methods, compounds, or experiments described herein. In using such information or methods they should be mindful of their own safety and the safety of others, including parties for whom they have a professional responsibility.

To the fullest extent of the law, neither the Publisher nor the authors, contributors, or editors, assume any liability for any injury and/or damage to persons or property as a matter of products liability, negligence or otherwise, or from any use or operation of any methods, products, instructions, or ideas contained in the material herein.

Library of Congress Cataloging-in-Publication Data
A catalog record for this book is available from the Library of Congress

British Library Cataloguing-in-Publication Data
A catalogue record for this book is available from the British Library

ISBN: 978-0-12-803547-4

For information on all Academic Press publications
visit our website at https://www.elsevier.com/

  Working together
to grow libraries in
developing countries

www.elsevier.com • www.bookaid.org

Publisher: Mica Haley
Acquisition Editor: Stacy Masucci
Editorial Project Manager: Sam W. Young
Production Project Manager: Lucía Pérez
Designer: Matthew Limbert

Typeset by Thomson Digital

Cancer and heart failure, two faces of the same deadly coin
One a failure of cellular self-renewal, the other cell growth gone wild
Cancer a problem of cells growing too much
Proliferating amok in lungs bone and such;
Powerful drugs are employed to keep in control
Cancerous stem cells grown too bold.
Treating the cancer may poison the heart
Toxicity and efficacy are parcel and part
Kinase signaling common to both, keeping heart cells alive
And causing cancer cells to replicatively thrive
The heart is a bystander who is stung by the arrows
Of off-target effects meant for bone marrow.
VEGF receptor and tyrosine kinase path blockers
Have serious consequences for the cardiac tick-tocker.
Cancer drugs that drive tumor regression
Inconveniently cause bad hypertension.
Other health issues are present in those who need chemo:
Obesity, atherosclerosis and all problems renal.
Oncologists must remember the tumor's a part
Of a patient who needs an operational heart.
And while the cardiologist might prefer to forbid
Radiation, doxorubicin, and imatinib,
To keep the heart well, we must ensure the cancer will go
Therefore the team must cardio-oncology know.
This book our knowledge of the state of the art
To curing cancer while protecting the heart.

Cancer the wild untrammeled growth
We seek to cure yet abide by our oath
First, do no harm.
In curing one, we cause alarm
The heart throbs and aches
And eventually breaks.
We must take care
To protect the heart and help repair
The damage done
By anticancer guns.

Roberta A. Gottlieb
July 14, 2016

Contents

List of Contributors

A. AlBadri, Barbra Streisand Women's Heart Center, Cedars-Sinai Heart Institute, Los Angeles, CA, United States

Z. Almuwaqqat, Division of Hospital Medicine, Department of Medicine, Emory University, Atlanta, GA, United States

O. Aseyev, Department of Medicine, Division of Medical Oncology, University of Ottawa, The Ottawa Hospital, Ottawa, ON, Canada

A. Asher, Cedars Sinai Medical Center, Los Angeles, CA, United States

S. Asier, Division of Cardiology, Emory University School of Medicine, Atlanta, GA, United States

G. Biasillo, Cardioncology Unit, European Institute of Oncology, IRCCS, Milan, Italy

E. Bronte, Department of Surgical, Oncological and Oral Sciences, Section of Medical Oncology, University of Palermo, Palermo, Italy

P.A. Cahill, Vascular Biology and Therapeutics Laboratory, School of Biotechnology Faculty of Science and Health, Dublin City University, Dublin, Ireland

D. Cardinale, Cardioncology Unit, European Institute of Oncology, IRCCS, Milan, Italy

J. Carver, Abramson Cancer Center of the University of Pennsylvania, Philadelphia, PA, United States

S. Chandra, Abramson Cancer Center of the University of Pennsylvania, Philadelphia, PA, United States

C.M. Cipolla, Cardiology Division, European Institute of Oncology, IRCCS, Milan, Italy

S. Dent, Department of Medicine, Division of Medical Oncology, University of Ottawa, The Ottawa Hospital, Ottawa, ON, Canada

R. Dhingra, The Institute of Cardiovascular Sciences, St. Boniface Hospital Albrechtsen Research Centre, Department of Physiology and Pathophysiology, Max Rady College of Medicine, Rady Faculty of Health Sciences, University of Manitoba, Winnipeg, MB, Canada

J. Dunhill, Cedars-Sinai Medical Center, Los Angeles, CA, United States

M.F. El-Chami, Emory University Hospital Midtown, Division of Cardiology-Section of Electrophysiology, Emory University School of Medicine, Atlanta, GA, United States

J. Engle, University of Texas MD Anderson Cancer Center, Houston, TX, United States

S. Fisher, University of Maryland School of Medicine, Baltimore, MD, United States

V.I. Franco, Department of Pediatrics, Wayne State University School of Medicine, Children's Hospital of Michigan, Detroit, MI, United States

A. Galvano, Department of Surgical, Oncological and Oral Sciences, Section of Medical Oncology, University of Palermo, Palermo, Italy

D. Geft, Cedars-Sinai Heart Institute, Los Angeles, CA, United States

N. Ghosh, Department of Medicine, Division of Medical Oncology, University of Ottawa, The Ottawa Hospital, Ottawa, ON, Canada

P.T. Gleason, Division of Cardiology, Emory University School of Medicine, Atlanta, GA, United States

D. Gupta, Division of Cardiology, Emory University School of Medicine, Atlanta, GA, United States

A. Hage, Cedars-Sinai Heart Institute, Los Angeles, CA, United States

M.A. Hamilton, Cedars-Sinai Medical Center, Los Angeles, CA, United States

O. Hung, Division of Cardiology, Department of Medicine, Emory University, Atlanta, GA, United States

M.M. Johl, Internal Medicine Department, Cedars-Sinai Medical Center, Los Angeles, CA, United States

C. Johnson, Department of Medicine, Division of Medical Oncology, University of Ottawa, The Ottawa Hospital, Ottawa, ON, Canada

L.A. Kirshenbaum, The Institute of Cardiovascular Sciences, St. Boniface Hospital Albrechtsen Research Centre, Department of Physiology and Pathophysiology, Max Rady College of Medicine, Rady Faculty of Health Sciences, University of Manitoba, Winnipeg, MB, Canada

M.M. Kittleson, Cedars-Sinai Heart Institute, Los Angeles, CA, United States

E.P. Kransdorf, Cedars-Sinai Heart Institute, Los Angeles, CA, United States

R.A. Kumbla, Department of Hematology/Oncology Samuel Oschin Comprehensive Cancer Institute Cedars-Sinai Medical Center, Los Angeles, CA, United States

A. Lajoie, Cedars-Sinai Medical Center, Los Angeles, CA, United States

C. Lally, Department of Mechanical and Manufacturing Engineering, School of Engineering, Trinity College Dublin, The University of Dublin, Dublin, Ireland

A. Law, Department of Medicine, Division of Medical Oncology, University of Ottawa, The Ottawa Hospital, Ottawa, ON, Canada

S. Lerakis, Division of Cardiology, Emory University School of Medicine, Atlanta, GA, United States

S.E. Lipshultz, Department of Pediatrics, Wayne State University School of Medicine, Children's Hospital of Michigan, Detroit, MI; Karmanos Comprehensive Cancer Center, Detroit, MI, United States

J.C. Lisko, Division of Cardiology, Emory University School of Medicine, Atlanta, GA, United States

V. Margulets, The Institute of Cardiovascular Sciences, St. Boniface Hospital Albrechtsen Research Centre, Department of Physiology and Pathophysiology, Max Rady College of Medicine, Rady Faculty of Health Sciences, University of Manitoba, Winnipeg, MB, Canada

P.K. Mehta, Division of Cardiology, Emory University School of Medicine, Atlanta, GA, United States

M. Mita, Department of Hematology/Oncology Samuel Oschin Comprehensive Cancer Institute Cedars- Sinai Medical Center, Los Angeles, CA, United States

M. Motwani, Cedars Sinai Medical Center, Los Angeles, CA, United States

R. Moudgil, Department of Cardiology, The University of Texas, MD Anderson Cancer Center, Houston, TX, United States

A. Ng, University of Texas MD Anderson Cancer Center, Houston, TX, United States

G. Novo, Department of Internal Medicine and Cardiovascular Disease, University of Palermo, Palermo, Italy

T.M. Okwuosa, Division of Cardiology, Rush University Medical Center, Chicago, IL, United States

A. Palomo, Rush University Medical Center, Chicago, IL, United States

S. Parashar, Division of Cardiology, Department of Medicine, Emory University, Atlanta, GA, United States

N. Patel, University of Maryland School of Medicine, Baltimore, MD, United States

E.M. Redmond, Department of Surgery, University of Rochester Medical Centre, Rochester, NY, United States

A. Russo, Department of Surgical, Oncological and Oral Sciences, Section of Medical Oncology, University of Palermo, Palermo, Italy

R. Sarbaziha, Barbra Streisand Women's Heart Center, Cedars-Sinai Heart Institute, and Department of Obstetrics and Gynecology, Division of Reproductive Endocrinology and Infertility, Cedars-Sinai Medical Center, Los Angeles, CA, United States

N. Sekhon, Department of Hematology/Oncology Samuel Oschin Comprehensive Cancer Institute Cedars- Sinai Medical Center, Los Angeles, CA, United States

S.L. Shiao, Department of Radiation Oncology, Cedars-Sinai Medical Center, Los Angeles, CA; Department of Biomedical Sciences, Cedars-Sinai Medical Center, Los Angeles, CA; Department of Medicine, University of California, Los Angeles, CA, United States

C.L. Shufelt, Barbra Streisand Women's Heart Center, Cedars-Sinai Heart Institute, and Department of Obstetrics and Gynecology, Division of Reproductive Endocrinology and Infertility, Cedars-Sinai Medical Center, Los Angeles, CA, United States

A. Silver, Rush University Medical Center, Chicago, IL, United States

M.P. Sittig, Department of Radiation Oncology, Cedars-Sinai Medical Center, Los Angeles, CA, United States

B.K. Tamarappoo, Cedars Sinai Medical Center, Los Angeles, CA, United States

R.H. Tank, Internal Medicine Department, Cedars-Sinai Medical Center, Los Angeles, CA, United States

T. Tejada, Electrophysiology Fellow, Emory University, Atlanta, GA, United States

L.E.J. Thomson, Cedars Sinai Medical Center, Los Angeles, CA, United States

D. Wall, Barbra Streisand Women's Heart Center, Cedars-Sinai Heart Institute, and Department of Obstetrics and Gynecology, Division of Reproductive Endocrinology and Infertility, Cedars-Sinai Medical Center, Los Angeles, CA, United States

E.T. Wang, Barbra Streisand Women's Heart Center, Cedars-Sinai Heart Institute, and Department of Obstetrics and Gynecology, Division of Reproductive Endocrinology and Infertility, Cedars-Sinai Medical Center, Los Angeles, CA, United States

J. Wei, Barbra Streisand Women's Heart Center, Cedars-Sinai Heart Institute, Los Angeles, CA, United States

E.T.H. Yeh, Department of Cardiology, The University of Texas, MD Anderson Cancer Center, Houston, TX, United States

Acknowledgments

We are grateful to the countless researchers and clinicians in cardio-oncology who have worked tirelessly to advance research and clinical care in this field. We deeply appreciate the authors for their contribution to this book, dedicated to cancer patients and their families.

Chapter 1

Current Trends in Cancer Therapy

N. Sekhon, R.A. Kumbla and M. Mita

Department of Hematology/Oncology Samuel Oschin Comprehensive Cancer Institute Cedars- Sinai Medical Center, Los Angeles, CA, United States

PI3K/AKT PATHWAY

Multiple studies have demonstrated that cellular development and proliferation are heavily dependent on their microenvironments and access to metabolites and growth factors. There are various signals both extracellular and intracellular that lead to a cascade of regulated events allowing for proliferation and growth. These intricate cascades are often suppressed or overexpressed in cancer biology. The goal of many novel cancer therapies is to exploit these pathways and alter signaling in order to turn off inappropriately activated kinases leading to tumorigenesis [1].

The phosphatidylinositol 3-kinase (PI3K) signaling pathway has been studied since the 1970s since the discovery of Rapamycin (see section, mTOR Pathway). The structure of the phosphatidylinositol and the phosphorylation of different moieties of the inositol ring by the phosphatidylinositol kinase leads to production of different phosphoinositides (PIs). The PIs, such as phosphatidylinositol (4,5) bisphosphate (PIP2) are important lipid messengers that interact with PI3K affecting downstream kinases and phosphatases that regulate cellular proliferation and apoptosis [2]. Thus, alterations and mutations of these kinases can have activating consequences on the pathway, resulting in tumorigenesis, but have also been implicated in other disease, such as cardiac hypertrophy where mouse cardiac myocytes have demonstrated to grow larger in the setting of constitutive PI3K expression [3]. Studies suggested that the PI3K pathway is the most frequently altered in human tumors [4]. Given the complexity of the pathway, the authors will discuss the important aspects that have become clinically relevant. PI3K activation begins with a ligand, such as a growth factor binding to the receptor tyrosine kinase that dimerizes and activates PI3K. The activated PI3K phosphorylates PIP2 and creates phosphatidylinositol (3,4,5) trisphosphate (PIP3). The activated PIP3 then serves to activate phosatidylinositol dependent kinase (PDK1). PDK1 phosphorylates and activates protein kinase B (also known as AKT) which directly regulates many downstream transcription factors via phos-

phorylation, such as FOXO (a family of proapoptotic genes), IKK (family of prosurvival genes), GSK3β (controls cell cycle progression, specifically cyclin D1), mTOR (kinase involved in protein synthesis and cell proliferation), and many others [4]. AKT activation therefore regulates cellular proliferation, nutrition, and survival. The PI3K pathway has multiple checkpoints including regulation by a combined protein/lipid phosphatase known as phosphatase and tensin homolog (PTEN) located on chromosome 10. PTEN protein is known as a tumor suppressor and serves as part of the negative feedback of the PI3K pathway, specifically by dephosphorylating PIP3 [5]. The PTEN gene has been found to be mutated in its phosphatase domain and these mutations and loss of copies of the gene determine activation of the PI3K pathway and were more frequently associated with malignancies, such as prostate cancer, glioblastoma multiforme, endometrial cancer, lung cancer, and even breast cancer. It is important to understand that the PI3K pathway is intertwined with other pathways, such as RAS (family of signal transduction proteins) and Mammalian Target of Rapamycin (mTOR) (see sections, Mitogen-Activated Protein Kinase Pathway and mTOR Pathway, in this chapter).

Idelelasib

Idalalisib, a PI3K small molecule inhibitor, specifically blocks the phosphatidylinositol-4, 5-bisphosphate 3-kinase catalytic subunit delta isoform (PI3Kδ). This drug is targeted specifically for relapsed chronic lymphocytic leukemia (CLL). The pathogenesis for CLL is through the B cell receptor and the PI3K pathway normally regulates this. The subunit PI3Kδ is highly expressed in malignant lymphoid cells, specifically in CLL [6]. As mentioned earlier, the PI3K pathway regulates proliferation and cellular growth and this may be altered with increased expression of this PI3Kδ subunit isoform. It is an oral drug generally started at 150 mg orally given twice daily until disease progression or acceptable toxicity.

Idelalisib has been studied in a phase III trial (Study 116) in which 220 patients with relapsed CLL and other comorbidities precluding standard chemotherapy were split into two arms: Rituximab plus placebo versus Rituximab plus idelalisib. The primary endpoint was progression free survival (PFS). The PFS for Rituximab plus placebo was 5.5 months and the trial was stopped early because of the significant benefit of idelalasib for extending PFS. The overall response was dramatic in the idelalisib group versus placebo group (81% vs. 13%). The secondary endpoint of overall survival in the idelalisib arm versus placebo arm was notable at 12 months (92% vs. 80%; Hazard ratio (HR) for death: 0.28; $p = 0.02$). A subgroup of patients with high-risk disease, harboring a p53 (17p deletion), benefited as well (HR for death 0.14). This PI3K inhibitor opens the door for a new treatment for patients not able to tolerate the older chemotherapeutic regimens and for patients with refractory disease.

There have been fatal or serious hepatotoxicity and diarrhea/colitis in 14% of patients treated with idelalisib. Additionally, fatal or serious neutropenia, pneumonitis, and intestinal perforation have been reported. In the case of any grade III or IV events, idelalisib should be discontinued. 40% of patients in idelalisib group had at least one serious event compared with 35% in the placebo group [7]. While on the drug, patients should be monitored for adverse events, such as leukopenia/neutropenia, anemia, rash, fatigue, and thrombocytopenia.

mTOR PATHWAY

The mTOR pathway was first discovered while researching rapamycin, an inhibitor of mTOR. The pathway serves in transmitting signals that control cell metabolism, growth, and survival. mTOR is a serine/threonine kinase (weight 289-kDa) belonging to the PI3K family. This kinase is part of two important protein complexes known as mTOR complex 1 (mTORC1) and mTOR complex 2 (mTORC2) [8]. mTORC1 involves mTOR being bound to Raptor (regulator associated protein of mTOR) and mTORC2 involves mTOR being bound to Rictor (rapamycin-insenstive companion of mTOR). mTOR signals downstream to mTORC1 leading to protein translation, lipid synthesis, oxygen level regulation, and overall regulation of cell growth. mTORC1 is negatively regulated by Tuberous Sclerosis Complex (TSC). When growth factors, such as insulin increase phosphorylation of TSC via AKT activation, mTORC1 is increasingly activated leading to further downstream effects. Furthermore, mTORC1 has also been implicated in negative feedback of the upstream PI3K pathway further delineating the complexity of these signals [9].

Mutations in TSC are known to cause tuberous sclerosis and are associated with increased rates of certain malignancies (e.g., kidney, brain, and soft tissues). For example, cytokines, such as tumor necrosis factor alpha (TNFα) have been shown to interact with TSC via phosphorylation and thereby inactivate TSC and activate mTORC1. This positive relationship between inflammation and mTORC1 is suggestive of its role in tumor angiogenesis. Additionally, mTOR activates hypoxia induced growth factor 1 alpha (HIF1α) which then stimulates production of VEGF; overexpression of HIF1α is also implicated in angiogenesis. mTOR has various mechanisms of tumorigenesis—via receptor tyrosine kinases, mutation of tumor suppressor genes as well as oncogenes [10]. Researchers have uncovered many details about the regulation and dysregulation of the PI3K/AKT/mTOR intricately intertwined pathways, but there is still a great deal we do not understand, as evidenced by the many targeted therapies that have been tested without significant clinical benefit. There has been some success in exploiting these pathways responsible for tumorigenesis with the development of temsirolimus and everolimus (mTOR inhibitors) as well as idelalisib (PI3K inhibitor).

mTOR Inhibitors

Temsirolimus

Rapamycin (the original mTOR inhibitor) was discovered in the soil in 1975 and used as an antifungal agent. It was soon found to have immunosuppressive properties that led to development of transplant rejection medications [11]. In renal cell carcinoma (RCC) tumors specifically, an overactive mTOR pathway leads to increased levels of HIF1α secondary to mutations in Von Hippel Lindau (VHL) tumor suppressor gene, allowing for increased angiogenesis. Temsirolimus is a prodrug of rapamycin. It has been shown to lead to cell cycle arrest specifically in the G1 phase as well as to inhibit tumor angiogenesis by blocking production of vascular endothelial growth factor (VEGF) [12,13]. Temsirolimus is approved for the treatment of metastatic renal cell carcinoma, although alternative targeted agents (discussed in section Antiangiogenic Agents) are generally preferred for the first and second line treatment.

Temsirolimus was studied in a large phase III trial of 626 previously untreated patients with metastatic renal cell carcinoma randomized to receive interferon alfa versus single agent temsirolimus versus combination therapy of interferon alfa plus temsirolimus. The primary end point of this study was overall survival. The single agent temsirolimus group was found to have a statistically significant overall survival compared to the interferon group (10.9 months vs. 7.3 months). The combination group of interferon and temsirolimus did not confer an advantage and significantly worsened toxicity [14]. Temsirolimus has been studied in the treatment of breast cancer; however, unfortunately it has not been of significant benefit.

The most common adverse events associated with temsirolimus are rash, nausea, edema, and anorexia (affected 30% of patients in the trial). Additionally, common lab abnormalities that are now monitored while on temsirolimus therapy include hyperlipidemia (specifically hypertriglyceridemia), elevated liver enzymes (aspartate transaminase and alkaline phosphatase), hyperglycemia, elevated creatinine, leukopenia, and anemia.

Everolimus

Everolimus is similar to temsirolimus in that it allosterically inhibits the mTOR pathway affecting tumor cell division and angiogenesis. The drug is given orally and generally dosed until disease progression or unacceptable toxicity. Everolimus is approved for the second line treatment of metastatic renal cell carcinoma, treatment of metastatic hormone positive breast cancer, advanced pancreatic neuroendocrine tumors, and subependymal giant cell astrocytoma. Similar to temsirolimus, with the approval of various targeted agents more effective in the treatment of metastatic RCC, use of everolimus in this setting has become less frequent.

The RECORD-1 trial randomized 416 previously treated patients with metastatic RCC to receive everolimus versus placebo plus best supportive care. Patients had been previously treated with sunitinib, sorafenib, or both sequentially. Median progression free survival was significantly improved in the everolimus arm (4.9 months vs. 1.9 months) [15]. Everolimus was compared against sunitinib (refer to VEGF TKI section) for first line treatment of metastatic RCC in the RECORD 3 trial. PFS was worse in the everolimus arm as compared to sunitinib (7.9 months vs. 10.7 months) [16].

Everolimus has been studied for the treatment of a rare tumor known as subependymal giant cell astrocytoma (SEGA) associated with tuberous sclerosis. A trial of 28 patients (age 3 and above) showed a benefit with everolimus in treatment of SEGA. At 6 months, nine patients (32%) had greater than a 50% reduction in tumor volume, and duration of response was a median of 266 days [17]. Given the limited treatment resources in this disease and significant benefit, the FDA granted expedited approved of everolimus for the treatment of SEGA. Subsequent data from the EXIST-1 trial showed similar response rates. The EXIST-2 trial demonstrated everolimus benefit in the treatment of renal angiomyolipomas, a noncancerous tumor also associated with tuberous sclerosis, and was subsequently approved by the FDA for this indication as well [18,19].

Everolimus was originally studied in the BOLERO-1 trial for advanced breast cancer. This study observed women with Human epidermal growth factor receptor 2 (Her2Neu) positive disease receiving trastuzumab (refer to section, Trastuzumab) and weekly Paclitaxel plus or minus everolimus. Unfortunately, results in this study did not reach statistical significance [20]. The approval for

everolimus came from a subsequent BOLERO-2 trial in which 724 postmenopausal women with advanced breast cancer and estrogen receptor positive (ER+), Her2Neu negative hormonal status who had previously failed letrozole and anastrozole were selected to receive everolimus with exemestane versus exemestane alone until time of progression or unacceptable toxicity. At interim analysis, both local investigators and central investigators noted improvement in PFS in the everolimus plus exemestane arm, (6.9 months vs. 2.8 months and 10.6 months vs. 4.1 months, respectively) [21]. Further evaluation of Her2Neu positive disease was examined in BOLERO-3. It is thought that the patients with Her2Neu positive disease develop a resistance to the monoclonal antibody, trastuzumab, after some time, although the mechanism is unclear and may be related to overexpression of the mTOR pathway. The BOLERO-3 trial involved 572 women with locally advanced or metastatic Her2Neu positive breast cancer who had previously progressed through taxane and trastuzumab. Patients were randomized to vinorelbine/trastuzumab plus placebo versus vinorelbine/trastuzumab plus everolimus. The median PFS for the vinorelbine/trastuzumab/everolimus group was 7 months versus 5.78 months for vinorelbine/trastuzumab/Placebo. The difference while statistically significant was marginal and overall survival data is not yet available [22].

Additionally, everolimus has proved beneficial in the realm of pancreatic neuroendocrine tumors (PNET). The Radiant-1 trial included 160 patients with advanced pancreatic neuroendocrine tumors who had progressive disease after cytotoxic chemotherapy. Patients who were not undergoing treatment were started on everolimus (45 patients) and others that were on long-acting octreotide were continued on long-acting octreotide with everolimus. The response rate for everolimus arm was 9.6% and 4.4% for patients receiving both everolimus and long acting octreotide. Median PFS was 9.7 months in the group receiving everolimus and 16.7 months in the arm receiving both everolimus and long acting octreotide [23]. This was followed by the Radiant-3 trial in which patients with advanced pancreatic neuroendocrine tumor (low and intermediate grade) were assigned to everolimus versus placebo. Long-acting octreotide could be used for treatment of symptoms from hormone secretion. In the everolimus arm the PFS was 11 months versus 4.6 months in the placebo arm. Additionally, the VEGF markers in these patients were studied and noted to be lower in the everolimus group suggesting the antiangiogenic effect of mTOR inhibitors. The prognostic value of these markers is yet to be determined [24]. The Radiant-2 trial assessed everolimus given with long-acting octreotide versus placebo with long-acting octreotide alone in advanced low grade or intermediate neuroendocrine tumors (carcinoid). 429 individuals were randomly assigned to each arm (of note 357 discontinued study treatment). Median progression free survival was 16.4 months in the everolimus arm versus 11.3 months in the placebo arm [25].

Everolimus most commonly associated adverse side effects of stomatitis, hypersensitivity pneumonitis, hyperglycemia, anemia, diarrhea, rash, and fatigue. Grade III and IV events were more common with everolimus versus placebo in the above trials. Holding the drug is of greatest benefit in these grade III and grade IV reactions and it is indicated to monitor blood sugars and liver function tests while on everolimus.

MITOGEN-ACTIVATED PROTEIN KINASE (MAPK) PATHWAY

Ras (rat sarcoma virus) oncogenes (HRAS, NRAS, KRAS) encompass a family of GTPases that help with intracellular signaling pathways and control cell growth, differentiation, and apoptosis. They were originally associated with human cancers beginning in 1982. RAS mutations are found in 33% of human malignancies, of which KRAS is the most common mutation especially in relation to lung, colon, and pancreatic cancer [26]. KRAS and its inhibition will be further discussed in the section, EGFR Pathway. The order of activation (Ras → Raf → MEK → ERK) is well studied. Several elements from this pathway represent targets for new therapies. It is also important to note that this pathway is not linear and Ras has other downstream effects on other pathways, such as PI3K pathway [27]. GTPases are active in the GTP bound state and inactive in the GDP bound state. The switching between the two is regulated by guanine nucleotide exchange factors (GEF). Ras is activated through epidermal growth factor (EGF) receptor tyrosine kinase (RTK). The RTK recruits a GEF protein known as Son-of-sevenless (SOS) that promotes the GTP-bound state allowing activation of Ras via RTK [28]. Ras is at the start of the mitogen activated protein kinase pathway (MAPK). The activation of Ras leads to further downstream direct activation of Raf serine/threonine kinase (activated via phosphorylation). Activated Raf subsequently turns on MEK1/2 protein kinase and then leads to activation of ERK1/2 that leads to intranuclear activation of transcription factors [29]. The activation of RAS via GEF is counteracted by GTPase activation proteins (GAP) that promote RAS moving back to a GDP-bound inactive state. With point mutations in the amino acids of the Ras proteins (Gly12 and Gln61), Ras becomes insensitive to GAP and persists in a GTP bound active state, leading to further downstream activation of the MAPK pathway. Ras has been found to be of high importance in cell signaling, given its multiple locations including not only the plasma membrane but also the endoplasmic reticulum, the Golgi apparatus, and the endosomes. This wide distribution reveals how it can have many roles controlling diverse cellular processes [30].

Ras has proven to be difficult to inhibit from a therapeutic standpoint as it transitions rapidly from GDP- to GTP-bound states and has no clear binding pocket where molecules attach. There has been much study in trying to restore the GAP regulation but this has unfortunately not proven fruitful for therapeutic intervention [31]. Therefore, given the difficulty targeting Ras, researchers have begun to focus on the downstream kinases as targets. Some of the promising results will be presented here.

RAF Inhibitors

Raf protein kinase is a family of kinases (A, B, and C). However BRAF has been the protein kinase found to be most frequently associated with malignancies. Specifically BRAF mutations are noted at codon 600 in which the valine residue is replaced with a glutamic acid residue (BRAFV600E) allowing the MAPK pathway to be constitutively activated and resistant to apoptosis [32]. This mutation is most notable in melanoma. Additionally there are other mutations noted at this residue, V600K and V600R, for example; however, these are not as common.

Vemurafenib

Vemurafenib is a selective BRAF kinase inhibitor specifically against the V600 mutation. This drug was studied in the BRIM-3 trial in which 675 patients with metastatic or stage IIIC melanoma were randomly assigned to vemurafenib versus dacarbazine chemotherapy until disease progression. The extended analysis yielded a median OS 13.6 versus 9.7 months and PFS 6.9 months versus 1.6 months in the vermurafenib group and the dacarbazine group, respectively. Specifically looking at the BRAFV600E disease, median OS was 13.3 months versus 10 months in the vermurafenib group versus the dacarbazine group. Of note, it also proved beneficial in the other BRAF mutation V600K [33].

At the time of progression, it was noted the MAPK pathway had further upregulation of expression leading to increased levels of ERK1/2 despite blocking BRAF. This was achieved through upregulation of the RTK, activation of RAS, activating mutations of MEK and several others [34]. This interesting data opened the door to other studies including new ERK inhibitors and combinations.

Dabrafenib

Dabrafenib is a selective BRAF inhibitor and has been studied in patients with stage III or IV melanoma with a BRAF V600E mutation in comparison to dacarbazine. PFS was increased in the dabrafenib group compared to the dacarbazine group (6.7 vs. 2.9 months). Overall survival data did not reach statistical significance but this may have been due to significant crossover allowed from the dacarbazine group to the dabrafenib group [35]. Dabrafenib was first approved for single agent treatment of BRAF V600E mutation positive unresectable or metastatic melanoma. Subsequently, it was FDA approved in combination with trametinib for treatment of BRAF V600E or V600K mutation in unresectable or metastatic melanoma (see section, Combination of MEK and BRAF Inhibitors). The most common adverse events with vemurafenib and dabrafenib were dermatologic in nature including rash, photosensitivity, and hyperkeratosis. Additionally, patients may experience nausea, diarrhea, arthralgias, and significant fatigue. While on these RAF inhibitors, patients have been reported to develop secondary cutaneous toxicities, such as squamous cell carcinomas, keratoacanthomas (25% of cases), and hyperkeratotic lesions. The treatment for most lesions is excision. Nonetheless, given that this can occur relatively early on in therapy, it appears beneficial to involve Dermatology in these patients early on to prevent disruption in RAF therapy at a later time. There are not set guidelines [36]. Specifically, while on vemurafenib, kidney function should be monitored especially in the first 2 months and it should be noted that there have been reports of prolonged QTc intervals with this medication [37]. In different studies, Dabrafenib was shown to have adverse events including febrile reactions and significant hyperglycemia.

Sorafenib

Sorafenib is a *nonselective* BRAF inhibitor and has other targets such as vascular endothelial growth factor (VEGFR) and platelet derived growth factor receptor β (PDGFR). It does not block the BRAF V600E mutation, however. Sorafenib has not been shown to have much benefit as a BRAF inhibitor in melanoma but has proved of some benefit in iodine refractory, locally advanced or metastatic differentiated thyroid cancer that can also have BRAF mutations. The Decision-3 trial demonstrated an improvement in PFS of 10.8 months versus 5.8 months in the Sorafenib versus placebo group, respectively. The drug was tolerated well with most notable reactions being hand foot skin rash, diarrhea, and alopecia [38]. Sorafenib gives another option for benefit given in the arena of metastatic thyroid cancer refractory to iodine therapy; there are very few options for therapy and clinical trial is often preferred.

MEK Inhibitors

Trametinib

Trametinib is a MEK1/MEK2 inhibitor and also shows efficacy in patients with a V600 BRAF mutation. It was initially studied as a single agent therapy in the METRIC trial in which 322 patients with advanced or metastatic melanoma were randomized to trametinib versus chemotherapy with dacarbazine or paclitaxel. All patients were noted to have a V600E or V600K BRAF mutation without prior

BRAF targeted therapy. PFS was significantly improved in the trametinib arm versus chemotherapy (4.8 months vs. 1.5 months).

Toxicities associated with trametinib were pyrexia, acneiform dermatitis, nausea, diarrhea, peripheral edema, uveitis, and rarely a reversible drop in cardiac ejection fraction and central serous retinopathy. No squamous cell carcinoma was observed with this population [39]. Patients receiving trametinib should be closely monitored for visual disturbances and ophthalmology should be involved early on in treatment course to survey visual acuity.

Combination of MEK and BRAF inhibitors

Two phase III trials have evaluated the combination of BRAF inhibitors and MEK inhibitors used together in patients with metastatic melanoma. In the COMBI-d trial, 423 patients with BRAF V600 mutations previously untreated were randomized to dabrafenib with trametinib or dabrafenib alone. The primary endpoint was PFS and results in the combination group versus the dabrafenib alone group, respectively were statistically significant (median 11.0 vs. 8.8 months). Of note, as a secondary endpoint, overall survival was also significant with the combination (median 25.1 vs. 18.7 months). Given the combination of two different MAPK pathway inhibitors, it is conceivable that toxicity would be considerably increased. The most common toxicities were diarrhea, pyrexia, and chills; these were significantly increased (almost double and often grade 3 events) in the combination group [40].

The coBRIM trial is evaluating vemurafenib with cobimetinib (MEK inhibitor) versus vemurafenib with placebo in 495 patients with advanced BRAF V600 mutated melanoma without previous treatment. The updated 14.2 months median follow up results for PFS were presented at the 2015 American Society of Clinical Oncology (ASCO) meeting and the extended analysis revealed 12.25 versus 7.2 months (vemurafenib with cobimetinib vs. vemurafenib with placebo). The adverse events were similarly increased as with the COMBI trial including diarrhea, nausea, photosensitivity, liver toxicity, and serous retinopathy but there were lower rates of squamous cell carcinomas and keratoacanthomas [41,42].

EGFR PATHWAY

Endothelial growth factor receptor (EGFR) is a member of the ErbB family of cell surface receptors known as tyrosine kinases. The ErbB family consists of ErbB4/Her4, ErbB3/HER3, ErbB2/Her2 (described in section, Human Epidermal Growth Factor Receptor 2), and ErBb1/EGFR/Her1. Endothelial growth factor (EGF) and transforming growth factor alpha (TGFα) serve as ligands for EGFR that bind and activate the receptor leading to dimerization. This results in autophosphorylation of tyrosine residues in the C terminal domain of the EGFR. The cascade continues with the activation of downstream MAPK and AKT/PI3K allowing for cellular proliferation [43].

Mutations in EGFR creating unregulated cellular proliferation have been associated most frequently with glioblastoma multiforme, colon cancer, and non-small cell lung carcinoma (NSCLC), particularly lung adenocarcinoma. Approximately 15% of NSCLC adenocarcinoma in the US is EGFR mutated. Patients of Asian descent, females and light or never smokers have increased incidence of the mutation. Thus, EGFR is considered an oncogene for which targeted therapies have been developed.

EGFR Tyrosine Kinase Inhibitors

Gefitinib

Gefitinib is a reversible tyrosine kinase inhibitor (TKI) with high binding affinity for EGFR exon 19 deletions and exon 21 (L858R) substitutions and to a lesser degree for EGFR wild type. Gefinitib was the first EGFR TKI studied in NSCLC. In the IPASS trial 1217 patients with advanced lung adenocarcinoma, of Asian descent and light or never smokers were randomized to receive gefitinib versus carboplatin and paclitaxel. The 12-month progression free rate of gefitinib compared with chemotherapy was found to be significantly better (25% vs. 7%) [44]. Among 437 evaluable patients, 60% had EGFR mutations. Further subgroup analysis noted that patients with EGFR mutations had significantly improved PFS while on gefitinib versus chemotherapy (9.5 vs. 6.3 months). Gefitinib was thus approved by the FDA for patients with metastatic NSCLC harboring and EGFR exon 19 or 21 mutation [45–47].

Erlotinib

Erlotinib is a reversible EGFR TKI that binds to the ATP site of the receptor inhibiting EGFR autophosphorylation, dimerization, and activation of the downstream cascade. Erlotinib has higher binding affinity for EGFR exon 19 deletions and exon 21 mutations. The drug was first studied in the SATURN trial in which 1949 patients with advanced NSCLC received platinum-based therapy followed by randomization of 889 patients without progressive disease to maintenance erlotinib versus placebo. PFS was significantly improved in the erlotinib group versus placebo group (12.3 months vs. 11.1 months, respectively) [48]. After comparison with placebo, erlotinib was compared in the first line metastatic setting against platinum-based chemotherapy in several phase III trials. In the EURTAC trial 174 patients with treatment naïve metastatic lung cancer harboring an EGFR exon 19 deletion or exon 21 substitution were randomized to receive erlotinib versus platinum-based chemotherapy. Erlotinib was associated with improved PFS (9.7 months vs. 5.2 months). Erlotinib has thus been approved as first line therapy for EGFR mutated advanced or metastatic NSCLC, refractory NSCLC, and as maintenance therapy for NSCLC [49].

Afatinib

Afatinib is an irreversible TKI that binds to the intracellular tyrosine kinase domain of EGFR, ErB2/Her2 and ErB4/Her4. In the Lux-Lung 3 trial 345 treatment naïve patients with metastatic EGFR mutated lung adenocarcinoma were randomized to afatinib versus cisplatin with pemetrexed resulting in an improved PFS (11.1 months—afatinib vs. 6.9 months—chemotherapy) [50]. Afatinib has been studied with similar results in the Lux-Lung 6 trial and meta-analysis of these trials revealed that afatinib improved overall survival in patients with exon 19 deletion but not L858R mutations. Afatinib is approved as first line treatment for patients with metastatic NSCLC harboring an EGFR exon 19 deletion or exon 21 substitution [51].

Resistance to these tyrosine kinase inhibitors has been demonstrated but is not completely understood. One mechanism is acquired mutation of EGFR that reduce binding of the TKI; the most common mutation is a substitution at the 790 position of methionine for threonine (T790M) [52]. Osimertinib is an irreversible EGFR TKI that binds to mutated EGFR with an exon 19 deletion, exon 21 substitution or T790M mutation and is currently the only approved TKI for metastatic NSCLC with an acquired T790M mutation. There are currently ongoing phase I/II studies looking into rociletinib as a therapy that may have activity in T790 mutated EGFR tumors [53]. Thus far there is no role for EGFR inhibitors combined with chemotherapy given trials without any significant overall survival [54].

Erlotinib, gefitinib, and afatinib are recommended as first line therapy for EGFR mutated metastatic lung cancer and should be continued until the patient experiences symptomatic disease progression. Progression of disease with one EGFR targeted agent does not preclude use of another agent in the same class or possible reuse at a later point in treatment. Osimertinib may be used in cases of disease progression due to acquired T790M mutation. Common side effects of these tyrosine kinase inhibitors include diarrhea, acneiform rash, and liver toxicity. Fatal lung toxicity was reported with erlotinib and gefitinib in the above trials.

EGFR Monoclonal Antibodies

EGFR activation has multiple downstream effects specifically on the RAS pathway. Mutations in the KRAS or NRAS members of the RAS family lead to constitutive activation of the RAS pathway and resultant cellular proliferation. KRAS mutations occur in 35–40% of patients with metastatic colorectal cancer, most commonly at exon 2. In colon cancer, KRAS wild type tumors have been shown to be responsive to targeted EGFR therapies [55,56].

Panitumumab

Panitumumab is a monoclonal antibody that binds to and prevents EGFR activation. Panitumumab combined with chemotherapy (FOLFIRI-5 fluorouracil, leucovorin, irinotecan) versus chemotherapy alone (5 fluorouracil, leucovorin, irinotecan) was studied in 1186 patients with metastatic colorectal cancer who had been treated with one prior regimen. Approximately 55% of patients had KRAS WT tumors and this subgroup of patients experienced an improvement in median PFS (5.9 months vs. 3.9 months, respectively) [57]. In the PRIME trial patients with RAS wild type metastatic colorectal cancer treated with FOLFIRI plus panitumumab had a PFS benefit compared to FOLFIRI alone (10.1 months vs. 7.9 months); however, it was found that despite KRAS exon 2 WT, mutations in KRAS exons 3,4 or NRAS exons 2, 3, or 4 conferred resistance to EGFR inhibition [58]. Panitumumab is approved for the treatment of metastatic RAS WT colorectal cancer in the first, second, or third line setting in combination with oxaliplatin- or irinotecan-based chemotherapy.

Cetuximab

Cetuximab is a monoclonal antibody which competitively binds to EGFR resulting in receptor internalization. The drug has been evaluated in the CRYSTAL trial in which patients with untreated metastatic colorectal carcinoma with EGFR overexpression (by immunohistochemistry) were randomized to FOLFIRI plus cetuximab versus FOLFIRI alone. There was a significant benefit in OS (23.5 vs. 20 months, respectively) and PFS (9.9 vs. 8.4 months, respectively). There have been subsequent trials OPUS and CELIM with conflicting data in which results are mixed with regards to PFS benefit with cetuximab in combination with an oxaliplatin-based regimen [59]. Cetuximab has also demonstrated activity in the treatment of metastatic head and neck squamous cell carcinoma. Currently Cetuximab is approved for the treatment of metastatic RAS WT colorectal carcinoma in combination with an irinotecan- or oxaliplatin-based regimen as well as metastatic head and neck carcinoma in combination with a platinum-based regimen or as a single agent.

Similar to TKIs, both panitumumab and cetuximab are associated with acneiform rash and diarrhea. Additionally, these agents are uniquely associated with significant hypomagnesemia and hypokalemia likely due to renal tubular dysfunction but the complete mechanism is not understood [60].

HUMAN EPIDERMAL GROWTH FACTOR RECEPTOR 2

Her2 (Neu, ERB2) is a member of the ErbB receptor tyrosine kinase family of proteins that are structurally related to EGFR. These proteins include Her1 (EGFR, ErbB1), Her2 (Neu, ERbB2), Her3 (ErbB3), and Her4 (ErbB4). The receptors exist as monomers on the cell membrane and include an extracellular binding domain, transmembrane domain, and intracellular domain with tyrosine kinase activity. Upon ligand binding, the receptors form homo- or heterodimers resulting in cross phosphorylation and tyrosine kinase mediated downstream signaling. Activated signaling pathways include PI3-K/Akt, MAPK, PLC-PKC, and JAK/STAT which results in cellular differentiation, proliferation, inhibition of apoptosis, and enhanced survival [61].

Her2 is a proto-oncogene located on chromosome 17q21 encoding the Her2 transmembrane tyrosine kinase receptor. In contrast to other members of the ErbB family, Her2 has no natural ligand and remains in a constitutively open conformation. Her2 acts as the preferred coreceptor for heterodimerization with Her1, Her3, and Her4. In particular, Her3 expression is commonly seen with Her2 and their dimerization has been identified as the most mitogenic in the Her family through enhanced PI3K signaling [62]. Her3 expression may also be a means of tumor cell developed resistance to Her2 blockade. Additionally, when Her2 is overexpressed it can undergo ligand independent activation via spontaneous homodimerization and autophosphorylation.

Her2 overexpression may occur through gene amplification or polysomy and is seen in a variety of malignancies including breast, gastric, ovarian, and head and neck carcinoma. Her2-directed therapy can target the ligand, extracellular or intracellular domains of the receptors, and downstream pathways. Development of novel targeted agents against Her2 has drastically changed patient management and outcomes particularly in the field of breast cancer where Her2 overexpression is identified in approximately 15–20% of patients. Currently, there are four FDA approved therapies targeting Her2, three of which are monoclonal antibodies and one small molecule tyrosine kinase inhibitor [63,64].

Trastuzumab

Trastuzumab is a recombinant humanized IgG1 monoclonal antibody targeting the extracellular portion of the Her2 receptor. This down regulates Her2 activity by preventing homo or heterodimerization, increasing endocytic destruction of the receptor, inhibiting shedding of the extracellular domain, and by inhibiting proliferation of cells overexpressing Her2 [64]. Trastuzumab is currently approved for the treatment of Her2 overexpressed breast cancer in the neoadjuvant, adjuvant, and metastatic setting and metastatic gastric cancer. The drug may be administered as a single agent or in combination with various chemotherapeutic agents and or antihormonal therapy.

Trastuzumab was the first FDA approved Her2 targeted agent after demonstrating activity in combination with paclitaxel in patients with metastatic breast cancer. A study in patients with Her2 overexpressed metastatic breast cancer randomized to receive standard chemotherapy alone (adriamycin and cyclophosphamide or single agent paclitaxel) or with trastuzumab demonstrated an increased PFS of 7.4 months versus 4.6 months in patients receiving trastuzumab [65]. Joint analysis of two studies NCCTG N9831 and NSABP B-31 demonstrated a 37% relative improvement in overall survival and increase in 10 year survival rate from 75.2% to 85% in patients who received adjuvant adriamycin and cyclophosphamide followed by paclitaxel and trastuzumab versus adriamycin and cyclophosphamide followed by paclitaxel alone in adjuvant setting [66]. A subsequent trial compared adjuvant adriamycin and cyclophosphamide followed by paclitaxel with or without trastuzumab and adjuvant docetaxel, carboplatin, and trastuzumab in patients with Her2 overexpressed breast cancer. Both trastuzumab containing arms were found to have improved overall survival compared to the chemotherapy only arm; however, the docetaxel, carboplatin, and trastuzumab arm had lower incidence of congestive heart failure (0.2% vs. 4%) and reduction in ejection fraction (EF) [67]. The HERA trial supported the continuation of trastuzumab for 1 year in the adjuvant setting versus 2 years where no added benefit was gained and there was greater cardiac toxicity [68]. Subsequently the PHARE trial confirmed that superiority of continuation of trastuzumab for 1 year in the adjuvant setting over 6 months [69]. Based upon these results, trastuzumab therapy is standard of care for treatment of localized Her2 positive breast cancer in the neoadjuvant or adjuvant setting in combination with adriamycin and cytoxan followed by paclitaxel or with taxotere and carboplatin with or without pertuzumab. Additionally, trastuzumab is continued after chemotherapy to complete in total 1 year of Her2 directed therapy. In the metastatic setting, trastuzumab is recommended first line with pertuzumab and taxotere or paclitaxel. Traztuzumab therapy may be continued with different chemotherapeutic agents after disease progression.

Trastuzumab is also approved for first line treatment of metastatic Her2 overexpressed gastric or gastroesophageal junction adenocarcinoma in combination with cisplatin and 5FU-based chemotherapy. This was based upon the results of the ToGA study which demonstrated an overall survival benefit of 13.8 months in the trastuzumab arm versus 11.1 months in the chemotherapy only arm [70].

Trastuzumab is generally well tolerated and the most common adverse effects are fever, fatigue, headache, diarrhea, rash, and infusion reactions. Significant toxicities associated with the medication are rare pulmonary toxicity and cardiotoxicity. Her2 signaling is involved in myocardial homeostasis and trastuzumab associated cardiotoxicity is typically an asymptomatic decrease in left ventricular ejection fraction (LVEF). Unlike cardiotoxicity associated with anthracyclines which cause permanent myocyte injury, cardiac dysfunction from trastuzumab is not dose dependent and may be associated with a reversible loss of contractility [71]. On a retrospective review of seven phase II and III trials containing trastuzumab, cardiac dysfunction was greatest in patients receiving a concomitant anthracycline (27%) versus concomitant paclitaxel (13%) or trastuzumab alone (3–7%). The majority of patients who developed cardiac toxicity were symptomatic; however, the majority (79%) showed improvement with appropriate management [72]. Additional risk factors for the development of trastuzumab associated cardiotoxicity include hypertension, age over 50 years, and diabetes mellitus. Treatment consists of conventional congestive heart failure management. It is recommended prior to the initiation of trastuzumab that all patients have a baseline echocardiogram. Frequency of further monitoring is not standardized, however, generally consists of repeat echocardiograms done every 3–6 months. The medication should be held for any patient developing symptomatic heart failure or asymptomatic heart failure with a significant decline in EF. After a month of medical management, treatment may be reinitiated should the patient's symptoms and EF improve. While trastuzumab induced cardiac dysfunction during adjuvant treatment may result in discontinuation of the medication, it is generally accepted in the metastatic setting that the benefit of continuation of therapy may outweigh the risk in patients with an asymptomatic decrease in EF [71].

Pertuzumab

Pertuzumab is a recombinant humanized monoclonal antibody targeting the extracellular dimerization domain of Her2. This inhibits Her2 dimerization with Her1, Her3, and Her4, and downstream activation of the PI3K and MAPK pathways. Specifically, pertuzumab counters increased Her2 and Her3 dimerization signaling associated with trastuzumab resistance and is used in combination with trastuzumab and chemotherapy. Pertuzumab is approved for the first line treatment of Her2 overexpressing metastatic breast cancer and for neoadjuvant and adjuvant treatment of Her2 positive breast cancer.

Pertuzumab is approved in combination with trastuzumab and docetaxel for the first line treatment of Her2 positive metastatic breast cancer. This was based upon the results of the CLEOPATRA study which demonstrated a progression free survival benefit of 7 months (19 vs. 14 months) in the pertuzumab containing arm. At study completion, the pertuzumab containing arm also demonstrated an overall survival benefit of 56.5 months versus 40.8 months. The combination Her2 blockade arm experienced greater toxicities of fatigue, rash, neutropenia, and diarrhea; however, there was no increase in incidence of decreased LVEF [73]. Accelerated approval for pertuzumab for Her2 positive breast cancer in the neoadjuvant setting was granted based upon results of the NeoSphere trial. Patients were randomized to receive four neoadjuvant cycles of A (trastuzumab plus docetaxel), B (pertuzumab and trastuzumab plus docetaxel), C (pertuzumab and trastuzumab), or D (pertuzumab plus docetaxel). Patients in the pertuzumab and trastuzumab plus docetaxel arm had a significantly improved pathologic complete response rate of 45.8% vs. 29% (A), 24% (C), and 16.8% (D) in the other arms, respectively. No increase in cardiac toxicity was seen in the combination Her2 blockade arms [74]. The TRY-PHAENA study was designed to evaluate the cardiac tolerability of neoadjuvant pertuzumab and trastuzumab given with standard anthracycline or platinum-based neoadjuvant chemotherapy for Her2 positive breast cancer. Patients were randomized to receive: A. 5-fluorouracil, epirubicin, cyclophosphamide (FEC) with pertuzumab and trastuzumab 3 times cycles followed by docetaxel plus pertuzumab and trastuzumab (THP) 3 times cycles; B. FEC 3 times followed by THP 3 times cycles; or C. docetaxel and carboplatin plus pertuzumab and trastuzumab 6 times cycles followed by surgery and adjuvant trastuzumab for 1 year. The primary end points of symptomatic of left ventricular systolic dysfunction (LVSD) and decline in EF greater than or equal to 10% were low and similar across all arms with overall 2 of 225 patients experiencing symptomatic LVSD and 11 of 225 experiencing a significant decline in EF. Furthermore, the secondary endpoint of pathologic CR was encouraging and similar across all arms ranging from 57% to 66% [75]. The most common adverse events associated with pertuzumab are fatigue, rash, and diarrhea. Combination pertuzumab and trastuzumab has not been shown to increase cardiac toxicity.

Lapatinib

Lapatinib is a small molecule dual tyrosine kinase inhibitor that has intracellular activity against both Her1 and Her2. Lapatinib potently and reversibly binds to the tyrosine kinase domain of Her1 and Her2 to prevent downstream MAPK and P13K signaling cell proliferation and survival [76]. Unlike the large monoclonal antibodies targeting the Her2 pathway, lapatinib is able to cross the blood–brain barrier and has demonstrated activity in patients with brain metastasis. Lapatinib is approved in combination with capecitabine for the treatment of metastatic Her2 overexpressed breast cancer after prior treatment with an anthracycline, taxane and trastuzumab. This was based upon a study comparing combination lapatinib and capecitabine versus capecitabine alone in patients with metastatic Her2 positive breast cancer previously treated with an anthracycline, taxane, and trastuzumab. Patients in the combination group had an increase in PFS by 4 months (8.4 months vs. 4.4 months) [77]. Combination therapy with lapatinib and trastuzumab for patients with metastatic Her2 positive

breast cancer with disease progression on prior trastuzumab therapy has also demonstrated superiority to treatment with lapatinib alone [78].

Similar to other tyrosine kinase inhibitors, toxicities associated with lapatinib include fatigue, palmar plantar erythrodysesthesia, rash, and diarrhea. In particular, lapatinib has been associated with severe deadly hepatotoxicity in less than 1% of patients. Cardiac toxicity associated with lapatinib is infrequent. A pooled analysis of 3,689 patients in clinical trials who had received lapatinib revealed an asymptomatic cardiac event in 1.4% of patients and symptomatic CHF in 0.2% of patients. The majority of cardiac events were reversible asymptomatic decreases in EF and the incidence did not increase when lapatinib was given after prior anthracycline or trastuzumab therapy [79]. Similar to treatment with trastuzumab or pertuzumab, baseline echocardiogram is recommended prior to initiation of lapatinib therapy and periodically during treatment. The medication should be held for symptomatic CHF or significant decline in EF for a minimum of two weeks. Subsequently, lapatinib may be resumed at a reduced dose.

Ado Trastuzumab Emtansine

Ado Trastuzumab Emtansine (T-DM1) is an antibody drug conjugate linking trastuzumab to the chemotherapeutic agent DM1. DM1 is a derivative of maysantine, a potent microtubule inhibitor associated with treatment-limiting diarrhea, neuropathy, and fatigue impeding its early clinical development. However, given as a conjugate with trastuzumab, DM1 is selectively delivered to tumor cells and thus better tolerated. T-DM1 binds to the extracellular domain of Her2 with the same potency as trastuzumab. This complex is subsequently endocytosed allowing for intracellular cytotoxic DM-1 activity and cell cycle arrest [80]. T-DM1 is approved for use in patients with Her2 overexpressed metastatic breast cancer previously treated with a taxane and trastuzumab. This was based upon the EMILIA study which randomized patients with Her2 positive metastatic breast cancer previously treated with trastuzumab and a taxane to receive T-DM1 or lapatinib and capecitabine. Patients receiving T-DM1 had an improved progression free survival of 9.6 versus 6.4 months and median overall survival of 30.9 months versus 25.1 months as well as a higher objective response rate. Consequently, T-DM1 is often that preferred second line agent for treatment of Her2 metastatic breast cancer over lapatinib [81]. The most common adverse events associated with T-DM1 are transaminase elevations and thrombocytopenia. Cardiac toxicity is rarely associated with T-DM1 and 97.1% of patients receiving T-DM1 in the EMILIA studied maintained an EF greater than or equal to 45%. Baseline echocardiogram and periodic monitoring is recommended.

ANAPLASTIC LYMPHOMA KINASE PATHWAY

The anaplastic lymphoma kinase (ALK) fusion gene codes for an oncogenic tyrosine kinase protein with constitutive activity resulting in cellular proliferation and enhanced survival. This gene has is a key oncogenic driver in certain lymphomas, in a subset of patients with non-small-cell lung cancer (NSCLC) and is mutually exclusive of an EGFR mutation. ALK gene fusion mutations are present in the vast majority (60–80%) of patients with anaplastic large cell lymphoma while point mutations occur in a subset (8–9%) of patients with neuroblastoma. ALK mutations have also less frequently been identified in esophageal squamous, colon, and anaplastic thyroid cancers. Approximately 2–7% of patients with metastatic NSCLC harbor an ALK mutation and these patients tend to be nonsmokers and have adenocarcinoma histology [82]. The development of targeted therapy for treatment of ALK mutated NSCLC has drastically changed the management and clinical course for these patients.

ALK is a transmembrane protein receptor with intracellular tyrosine kinase activity and is part of the insulin receptor tyrosine kinase family. Echinoderm microtubule associated protein-like 4 (EML4) is a cytoplasmic protein required for microtubule formation. The EML4 and ALK genes are closely located on the short arm of chromosome 2. A characteristic inversion of the short arm of chromosome 2 inv(2)(p21p23) results in a fusion EML4-ALK gene encoding a protein with the 5′ amino terminal half of EML4 ligated to the 3′ intracellular tyrosine kinase receptor region of ALK. The EML4 portion of the protein contains a coiled-coil domain that mediates the constitutive dimerization and thus activation of the tyrosine kinase receptor portion of ALK. ALK mediates signaling via the Ras/MAPK, P13K, Jak/STAT, and PLC gamma pathways resulting in cellular proliferation, differentiation, and survival. There are multiple variants of the EML4-ALK fusion gene, formed from exon 20 of the ALK gene joined with variable truncations of the EML4 gene (at exons 2,6,13,14,15,18, and 20). These all contain the tyrosine kinase domain of ALK and the coiled coil domain of EML4 [83–85].

Crizotinib

Crizotinib is a small molecule multitargeted tyrosine kinase receptor inhibitor targeting ALK, MET, and ROS1 kinases. By inhibiting ALK tyrosine kinase activity, crizotinib inhibits cell proliferation, induces G1-S phase cell cycle arrest and apoptosis [86]. Crizotinib is approved for the first line treatment of metastatic NSCLC with an ALK mutation.

The PROFILE 1007 trial compared crizotinib to chemotherapy in patients with metastatic ALK mutated NSCLC who had disease progression on prior platinum-based chemotherapy (docetaxel or pemetrexed) [87]. Patients in the crizotinib arm had an improved progression free survival of 7.7 months versus 3 months and a response rate of 65% versus 20%. There was no benefit in overall survival, likely because of the crossover design. Subsequently the PROFILE 1014 trial randomized patients with previously untreated metastatic ALK mutated NSCLC to receive crizotinib or standard first line chemotherapy with carboplatin and pemetrexed. The crizotinib arm had an improved progression free survival of 3.9 months (10.9 months vs. 7.0 months) and an objective response rate of 74% vs. 45% [88]. Retrospective analysis of clinical trials with crizotinib has revealed poor intracranial response rates and overall poor central nervous system penetration [89].

The most common adverse events associated with crizotinib are vision disorder, diarrhea, and edema. The majority of adverse effects are grade 1 and grade 2, with grade 3 and 4 toxicities being infrequent and most often transaminase elevations or neutropenia. Crizotinib is also associated with QT prolongation and bradycardia. QT prolongation has been observed however without associated arrhythmias. Patients should have baseline and periodic monitoring of EKGs and electrolytes. Bradycardia is typically grade 1 or 2 and is asymptomatic sinus bradycardia without associated EKG changes [90].

Despite promising response rates, tumors inevitably acquire resistance to crizotinib, usually within 1 year. Mechanisms of resistance include mutations in ATP binding pocket of the tyrosine kinase domain of ALK. Specific mutations include G1202R, S1206Y which result in decreased binding capacity of crizotinib, L1196M gatekeeper mutation, G1269A and 1151Tins which affects the affinity of ALK to ATP. Tumors may also develop resistance via amplification of ALK and bypassing the pathway via aberrant activation of other kinase signaling pathways such as KIT, KRAS, and EGFR [91]. Second generation ALK inhibitors have been developed to overcome crizotinib resistance.

Ceritinib

Ceritinib is a second generation small molecule tyrosine kinase activity with increased ALK selectivity approximately 20 times more potent than crizotinib. The chemical structure of ceritinib is modified so that it has activity against several ALK resistance mutations including L1196M, G1269A, and S1206Y. Ceritinib does not however overcome the G1202R ALK resistance mutation [92]. Ceritinib is approved for the treatment of metastatic ALK mutated NSCLC in patients who are unable to tolerate or have progressed on prior crizotinib therapy.

Ceritinib received accelerated approval for the treatment of ALK mutated metastatic NSCLC after disease progression on crizotinib based upon the results of the ASCEND 1 trial. In this trial, patients who had previously received crizotinib for metastatic ALK mutated NSCLC had an overall response rate of 56% and median progression free survival of 6.9 months [93]. Ceritinib is fairly well tolerated with most frequent adverse effects being grade 1 to 2 nausea, vomiting, diarrhea, and fatigue. Grade 3 and 4 toxicities reported were most commonly a rise in liver function tests and diarrhea. Serious adverse effects include pneumonitis and interstitial lung disease. Concentration dependent QTc prolongation has also been reported.

ANTIANGIOGENIC AGENTS

Tumor angiogenesis allows for supply of oxygen, nutrients, growth factors, and tumor dissemination to distant sites. Sprouting vessels are formed from existing blood vessels through the proliferation of endothelial progenitors into the surrounding matrix in response to an angiogenic stimulus. Angiogenesis is regulated by pro and antiangiogenic molecules and tumors cells develop a "switch" angiogenic phenotype during which proangiogenic mechanisms overwhelm negative regulation [94]. As a result endothelial cells are switched from a resting state to a rapid growth phase. Pro-angiogenic molecules upregulated during this process include vascular endothelial growth factor (VEGF), fibroblast growth factor 2 (FGF-2), interleukin-8 (IL-8), placental growth factor (PIGF), transforming growth factor beta (TGF beta), and platelet derived growth factor (PDGF) among others. The switch may also cause downregulation of negative regulatory molecules, such as endostatin, angiostatin, or thrombospondin [95]. As such, tumor angiogenesis has long been an area of interest for targeted therapy.

VEGF PATHWAY

The vascular endothelial growth factor pathway is the predominant regulator of physiologic and pathogenic angiogenesis. Activation of the pathway results in endothelial cell survival, migration, differentiation, and mobilization of endothelial progenitor cells from the bone marrow to the peripheral circulation [94]. VEGF activation also results in increased vascular permeability and secretion of proteases involved in extracellular matrix degradation thus facilitating endothelial cell migration. The pathway is highly regulated by hypoxia which results in increased production of VEGF and neoangiogenesis. Under normal conditions, autocrine release of VEGF by endothelial cells maintains vascular homeostasis [96]. However, as malignant cells grow and central tumor cells become hypoxic, paracrine VEGF release in response to hypoxia results in tumor angiogenesis [97].

The VEGF family of angiogenic and lymphoangiogenic growth factors is comprised of the six glycoproteins VEGF-A, VEGF-B, VEGF-C, VEGF-D, VEGF-F, and PIGF [94]. These growth factors may be produced by a variety of cells and act exclusively on endothelial cells. VEGF-A is the predominant growth factor involved in angiogenesis and studied for targeted therapy. VEGF proteins bind to specific receptors on endothelial cells with intracellular tyrosine kinase activity known as vascular endothelial growth factor receptors (VEGFR). VEGF-A binds to VEGFR1 (Flt-1) and VEGR2 (Fflk-1/KDR), which is coupled with the coreceptor neuropilin 1 (NRP1). VEGFR2 plays the central role in mediating angiogenesis stimulated by VEGF-A, and activating mutations in VEGFR2 have been associated with vascular tumors. VEGFR1 has weak tyrosine kinase activity and its role in angiogenesis is unclear. Signaling activity of VEGFR1 and 2 promote vasculogenesis while VEGFR3 promotes lymphangiogenesis. Several additional growth factors, transcription factors, oncogenes, and tumor suppressor genes, including RAS, Her2, PTEN, and p53 have also been implicated in increased VEGF expression.

Tumor cells, stroma, or endothelial cells may secrete VEGF-A. Through alternative RNA splicing, several isoforms of the various VEGF proteins exist. Smaller isoforms are freely excreted and promote vessel enlargement while larger isoforms remain in the extracellular matrix and stimulate vessel branching. VEGF-A isoforms include 121, 165, 189, and 206 amino acids. VEGF 165 is the predominant isoform and is overexpressed in several solid tumors [98]. VEGF-B and PIGF also bind to VEGF1, while VEGF-E binds to VEGFR2. VEGF-C and VEGF-D bind to VEGFR3 (Flt-4) and its coreceptor NRP-2. Tip cells, or the leading cells on an angiogenic sprout, express higher levels of VEGFR3. Tissue hypoxia results in stabilization of hypoxia inducible transcription factor (HIF1α) which binds to the VEGF promoter, causing increased VEGF transcription.

VEGF Monoclonal Antibodies

Bevacizumab

Bevacizumab is a humanized IgG monoclonal antibody targeting VEGF-A. The drug irreversibly binds to all isoforms of VEGF-A, inhibiting binding of the ligand to VEGFR1 or VEGFR2, thus preventing and causing regression of tumor neovascularization. It may also improve the delivery of concurrent chemotherapy by normalizing tumor vasculature [99]. Efficacy of bevacizumab was first demonstrated in the treatment of metastatic colorectal cancer. Since that time it has gained approval for first line treatment of metastatic non squamous NSCLC, first line treatment of metastatic renal cell carcinoma, treatment for recurrent platinum resistant epithelial ovarian, fallopian tube and primary peritoneal carcinoma, recurrent or persistent metastatic cervical carcinoma, and for the treatment of glioblastoma in the second line setting.

Bevacizumab is approved for the first and second line treatment of metastatic colorectal cancer based upon the results of several large studies. The AVF2107g trial randomized 813 patients with treatment naive metastatic colorectal carcinoma to receive IFL (irinotecan, leucovorin, and 5-fluorouracil) alone or in combination with bevacizumab.

Overall survival (20.3 vs. 10.6 months) and progression free survival (15.6 vs. 6.2 months) were significantly improved in the bevacizumab arm versus the chemotherapy only arm. Additionally, the bevacizumab arm had an overall response rate of 44.8% versus 34.4% in the chemotherapy only arm [100]. Since this time, other chemotherapeutic regimens have emerged as superior to IFL and bevacizumab is often added to these (FOLFOX4: 5-fluorouracil/oxaliplatin; FOLFIRI: 5-fluorouracil/oxaliplatin/irinotecan; 5FU/LV: 5-fluorouracil/leucovorin). The E3200 trial compared FOLFOX 4 with bevacizumab versus FOLFOX 4 alone versus bevacizumab alone in patients with metastatic colorectal carcinoma previously treated with a fluoropyrimidine and irinotecan. Patients in the combination arm had an improvement in overall survival of 12.9 versus 10.8 months in the chemotherapy arm and 10.2 months for bevacizumab alone. Overall response rates were 22.7% versus 8% versus 3.3% [101]. The ML18147 trial evaluated use of bevacizumab in combination with second line chemotherapy in patients with metastatic colorectal cancer who had progressed on first line bevacizumab based treatment. Patients receiving second line bevacizumab were found to have a median overall survival benefit of 11.2 versus 9.8 months in the chemotherapy only arm [102]. Based upon this, bevacizumab may also be continued in the second line setting; however, if the tumor is KRAS wild type, targeted therapy with an EGFR antibody is generally preferred.

Bevacizumab is also approved for treatment in the first line setting for locally advanced, recurrent or metastatic nonsquamous NSCLC in combination with carboplatin and paclitaxel. This was based upon the E4599 trial in which the addition of bevacizumab resulted in a two months overall survival benefit [103]. Bevacizumab was approved for treatment of metastatic renal cell carcinoma after a study demonstrated that bevacizumab combined with interferon alpha versus interferon alone resulted in a three month improvement in progression free survival [104]. Phase II trials have also demonstrated efficacy of bevacizumab in second line treatment of glioblastoma.

Bevacizumab therapy is frequently associated with hypertension and proteinuria. Hypertension is often medically managed and proteinuria in nephrotic range is rare. Significant toxicities associated with bevacizumab include hemorrhage, poor wound healing, thrombosis, and cardiac dysfunction. Hemorrhage and bleeding has been particularly associated lung squamous cell histology leading to the use of bevacizumab in nonsquamous NSCLC only. Caution should also be used in patients with pretreatment hemoptysis or brain metastases. By inhibiting neovascularization, treatment also impairs wound healing. Thus the medication should be discontinued 28 days prior to a procedure and resumed 28 days post procedure. Bevacizumab has also been associated with increased risk of thromboembolism, particularly in patients greater than the age of 65 and with

prior thrombus [105]. Use of the medication in patients with existing thrombus on anticoagulation is generally avoided. Anti-VEGF therapy has also been associated with congestive heart failure for which the medication should be discontinued. Use in patients with preexisting congestive heart failure is not studied.

Ramucirumab

Ramucirumab is a fully human IgG1 monoclonal antibody targeting VEGFR2 thus inhibiting downstream signaling promoting angiogenesis. Ramucirumab is approved for treatment of advanced gastric or gastroesophageal carcinoma in the second line setting where it has demonstrated efficacy both as monotherapy and in combination with paclitaxel [106]. The REGARD trial compared best supportive care plus placebo versus ramucirumab. Patients receiving ramucirumab had a modest overall survival benefit of 1.4 months (5.2 vs. 3.8 months) [107]. Subsequently, the RAINBOW trial randomized patients with advanced gastric or gastroesophageal junction carcinoma who had progressed on prior platinum or 5 FU based therapy to receive weekly paclitaxel days 1, 8 and 15 of a 4 week cycle with or without ramucirumab. Patients who received ramucirumab had an overall survival benefit of 2.2 months (9.6 vs. 7.4 months) [108]. Most recently ramucirumab was approved for the second line treatment of NSCLC in combination with docetaxel and second line treatment of metastatic colorectal cancer after disease progression on combination therapy with bevacizumab. In both cases the addition of ramucirumab resulted in a modest overall survival benefit of 1.4 and 1.6 months, respectively [109,110]. Similar to bevacizumab, common toxicities associated with ramucirumab include hypertension and proteinuria. Significant side effects include hemorrhage, obstruction, and thromboembolic events. Gastrointestinal perforation is rare.

VEGF Tyrosine Kinase Inhibitors

Tyrosine kinase inhibitors are oral small molecules with intracellular activity against multiple protein kinases including VEGFR. These drugs competitively inhibit tyrosine kinase activity by binding to the ATP binding site of the receptors. By inhibiting VEGFR and PDGFR these medications act as antiangiogenic agents. Additionally, by inhibiting other protein kinases, such as c-kit, RAS, and RET, treatment also targets tumor cell proliferation. Tyrosine kinase inhibitors have activity in various malignancies, most notably renal cell carcinoma of clear cell histology, sarcoma, medullary thyroid carcinoma, hepatocellular carcinoma, and colorectal cancer.

Sunitinib

Sunitinib is an oral multityrosine kinase inhibitor with activity against the stem cell factor receptor (c-kit), PDGFR alpha, beta, VEGFR-1,2,3, colony-stimulating factor 1 receptor (CSF1R), and fms-like tyrosine kinase receptor (FLT3). Studies have shown that sunitinib has the best binding potency for VEGFR and PDGFR [111].

A large phase III study demonstrated superior efficacy of sunitinib over interferon alpha for treatment naive metastatic clear cell renal cell carcinoma with a 4 month improvement in progression free survival (11 vs. 6 months) and response rate of 31% (vs. 6%). Sunitinib was also better tolerated than interferon alpha [112]. A trial comparing sunitinib to placebo for treatment of unresectable imatinib-resistant gastrointestinal stromal tumor (GIST) showed a 21 week improvement in time to tumor progression, leading to its approval [113]. Sunitinib was subsequently approved for the treatment of advanced well differentiated neuroendocrine carcinoma. This was based upon a study comparing continuous dosing of sunitinib versus placebo with somatostatin analogs continued at investigators discretion. The trial was discontinued early as more serious adverse events were observed in the placebo arm and the sunitinib arm was found to have a progression free interval of 11.4 versus 5.5 months in the placebo [114]. Sunitinib is approved for use in first line treatment of metastatic renal cell carcinoma, advanced pancreatic neuroendocrine tumor, and GIST after disease progression or intolerance to imatinib.

Sorafenib

Sorafenib is a small oral serine threonine and tyrosine kinase inhibitor that has activity against VEGF-2,3 PDGFR beta, c-kit, FLT-3, Raf, and RET. As such, angiogenesis is inhibited through targeting VEGF and PDGFR while cell proliferation is targeted through the RAF pathway. Sorafenib is currently approved for the second line treatment of advanced renal cell carcinoma, unresectable hepatocellular carcinoma, and advanced thyroid carcinoma unresponsive to treatment with radioactive iodine ablation.

Sorafenib has been studied in multiple different tumor types with notable advances in advanced hepatocellular carcinoma and renal cell carcinoma. The SHARP trial evaluated patients with nonsurgical hepatocellular carcinoma with Child Pugh liver function class A cirrhosis and randomized them to sorafenib versus placebo. An improved overall survival was demonstrated in the sorafenib arm versus placebo arm (10.7 vs. 7.9 months, respectively). Significant adverse events included diarrhea and palmar plantar erythrodysesthesia [115]. The drug's FDA approval does not specify patient Child Pugh class, however there is limited safety data in the more advanced B and C classes. Smaller studies including patients of Childs Pugh class B often had more adverse events and shorter time to progression [116]. The TARGET trial randomized 903 patients with advanced renal cell carcinoma and disease progression after prior cytokine therapy to receive sorafenib versus placebo. Median PFS was notably longer in sorafenib group compared with

placebo (5.5 vs. 2.8 months). A second analysis of this trial also noted increased benefit of sorafenib therapy in previously treated elderly patients, specifically those greater than 70 years old [117].

Pazopanib

Pazopanib is a second generation tyrosine kinase inhibitor targeting VEGFR1, VEGFR2, VEGFR3, PDGFR alpha, PDGFR beta, FGFR1, FGFR2, c-kit, and with modest activity against c-FMS1. Pazopanib works through ATP competitive inhibition of tyrosine kinase activity and is approved for the treatment of therapy naïve advanced renal cell carcinoma and advanced sarcoma after disease progression on chemotherapy.

The approval of pazopanib for treatment of advanced or metastatic renal cell carcinoma is based upon a large study comparing pazopanib versus placebo in patients with advanced clear cell renal carcinoma who were untreated or had progressed on prior cytokine treatment. The primary end point of the study revealed a 5 month increase in progression free survival (9.2 vs. 4.2 months) [118]. The PISCES III study demonstrated noninferiority of pazopanib in comparison to sunitinib for treatment of advanced renal cell carcinoma. Subsequent studies comparing pazopanib and sunitinib for the treatment of advanced renal cell carcinoma have yielded a similar progression free survival; however, better tolerability and quality of life were reported by patients on the pazopanib arm. Patients who received sunitinib experienced more fatigue, palmar plantar erythrodysesthesia, thrombocytopenia, and decreased quality of life versus patients who received pazopanib and experienced increased transaminitis [119]. Results of the PALETTE trial demonstrated efficacy of pazopanib in metastatic soft tissue sarcomas of various subtypes (excluding GI stromal tumors) who had disease progression on prior anthracycline-based chemotherapy. Median progression free survival in the pazopanib arm was 4.6 months compared to 1.6 months for the placebo arm. There was no statistically significant difference in overall survival [120].

Axitinib

Axitinib is a second generation tyrosine kinase inhibitor with greater selective inhibition of VEGF1, VEGF2, and VEGF3 only. Axitinib has a higher potency of inhibition in comparison to first generation tyrosine kinase inhibitors or pazopanib which may contribute to its better therapeutic window and decreased incidence of adverse effects. Axitinib is approved for the second line treatment of advanced renal cell carcinoma

The AXIS trial compared axitinib versus sorafenib for the second line treatment of patients with advanced renal clear cell carcinoma. Patients receiving axitinib were found to have a statistically significant improvement in progression free survival of 6.7 versus 4.7 months and an increase in response rate and stable disease. There was no difference in overall survival [121].

Vandetinib

Vandetinib is a tyrosine kinase inhibitor with activity against VEGF2, VEGF3, EGFR, RET, and to a lesser extent VEGF1. Vandetinib is approved for the treatment of symptomatic or progressive advanced, unresectable medullary thyroid carcinoma. The ZETA trial randomized patients with advanced medullary thyroid carcinoma to receive vandetinib versus placebo. At time of analysis, the progression free survival had not been reached for the vandetinib arm, with a predicted 30.5 versus 19.3 months in the placebo arm. Overall survival data was immature [122]. The vandetinib arm experienced considerable more toxicity, with the majority requiring a dose reduction. Vandetinib was also associated with QTc prolongation and torsades de pointes.

Cabozantinib

Cabozantinib is a small molecule tyrosine kinase inhibitor targeting VEGF1, 2, cMET, and RET. The EXAM trial demonstrated a progression free survival of 11.2 months in patients receiving cabozantinib versus 4.0 months in the placebo arm [123]. Cabozantinib is approved for the treatment of progressive metastatic medullary thyroid cancer.

Regorafenib

Regorafenib inhibits multiple kinases including VEGF1, VEGF2, VEGF3, PDGFR, FGFR involved in tumor angiogenesis and KIT, RET, RAF-1, BRAF involved in oncogenesis. Regorafenib is approved for the treatment of metastatic colorectal carcinoma refractory to several prior lines of treatment including fluoropyrimidine, oxaliplatin, or irinotecan-based chemotherapy with an VEGR inhibitor and anti-EGFR therapy if KRAS wild type. The COR-RECT study evaluated patients with metastatic colorectal carcinoma and disease progression on prior lines of therapy received regorafenib versus best supportive care. The regorafenib arm had an overall survival of 6.4 versus 5 months [124]. Regorafenib is also approved for third line treatment of advanced GIST after disease progression on imatinib or sunitinib.

IMMUNOTHERAPY

The immune system plays a pivotal role in the regulation of tumor growth. Due to multiple somatic mutations and epigenetic dysregulation, tumor cells produce foreign antigens that may be recognized and eliminated through immune surveillance [125]. However, it is clear that the relationship between the immune system and cancer cells is complex. Under the pressure of immune surveillance, tumor cells develop means to evade and exploit the immune response and thus proliferate. This is done through several mechanisms including downregulation of tumor associated antigens, exploitation of immune checkpoint pathways, and development of resistance. Additionally, expanding tumors contain tumor infiltrating lymphocytes that are rendered ineffective by suppressive elements in the tumor microenvironment, such as regulatory T cells, myeloid-derived suppressor cells, soluble factors, VEGF, TGF beta, and ligands for T cell coinhibitory receptors [126,127].

Immunotherapy aims at boosting the innate and adaptive immune response against proliferating tumor cells. Traditionally therapy has been geared toward increasing tumor-specific adaptive immunity as a means to establish long-term memory and durable response. Approaches to do so include administration of therapeutic vaccines, tumor specific monoclonal antibodies, and adoptive transfer of tumor-specific activated T or NK cells. Although promising, until recently the majority of these techniques have not yielded exciting results [128]. With the advent of immune checkpoint inhibition a new era in cancer treatment has begun and interest in immune therapy has been revitalized.

Cancer Vaccines

Cancer vaccines have long been viewed as a means of increasing tumor specific T and B cells, thus bolstering adaptive immunity. Tumor specific T cells serve the dual purpose of reducing tumor cell proliferation and acting as memory T cells that can control tumor relapse. Various immunization strategies have been employed and antigens may be in the form of whole tumor cells, peptides, proteins, recombinant viruses, or DNA/mRNA encoding tumor antigens [129,130]. Dendritic cells are the most potent antigen presenting cells and serve to bridge innate and adaptive immunity. Optimal T cell activation occurs when the tumor specific antigen is presented by dendritic cells which provide the proper costimulatory signals. Tumor-associated antigens may be delivered alone to activate dendritic cells in vivo or loaded ex vivo onto antigen presenting cells, such as dendritic cells.

Sipuleucel-T

Sipuleucel-T is an autologous dendritic cell vaccine that is produced by exposure and activation of the patient's peripheral blood mononuclear cells to PAP (prostate acid phosphatase), a tumor associated antigen. The activated dendritic cells are then infused back into the patient where they travel to lymph nodes and present processed antigen to T cells along with costimulatory signals to develop an immune response.

Sipuleucel-T was approved based upon the results of the IMPACT trial including patients with minimally symptomatic metastatic castrate resistant prostate cancer randomized

2:1 to receive either sipuleucel-T or placebo. There was a modest but statistically significant improvement in the primary endpoint of median overall survival of 25.8 months in the vaccine group versus 21.7 months in the placebo arm. However, sipuleucel-T did not improve progression free survival and rarely induced disease regression or changes in PSA level [131]. Sipuleucel-T was approved by the FDA in 2010 for the treatment of asymptomatic or minimally symptomatic metastatic castrate resistant prostate cancer and remains the only FDA approved cancer vaccine to date.

Adoptive T Cell Immunotherapy

Adoptive T cell immunotherapy involves ex vivo activation and expansion of tumor specific T lymphocytes which are infused into cancer patients. Several sources for T lymphocytes have been used including tumor infiltrating lymphocytes (TIL), engineered T cells which express a cancer specific T cell receptor (TCR), and engineered T cells expressing a chimeric antigen receptor (CARs) [126]. TILs are isolated from patient tumor samples and expanded ex vivo. However, there is often difficulty obtaining adequate amounts of TILs and the procedure is costly. Subsequently, use of engineered T cells was explored via transfer of tumor antigen-specific TCR genes into T cells isolated from the peripheral blood. These genetically engineered T cells are cultured and expanded in vitro prior to adaptive transfer. CAR modified T cells express an immunoglobulin based fusion protein. This fusion protein is composed of an extracellular targeting site, (often the antigen reactive portion of the immunoglobulin chains), fused with the T cell intracellular signaling domain. While TCRs target specific HLA complexes, CAR T cells recognize antigens independent of HLA complexes thus have the added benefit of a larger spectrum of tumor antigen recognition. Lymphodepletion, to deplete negative regulators of TILs, such as regulatory T lymphocytes (TREGs), prior to adoptive T cell transfer or concomitant use of IL-2 have also been used to improve efficacy [126,129].

Although adaptive T cell immunotherapy has shown promise, particularly for the treatment of metastatic melanoma, synovial sarcoma and cervical cancer, significant toxicity which is amplified by coadministration of IL-2 remains. Additionally, lymphodepletion prior to T cell administration causes a brief period of neutropenia at which time patients are at increased risk for infection. Sepsis is the main cause of a 1–2% rate of treatment-related mortality with T cell administration following lymphodepletion. Similar to IL-2, adoptive T cell therapy results in a cytokine release syndrome resembling sepsis with symptoms of fever, vascular leak syndrome, hypotension, oliguria, and possible multiorgan failure. Autoimmune type symptoms may develop if adoptive T cells react with normal tissue. Life-threatening toxicities have been reported when adoptive T

cells react with an unrecognized antigen at a critical site or unexpectedly develop specificity for antigens other than the prespecified target. Life-threatening toxicities are managed with high dose steroids, alemtuzumab and variably the addition of suicide genes to transferred T cells [132].

Immune Checkpoint Blockade

While previous immune therapy has focused on enhancing adaptive immunity, it has become clear that these methods are inadequate to maintain an effective antitumor response. Most recently, immune checkpoint inhibitors have yielded promising results in historically treatment-resistant malignancies. Immune checkpoint pathways exist as a means to dampen T cell activity to prevent autoimmunity and maintain immunologic homeostasis. Tumor cells hijack these pathways in order to evade immune regulation by downregulating T cell activity [133]. Checkpoint blockade uses monoclonal antibodies to reactivate T cells and recover their antitumor activity. Currently, antibodies targeting two immune checkpoint pathways—cytotoxic T lymphocyte associated antigen 4 (CTLA 4) and programmed death receptor 1 (PD1)—have been employed for various malignancies.

Antibodies targeting negative T cell regulatory pathways of CTLA-4 and PD-1 help to reactivate immune surveillance against foreign tumor antigens. CTLA-4 (CD165) is a cell surface protein is expressed and up regulated on activated CD4+ T cells. CTLA-4 inhibition occurs largely in the lymphoid organs. Mechanisms of CTLA-4 inhibitory activity are competitive binding for costimulation, negative signaling, and B7.1 and B7.2 transcytosis. CTLA-4 has a 10–100-fold higher affinity for and competes with CD28 for binding to B7.1 and B7.2. Once a T cell is activated CTLA-4 is upregulated and binds to B7 to dampen T cell activity [134]. PD-1 is a T cell surface receptor protein activated by ligands PDL-1 and PDL-2. Activation of the PD1 pathway promotes T cell death. T cell activity is restored with monoclonal blockade of CTLA4 and PD1 (anti-PD-1 and anti-CTLA4).

CTLA-4 Inhibition

Immune activation involves the complex interaction of antigen presenting cells (APC), such as dendritic cells with T cells and requires specific costimulatory pathways. Antigen presenting cells recognize, process, and display tumor antigens on major histocompatibility complex (MHC) molecules. This also results in the expression of B7.1 (CD80) and B7.2 (CD86) proteins on the APC cell surface. These cells subsequently migrate to lymph nodes with resting T cells. Helper T cell activation requires not only interaction between the MHC class II and tumor cell receptor (TCR) but also costimulation via interaction between B7.1 and B7.2 with CD28 on T cells. Activation of CD4+ T cells results in secretion of cytolytic enzymes perforin and granzyme, cytokines, such as TNF alpha, interferon gamma, and IL-2, resulting in proliferation and recruitment of immunoregulatory cells [133,135]. CTLA 4 (CD165) is a cell surface protein expressed on CD4+ T cells that competitively binds B7.1 and B7.2 to downregulate T cell activity.

Activation of CTLA-4 results in transduction of inhibitory signals through protein phosphatases and there is suggestion that CTLA-4 may compete with CD28 for activation of the PI3K pathway. It has also been postulated the CTLA-4 results in phosphorylation and attenuation of TCR activity. Additionally, CTLA-4 on TREGS removes B7.1 and B7.2 from APCs and internalizes them into the T cell to prevent helper T cell activation [135].

Ipilimumab

Ipilimumab is an IgG1 CTLA-4 monoclonal antibody approved for treatment of unresectable or metastatic melanoma. Ipilimumab was the first checkpoint inhibitor initially developed after preclinical studies in the mid-1990s revealed increased T cell response with CTLA-4 inhibition. Ipilimumab is approved for the treatment of unresectable or metastatic melanoma at a dose of 3 mg/kg and in the adjuvant setting for stage III disease at 10 mg/kg. The MDX010-20 trial randomized patients to receive ipilimumab plus a peptide vaccine glycoprotein 100 (gp100), ipilimumab alone or gp100 alone in patients with previously treated metastatic melanoma. Median overall survival was 10 months in the ipilimumab arms versus 6.4 months in the gp100 arm. More impressively, 20% of patients in the ipilimumab arm were alive at 3 years, with the longest reported survival reaching 10 years [136]. Subsequently the CA 184-024 trial was published, comparing ipilimumab to traditional chemotherapy in patients with treatment naïve BRAF wild type unresectable or metastatic melanoma. Patients were randomized to receive ipilimumab followed by dacarbazine or dacarbazine alone with placebo. Median overall survival was significantly longer in the ipilimumab group by 2 months (11.2 vs. 9.1 months). Similarly 28.8% of patients in the ipilimumab arm were alive at 3 years opposed to 12.2% in the dacarbazine arm [137]. In both trials, the ipilimumab arms experienced greater toxicity, with grade 3 and grade 4 reactions being seen in approximately 50% of patients in the CA 184-024 trial. As seen in previous trials with checkpoint inhibitors, toxicities were largely autoimmune in nature with the most common being rash, colitis, diarrhea, and nausea. In the EORTC 1871 trial, patients with stage III melanoma who had undergone wide local excision followed by axillary lymph node dissection were randomized to adjuvant ipilimumab versus placebo. Ipilimumab was given at a dose of 10 mg/kg every 3 weeks for four doses followed by every 3 months for up to 3 years. PFS was 26.2 months in the ipilimumab group versus 17.1 months with a trend toward benefit in patients with more advanced or stage IIIC disease. There was, however, a significant amount of treatment toxicity, with a 52% discontinuation rate secondary to adverse events and 5 treatment related deaths (3 due to colitis, 1 due to myocarditis, 1 due to Guillain-Barre syndrome) [138].

Ipilimumab has also been studied for use in other malignancies, specifically in metastatic castrate resistant prostate cancer and in combination with GVAX (granulocyte-macrophage colony-stimulating factor) for pancreatic cancer. While a phase III study showed no benefit in metastatic castrate resistant prostate cancer, ipilimumab has shown promising results for NSCLC and pancreatic cancer. Another CTLA-4 blocking antibody, tremelimumab had encouraging results in initial studies for treatment of metastatic melanoma; however, it failed to improve overall survival in a phase III study. Despite that, tremelimumab is being studied in several malignancies including hepatocellular carcinoma, mesothelioma, and colorectal cancer [139].

PD1/PDL1/PDL2 Inhibition

PD1 (programmed cell death 1, CD279) is an immunoglobulin cell surface protein expressed on activated T cells, B lymphocytes, and macrophages. PD1 is a member of the CD28/CTLA-4 family of T cell regulators and is composed of an extracellular IgV domain, transmembrane region and intracellular tail containing phosphorylation sites. Activation of PD1 recruits tyrosine phosphatases SHP-1 and SHP-2 resulting in signaling events which deactivate the TCR complex and promote apoptosis of activated T cells while reducing apoptosis of Tregs [134].

The ligands identified for PD1 are members of the B7 family, PDL1 (B7H1, CD274) and PDL2 (B7DC, CD273). PDL1 is expressed on various hematopoietic and tissue cells and is highly inducible by interferon gamma. PDL2 is almost exclusively expressed by antigen presenting dendritic cells. Thus, PDL1 expression is seen in several tumor types while PDL2 expression is less common. Tumor cell PDL1 expression may be driven by interferon gamma secretion by the tumor microenvironment or oncogenic production of excess PDL1. In contrast to CTLA4, PD1 has more of a role in modulating T cell activity in peripheral tissues and organs during inflammatory responses to prevent host tissue damage. Additionally, while CTLA-4 plays a role earlier in the process of T cell deactivation, PD1 plays a role later in this process after T cells have migrated to the tumor microenvironment [133]. Monoclonal antibodies have been developed against PD1, thus disrupting the interaction with ligands PDL1 or PDL2, and against PDL1, thus blocking its binding to PD1. There is evidence that PDL-1 also binds to B7.1 downregulate T cell activation.

Nivolumab

Nivolumab is an IgG4 fully human antibody targeting PD1 that is approved for unresectable or metastatic melanoma, metastatic NSCLC after platinum-based chemotherapy, and metastatic renal cell carcinoma in the second line setting, at a dose of 3 mg/kg. In Checkmate 037, patients with metastatic melanoma previously treated with CTLA-4 or BRAF inhibition if BRAF mutated were randomized to receive nivolumab or chemotherapy (dacarbazine or carboplatin plus paclitaxel). The study yielded an overall response rate of 38% in the nivolumab arm versus 5% in the chemotherapy arm with a longer median duration of response [140]. CheckMate 066 compared nivolumab to dacarbazine in patients with previously untreated BRAF wild type advanced melanoma. Patients treated with nivolumab had an improved overall survival for 73% at 1 year versus 42% on the dacarbazine arm [141]. In CheckMate 017, patients with metastatic squamous NSCLC with disease progression on platinum-based chemotherapy were randomized to receive nivolumab or docetaxel. Median overall survival was 9.3 months in the nivolumab versus 6 months in the docetaxel [142]. Additionally, nivolumab was better tolerated. CheckMate057 randomized 588 patients with nonsquamous NSCLC with disease progression on prior platinum-based therapy to receive nivolimab versus taxotere. Patients in the nivolumab arm experienced improved OS (12.2 vs. 9.4 months) regardless of PDL1 expression and with less toxicity than observed in the taxotere arm [143]. In CheckMate 25, 821 patients with metastatic renal cell carcinoma and disease progression on 1–2 prior antiangiogenic agents were randomized to receive nivolumab versus everolimus. Median OS was 25 months in the nivolumab arm versus 19.6 months in the everolimus arm [144].

Pembroluzimab

Pembroluzimab is a humanized IgG4 monoclonal antibody to PD1 approved for treatment of metastatic melanoma and for PDL1 positive advanced NSCLC at a dose of 2 mg/kg. In KEYNOTE 002 trial, 540 patients with ipilimumab refractory advanced melanoma were randomized to receive pembroluzimab 2 mg/kg every 2 weeks, 10 mg/kg every 2 weeks, or chemotherapy. The pembroluzimab arms had 6 month progression free survivals of 34% and 38% as opposed to 16% in the chemotherapy arm. The 2 mg/kg and 10 mg/kg dose of pembroluzimab had similar efficacy [145]. The KEYNOTE 010 study randomized patients with previously treated PDL1 positive (greater than 1% by immunohistochemistry) NSCLC to receive pembroluzimab 2 mg/kg versus 10 mg/kg every 2 weeks versus docetaxol. Median OS was 10.4 and 12.7 months in the pembroluzimab arms versus 8.5 months in the docetaxel arm, respectively [146]. Use of pembroluzimab is also being investigated in head and neck, esophageal, colorectal, and ovarian carcinoma [147].

Toxicities of Immune Checkpoint Inhibitions In keeping with their mechanism of action, the toxicities of checkpoint inhibition are T cell mediated autoimmune events. Normal tissue damage occurs due to increased cytokine release from CD4 helper T cells and increased migration of cytolytic CD8 T cells. It is important that the practitioner be able to recognize and treat these side effects in a timely manner. The most common adverse events of any grade for all checkpoint inhibitors are rash, fatigue and pruritus. Other toxicities include colitis, pneumonitis, drug related hepatitis and autoimmune mediated endocrinopathies, such as thyroiditis, hypophysitis, and adrenal insufficiency. Rare immune related hematologic and neurologic toxicities, such as encephalitis, Guillain-Barre syndrome, autoimmune thrombocytopenia, and leukopenia may occur. In general, dermatologic and GI toxicity is seen early, while liver toxicity and endocrinopathies are seen later in the treatment course. Most adverse events are seen by week 24 and may take longer to resolve for PD1/PDL1 inhibition than with CTLA4 inhibition, requiring a steroid taper. Patients receiving immune checkpoint inhibitors should have routine complete blood counts, liver function tests, metabolic panel, and thyroid function tests at intervals of 6–12 months continuing until 6 months posttreatment. Adrenocorticotropic hormone, cortisol, and testosterone may be checked for symptoms of fatigue or nonspecific symptoms [132].

Checkpoint inhibitors should be held and steroids initiated for any grade 3 or 4 or prolonged grade2 adverse event. Initiation of steroids has not been associated with decreased response and it is not uncommon for continued response after drug withdrawal. Colitis is more common in ipilimumab occurring in 6–14% of patients versus less than 1% of patients receiving PD1 inhibition. Obstruction and bowel perforation remain life-threatening complications of severe colitis. High dose steroids should be immediately initiated and if symptoms do not improve within three days or relapse after steroid taper, infliximab should be given. Pneumonitis is less common with ipilimumab than with PD1 blockade, where patients may present with shortness of breath, fevers, chest pain, and diffuse infiltrates on chest X-ray. Treatment with high dose steroids typically results in resolution of symptoms; however time to recovery may be prolonged. Although there is evidence that thyroid function may improve with time, endocrinopathies are for the large part irreversible. Combination CTLA4 and PD1/PDL1 blockade results in similar autoimmune toxicities with additive effect [132,139].

Monitoring Response in Checkpoint Inhibition It has become clear that the traditional Response Evaluation Criteria in Solid Tumors (RECIST) do not adequately reflect immune checkpoint response [133]. Patients may initially have evidence of disease progression (tumor enlargement) but ultimately achieve disease response, which is known as pseudo-progression. Additionally, a reduction of total tumor burden despite appearance of new lesions may be observed. Consequently, an alternative means of assessing response known as the immune related response criteria (iRC) has been established. Progressive disease by iRC is defined as a greater than or equal to 25% increase in tumor burden including new lesions added to tumor burden and requires confirmation on repeat interval imaging at least 4 weeks apart to differentiate from pseudo-progression.

Combination Therapy

Combination CTLA4 and PD1/PDL1 inhibition is now being explored. It has been established that PD1/PDL1 inhibition is effective after disease progression on CTLA4 inhibition. Additionally, CTLA4 inhibition occurs early in the immune response in the lymphatics while PD1/PDL1 inhibition occurs later at the site of the tumor microenvironment, thus they may work synergistically. Most recently, this has been demonstrated in CheckMate 067 which compared combination therapy with ipilimumab and nivolumab and nivolumab alone versus ipilimumab alone in patients with BRAF wild type advanced melanoma. Patients in both the combination and nivolumab arm were found to have an improvement in progression free survival of 11.5 and 6.9 months opposed to 2.9 months in the ipilimumab alone arm. Specifically patients with low PDL1 tumor expression had greater benefit from combination therapy [148]. This supports the concept that administration of a CTLA-4 inhibitor can activate peripheral T cells and recruit them to the tumor microenvironment, thus increasing tumor immunogenicity and response to PD1/PDL1 inhibition

Future Directions

The use of immune checkpoint inhibitors is undergoing evaluation is several malignancies including NSCLC, prostate cancer, ovarian cancer, urothelial carcinoma, cholangiocarcinoma, Hodgkins lymphoma, and colorectal cancer among others. Immune checkpoint inhibition may be more effective in malignancies with a high mutational burden as is seen in melanoma and lung cancer, as these tumors have a more immunogenic or inflammatory tumor microenvironment. It has been demonstrated that patients with microsatellite instability (MSI) high colorectal cancers and thus higher mutational burden attain greater benefit from PD1 blockade than patients with intact mismatch repair [147].

As the role of immune checkpoint inhibition continues to broaden, several issues remain to be explored and delineated. Specifically, the optimal dose and scheduling of these medications remains unclear. The role of biomarkers to identify patients most likely to benefit from checkpoint inhibition is also undergoing study. Furthermore, the standardization of such assays remains to be determined [139]. There has also been a significant concern in use of nivolumab and ipilimumab especially in combination due to increased cost. As the increasing use of these medications is anticipated, these issues remain to be clarified.

CYCLIN DEPENDENT KINASES AND THEIR PATHWAYS

The cell cycle has long been known to have multiple checkpoints that allow a cell to transition from growth phase (G1) to replication phase (S) to division phase, mitosis (M).

These checkpoints are a family of proteins known as cyclin dependent serine/threonine kinases (CDK) and are activated by the binding of different cyclins. Furthermore, it has also been discovered that multiple cyclin CDK inhibitor proteins (CDI) regulate the transition from one phase to another of the cell cycle. The specific checkpoint that has been implicated in tumorigenesis is known as the START checkpoint that has been found in mammalian cells to be a regulator of transition from G1 phase to S phase.

The START checkpoint is altered via changes in the CDK complexes (most commonly CDK4 and CDK6) allowing the cell to proceed to the S phase of replication without any regulation and thus replicating possible unrepaired mutations creating genetic alterations of a specific tumor type [149]. The cyclins typically associated with CDK4 and CDK6 are known as the D cyclins (D1, D2, D3) and allow the cell to move from G1 phase (late) through the START checkpoint to S phase [150].

Research of the CDIs has revealed multiple families of protein inhibitors however one in particular is pivotal to the development of important CDK inhibitors. The family of proteins known as $p16^{INK4a}$, $p15^{INK4b}$, $p18^{INK4c}$, $p19^{INK4d}$ are translated from the INK4 locus and serve as specific inhibitors of the aforementioned D cyclins and CDKs [151].

The D type cyclins play a role in tumorigenesis via association with the retinoblastoma tumor suppressor gene, Rb. Rb is controlled through phosphorylation via cyclin/CDK complexes. When Rb is underphosphorylated, the cell is halted in the G1 phase (a protective mechanism) but phosphorylation leads to Rb inactivation, allowing the cell to proceed into S phase and further on to the M phase [152]. Overexpression of this pathway, leads to cellular proliferation without significant regulation and thus tumorigenesis. Cyclin D1 overexpression has been associated with estrogen (ER) positive breast cancer [153]. It is even suggested that there may be an independent interaction between the two, allowing for activation of ER independent of phosphorylated Rb and CDK [154].

Increasing knowledge of cyclin/CDK complexes and mechanisms has led to the investigation of cell cycle checkpoint control as a means of targeted antineoplastic therapy. Given the knowledge of the tumor suppressor gene Rb, the study of CDK4/CDK6 inhibition has proven of clinical benefit in hormonal positive metastatic breast cancer.

Palbociclib

Palbociclib is a CDK4/6 inhibitor which prevents cellular transcription by blocking advancement from G1 to S phase during cell cycle division. It was initially evaluated in the PALOMA-1 trial in which patients were randomized to letrozole versus letrozole in combination with palbociclib. This drug was tested in metastatic setting as first line treatment specifically in ER positive, Her2/Neu negative patients. The primary endpoint was progression free survival. The letrozole group had progression free survival (PFS) of 10.2 months versus the combination group with PFS of 20.2 months. The results were statistically significant. Overall survival data were promising but has yet to mature [155].

Subsequently, the PALOMA-3 trial examined patients with advanced metastatic breast cancer who had relapsed or had progression on prior endocrine therapy. 521 patients were randomized to palbociclib with fulvestrant versus fulvestrant with placebo. Palbociclib was given 125 mg/day orally for 3 weeks followed by 1 week off and fulvestrant was given 500 mg standard dosing. The primary endpoint in this study was PFS with several secondary endpoints including overall survival, tolerability, and response assessment. Of note, in the demographics of these women, 79% were postmenopausal; 60% had visceral disease; and 33% had prior chemotherapy. At the time of interim analysis, the primary endpoint had been met with the PFS in the palbociclib group at 9.2 months versus the fulvestrant/placebo group at 3.8 months. This difference is significant and was noted in both premenopausal and postmenopausal women [156].

Notable side effects observed with palbociclib are neutropenia and leukopenia. Additionally, patients reported significant fatigue in the combination groups versus the single agent. Given CDK inhibition at the level of the cell cycle with resulting inhibition of progenitor cells this was an anticipated side effect. Most common adverse events outside of neutropenia were thrombocytopenia and anemia. Grade 3 and 4 events occurred with an incidence less than 4%.

POLY ADP RIBOSE POLYMERASE INHIBITION

Poly ADP ribose polymerase (PARP) inhibitors have long been studied as a potential cancer therapy specifically in breast, prostate and ovarian cancer. Thus far, it has only proven beneficial in ovarian cancer which will be further discussed in this section.

PARP proteins are a family importantly involved in repair of single strand breaks. The specific mechanism involves PARP proteins binding to DNA at the site of single strand breaks, making polymers of ADP-ribose, and recruiting DNA repair proteins to the site. Many ovarian cancers are associated with BRCA germline mutations. Wild type BRCA1/2 genes have a significant role in DNA repair and serve as tumor suppressors regulating the cell cycle [157]. BRCA wild type tumors have not been associated with significant response to PARP inhibitors likely due to intact DNA repair capabilities [158]. BRCA mutations in malignant cells impair their ability to accomplish error-free DNA repair. PARP inhibitors prevent repair proteins from being recruited to sites of DNA breaks, stalling DNA replication forks. The resulting double-strand breaks culminate in apoptosis.

Olaparib

Olaparib is the first FDA approved PARP inhibitor in metastatic ovarian cancer. It has been studied in breast cancer without significant results thus far; therefore, it will be discussed here in the context of ovarian cancer. Study 19 involved 265 patients with platinum sensitive disease randomized to olaparib versus placebo. Primary endpoint in this study was PFS. Results in the olaparib versus placebo groups were promising with PFS 8.4 months vs. 4.8 months, respectively. As a secondary endpoint, overall survival (OS) at interim analysis was without significant benefit. Subgroup retrospective analysis of Study 19 looking at BRCA mutated patients showed significant clinical benefit in this group (PFS 11.2 months vs. 4.3 months). There was less of an advantage for wild type BRCA group. Common adverse events included nausea, vomiting, fatigue, anemia, diarrhea, and headache [159].

To further evaluate the BRCA subpopulation prospectively, Study 42 administered olaparib to patients with advanced breast, prostate, pancreatic and ovarian cancers with BRCA mutations. The results most clinically significant were the 137 ovarian cancer patients with at least 3 lines of prior therapy who had objective response rate of 34% and median duration of response of 7.9 months. Study 42 also noted 3.1% incidence of myelodysplastic syndrome on olaparib, but given limited options of therapy in this population, the FDA panel agreed that benefits outweighed risks in this population [160].

These two studies led to the FDA approval for olaparib in BRCA mutated patients with platinum sensitive recurrent disease after at least three lines of therapy. Currently, phase III SOLO trials I, II, III are evaluating olaparib and results are pending. Additionally, olaparib is currently being evaluated in conjunction with cediranib, a vascular endothelial growth factor (VEGF) inhibitor in the treatment of ovarian cancer, with phase II data looking promising [161].

CONCLUSIONS

With increased knowledge of tumor cell biology, a new era of cancer therapeutics has evolved that are vastly different from conventional cytotoxic chemotherapy. Greater understanding of mechanisms of cellular proliferation, oncogenic molecular mutations, importance of tumor bed vasculature, and the intricate balance between the immune system and tumor cells has allowed for tailored therapy guided by underlying pathology. Such treatments have resulted not only in a significant improvement in efficacy and overall survival but for the large part an improvement in patient tolerability and quality of life. Toxicities with many of these agents are unique and differ from those seen with chemotherapy, requiring practitioners to be familiar with different classes of drugs.

The above described new agents in oncology are approved and considered standard treatments at this moment. In parallel there is still an immense research effort ongoing to obtain better drugs with fewer side effects, and many targeted therapies are now in clinical studies as 2nd or 3rd generation therapeutics. We are in an era of spectacular discoveries and we will continue to see new drugs added to the armamentarium for cancer treatment. It is clear that the landscape for cancer therapy is rapidly changing and novel practice-changing therapies are anticipated in the near future.

REFERENCES

[1] Pópulo H, Lopes J, Soares P. The mTOR signalling pathway in human cancer. Int J Mol Sci 2012;13(2):1886–918.

[2] Davis WJ, Lehmann PZ, Li W. Nuclear PI3K signaling in cell growth and tumorigenesis. Front Cell Dev Biol 2015;3:24.

[3] Proud CG. Ras, PI3-kinase and mTOR signaling in cardiac hypertrophy. Cardiovasc Res 2004;63(3):403–13.

[4] Cully M, You H, Levine AJ, Mak TW. Beyond PTEN mutations: the PI3K pathway as an integrator of multiple inputs during tumorigenesis. Nat Rev Cancer 2006;6(3):184–92.

[5] Fruman DA, Rommel C. PI3K and cancer: lessons, challenges and opportunities. Nat Rev Drug Discov 2014;13:140–56.

[6] Blanco-Aparicio C, Renner O, Leal JF, Carnero A. PTEN, more than the AKT pathway. Carcinogenesis 2007;28(7):1379–86.

[7] Okkenhaug K, Vanhaesebroeck B. PI3K in lymphocyte development, differentiation and activation. Nat Rev Immunol 2003;3:317–30.

[8] Furman RR, Sharman JP, Coutre SE, et al. Idelalisib and rituximab in relapsed chronic lymphocytic leukemia. N Eng J Med 2014;370(11):997–1007.

[9] Guertin DA, Sabatini DM. Defining the role of mTOR in cancer. Cancer Cell 2007;12:9–22.

[10] Laplante M, Sabatini DM. mTOR signaling in growth control and disease. Cell 2012;149(2):274–93.

[11] Strimpakos AS, Karapanagiotou EM, Saif M, Wasif S, Kostas N. The role of mTOR in the management of solid tumors: An overview. Cancer Treat Rev 2009;35(2):148–59.

[12] Wan X, Shen N, Mendoza A, Khanna C, Helman LJ. CCI-779 inhibits rhabdomyosarcoma xenograft growth by an antiangiogenic mechanism linked to the targeting of mTOR/Hif-1α/VEGF signaling. Neoplasia 2006;8(5):394–401.

[13] Thomas GV, Tran C, Mellinghoff IK, Welsbie DS, Chan E, Fueger B, Czernin J, Sawyers CL. Hypoxia-inducible factor determines sensitivity to inhibitors of mTOR in kidney cancer. Nat Med 2005;12(1):122–7.

[14] Hudes G, Carducci M, Tomczak P, Dutcher J, Figlin R, Kapoor A, et al. Temsirolimus, interferon alfa, or both for advanced renal-cell carcinoma. N Engl J Med 2007;356:2271–81.

[15] Motzer RJ, Escudier B, Oudard S, Hutson TE, Porta C, Bracarda S, et al. Phase 3 trial of everolimus for metastatic renal cell carcinoma: final results and analysis of prognostic factors. Cancer 2010;116:4256–65.

[16] Motzer RJ, Barrios CH, Kim TM, Falcon S, Cosgriff T, Harker WG, et al. Phase II randomized trial comparing sequential first-line everolimus and second-line sunitinib versus first-line sunitinib and second-line everolimus in patients with metastatic renal cell carcinoma. J Clin Oncol 2014;32:2765–72.

[17] Krueger DA, Care MM, Holland K, Agricola K, Tudor C, Mangeshkar P, et al. Everolimus for subependymal giant-cell astrocytomas in tuberous sclerosis. N Engl J Med 2010;363:1801–11.

[18] Bissler J, et al. Everolimus for angiomyolipoma associated with tuberous sclerosis complex or sporadic lymphangioleiomyomatosis: a multicentre, randomised, double-blind, placebo-controlled trial. Lancet 2013;381:817–24.

[19] Franz D, et al. Efficacy and safety of everolimus for subependymal giant cell astrocytomas associated with tuberous sclerosis complex (EXIST-1): a multicentre, randomised, placebo-controlled phase 3 trial. Lancet 2013;381(9861):125–32.

[20] Hurvitz SA, et al. Combination of everolimus with trastuzumab plus paclitaxel as first-line treatment for patients with HER2-positive advanced breast cancer (BOLERO-1): a phase 3, randomised, double-blind, multicentre trial. Lancet Oncol 2015;16(7):816–29.

[21] Beaver JA, Park BH. The BOLERO-2 trial: the addition of everolimus to exemestane in the treatment of postmenopausal hormone receptor-positive advanced breast cancer. Future Oncol 2012;8(6):651–7.

[22] André F, O'Regan R, Ozguroglu M, et al. Everolimus for women with trastuzumab-resistant, her2-positive, advanced breast cancer (bolero-3): a randomized, double-blind, placebo-controlled phase 3 trial. Lancet Oncol 2014;15:580–91.

[23] Yao JC, Lombard-Bohas C, Baudin E, et al. Daily oral everolimus activity in patients with metastatic pancreatic neuroendocrine tumors after failure of cytotoxic chemotherapy: A phase II trial. J Clin Oncol 2010;28:69–76.

[24] Yao JC, Shah MH, Ito T, et al. Everolimus for advanced pancreatic neuroendocrine tumors. N Engl J Med 2011;364(6):514–23.

[25] Pavel, Marianne E, et al. Everolimus plus octreotide long-acting repeatable for the treatment of advanced neuroendocrine tumours associated with carcinoid syndrome (RADIANT-2): a randomised, placebo-controlled, phase 3 study. Lancet 2011;378(9808):2005–12.

[26] Baines AT, Xu D, Der CJ. Inhibition of Ras for cancer treatment: the search continues. Future Med Chem 2011;3(14):1787–808.

[27] Knrnoub AE, Weinberg RA. Ras onco-genes: split personalities. Nat Rev Mol Cell Biol 2008;9:517–31.

[28] Fumi S, Shigeyuki M, Yoko Y, Takashi K, Masayuki I, Tohru K. Current status of the development of Ras inhibitors. J. Biochem 2015;158(2):mvv060.

[29] Wennerberg K, Rossman KL, Der CJ. The Ras superfamily at a glance. J Cell Sci 2005;118:843–6.

[30] Fehrenbacher N, Bar-Sagi D, Philips M. Ras/MAPK signaling from endomembranes. Mol Oncol 2009;3(4):297–307.

[31] Gysin S, Salt M, Young A, McCormick F. Therapeutic strategies for targeting ras proteins. In: Santos E, editor. Genes Cancer 2011;2(3):359–72.

[32] Wong KK. Recent developments in anti-cancer agents targeting the Ras/Raf/ MEK/ERK pathway. Recent Pat Anticancer Drug Discov 2009;4(1):28–35.

[33] Chapman PB, Hauschild A, Robert C, et al. Improved survival with vemurafenib in melanoma with BRAF V600E mutation. NEJM 2011;364(26):2507–16.

[34] Sosman JA, Pavlick AC, Schuchter LM, et al. Analysis of molecular mechanisms of response and resistance to vemurafenib in BRAF V600E melanoma. J Clin Oncol 2012;30 (Suppl; abstr 8503).

[35] Menzies AM, Long GV, Murali R. Dabrafenib and its potential for the treatment of metastatic melanoma. Drug Des Dev Ther 2012;6:391–405.

[36] Anforth R, Fernandez-Peñas P, Long GV. Cutaneous toxicities of RAF inhibitors. Lancet Oncol 2013;14(1):e11–8.

[37] Su F, Viros A, Milagre C, et al. RAS mutations in cutaneous squamous-cell carcinomas in patients treated with BRAF inhibitors. N Engl J Med 2012;366(3):207–15.

[38] Brose MS, Nutting CM, Jarzab B, et al. Sorafenib in radioactive iodine refractory locally advanced or metastatic differentiated thyroid cancer: a randomised, double blind phase 3 trial. Lancet 2014;384(9940):319–28.

[39] Flaherty KT, Robert C, Hersey P, Nathan P, Garbe C, Milhem M, et al. Improved survival with MEK inhibition in BRAF-mutated melanoma. N Engl J Med 2012;367(2):107–14.

[40] Georgina VL, Daniil S, Helen G, Evgeny L, et al. Dabrafenib and trametinib versus dabrafenib and placebo for Val600 BRAF-mutant melanoma: a multicentre, double-blind, phase 3 randomised controlled trial. Lancet 2015;386(9992):444–51.

[41] Larkin JMG, Yan Y, McArthur GA, et al. Update of progression-free survival (PFS) and correlative biomarker analysis from coBRIM: phase III study of cobimetinib (cobi) plus vemurafenib (vem) in advanced BRAF-mutated melanoma. J Clin Oncol 2015;33. (suppl; abstr 9006).

[42] Larkin JMG, Ascierto PA, Dréno B, et al. Combined vemurafenib and cobimetinib in BRAF-mutated melanoma. N Engl J Med 2014;371(20):1867–76.

[43] Downward J, Parker P, Waterfield MD. Autophosphorylation sites on the epidermal growth factor receptor. Nature 1984;311(5985):483–5.

[44] Mok TS, Wu YL, Thongprasert S, et al. Gefitinib or carboplatin-paclitaxel in pulmonary adenocarcinoma. N Engl J Med 2009;361(10):947–57.

[45] Maemondo M, et al. Gefitinib or chemotherapy for non-small-cell lung cancer with mutated EGFR. N Engl J Med. 2010;362:2380–8.

[46] Fukuoka M, Wu YL, Thongprasert S, et al. Biomarker analyses and final overall survival results from a phase III, randomized, open-label, first-line study of gefitinib versus carboplatin/paclitaxel in clinically selected patients with advanced non-small-cell lung cancer in Asia (IPASS). J Clin Oncol 2011;29(21):2866–74.

[47] Pak MG, Lee C-H, Lee W-J, Shin D-H, Roh M-S. Unique microRNAs in lung adenocarcinoma groups according to major TKI sensitive EGFR mutation status. Diagn Pathol 2015;10:99.

[48] Neal JW. The SATURN trial: the value of maintenance erlotinib in patients with non-small-cell lung cancer. Future Oncol 2010;6(12):1827–32.

[49] Rosell R, Carcereny E, Gervais R, Vergnenegre A, Massuti B, Felip E, et al. Erlotinib versus standard chemotherapy as first-line treatment for European patients with advanced EGFR mutation-positive non-small-cell lung cancer (EURTAC): a multicentre, open-label, randomised phase 3 trial. Lancet Oncol 2012;13(3):239–46.

[50] Sequist LV, Yang JC, Yamamoto N, et al. Phase III study of afatinib or cisplatin plus pemetrexed in patients with metastatic lung adenocarcinoma with EGFR mutations. J Clin Oncol 2013;31(27):3327–34.

[51] Yang JC, Wu YL, Schuler M, et al. Afatinib versus cisplatin-based chemotherapy for EGFR mutation-positive lung adenocarcinoma (LUX-Lung 3 and LUX-Lung 6): analysis of overall survival data from two randomised, phase 3 trials. Lancet Oncol 2015;16:141–51.

[52] Balak MN, Gong Y, Riely GJ, Somwar R, Li AR, Zakowski MF, et al. Novel D761Y and common secondary T790M mutations in epidermal growth factor receptor-mutant lung adenocarcinomas with acquired resistance to kinase inhibitors. Clin Cancer Res 2006;12:6494–501.

[53] Sequist LV, Soria J-C, Goldman JW, Wakelee HA, Gadgeel SM, Varga A, et al. Rociletinib in EGFR-mutated non-small-cell lung cancer. N Engl J Med 2015;372(18):1700–9.

[54] Herbst RS, Prager D, Hermann R, Fehrenbacher L, Johnson BE, Sandler A, et al. TRIBUTE: a phase III trial of erlotinib hydrochloride (OSI-774) combined with carboplatin and paclitaxel chemotherapy in advanced non-small-cell lung cancer. J Clin Oncol 2005;23:5892–9.

[55] Jimeno A, Messersmith WA, Hirsch FR, Franklin WA, Eckhardt SG. KRAS mutations and sensitivity to epidermal growth factor receptor inhibitors in colorectal cancer: practical application of patient selection. J Clin Oncol 2009;27:1130–6.

[56] Peeters M, Price TJ, Cervantes A, et al. Randomized phase III study of panitumumab with fluorouracil, leucovorin, and irinotecan (FOLFIRI) compared to FOLFIRI alone as second-line treatment in patients with metastatic colorectal cancer. J Clin Oncol 2010;28:4706–13.

[57] Douillard JY, Oliner KS, Siena S, Tabernero J, Burkes R, Barugel M, et al. Panitumumab-FOLFOX4 treatment and RAS mutations in colorectal cancer. N Engl J Med 2013;369(11):1023–34.

[58] Van Cutsem E, Köhne CH, Láng I, et al. Cetuximab plus irinotecan, fluorouracil, and leucovorin as first-line treatment for metastatic colorectal cancer: updated analysis of overall survival according to tumor KRAS and BRAF mutation status. J Clin Oncol 2011;29(15):2011–9.

[59] Salem B, Hmouda H, Bouraoi K. Drug induced hypokalemia. Curr Drug Saf 2009;4(1):55–61.

[60] Koutras AK, Evans TR. The epidermal growth factor receptor family in breast cancer. Onco Targets Ther 2008;1:5–19.

[61] Ahmed KM, Cao N, Li JJ. HER-2 and NF-kappaB as the targets for therapy-resistant breast cancer. Anticancer Res 2006;26:4235–43.

[62] Eroglu Z, Tagawa T, Somlo G. Human epidermal growth factor receptor family-targeted therapies in the treatment of HER2-overexpressing breast cancer. Oncologist 2014;19:135–50.

[63] Giordano SH, Temin S, Kirshner JJ, et al. Systemic therapy for patients with advanced human epidermal growth factor receptor 2-positive breast cancer: American Society of Clinical Oncology clinical practice guideline. J Clin Oncol 2014;32:2078–99.

[64] Hudis CA. Trastuzumab—mechanism of action and use in clinical practice. N Engl J Med 2007;357(1):39–51.

[65] Slamon DJ, Leland-Jones B, Shak S, et al. Use of chemotherapy plus a monoclonal antibody against metastatic breast cancer that overexpresses her2. N Eng J Med 2001;344(11):783–92.

[66] Perez EA, Romon EH, Suman VJ. Trastuzumab plus adjuvant chemotherapy of human epidermal growth factor receptor 2-positive breast cancer: planned joint analysis of overall survival from NSABP B-31 and NCCTG N9831. J Clin Oncol 2014;32(33):3744–52.

[67] Slamon D, Eiermann W, Robert N, et al. Adjuvant trastuzumab in her2-positive breast cancer. N Engl J Med 2011;365(14):1273–83.

[68] Goldhirsch A, et al. 2 years versus 1 year of adjuvant trastuzumab for HER2-positive breast cancer (HERA): an open-label, randomised controlled trial. Lancet 2013;382(9897):1021–8.

[69] Pivot X, et al. 6 months versus 12 months of adjuvant trastuzumab for patients with HER2-positive early breast cancer (PHARE): a randomised phase 3 trial. Lancet Oncol 2013;14(8):741–8.

[70] Bang YJ, Van Cutsem E, Feyereislova A. Trastuzumab in combination with chemotherapy versus chemotherapy alone for treatment of her2-positive advanced gastric or gastroesophageal junction cancer ToGA: a phase 3 open label randomized control trial. Lancet 2010;376(9742):687–97.

[71] Perez E, Rodeheffer R. Clinical cardiac tolerability of trastuzumab. J Clin Oncol 2004;22(2):322–9.

[72] Seidman A, Hudis C, Pierri MK, et al. Cardiac dysfunction in the trastuzumab clinical trials experience. J Clin Oncol 2002;20(5):1215–21.

[73] Swain SM, Baselga J, Kim SB. Pertuzumab trastuzumab and docetaxel in her2-positive metastatic breast cancer. N Engl J Med 2015;372(8):724–34.

[74] Gianni L, Pienkowski T, Im YH, et al. Efficacy and safety of neoadjuvant pertuzumab and trastuzumab in women with locally advanced, inflammatory, or early her2-positive breast cancer (neosphere): a randomised multicentre, open-label, phase 2 trial. Lancet Oncol 2012;13(1):25–32.

[75] Schneeweiss A, Chia S, Hickish T. Pertuzumab plus trastuzumab in combination with standard neoadjuvant anthracycline-containing and anthracycline-free chemotherapy regimens in patients with her-2 positive early breast cancer: a randomized phase ii cardiac safety study (TRYPHAENA). Ann Oncol 2013;24(9):2278–84.

[76] Tevaarwerk AJ, Kolesar JM. Lapatinib: a small-moledule inhibitor of epidermal growth factor receptor and human epidermal growth factor receptor-2 tyrosine kinases used in the treatment of breast cancer. Clin Ther 2009;31(Pt. 2):2332–48.

[77] Geyer C, Forster J, et al. Lapatinib plus Capecitabine for HER2-Positive Advanced Breast Cancer. J Engl J Med 2006;355(26):2733–43.

[78] Blackwell KL, Burnstein HJ, et al. Overall survival benefit with lapatinib in combination with trastuzumab for patients with human epidermal growth factor receptor 2-positive metastatic breast cancer: final results from the egf104900 study. J Clin Oncol 2012;30(21):2585.

[79] Perez EA, Koehler M, et al. Cardiac safety of lapatinib: pooled analysis of 3689 patients enrolled in clinical trials. Mayo Clin Proc 2008;83(6):679–86.

[80] Wong DJ, Hurvitz SA. Recent advances in the development of anti-HER12 antibodies and antibody-drug conjugates. Ann Transl Med 2014;2(12):122.

[81] Verma S, Miles D, et al. Trastuzumab emtansine for HER2-positive advanced breast cancer. N Engl J Med 2012;367:1783–91.

[82] Casaluce F, Sgambato A, Maione P, Rossi A, Ferrara C, Napolitano A, et al. ALK inhibitors: a new targeted therapy in the treatment of advanced NSCLC. Target Oncol 2013;8:55–67.

[83] Mano H. Non-solid oncogenes in solid tumors: EML4-ALK fusion genes in lung cancer. Cancer Sci 2008;99(12):2349–55.

[84] Palmer RH, Vernersson E, Grabbe C, Hallberg B. Anaplastic lymphoma kinase: signalling in development and disease. Biochem J 2009;420:345–61.

[85] Choi YL, Takeuchi K, Soda M, et al. Identification of novel isoforms of the EML4-ALK transforming gene in non-small cell lung cancer. Cancer Res 2008;68:4971–6.

[86] Horn L, Pao W. EML4-ALK: honing in on a new target in non-small-cell lung cancer. J Clin Oncol 2009;27:4232–5.

[87] Shaw AT, Kim DW, Nakagawa K, Seto T, Crino L, Ahn MJ, et al. Crizotinib versus chemotherapy in advanced ALK-positive lung cancer. N Engl J Med 2013;368(25):2385–94.

[88] Solomon BJ, Mok T, Kim DW, et al. PROFILE 1014 investigators: first-line crizotinib versus chemotherapy in ALK-positive lung cancer. N Engl J Med 2014;371:2167–77.

[89] Shaw AT, Engelman JA. ALK in lung cancer: past, present, and future. J Clin Oncol 2013;31(8):1105–11.

[90] Rothenstein JM, Letarte N. Managing treatment-related adverse events associated with Alk inhibitors. Curr Oncol 2014;21:19–26.

[91] Katayama R, Shaw AT, Khan TM, Mino-Kenudson M, Solomon BJ, Halmos B, et al. Mechanisms of acquired crizotinib resistance in ALK-rearranged lung cancers. Sci Transl Med 2012;4:120ra117.

[92] Massarelli E, Papadimitrakopoulou V. Ceritinib for the treatment of late-stage (metastatic) non-small cell lung cancer. Clin Cancer Res 2015;21(40):670–4.

[93] Shaw AT, Kim DW, Mehra R, et al. Ceritinib in ALK-rearranged non-small-cell lung cancer. N Engl J Med 2014;370(26):1189–97.

[94] Hicklin DJ, Ellis LM. Role of the vascular endothelial growth factor pathway in tumor growth and angiogenesis. J Clin Oncol 2005;23:1011–27.

[95] Wang Z, Dabrosin C, Yin X, et al. Broad targeting of angiogenesis for cancer prevention and therapy. Semin Cancer Biol 2015;35(Suppl.):S224–43.

[96] Samant RS, Shevde LA. Recent advances in anti-angiogenic therapy of cancer. Oncotarget 2011;2:122–34.

[97] Carmeliet P, Jain RK. Molecular mechanisms and clinical applications of angiogenesis. Nature 2011;473(7347):298–307.

[98] Grothey A, Ellis LM. Targeting angiogenesis driven by vascular endothelial growth factors using antibody-based therapies. Cancer J 2008;14(3):170–7.

[99] Keating GM. Bevacizumab: a review of its use in advanced cancer. Drugs 2014;74:1891–925.

[100] Hurwitz H, Fehrenbacher L, Novotny W, Cartwright T, Hainsworth J, Heim W, Berlin J, Baron A, Griffing S, Holmgren E, et al. Bevacizumab plus irinotecan, fluorouracil, and leucovorin for metastatic colorectal cancer. N Engl J Med 2004;350:2335–42.

[101] Giantonio BJ, Catalano PJ, et al. Bevacizumab in combination with oxaliplatin, fluorouracil, and leucovorin (FOLFOX4) for previously treated metastatic colorectal cancer: results from the Eastern Cooperative Oncology Group Study E3200. J Clin Oncol 2007;25(12):1539–44.

[102] Bennouna J, Sastre J, Arnold D, Österlund P, Greil R, Van Cutsem E, von Moos R, Viéitez JM, Bouché O, Borg C, et al. Continuation of bevacizumab after first progression in metastatic colorectal cancer (ML18147): a randomised phase 3 trial. Lancet Oncol 2013;14:29–37.

[103] Sandler A, Gray R, Perry MC, Brahmer J, Schiller JH, Dowlati A, et al. Paclitaxel-carboplatin alone or with bevacizumab for non-small-cell lung cancer. N Engl J Med 2006;355:2542–50.

[104] Rini BI, et al. Bevacizumab plus interferon alfa compared with interferon alfa monotherapy in patients with metastatic renal cell carcinoma: CALGB 90206. J Clin Oncol 2008;26(22):5422.

[105] Gressett SM, Shah SR. Intricacies of bevacizumab -induced toxicities and their management. Ann Pharmacother 2009;43(3):490–501.

[106] Shah M. Update on metastatic gastric and esophageal cancers. J Clin Oncol 2015;33(16):1760–6.

[107] Fuchs CS, Tomasek J, Yong CJ, Dumitru F, Passalacqua R, Goswami C, et al. Ramucirumab monotherapy for previously treated advanced gastric or gastro-oesophageal junction adenocarcinoma (REGARD): an international, randomised, multicentre, placebo-controlled, phase 3 trial. Lancet 2014;383(9911):31–9.

[108] Wilke H, Muro K, Van Cutsem E, Oh S, Bodoky G, Shimada Y, et al. Ramucirumab plus paclitaxel versus placebo plus paclitaxel in patients with previously treated advanced gastric or gastro-oesophageal junction adenocarcinoma (RAINBOW): a double-blind, randomised phase 3 trial. Lancet Oncol 2014;15:1224–35.

[109] Garon EB, Ciuleanu TE, Arrieta O, et al. Ramucirumab plus docetaxel versus placebo plus docetaxel for second-line treatment of stage IV non-small-cell lung cancer after disease progression on platinum-based therapy (REVEL): a multicentre, double-blind, randomized phase 3 trial. Lancet 2014;384(9944):665–73.

[110] Tabernero J, Yoshino T, Cohn AL, et al. Ramucirumab versus placebo in combination with second-line FOLFIRI in patients with metastatic colorectal carcinoma that progressed during or after first-line therapy with bevacizumab, oxaliplatin, and a fluoropyrimidine (RAISE): A randomised, double-blind, multicentre, phase 3 study. Lancet Oncol 2015;5:499–508.

[111] Kim S, Ding W, et al. Clinical response to sunitinib as a multi-targeted tyrosine-kinase inhibitor (TKI) in solid cancers: a review of clinical trials. Onco Targets Ther 2014;7:719–28.

[112] Motzer RJ, Hutson TE, Tomczak P, et al. Sunitinib versus interferon alfa in metastatic renal-cell carcinoma. N Engl J Med 2007;356:115–24.

[113] Demetri GD, van Oosterom AT, Garrett CR, et al. Efficacy and safety of sunitinib in patients with advanced gastrointestinal stromal tumour after failure of imatinib: a randomised controlled trial. Lancet 2006;368(9544):1329–38.

[114] Raymond E, Dahan L, Raoul JL, Bang YJ, Borbath I, Lombard-Bohas C, et al. Sunitinib malate for the treatment of pancreatic neuroendocrine tumors. N Engl J Med 2011;364(6):501–13.

[115] Llovet JM, Ricci S, Mazzaferro V, et al. Sorafenib in advanced hepatocellular carcinoma. N Engl J Med 2008;359(4):378.

[116] Lencioni R, Kudo M, Ye SL, et al. First interim analysis of the GIDEON (Global Investigation of therapeutic decisions in hepatocellular carcinoma and of its treatment with sorafenib) non-interventional study. Int J Clin Pract 2012;66(7):675–83.

[117] Escudier B, Eisen T, Stadler WM, et al. Sorafenib for treatment of renal cell carcinoma: final efficacy and safety results of the phase III treatment approaches in renal cancer global evaluation trial. J Clin Oncol 2009;27(20):3312–8.

[118] Sternberg CN, Davis ID, Mardiak J, et al. Pazopanib in locally advanced or metastatic renal cell carcinoma: results of a randomized phase III trial. J Clin Oncol 2010;28(6):1061–8.

[119] Escudier B, Porta C, Bono P, Powles T, Eisen T, Sternberg CN, et al. Randomized, controlled, double-blind, cross-over trial assessing treatment preference for pazopanib versus sunitinib in patients with metastatic renal cell carcinoma: PISCES study. J Clin Oncol 2014;32:1412.

[120] Van der Graaf Winette TA, Blay J, Chawla SP, Kim D, Bui-Nguyen B, Casali PG, Schöffski P, Aglietta M, Staddon AP, Beppu Y, Le Cesne A, Gelderblom H, Judson IR, Araki N, Ouali M, Marreaud S, Hodge R, Dewji MR, Coens C, Demetri GD, Fletcher CD, Dei Tos Angelo P, Hohenberger P. Pazopanib for metastatic soft-tissue sarcoma (PALETTE): a randomised, double-blind, placebo-controlled phase 3 trial. Lancet 2012;379:1879–86.

[121] Ueda T, Uemura H, Tomita Y, Tsukamoto T, Kanayama H, Shinohara N, et al. Efficacy and safety of axitinib versus sorafenib in metastatic renal cell carcinoma: subgroup analysis of Japanese patients from the global randomized Phase 3 AXIS trial. Jpn J Clin Oncol 2013;43:616–28.

[122] Wells SA Jr, Robinson BG, Gagel RF, et al. Vandetanib in patients with locally advanced or metastatic medullary thyroid cancer: a randomized, double-blind phase III trial. J Clin Oncol 2012;30(2):134–41.

[123] Elisei R, Schlumberger MJ, Müller SP, et al. Cabozantinib in progressive medullary thyroid cancer. J Clin Oncol 2013;31(29):3639–46.

[124] Grothey A, Van Cutsem E, Sobrero A, Siena S, Falcone A, Ychou M, Humblet Y, Bouché O, Mineur L, Barone C, et al. Regorafenib monotherapy for previously treated metastatic colorectal cancer (CORRECT): an international, multicentre, randomised, placebo-controlled, phase 3 trial. Lancet 2013;381:303–12.

[125] Disis ML. Mechanism of action of immunotherapy. Semin Oncol 2014;41(5):53–9.

[126] Goel G, Sun W. Cancer immunotherapy in clinical practice—the past, present and future. Chin J Cancer 2014;33(9):445–57.

[127] Weber J. Current perspectives on immunotherapy. Semin Oncol 2014;41(5):14–29.

[128] Kirkwood J, Butterfield L, Tarhini AA, Zarour H, Kalinski P, Ferrone S. Immunotherapy of cancer in 2012. Ca Caner J Clin 2012;62:309–28.

[129] Chunging G, Masoud HM, Subjeck JR, Sarkar D, Fisher PB, Wang X. Therapeutic cancer vaccines: past, present and future. Adv Cancer Res 2013;119:421–75.

[130] Topalian SL, Weiner GJ, Pardoll DM. Cancer immunotherapy comes of age. J Clin Oncol 2011;29(36):4828–36.

[131] Kantoff PW, et al. Sipuleucl-T immunotherapy for castrate resistant prostate cancer. N Engl J Med 2010;363(5):411–9.

[132] Weber J, Yang J, Atkins M, Disis M. Toxicities of immunotherapy for the practitioner. J Clin Oncol 2015;33(18):2092–9.

[133] Shih K, Arkenau H, Infante J. Clinical impact of checkpoint inhibitors as novel cancer therapies. Drugs 2014;74:1993–2013.

[134] Perez-Garcia JL, Labiano S, et al. Orchestrating imune check-point blockade for cancer immunotherapy in combinations. Curr Opin Immunol 2014;27:89–97.

[135] Krummel M, Allison J. CD28 and CTLA-4 have opposing effects on the response of T cells to stimulation. J Immunol 2011;187:3459–65.

[136] Hodi FS, O'Day SJ, McDermott DF, Weber RW, Sosman JA, Haanen JB, et al. Improved survival with ipilimumab in patients with metastatic melanoma. N Engl J Med 2010;363:711–23.

[137] Robert C, Thomas L, Bondarenko I, et al. Ipilimumab plus dacarbazine for previously untreated metastatic melanoma. N Engl J Med 2011;364:2517–26.

[138] Eggermont AMM, et al. Adjuvant ipilimumab versus placebo after complete resection of high risk stage III melanoma (EORTC 18071): a randomized, double blind, phase 3 trial. Lancet Oncol 2015;16(5):522–30.

[139] Postow MA, Callahan MK, Wolchok JD. Immune checkpoint blockade in cancer therapy. J Clin Oncol 2015;33(17):1974–82.

[140] Weber JS, D'Angelo SP, Minor D, Hodi FS, Gutzmer R, Neyns B, et al. Nivolumab versus chemotherapy in patients with advanced melanoma who progressed after anti-CTLA-4 treatment (CheckMate 037): a randomised, controlled, open-label, phase 3 trial. Lancet Oncol 2015;16(4):375–84. 10.

[141] Robert C, et al. Nivolumab in previously untreated melanoma without BRAF mutation. N Engl J Med 2015;372:320–30.

[142] Brahmer J, et al. Nivolumab versus docetaxel in advanced squamous-cell non-small-cell lung cancer. The N Engl J Med 2015;373:123–35.

[143] Paz-Ares L, et al. Phase III randomized trial (CheckMATE 057) of nivolumab versus docetaxel in advanced non squamous cell non small cell lung cancer. J Clin Oncol 2015;33. (Suppl; abstr LBA109).

[144] Motzer RJ, et al. Nivolumab versus everolimus n advanced renal-cell carcinoma. N Eng J Med 2015;373:1803–13.

[145] Ribas A, et al. Pembrolizumab versus investigator-choice chemotherapy for ipilimumab-refractory melanoma (KEYNOTE-002): a randomized, controlled, phase 2 trial. Lancet Oncol 2015;16(8): 908–18.

[146] Herbst RS, et al. Pembroluzimab versus docetaxel for previously treated, PD-L1-positive, advanced non-small-cell lung cancer (KEYNOTE-010): a randomized control trial. Lancet Oncol 2016;387(10027):1540–50.

[147] Allison, J.P. Immune checkpoint blockade in cancer therapy: new insights, opportunities, and prospects for a cure. Presented at ASCO 2015 annual meeting.

[148] Postow M, et al. Nivolumab and ipilimumab versus ipilimumab in untreated melanoma. N Eng J Med 2015;372:2006–17.

[149] Hunter T, Pines J. Cyclins and cancer. II: cyclin D and CDK inhibitors come of age. Cell 1994;79(4):573–82.

[150] Besson A, Dowdy SF, Roberts JM. CDK inhibitors: cell cycle regulators and beyond. Dev Cell 2008;14(2):159–69.

[151] Sherr CJ, Roberts JM. CDK inhibitors: positive and negative regulators of G1-phase progression. Genes Dev 1999;13:1501–12.

[152] Hinds PW, Dowdy SF, Eaton EN, Arnold A, Weinberg RA. Function of a human cyclin gene as an oncogene. Proc Natl Acad Sci USA 1994;97:709–13.

[153] Butt AJ, McNeil CM, Musgrove EA, Sutherland RL. Downstream targets of growth factor and oestrogen signalling and endocrine resistance: the potential roles of c-Myc, cyclin D1 and cyclin E. Endocr Relat Cancer 2005;12(Suppl. 1):S47–59.

[154] Zukerberg LR, Yang WI, Gadd M, Thor AD, Koerner FC, Schmidt EV, Arnold A. Cyclin D1 (PRAD1) protein expression in breast cancer: approximately one-third of infiltrating mammary carcinomas show overexpression of the cyclin D1 oncogene. Mod Pathol 1995;8:560–7.

[155] Finn RS, et al. Final results of a randomized Phase II study of PD 0332991, a cyclin-dependent kinase (CDK)-4/6 inhibitor, in combination with letrozole vs letrozole alone for first-line treatment of ER+/HER2- advanced breast cancer (PALOMA-1; TRIO-18). AACR Annual Meeting. Abstract CT101. Presented April 6, 2014. San Diego, California.

[156] Nicholas CT, Jungsil R, Fabrice A, Sherene L, Sunil V, Hiroji I, Nadia H, Sibylle L, Cynthia HB, Ke Z, Carla G, Sophia R, Maria K, Massimo C. PALOMA3: a double-blind, phase III trial of fulvestrant with or without palbociclib in pre- and post-menopausal women with hormone receptor-positive, HER2-negative metastatic breast cancer that progressed on prior endocrine therapy. J Clin Oncol 2015;33(suppl; abstr LBA502), ASCO Annual Meeting. Presented June 1, 2015. Chicago, Illinois.

[157] Liu N-A, Jiang H, Ben-Shlomo A, Wawrowsky K, Fan X-M, Lin S, Melmed S. Targeting zebrafish and murine pituitary corticotroph tumours with a cyclin-dependent kinase (CDK) inhibitor. PNAS 2011;108(20):8414–9.

[158] Tewari KD, Eskander RN, Monk BJ. Development of olaparib for BRCA-deficient recurrent epithelial ovarian cancer. Clin Cancer Res 2015;21(17):3829–35.

[159] Ledermann J, Harter P, Gourley C, et al. Olaparib maintenance therapy in platinum-sensitive relapsed ovarian cancer. N Engl J Med 2012;366:1382–92.

[160] Kaufman B, Shapira-Frommer R, Schmutzler RK, Audeh MW, Friedlander M, Balmana J, et al. Olaparib monotherapy in patients with advanced cancer and a germline BRCA 1/2 mutation. J Clin Oncol 2015;33:244–50.

[161] Liu J, Barry WT, Birrer MJ, et al. A randomized phase 2 trial comparing efficacy of the combination of the PARP inhibitor olaparib and the antiangiogenic cediranib against olaparib alone in recurrent platinum-sensitive ovarian cancer. J Clin Oncol 2014;32. 5s.(suppl; abstr LBA5500).

Chapter 2

Molecular Mechanisms Underlying Anthracycline Cardiotoxicity: Challenges in Cardio-Oncology

R. Dhingra, V. Margulets and L.A. Kirshenbaum

The Institute of Cardiovascular Sciences, St. Boniface Hospital Albrechtsen Research Centre, Department of Physiology and Pathophysiology, Max Rady College of Medicine, Rady Faculty of Health Sciences, University of Manitoba, Winnipeg, MB, Canada

INTRODUCTION

Anthracycline antibiotics were first isolated from fungi *Streptomyces peucetius* and *Streptomyces caesius* and were introduced into clinical oncology in 1960s and still continue as key components of cancer treatment regimen [1]. In principle these drugs are effective antiproliferative agents because they inhibit topoisomerase I and II, which are critical for DNA replication and thus interfere with helical unwinding of DNA. Anthracyclines are widely used to treat leukemia, breast cancers, aggressive lymphomas, lung cancers, non-Hodgkin's lymphoma, and many hematologic and solid malignancies. On the basis of the level and extent of cardiotoxicity induced by these agents, chemotherapeutic drugs are classified into two general types, type-I agents which include the agents that cause dose-dependent and irreversible cardiac damage; and type-II agents that induce reversible cardiotoxic side effects and are not dose dependent. Anthracyclines belong to type-I category and induce cellular defects that include disrupted sarcomeres, mitochondrial perturbations, oxidative stress from reactive oxygen species (ROS) generation, lipid and proteotoxic stress, which culminate in cell death [2,3].

These cellular defects evoke both acute and chronic cardiac abnormalities, such as ventricular arrhythmias, ventricular repolarization defects, electrocardiographic QT-interval changes that develop within days of chemotherapy treatment. In contrast, chronic anthracycline cardiotoxicity is related to the cumulative dose of the drug temporally that manifests as impaired contractile performance and heart failure after several years of chemotherapy treatment [4]. There are a number of anthracycline antibiotics currently used for treating variety of cancers, such as doxorubicin and its analogs daunorubicin, epirubicin, idarubicin, and mitoxantrone [5]. Unfortunately doxorubicin and its analogs are associated with severe cardiotoxicity [6–8] (Table 2.1). Both animal and clinical research demonstrate that anthracyclines induce cardiac damage and cardiac myocyte death when cumulative dose exceeds 500 mg/m^2 in the case of doxorubicin or 950 mg/m^2 in the case of epirubicin [7–9]. Notably, doxorubicin remains an important component of cancer therapy despite its known cardiotoxic effects.

Though multiple theories have been proposed, a cogent explanation of the cardiotoxic effects of doxorubicin has not been provided to date. At the cellular level increased oxidative stress together with mitochondrial perturbations including impaired respiration, iron and calcium overload, and altered gene expression have been proposed as common underlying defects associated with doxorubicin toxicity [10,11] (Fig. 2.1). Notably, the mitochondrion is a major organelle affected by doxorubicin treatment. Given that the cardiac muscle is abundantly rich in mitochondria, it would stand to reason that abnormalities in mitochondrial function that affect electron transport within the respiratory chain complexes would impair ATP synthesis required for normal cardiac function. The loss of ATP would lead to the eventual demise of the cell by apoptosis or necrosis and contractile failure (Fig. 2.2). This raises the question: What are the critical signaling events that lead to mitochondrial abnormalities and oxidative stress injury in the hearts of patients treated with doxorubicin?

IMPAIRED REDOX SIGNALING

Recent advances have implicated impaired redox signaling and downregulation of antioxidant pathways in anthracycline cardiotoxicity, but the precise mechanism underlying mitochondrial oxidative stress are unclear. Extensive

TABLE 2.1 Cardiotoxicity Induced by Anthracyclines

Anthracycline Drugs	Acute Effects	Chronic Effects
Doxorubicin	Arrhythmias, QT interval changes, pericarditis/myocarditis, sudden cardiac death	Decline in left ventricle function, progression to heart failure
Daunorubicin		
Epirubicin		
Idarubicin		
Mitoxantrone		

The importance of antioxidants in reducing oxidative stress and cytotoxicity is proved in in vitro studies where use of antioxidant *N*-acetylcysteine (NAC) demonstrate a protective effect on doxorubicin-treated cells, suggesting that shifting the balance in favor of antioxidant can mitigate the injury. Nuclear factor erythroid 2-related factor 2 (Nrf2) is a master regulator and key redox-sensitive transcription factor that regulates transcription of genes involved in antioxidant signaling, such as heme oxygenase-1 (HO-1) and NAD(p)H: quinone oxidoreductase-1 (NQO-1) [13]. Notably, inactivation of Nrf2 evidenced by loss of nuclear Nrf2 binding in doxorubicin-treated hearts was associated with increased lipid peroxidation and oxidative stress. Furthermore, restoration of Nrf2 signaling and activation of downstream targets resulted in decreased lipid peroxidation evidenced by decreased 4-hydroxynonenal (4-HNE)

investigations into doxorubicin cardiotoxicity point toward the downregulation of the antioxidant defense system as a key point that shifts the balance in favor of oxidants and therefore renders the heart sensitive to oxidative stress [12].

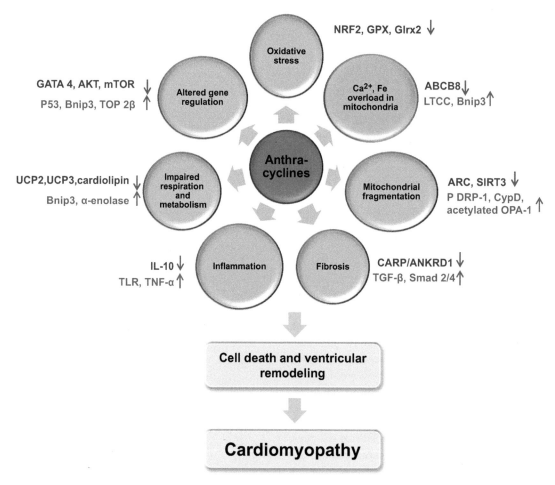

FIGURE 2.1   **Diagrammatic representation of signaling pathways implicated in anthracycline-induced cardiotoxicity.** Anthracyclines are believed to alter expression of genes involved in several cellular processes including critical genes associated with oxidative stress, mitochondrial defects, such as calcium (Ca^{2+}), iron (Fe) overload, impaired respiration, and mitochondrial fragmentation. *NRF2*, Nuclear factor erythroid 2-related factor 2; *GPX*, glutathione peroxidase; *Glrx2*, glutaredoxin 2; *ABCB8*, ATP-binding cassette subfamily B member 8; *LTCC*, L-type Ca^{2+} channel; *Bnip3*, Bcl2/adenovirus E1B 19 kDa interacting protein 3; *ARC*, apoptosis repressor with caspase recruitment domain; *SIRT3*, sirtuin 3; *DRP-1*, dynamin related protein 1; *CypD*, cyclophilin D; *OPA1*, optic atrophy 1; *CARP/ANKRD1*, cardiac ankyrin repeat protein; *TGF-β*, transforming growth factor-β; *mTOR*, mammalian target of rapamycin; *TOP 2β*, topoisomerase 2β; *UCP2* and *UCP3*, uncoupling protein 2 and uncoupling protein 3; *IL-10*, interleukin 10; *TLR*, toll-like receptor; *TNFα*, tumor necrosis factor-α.

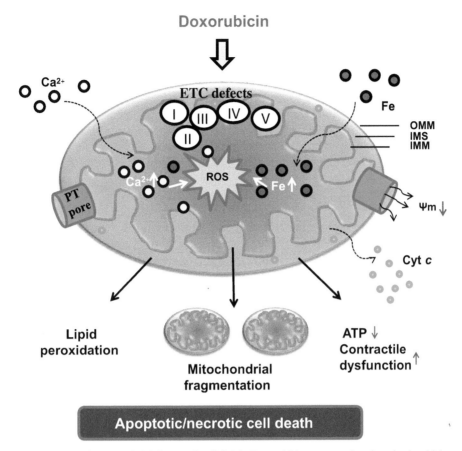

FIGURE 2.2 Doxorubicin induced mitochondrial defects and cell death. Doxorubicin treatment impairs mitochondrial respiration by disrupting electron transport chain *(ETC)*, resulting in loss of ATP and therefore contractile dysfunction of cardiomyocytes. Doxorubicin treatment provokes lipid peroxidation, mitochondrial permeability transition pore opening *(PT)*, and loss of mitochondrial membrane potential *(Ψm)* resulting in permeability changes of mitochondrial membranes, release of cytochrome *c* from IMS, and mitochondrial calcium *(Ca²⁺)* and iron *(Fe)* overload. Damaged mitochondria undergo fission resulting in fragmentation and apoptotic/necrotic cell death. *OMM,* Outer mitochondrial membrane; *IMS,* intermembrane space; *IMM,* inner mitochondrial membrane, ETC I, II, III, IV, and V, electron transport chain complexes I, II, III, IV, and V.

accumulation, and improved mitochondrial respiration and cardiac function [14]. Moreover, the role of Nrf2 in regulating doxorubicin-induced oxidative stress was substantiated by studies in which Nrf2 knockout mice were found to be more sensitive than wild-type littermates to ROS and doxorubicin toxicity [15]. Moreover, a role for oxidative stress as an underlying cause of doxorubicin toxicity was provided by studies in which the effects of doxorubicin were tested in transgenic mice hearts expressing glutathione peroxidase (Gpx1). In contrast to nontransgenic mice treated with doxorubicin, which demonstrated impaired state-3 mitochondrial respiration, reduced contractility, and coronary flow rate, Gpx1 overexpressing mice were resistant to the cytotoxic effects and cardiac dysfunction induced by doxorubicin [16]. Similarly overexpression of glutaredoxin 2 (Glrx2), a thioltransferase, also exerted a protective effect by increasing protein S-glutathionylation of heart mitochondrial proteins resulting in improved respiratory parameters and cardiac performance [17]. Beside disturbed oxidant and antioxidant balance, defects in mitochondrial

respiration can also trigger ROS production [11]. Uncoupling proteins (UCP) that regulate mitochondrial membrane potential and ATP production have recently been demonstrated to protect from mitochondrial ROS by preventing the build-up of excess protons in the intermembrane space of mitochondria. Therefore, a decline in levels of cardiac UCP2 and UCP3 after doxorubicin treatment may have predisposed mitochondria to oxidative stress injury [18].

However, despite these overwhelming studies demonstrating a therapeutic benefit of antioxidant therapy, many of the clinical trials failed to show any benefit to cardiac function and long-term outcome [19]. For example, a randomized trial was conducted in soft-tissue sarcoma patients treated with doxorubicin. In this study, NAC was tested for cardioprotection, but no difference in left ventricular ejection fraction (LVEF) was observed and both groups developed overt congestive heart failure in a similar fashion [20]. Further, antioxidant therapy using the semisynthetic flavonoid 7-monohydroxyethylrutoside (monoHER) in conjunction with doxorubicin did not show beneficial effects but instead exacerbated cardiotoxicity in a phase-II trial in patients with metastatic cancer [21]. More importantly, a database search done from registered clinical trials [Cochrane Central Registry of Controlled Trials (CENTRAL, issue 2, 2007), MEDLINE (1966 to April 2007), and EMBASE (1980 to 2007)] revealed that the cardioprotective agents established in preclinical studies, such as NAC, phenethylamines, coenzyme Q10, combinations of vitamin C and E, L-carnitine, and carvedilol, did not demonstrate cardioprotective effects in patients receiving chemotherapy in clinical trials [22]. Protective effects of antioxidants were further challenged by a study that tested cardioprotective effects of free radical scavenger super oxide dismutase (SOD) in a clinical trial conducted in female breast-cancer patients receiving four to five courses of adjuvant doxorubicin and cyclophosphamide chemotherapy. In this trial, 80 women receiving adjuvant chemotherapy were randomly assigned to receive 80 mg of lecithin-bound human recombinant SOD (PC-SOD) or placebo and were analyzed for echocardiography, QT assessment, biochemical markers for heart function, oxidative stress, and inflammation before, during, and after each course. Surprisingly, cardiotoxicity was similar in the groups receiving or not receiving SOD and suggest that oxidative stress may not be the only factor underlying anthracycline cardiotoxicity [23].

However, where most of the studies reveal failure of antioxidants to suppress anthracycline-induced cardiotoxicity in clinical trials, salidroside, [2-(4-hydroxyphenyl)ethyl-β-D-glucopyranoside], the principal ingredient extracted from the plant *Rhodiola rosea*, also known for antioxidant and cardioprotective properties, provided cardioprotection from epirubicin-induced early left ventricular regional systolic dysfunction in breast cancer patients [24]. Although these clinical trials disappointingly failed to equivocally show any benefit of antioxidant therapy against anthracycline-induced myocardial injury, lessons learned from these studies demonstrate that cellular defects in addition to oxidative stress may contribute to cardiac dysfunction and doxorubicin cardiotoxicity in humans.

IRON OVERLOAD IN MITOCHONDRIA

A role for iron overload in doxorubicin cardiotoxicity was established several years ago and largely substantiated by studies showing that elevated circulating plasma iron exacerbated cellular injury induced by doxorubicin. This was attributed to biological Fenton reaction and cycling of iron between oxidized and reduced states generating H_2O_2 and ROS in the process [25,26]. Further iron chelation with dexrazoxane was shown to reduce doxorubicin-induced cardiotoxicity, supporting a role for aberrant iron regulation in doxorubicin toxicity.

Notably, ATP-binding cassette subfamily B member 8 (ABCB8) is a mitochondrial transport protein that facilitates iron transport; downregulation or inactivation of ABCB8 was shown to impair iron export resulting in mitochondrial iron overload. Recently, Ichikawa et al. [25] demonstrated that cardiac-restricted downregulation of ABCB8 corresponded with an increase in accumulation of mitochondrial iron. Moreover, transgenic mice overexpressing ABCB8 demonstrated a reduction in mitochondrial iron, less ROS production, and markedly improved cardiac function compared to wild type mice treated with doxorubicin [25]. Furthermore, mitochondrial iron overload in doxorubicin cardiomyopathy was confirmed in studies in which iron chelation with dexrazoxane was shown to decrease mitochondrial iron accumulation and doxorubicin toxicity in vitro and in clinical studies. Meta-analysis of data from six clinical trials investigating cardiotoxic effects of doxorubicin verified the protective effects of dexrazoxane against doxorubicin and epirubicin, respectively. In this regard, dexrazoxane is recommended as an adjunctive therapy to the patients where the cumulative dose of doxorubicin approaches 300 mg/m^2. Interestingly, although preclinical studies showed dexrazoxane mediated protection against doxorubicin, it conferred little protection against other anthracycline agents, such as mitoxantrone [27–29] suggesting that mode of cytotoxicity might be different in these anthracyclines. Furthermore, cardiac fibrosis and ventricular matrix remodeling was inhibited by iron chelator, deferoxamine (DFX) cotreatment with doxorubicin evidenced by a reduction in TGF-β, Smad2/4 signaling pathway [26]. These studies highlight that doxorubicin may also induce critical changes in fibrosis signaling that contribute to cardiac remodeling and dysfunction.

CALCIUM OVERLOAD IN MITOCHONDRIA

Over the past 5 decades' advances in cardiovascular biology have implicated that Ca^{2+} overload or alterations in Ca^{2+} metabolism are underlying trigger of necrotic cell death of cardiomyocytes. In this regard, Nakayama et al. showed that increased Ca^{2+} influx through enhanced L-type Ca^{2+} channel (LTCC) activity contributed to cardiac dysfunction and premature necrotic death of cardiomyocytes that could be rescued by LTCC blockade or β-adrenergic receptor antagonists [30]. The cellular and molecular effectors that underlie abnormalities in Ca^{2+} handling in doxorubicin-induced cardiomyopathy remain cryptic. The inducible BH3 domain-only, *B*cl-2 *N*ineteen kilodalton *I*nteracting *P*rotein 3 (Bnip3), is a member of the Bcl-2 gene family recently implicated as an effector of doxorubicin-induced mitochondrial defects and Ca^{2+} overload [11]. Notably, knockdown of Bnip3 or a Bnip3 mutant lacking its mitochondrial targeting sequence prevented both mitochondrial Ca^{2+} overload and necrotic cell death of ventricular myocytes [11]. These studies highlight a novel role of Bnip3 as a molecular effector of doxorubicin-mediated mitochondrial injury and

Ca^{2+} overload. Details regarding Bnip3 as a critical effector of doxorubicin cardiotoxicity will be illustrated in greater detail in the subsequent sections.

ALTERED MITOCHONDRIAL DYNAMICS IN ANTHRACYCLINES

The cellular mitochondrial network is dynamically regulated by mitochondria continually undergoing fusion and fission events which ensure adequate mitochondrial quality control. Maintaining healthy mitochondria is crucial for the normal cellular function and tissue homeostasis. In this regard, altered balance between mitochondrial fission and fusion (too little or too much) has been linked to a number of pathological conditions, such as myocardial infarction, cancers, and neurodegenerative diseases [31–34]. Cardiotoxicity induced by anthracyclines has been associated with disruption of mitochondrial networks and fragmentation from increased fission (Fig. 2.2). Mitochondrial fission is regulated by the large GTPase motor protein *Dynamin related protein* 1 (Drp1) [33–35]. Drp1 is cytosolic under basal conditions but translocates to and binds to the outer mitochondrial membrane (OMM) where it promotes mitochondrial fission [36,37]. Recently doxorubicin cardiotoxicity has been linked to increased mitochondrial fission and is supported by the study demonstrating reduced cardiotoxicity upon Drp-1 inactivation. In cotreatment with the Drp-1 inhibitor, mitochondrial division inhibitor (mdivi-1) attenuated mitochondrial fission and the detrimental effects of doxorubicin on mitochondrial depolarization and hypercontracture of cardiac myocytes [38]. Recently, the antideath protein apoptosis repressor with caspase recruitment domain (ARC) has also been demonstrated to be a critical regulator of mitochondrial fission and doxorubicin-induced cell death. ARC downregulation in ventricular myocytes treated with doxorubicin was associated with accumulation of mitochondrial Drp1 and increased cell death. A link between ARC and Drp1 is further extended by identification of microRNA-532-3p (miR-532-3p) that targets and inactivates ARC gene, thus promoting apoptotic cell death. Moreover, overexpression of ARC is sufficient to prevent mitochondrial fission and cell death [39].

In addition, mitochondrial fragmentation could also arise from inactivation or posttranslational modifications of the proteins of mitochondrial fusion machinery. It is well known that posttranslational modifications, such as phosphorylation, methylation, acetylation, or SUMOylation can alter the functional activity of mitochondrial fusion proteins resulting in fission [40]. A study conducted in isolated ventricular myocytes demonstrated that posttranslational modification of fusion protein OPA-1 by sirtuin 3 (SIRT3)-regulated fusion/fission events and indirectly mitochondrial function. In that study hyperacetylation and inactivation of OPA-1 in cardiac myocytes treated with doxorubicin was similar to the increased mitochondrial fragmentation and loss of cell viability in SIRT3-deficient cells. Importantly, activation of SIRT3 in cardiac myocytes was treated with doxorubicin deacetylated OPA-1, preserving the mitochondrial network and cell viability [41].

Mitochondrial fragmentation is also regulated at the level of the permeability transition pore (PT-pore). Although the structural details regarding the mitochondrial PT-pore composition are not completely understood, the existing literature suggests PT-pore can be regulated by cyclophilin D (CypD) and F1/F0ATPase [42,43]. Interestingly, doxorubicin-induced mitochondrial fragmentation, impaired cardiac function, and mortality were attenuated with cyclosporin A (CsA), which binds to and inhibits CypD and mitochondrial PT-pore opening, in both acute and chronic models of doxorubicin cardiotoxicity. Furthermore CsA derivative tacrolimus (FK506), which has no effect on the mitochondrial PT-pore, did not prevent mitochondrial fragmentation or improve cardiac function or mortality rates, suggesting that mitochondrial PT-pore opening may underlie mitochondrial fragmentation associated with doxorubicin toxicity [44]. The role of CypD in regulation of mitochondrial PT-pore was further confirmed by the studies conducted in $Ppif^{-/-}$ mice (the gene that encode CypD), were relatively more resistant to doxorubicin-induced myocardial injury than corresponding wild-type mice [30].

RESPIRATORY DEFECTS AND ALTERED METABOLISM IN ANTHRACYCLINE CARDIOTOXICITY

Anthracyclines have also been demonstrated to impair metabolism and mitochondrial respiration [11]. Because the heart largely depends on oxidative processes for ATP generation for maintaining ventricular function, mitochondrial respiratory defects that impair ATP synthesis invariably compromise cardiac performance resulting in heart failure. Recently, our laboratory established Bnip3 to be crucial for provoking mitochondrial perturbations and respiratory chain defects resulting in necrotic cell death of cardiac myocytes treated with doxorubicin. In this study, we showed that mitochondrial targeting of Bnip3, was associated with severe mitochondrial abnormalities that impaired respiration both in vitro and in vivo [11]. Moreover interaction between respiratory chain complex IV subunit 1 (COX1) and uncoupling protein 3 (UCP3) was abundant in normal respiring cardiomyocytes, but was completely disrupted in cardiac myocytes treated with doxorubicin, resulting in impaired respiration. The significance of UCP3 and COX1 interaction for normal respiration and mitochondrial function is unknown, however, our data would argue its importance for normal complex-IV activity. However, mice hearts genetically ablated for Bnip3 were resistant to doxorubicin-induced mitochondrial respiratory defects and necrosis, evidenced by reduced LDH and troponin-T release and lowered mortality [11]. In addition to UCP's role in normal respiration and ATP synthesis, it also protects cardiomyocytes from exogenous as well as mitochondrial ROS production; a decline in UCP2 and UCP3 sensitizes mitochondria to oxidative stress and increased ROS production [18].

Anthracyclines also alter cellular metabolism by affecting several genes involved in glycolytic and oxidative metabolism. In this regard, Gao et al. [45] demonstrated that mitochondrial defects, such as reduced ATP and cell death were associated with an increased expression of glycolytic enzyme, α-enolase in doxorubicin treated cardiomyocytes in vitro and in vivo. Importantly, doxorubicin-induced mitochondrial dysfunction, ATP production defects, and apoptosis were suppressed in cells and hearts depleted of α-enolase [45]. Interestingly, altered metabolism of phospholipids, such as cardiolipins may also result in defective mitochondrial function and energy metabolism. Cardiolipins are major lipids in the inner mitochondrial membrane and have a key role in assembly and function of mitochondrial inner membrane proteins of the oxidative phosphorylation complexes [46].

AUTOPHAGY IN ANTHRACYCLINE CARDIOTOXICITY

Autophagy is a highly regulated catabolic process which is essential for removing damaged proteins and macromolecular structure and serves as quality control for cellular homeostasis and cell survival [47–49]. Autophagy can also involve chaperone proteins that facilitate removal of damaged proteins by association with heat shock cognate (HSC) protein. Defects in autophagy and proteasomal machinery results in the accumulation of damaged and misfolded proteins as well as organelles, such as damaged mitochondria that negatively impact cell metabolism and function. Autophagy is an extremely balanced process and considered crucial for cell survival. However, autophagy is a double-edged sword, since in some instances excessive or maladaptive autophagy can be detrimental and promote cell death [50]. Autophagic cell death is also referred to as type-II programmed cell death.

Notably, doxorubicin-treated cardiomyocytes and mice display an extensive vacuolization and increased autophagic flux [51]. In the context of doxorubicin toxicity there have been several conflicting reports suggesting autophagy on the one hand to be maladaptive and promote cell death, whereas on the other hand to be protective and promote cell survival. In separate studies, Zhang et al. demonstrated multiple genes and signaling pathways as key regulators of autophagy [39]. For example, autophagy was reportedly increased in H9c2 cells and hearts of mice treated with doxorubicin. In this case, the observed autophagy was attributed

to increased levels of c-Jun N-terminal kinase (JNK) and ROS production [50,52,53]. Moreover ophiopogonin D (OP-D), a steroidal glycoside, partially protected cardiac myocytes and mice hearts by preventing ROS production, loss of mitochondrial membrane potential, and autophagy. This was attributed to the downregulation of JNK and extracellular signal-regulated kinase (ERK) signaling pathways [39]. The maladaptive nature of autophagy was further supported in studies conducted in doxorubicin-treated H2c2 cells, which exhibited increased LDH release and cell death that could be abrogated by autophagy inhibitor 3-methyl adenine (3MA) or ghrelin, a multifunctional peptide hormone. Furthermore, ghrelin increased mTOR activity by decreasing AMPK and reduced autophagy [50]. Moreover, genetic approaches or drugs that increased autophagy further aggravated cell death, supporting a maladaptive role for autophagy in the context of doxorubicin cardiotoxicty. Further, the downregulation of transcription factor GATA4 in cells treated with doxorubicin was proposed as an underlying cause of excessive autophagy. Importantly, GATA4 overexpression upregulated Bcl-2, suppressing doxorubicin-induced autophagy and cardiomyocyte death [51]. Yet other studies linked mitochondrial aldehyde dehydrogenase (ALDH2) to cardioprotection via suppression of 4-hydroxynonenal (4-HNE), ROS, and autophagy. ALDH2 knockout mice displayed increased ROS production, autophagy, and deteriorated cardiac function. Restoration of ALDH2 activated survival kinase Akt and suppressed 4-HNE and autophagy [54]. Another study linked neuregulin (NRG)-1, a member of the NRG family, essential for embryonic cardiac development and cardiac function in the postnatal heart, to autophagy. Interestingly, recombinant neuregulin-1 (rhNRG-1) suppressed pathological cardiac remodeling and cardiac dysfunction by inhibiting doxorubicin-induced autophagy. Furthermore rhNRG-1-mediated inhibition of autophagy involved activation of Akt and Bcl-2 [55].

In contrast to aforementioned reports suggesting autophagy to be a detrimental process leading to cell death or heart failure, several studies have found the contrary to be true. For example, doxorubicin-induced mitochondrial defects, ROS production, and cell death were suppressed by the mTOR inhibitor rapamycin, which presumably would promote autophagy [56,57]. Further, impaired autophagic flux and accumulation of polyubiquitinated proteins were suggested to be an underlying cause of increased oxidative stress, cardiomyocyte necrosis, and cardiac dysfunction in acute mouse model of doxorubicin toxicity. Notably, Nrf2 knockout mice which exhibited a lower level of autophagy were more sensitive to doxorubicin cytotoxicity and Nrf2 overexpression restored autophagy flux, and decreased the accumulation of protein aggregates and doxorubicin cardiotoxicity. On the basis of these studies, one could argue that in addition to regulating cellular antioxidant status, Nrf2 is a key regulator of autophagy in the heart [10]. In another study, cytosolic p53 has been linked to impaired autophagy, mitochondrial dysfunction, and heart failure following doxorubicin treatment. According to this study, cytosolic p53 binds to Parkin, an E3-ligase essential for mitochondrial turnover and quality control, and prevents its translocation to damaged mitochondria, thereby impairing their clearance by mitophagy [31]. Negative regulation of mitophagy by p53 is further confirmed in p53-deficient mice which demonstrated increased mitophagy, preserved mitochondrial integrity, and cardiac function [57]. However, whether autophagy is adaptive, maladaptive, or a homeostatic response in heart following doxorubicin treatment, may depend on the spatial and temporal activation of autophagy in a cell type and context specific manner.

DEREGULATED MOLECULAR SIGNALING PATHWAYS IN ANTHRACYCLINE CARDIOTOXICITY

Altered expression of several critical genes and signaling pathways have been linked to anthracycline-induced myocardial injury. The majority of studies conducted on anthracycline toxicities have been linked to the genes and signaling pathways that impinge on mitochondrial function, oxidative stress, apoptosis, necrosis, or autophagy, where gain or loss of function of a genetic pathway predisposes cardiomyocytes to anthracycline toxicity (Fig. 2.1). For example, downregulation of GATA4 predisposes cardiomyocytes to autophagic cell death through loss of balance between Bcl-2 and Beclin-1 [51]. Moreover, acetylation of p53 protein on K379 residue has been shown to be critical for induction of Bax, cytochrome *c* release and caspase 3 and 9 activation. Importantly, acetylation of p53 and apoptotic cell death is regulated by interaction of p53 with sirtuin 1 (SIRT1) [52,58]. Interestingly, GATA4 has been shown to be downregulated by p53. Notably, p53 suppresses GATA4 transcription by inhibiting CBF/NF-Y (the CCAAT-binding factor/nuclear factor-Y) binding to the CCAAT box in GATA4 promoter and therefore inhibiting GATA4's ability to activate transcription; this presumably would result in loss of Bcl-2 and other GATA4-dependent genes required for cell survival [59].

Notably, as stated previously, mitochondrial targeting of Bnip3 disrupted interaction between UCP3 and COX1 consistently with defective mitochondrial respiration. Remarkably, doxorubicin-induced cardiomyocte injury was prevented with loss of function mutations of Bnip3 defective for mitochondrial targeting or following Bnip3 knockdown. Furthermore, in contrast to wild-type mice, which displayed severe mitochondrial abnormalities and extensive cardiac injury typical of doxorubicin toxicity, Bnip3 knockout mice were resistant to the cytotoxic effects of doxorubicin displaying normal mitochondrial respiration, cardiac function,

and reduced mortality. [11]. These findings collectively support the notion that Bnip3 is a critical downstream effector of doxorubicin cardiotoxicity.

Further evidence suggests that mitochondrial defects are secondary events linked to doxorubicin-induced DNA double-strand breaks and transcriptome changes by topoisomerase-IIβ (TOP2β). Following doxorubicin treatment, a TOP2β–doxorubicin–DNA ternary cleavage complex is formed which can induce DNA double strand breaks, trigger apoptotic signaling and alterations in the transcriptome that affects processes, such as oxidative phosphorylation and mitochondrial biogenesis in cardiomyocytes, subsequently leading to cell death. Moreover, cardiomyocyte-specific deletion of Top2β protected mice from developing cardiac dysfunction [60]. These studies reveal the interrelationship and intracellular cross-talk between nuclear DNA and mitochondrial dysfunction that underlie the cytotoxic effects of doxorubicin.

GENDER-SPECIFIC CARDIOTOXIC EFFECTS OF ANTHRACYCLINE

Notably, gender differences also play a role in the sensitivity to doxorubicin-induced myocardial injury. Surprisingly, men were found to be more susceptible to doxorubicin cardiotoxicity than women [61]. The mechanisms underlying this sexual dimorphism remain unclear but are believed to be related to altered mitochondrial metabolism between men and women. For instance, cardiolipin content, which is a major component of the inner mitochondrial membrane, was found to be markedly reduced in men versus women treated with doxorubicin [46].

Cardiolipins play a key role in assembly and function of mitochondrial membrane proteins for oxidative phosphorylation. Interestingly, altered metabolism of cardiolipins also resulted in mitochondrial dysfunction and impaired energy metabolism. Cardiac phospholipid profile of chemotherapy receiving men and women demonstrated that women had significantly higher cardiolipin species with longer acyl chains compared to men after dox-treatment. Remodeling in cardiolipin-acyl chains in females may have provided better protection from anthracyclines toxicity; however, this finding requires more detailed investigation [46].

ANTHRACYCLINES AND CARDIAC REMODELING

The electron micrographs and histological analysis of the myocardium of animals treated with doxorubicin revealed severe vacuolization, interstitial fibrosis, and loss of myofibrils, indicative features of pathological cardiac remodeling. Inflammation also initiates a cascade of events leading to adverse remodeling and cardiomyopathy. Proinflammatory cytokines TNF-α and IL-6 were elevated within the first

24 h of doxorubicin treatment and coincided with reduction of antiinflammatory cytokine IL-10. TNF-α–IL-10 balance has been shown to be critical for regulating cell survival in other conditions [62].

These acute changes in cytokine expression likely support the underlying cellular defects and progression of doxorubicin-induced cardiomyopathy. Toll-like receptors (TLRs) are an integral part of the innate immune system, play a critical role in cardiac inflammatory signaling, and have also been implicated in the cellular responses associated with doxorubicin-induced cardiomyopathy. This is evidenced by a recent study demonstrating increased TNFα, apoptosis, and defects in ventricular function in doxorubicin-treated wild-type mice. In contrast, TLR-deficient mice displayed reduced oxidative and inflammatory responses, expressed increased levels of GATA-4, and had better survival, suggesting a role for TLR receptors in doxorubicin cardiotoxicity [63].

Deposition of excessive extracellular matrix and fibrosis are important characteristics of pathological cardiac remodeling. In pathological settings, cardiac fibroblasts proliferate and differentiate into myofibroblasts and secrete collagen and fibronectin. The resulting ventricular wall stiffness eventually leads to arrhythmias and contractile dysfunction. TGF-β/SMAD3 signaling pathway is critical for initiating cardiac fibrosis and remodeling. Increased levels of TGF-β and Smad2/4 have been reported in cardiac myocytes treated with doxorubicin [26]. Activation of SIRT3 decreased TGF-β/SMAD3 signaling and reduced fibrosis and myocardial remodeling in doxorubicin-treated mice. However, which specific protein SIRT3 targets within TGF-β/SMAD3 signaling pathway is presently unclear. Matrix metalloproteinases (MMPs), which are responsible for degrading extracellular matrix components, have also been implicated in adverse cardiac remodeling after doxorubicin treatment [64]. Doxorubicin cardiotoxicity is associated with widespread sarcomere disarray and loss of myofilaments. Recently, cardiac ankyrin repeat protein (CARP, ANKRD1) has been linked to transcriptional regulation of myofilament genes. Notably, doxorubicin treatment resulted in depletion of CARP consistent with sarcomere disarray, whereas reestablishment of CARP restored sarcomere structure, verifying the role of CARP in maintaining sarcomere structure. Notably, CARP is regulated by GATA4 which binds to the proximal CARP promoter to activate it [65].

STRATEGIES TO PREVENT DOXORUBICIN CARDIOTOXICITY

To reduce doxorubicin cardiotoxicity and enhance its overall clinical benefit, selective delivery of doxorubicin to tumor cells by anthracycline formulations with comparable efficacy and improved safety are being tested. For example, polyethylene-conjugated liposomes containing doxorubicin (PLD) have been tested for greater specificity of doxorubicin tissue targeting with less cardiotoxicity. In phase-I and -II clinical trials the efficacy of PLD was tested in patients with solid tumors including breast cancer. The positive outcome showing efficacy of the drug in eradicating the tumor without causing cardiotoxicity led to phase-III clinical trials conducted in ovarian cancer patients. A phase-III trial also produced results similar to phase-I and -II and support the use of PLD for treating metastatic cancers [6].Several other strategies are under consideration to target doxorubicin to specific regions within the tumor by modulating pH or by biochemical targeting of cancer cell receptors [66].

CONCLUSIONS

Doxorubicin and related anthracycline agents are highly effective chemotherapeutic agents that unfortunately exhibit cardiotoxic effects that lead to cell death and ultimately cardiac failure. Understanding the underlying signaling pathways that mediate anthracycline toxicity is of paramount importance in this emerging new field of cardio-oncology toward the ultimate therapeutic goal in reducing the cardiotoxic effects of these compounds without compromising their efficacy as cancer therapies. The development of adjunctive therapies that can mitigate the off-target effects of doxorubicin particularly on mitochondrial function and respiration hold promise in reducing cardiac morbidity and mortality in cancer patients treated with these compounds.

REFERENCES

[1] Yeh ET, Tong AT, Lenihan DJ, Yusuf SW, Swafford J, Champion C, Durand JB, Gibbs H, Zafarmand AA, Ewer MS. Cardiovascular complications of cancer therapy: diagnosis, pathogenesis, and management. Circulation 2004;109:3122–31.

[2] Eschenhagen T, Force T, Ewer MS, de Keulenaer GW, Suter TM, Anker SD, Avkiran M, de AE, Balligand JL, Brutsaert DL, Condorelli G, Hansen A, Heymans S, Hill JA, Hirsch E, Hilfiker-Kleiner D, Janssens S, de JS, Neubauer G, Pieske B, Ponikowski P, Pirmohamed M, Rauchhaus M, Sawyer D, Sugden PH, Wojta J, Zannad F, Shah AM. Cardiovascular side effects of cancer therapies: a position statement from the Heart Failure Association of the European Society of Cardiology. Eur J Heart Fail 2011;13:1–10.

[3] Minotti G, Menna P, Salvatorelli E, Cairo G, Gianni L. Anthracyclines: molecular advances and pharmacologic developments in antitumor activity and cardiotoxicity. Pharmacol Rev 2004;56:185–229.

[4] Ewer MS, Von Hoff DD, Benjamin RS. A historical perspective of anthracycline cardiotoxicity. Heart Fail Clin 2011;7:363–72.

[5] Schimmel KJ, Richel DJ, van den Brink RB, Guchelaar HJ. Cardiotoxicity of cytotoxic drugs. Cancer Treat Rev 2004;30:181–91.

[6] O'Brien ME, Wigler N, Inbar M, Rosso R, Grischke E, Santoro A, Catane R, Kieback DG, Tomczak P, Ackland SP, Orlandi F, Mellars L, Alland L, Tendler C. Reduced cardiotoxicity and comparable efficacy in a phase III trial of pegylated liposomal doxorubicin HCl (CAELYX/Doxil) versus conventional doxorubicin for first-line treatment of metastatic breast cancer. Ann Oncol 2004;15:440–9.

[7] Sawyer DB, Fukazawa R, Arstall MA, Kelly RA. Daunorubicin-induced apoptosis in rat cardiac myocytes is inhibited by dexrazoxane. Circ Res 1999;84:257–65.

[8] Unverferth DV, Magorien RD, Unverferth BP, Talley RL, Balcerzak SP, Baba N. Human myocardial morphologic and functional changes in the first 24 hours after doxorubicin administration. Cancer Treat Rep 1981;65:1093–7.

[9] Ryberg M, Nielsen D, Skovsgaard T, Hansen J, Jensen BV, Dombernowsky P. Epirubicin cardiotoxicity: an analysis of 469 patients with metastatic breast cancer. J Clin Oncol 1998;16:3502–8.

[10] Li S, Wang W, Niu T, Wang H, Li B, Shao L, Lai Y, Li H, Janicki JS, Wang XL, Tang D, Cui T. Nrf2 deficiency exaggerates doxorubicin-induced cardiotoxicity and cardiac dysfunction. Oxid Med Cell Longev 2014;2014:748524.

[11] Dhingra R, Margulets V, Chowdhury SR, Thliveris J, Jassal D, Fernyhough P, Dorn GW, Kirshenbaum LA. Bnip3 mediates doxorubicin-induced cardiac myocyte necrosis and mortality through changes in mitochondrial signaling. Proc Natl Acad Sci USA 2014;111: E5537–44.

[12] Kumar D, Kirshenbaum LA, Li T, Danelisen I, Singal PK. Apoptosis in adriamycin cardiomyopathy and its modulation by probucol. Antioxid Redox Signal 2001;3:135–45.

[13] Wang JX, Zhang XJ, Feng C, Sun T, Wang K, Wang Y, Zhou LY, Li PF. MicroRNA-532-3p regulates mitochondrial fission through targeting apoptosis repressor with caspase recruitment domain in doxorubicin cardiotoxicity. Cell Death Dis 2015;6:e1677.

[14] Singh P, Sharma R, McElhanon K, Allen CD, Megyesi JK, Benes H, Singh SP. Sulforaphane protects the heart from doxorubicin-induced toxicity. Free Radic Biol Med 2015;86:90–101.

[15] Li DL, Hill JA. Cardiomyocyte autophagy and cancer chemotherapy. J Mol Cell Cardiol 2014;71:54–61.

[16] Xiong Y, Liu X, Lee CP, Chua BH, Ho YS. Attenuation of doxorubicin-induced contractile and mitochondrial dysfunction in mouse heart by cellular glutathione peroxidase. Free Radic Biol Med 2006;41:46–55.

[17] Diotte NM, Xiong Y, Gao J, Chua BH, Ho YS. Attenuation of doxorubicin-induced cardiac injury by mitochondrial glutaredoxin 2. Biochim Biophys Acta 2009;1793:427–38.

[18] Bugger H, Guzman C, Zechner C, Palmeri M, Russell KS, Russell RR III. Uncoupling protein downregulation in doxorubicin-induced heart failure improves mitochondrial coupling but increases reactive oxygen species generation. Cancer Chemother Pharmacol 2011;67:1381–8.

[19] Simunek T, Sterba M, Popelova O, Adamcova M, Hrdina R, Gersl V. Anthracycline-induced cardiotoxicity: overview of studies examining the roles of oxidative stress and free cellular iron. Pharmacol Rep 2009;61:154–71.

[20] Dresdale AR, Barr LH, Bonow RO, Mathisen DJ, Myers CE, Schwartz DE, d'Angelo T, Rosenberg SA. Prospective randomized study of the role of N-acetyl cysteine in reversing doxorubicin-induced cardiomyopathy. Am J Clin Oncol 1982;5:657–63.

[21] Bruynzeel AM, Niessen HW, Bronzwaer JG, van der Hoeven JJ, Berkhof J, Bast A, van der Vijgh WJ, van Groeningen CJ. The effect of monohydroxyethylrutoside on doxorubicin-induced cardiotoxicity in patients treated for metastatic cancer in a phase II study. Br J Cancer 2007;97:1084–9.

[22] van Dalen EC, Caron HN, Dickinson HO, Kremer LC. Cardioprotective interventions for cancer patients receiving anthracyclines. Cochrane Database Syst Rev 2008;2:CD003917.

[23] Broeyer FJ, Osanto S, Suzuki J, de JF, van SH, Tanis BC, Bruning T, Bax JJ, Ritsema van Eck HJ, de Kam ML, Cohen AF, Mituzhima Y, Burggraaf J. Evaluation of lecithinized human recombinant super oxide dismutase as cardioprotectant in anthracycline-treated breast cancer patients. Br J Clin Pharmacol 2014;78:950–60.

[24] Zhang S, Liu X, Bawa-Khalfe T, Lu LS, Lyu YL, Liu LF, Yeh ET. Identification of the molecular basis of doxorubicin-induced cardiotoxicity. Nat Med 2012;18:1639–42.

[25] Ichikawa Y, Ghanefar M, Bayeva M, Wu R, Khechaduri A, Naga Prasad SV, Mutharasan RK, Naik TJ, Ardehali H. Cardiotoxicity of doxorubicin is mediated through mitochondrial iron accumulation. J Clin Invest 2014;124:617–30.

[26] Al-Shabanah OA, Aleisa AM, Hafez MM, Al-Rejaie SS, Al-Yahya AA, Bakheet SA, Al-Harbi MM, Sayed-Ahmed MM. Desferrioxamine attenuates doxorubicin-induced acute cardiotoxicity through TFG-beta/Smad p53 pathway in rat model. Oxid Med Cell Longev 2012;2012:619185.

[27] Seymour L, Bramwell V, Moran LA. Use of dexrazoxane as a cardioprotectant in patients receiving doxorubicin or epirubicin chemotherapy for the treatment of cancer. The Provincial Systemic Treatment Disease Site Group. Cancer Prev Control 1999;3:145–59.

[28] Hasinoff BB, Herman EH. Dexrazoxane: how it works in cardiac and tumor cells. Is it a prodrug or is it a drug? Cardiovasc Toxicol 2007;7:140–4.

[29] Swain SM, Vici P. The current and future role of dexrazoxane as a cardioprotectant in anthracycline treatment: expert panel review. J Cancer Res Clin Oncol 2004;130:1–7.

[30] Nakayama H, Chen X, Baines CP, Klevitsky R, Zhang X, Zhang H, Jaleel N, Chua BH, Hewett TE, Robbins J, Houser SR, Molkentin JD. Ca2+− and mitochondrial-dependent cardiomyocyte necrosis as a primary mediator of heart failure. J Clin Invest 2007;117:2431–44.

[31] Song M, Gong G, Burelle Y, Gustafsson AB, Kitsis RN, Matkovich SJ, Dorn GW. Interdependence of Parkin-mediated mitophagy and mitochondrial fission in adult mouse hearts. Circ Res 2015;117: 346–51.

[32] Morais VA, Verstreken P, Roethig A, Smet J, Snellinx A, Vanbrabant M, Haddad D, Frezza C, Mandemakers W, Vogt-Weisenhorn D, Van CR, Wurst W, Scorrano L, De SB. Parkinson's disease mutations in PINK1 result in decreased Complex I activity and deficient synaptic function. EMBO Mol Med 2009;1:99–111.

[33] Narendra D, Tanaka A, Suen DF, Youle RJ. Parkin is recruited selectively to impaired mitochondria and promotes their autophagy. J Cell Biol 2008;183:795–803.

[34] Narendra DP, Jin SM, Tanaka A, Suen DF, Gautier CA, Shen J, Cookson MR, Youle RJ. PINK1 is selectively stabilized on impaired mitochondria to activate Parkin. PLoS Biol 2010;8:e1000298.

[35] Martinou JC, Youle RJ. Mitochondria in apoptosis: Bcl-2 family members and mitochondrial dynamics. Dev Cell 2011;21:92–101.

[36] Cribbs JT, Strack S. Reversible phosphorylation of Drp1 by cyclic AMP-dependent protein kinase and calcineurin regulates mitochondrial fission and cell death. EMBO Rep 2007;8:939–44.

[37] Ingerman E, Perkins EM, Marino M, Mears JA, McCaffery JM, Hinshaw JE, Nunnari J. Dnm1 forms spirals that are structurally tailored to fit mitochondria. J Cell Biol 2005;170:1021–7.

[38] Gharanei M, Hussain A, Janneh O, Maddock H. Attenuation of doxorubicin-induced cardiotoxicity by mdivi-1: a mitochondrial division/mitophagy inhibitor. PLoS One 2013;8:e77713.

[39] Zhang C, Qu S, Wei X, Feng Y, Zhu H, Deng J, Wang K, Liu K, Liu M, Zhang H, Xiao X. HSP25 down-regulation enhanced p53 acetylation

by dissociation of SIRT1 from p53 in doxorubicin-induced H9c2 cell apoptosis. Cell Stress Chaperones 2015;21(2):251–60.

[40] Dhingra R, Kirshenbaum LA. Regulation of mitochondrial dynamics and cell fate. Circ J 2014;78:803–10.

[41] Samant SA, Zhang HJ, Hong Z, Pillai VB, Sundaresan NR, Wolfgeher D, Archer SL, Chan DC, Gupta MP. SIRT3 deacetylates and activates OPA1 to regulate mitochondrial dynamics during stress. Mol Cell Biol 2014;34:807–19.

[42] Giorgio V, von SS, Antoniel M, Fabbro A, Fogolari F, Forte M, Glick GD, Petronilli V, Zoratti M, Szabo I, Lippe G, Bernardi P. Dimers of mitochondrial ATP synthase form the permeability transition pore. Proc Natl Acad Sci USA 2013;110:5887–92.

[43] Baines CP, Kaiser RA, Purcell NH, Blair NS, Osinska H, Hambleton MA, Brunskill EW, Sayen MR, Gottlieb RA, Dorn GW, Robbins J, Molkentin JD. Loss of cyclophilin D reveals a critical role for mitochondrial permeability transition in cell death. Nature 2005;434:658–62.

[44] Marechal X, Montaigne D, Marciniak C, Marchetti P, Hassoun SM, Beauvillain JC, Lancel S, Neviere R. Doxorubicin-induced cardiac dysfunction is attenuated by ciclosporin treatment in mice through improvements in mitochondrial bioenergetics. Clin Sci (Lond) 2011;121:405–13.

[45] Gao S, Li H, Feng XJ, Li M, Liu ZP, Cai Y, Lu J, Huang XY, Wang JJ, Li Q, Chen SR, Ye JT, Liu PQ. alpha-Enolase plays a catalytically independent role in doxorubicin-induced cardiomyocyte apoptosis and mitochondrial dysfunction. J Mol Cell Cardiol 2015;79:92–103.

[46] Moulin M, Piquereau J, Mateo P, Fortin D, Rucker-Martin C, Gressette M, Lefebvre F, Gresikova M, Solgadi A, Veksler V, Garnier A, Ventura-Clapier R. Sexual dimorphism of doxorubicin-mediated cardiotoxicity: potential role of energy metabolism remodeling. Circ Heart Fail 2015;8:98–108.

[47] Gottlieb RA, Mentzer RM. Autophagy during cardiac stress: joys and frustrations of autophagy. Annu Rev Physiol 2010;72:45–59.

[48] Kroemer G, Levine B. Autophagic cell death: the story of a misnomer. Nat Rev Mol Cell Biol 2008;9:1004–10.

[49] Levine B. Cell biology: autophagy and cancer. Nature 2007;446:745–7.

[50] Wang X, Wang XL, Chen HL, Wu D, Chen JX, Wang XX, Li RL, He JH, Mo L, Cen X, Wei YQ, Jiang W. Ghrelin inhibits doxorubicin cardiotoxicity by inhibiting excessive autophagy through AMPK and p38-MAPK. Biochem Pharmacol 2014;88:334–50.

[51] Kobayashi S, Volden P, Timm D, Mao K, Xu X, Liang Q. Transcription factor GATA4 inhibits doxorubicin-induced autophagy and cardiomyocyte death. J Biol Chem 2010;285:793–804.

[52] Zhang YY, Meng C, Zhang XM, Yuan CH, Wen MD, Chen Z, Dong DC, Gao YH, Liu C, Zhang Z. Ophiopogonin D attenuates doxorubicin-induced autophagic cell death by relieving mitochondrial damage in vitro and in vivo. J Pharmacol Exp Ther 2015;352:166–74.

[53] Smuder AJ, Kavazis AN, Min K, Powers SK. Doxorubicin-induced markers of myocardial autophagic signaling in sedentary and exercise trained animals. J Appl Physiol (1985) 2013;115:176–85.

[54] Sun A, Cheng Y, Zhang Y, Zhang Q, Wang S, Tian S, Zou Y, Hu K, Ren J, Ge J. Aldehyde dehydrogenase 2 ameliorates doxorubicin-induced myocardial dysfunction through detoxification of 4-HNE and suppression of autophagy. J Mol Cell Cardiol 2014;71:92–104.

[55] An T, Huang Y, Zhou Q, Wei BQ, Zhang RC, Yin SJ, Zou CH, Zhang YH, Zhang J. Neuregulin-1 attenuates doxorubicin-induced autophagy in neonatal rat cardiomyocytes. J Cardiovasc Pharmacol 2013;62:130–7.

[56] Sishi BJ, Loos B, van RJ, Engelbrecht AM. Autophagy upregulation promotes survival and attenuates doxorubicin-induced cardiotoxicity. Biochem Pharmacol 2013;85:124–34.

[57] Hoshino A, Mita Y, Okawa Y, Ariyoshi M, Iwai-Kanai E, Ueyama T, Ikeda K, Ogata T, Matoba S. Cytosolic p53 inhibits Parkin-mediated mitophagy and promotes mitochondrial dysfunction in the mouse heart. Nat Commun 2013;4:2308.

[58] Shizukuda Y, Matoba S, Mian OY, Nguyen T, Hwang PM. Targeted disruption of p53 attenuates doxorubicin-induced cardiac toxicity in mice. Mol Cell Biochem 2005;273:25–32.

[59] Park AM, Nagase H, Liu L, Vinod KS, Szwergold N, Wong CM, Suzuki YJ. Mechanism of anthracycline-mediated down-regulation of GATA4 in the heart. Cardiovasc Res 2011;90:97–104.

[60] Zhang H, Shen WS, Gao CH, Deng LC, Shen D. Protective effects of salidroside on epirubicin-induced early left ventricular regional systolic dysfunction in patients with breast cancer. Drugs R D 2012;12:101–6.

[61] Moulin M, Solgadi A, Veksler V, Garnier A, Ventura-Clapier R, Chaminade P. Sex-specific cardiac cardiolipin remodelling after doxorubicin treatment. Biol Sex Differ 2015;6:20.

[62] Dhingra S, Sharma AK, Arora RC, Slezak J, Singal PK. IL-10 attenuates TNF-alpha-induced NF kappaB pathway activation and cardiomyocyte apoptosis. Cardiovasc Res 2009;82:59–66.

[63] Riad A, Bien S, Gratz M, Escher F, Westermann D, Heimesaat MM, Bereswill S, Krieg T, Felix SB, Schultheiss HP, Kroemer HK, Tschope C. Toll-like receptor-4 deficiency attenuates doxorubicin-induced cardiomyopathy in mice. Eur J Heart Fail 2008;10:233–43.

[64] Polegato BF, Minicucci MF, Azevedo PS, Carvalho RF, Chiuso-Minicucci F, Pereira EJ, Paiva SA, Zornoff LA, Okoshi MP, Matsubara BB, Matsubara LS. Acute doxorubicin-induced cardiotoxicity is associated with matrix metalloproteinase-2 alterations in rats. Cell Physiol Biochem 2015;35:1924–33.

[65] Chen B, Zhong L, Roush SF, Pentassuglia L, Peng X, Samaras S, Davidson JM, Sawyer DB, Lim CC. Disruption of a GATA4/Ankrd1 signaling axis in cardiomyocytes leads to sarcomere disarray: implications for anthracycline cardiomyopathy. PLoS One 2012;7:e35743.

[66] Luo Y, Bernshaw NJ, Lu ZR, Kopecek J, Prestwich GD. Targeted delivery of doxorubicin by HPMA copolymer-hyaluronan bioconjugates. Pharm Res 2002;19:396–402.

Chapter 3

Common Pathways in Cancer, Tumor Angiogenesis and Vascular Disease

E.M. Redmond*, C. Lally** and P.A. Cahill†

*Department of Surgery, University of Rochester Medical Centre, Rochester, NY, United States; **Department of Mechanical and Manufacturing Engineering, School of Engineering, Trinity College Dublin, The University of Dublin, Dublin, Ireland; †Vascular Biology and Therapeutics Laboratory, School of Biotechnology Faculty of Science and Health, Dublin City University, Dublin, Ireland

INTRODUCTION

Vascular disease and cancer together account for the greatest burden on global health in terms of mortality and overall healthcare costs. Numerous mechanisms and pathways involved in cancer have also been implicated in cardiovascular disease, with several important common pillar properties that enable a normal cell to proliferate and ultimately become malignant [1]. Specifically, cancer cells have the ability to sustain growth; evade growth suppressors; resist apoptosis; enable replicative immortality; induce angiogenesis; activate invasion and metastasis; reprogram energy metabolism; and evade immune destruction [1]. Moreover, cancer is a disease of aging, as older adults are much more likely to develop the disease when compared with their younger counterparts [2]. Similarly, vascular cells of the blood vessel wall can become proliferative and migratory and ultimately contribute to vascular disease progression through an orchestrated process associated with aging [3]. Importantly, both diseases share several modifiable risk factors including sedentary lifestyle, obesity, smoking, unhealthy diet, and alcohol abuse [4].

Emerging evidence of a commonality of cellular and molecular pathways dictating cancer and vascular cell fate during disease progression suggest that they are far more closely aligned than previously thought. Fundamental changes in the function of key cell-proliferation regulatory pathways, including genes involved in the G1S checkpoint (p15, p16, p53, pRb and cyclins A, D, E, and cdk) are indicative of both conditions [5,6]. So too are key alterations in adhesion molecules [7,8], oxidative stress, and the associated cellular damage [9,10]. In addition, certain ligand-growth factor receptor interactions and nuclear transcription factors have been associated with the initiation, development, and progression of both conditions [11–13].

Although tumor angiogenesis is fundamental to cancer progression, angiogenic modulators have also recently been linked to atherosclerotic plaque expansion and restenosis after iatrogenic intervention [14–16]. Common disease treatments, such as antimitotic inhibitors and radiation treatment, first established as anticancer treatments, have since been introduced into atherosclerosis therapeutic strategies to prevent restenosis after angioplasty and endarterectomy [17].

Recent functional genomic and proteomic studies of tumor development have revealed the existence of a unique niche of tumor cells that possess distinctive self-renewal, proliferation, and differentiation capabilities, called cancer stem(-like) cells (CSCs) or tumor-initiating cells (TICs) [1,18]. As some tissue types are far more susceptible to cancer than others, a provocative new analysis has been recently put forward purporting that a large percentage of cancers may be due to "bad luck" as a result of stochastic random mutation events during DNA replication in normal, noncancerous resident tissue stem cells [19]. This paradigm shift, although controversial, raises not only important questions about the etiology of this disease but also about strategies for designing therapeutics to limit its high mortality rates. Moreover, it is now clear that in many cancers, such as multiple myelomas, a small fraction of clonogenic stem cell-like cells exhibit not only pronounced self-renewal and differentiation capacities but also pronounced drug resistance. Several markers including CD138$^-$ and ALDH1$^+$ have been used to identify this particular niche and they rely on self-renewal and prosurvival stimuli from AKT, Wnt/β-catenin, Notch, and Hedgehog signaling pathways. This neoplastic "stemness" and their interactions with the bone marrow microenvironment are also thought to promote drug resistance [20–22].

Similarly, an important paradigm shift has been proposed to explain the etiology of vascular diseases, including arteriosclerosis, atherosclerosis, and in-stent restenosis, which involve proliferative vascular smooth muscle cells (vSMCs) [23]. Activation of resident multipotent vascular stem cells or vascular progenitors (instead of, or in addition to, vSMC de-differentiation [24]), results in transition of resident stem cells down a vascular lineage and accumulation of proliferative synthetic vSMCs within the vessel wall. These stem cells are normally embedded within the vessel wall for normal homeostasis and tissue regeneration [23]. However, their activation by known risk factors for vascular disease can occur as a result of inductive signaling pathways, such as Hedgehog, Wnt/β-catenin, Notch and TGFβ-1, and lead to the accumulation of stem-cell derived vSMCs within the diseased vessel. These resident vascular stem cells may soon be recognized not only as important players in the etiology and development of several vascular diseases phenotypes [23,25–28] but also as important targets for therapeutic intervention. These pathways of vascular "stemness" can also promote a similar drug resistance to vascular antimitotic treatments as to those observed in cancer CCSs [29–31]. Both these paradigm shifts are predicted to have a transformative impact on our understanding of cancer and vascular disease etiology, and further, lead to the development of novel targeted molecular therapies against these tissue/resident stem cells. Although the origin and plasticity of CSCs and resident vascular stem cells remain controversial, the cellular heterogeneity and the presence of small populations of cells with stem-like characteristics is now well established in most malignancies and vascular lesions [19].

The prognosis for cancer has improved considerably with the advent of targeted molecular therapy. However, as higher survival rates emerge, many cancer survivors acquire a higher risk of cardiovascular disease than of relapse [32,33]. Indeed, clear associations between chemotherapy/radiotherapy treatments and the deterioration of vascular health, including hypertension, stroke, and atherosclerosis have been widely reported and are primarily due to the use of angiogenesis inhibitors (bevacizumab, sorafenib, and sunitinib), corticosteroids, erythropoietin, and nonsteroidal antiinflammatory drugs [17,34,35]. Morbidity increases in patients with cancer and associated hypertension without proper antihypertensive treatment. This underscores the unmet clinical need for early diagnosis, effective monitoring, and treatment strategies for in these hypertensive patients with cancer, in order to reduce cardiovascular mortality [33,34,36].

HEDGEHOG SIGNALING

Malignant tissue and vascular lesions both display many features of embryonic or tissue stem cells, and typically exhibit persistent activation of one or more highly conserved signal transduction pathways involved in embryonic development and tissue homeostasis, including Hedgehog (Hh), Notch, and Wnt pathways [37,38].

Discovered by Nusslein-Volhard et al., in 1980, Hh signaling is known as a key mediator of many cellular and developmental processes [31,39]. The Hh protein family consists of morphogenic molecules that are crucial in embryogenesis, postnatal morphogenesis, and general tissue homeostasis, acting in a dose-dependent manner or as inducing factors to control cell fate, proliferation, patterning, and survival. Three Hh ligand proteins have been described in vertebrates, Sonic (SHh), Indian (Ihh), and Desert hedgehog (Dhh). Although there is some redundancy, each ligand almost exclusively mediates one or more of particular developmental processes, such as neural tube patterning, endochondral skeletal development, and spermatogenesis through the regulation of stem cell populations [31,39].

The Hh gene family encodes precursor proteins that are processed to produce an N-terminal fragment (Hh-N) that is covalently bound to a cholesterol molecule. Hh-N undergoes further lipid modification to increase the hydrophobicity of the Hh protein and allow lipid tethering on the outer leaflet of the cell membrane. Hh ligand secretion is accomplished via two distinct and synergistic cholesterol-dependent binding events, mediated by two proteins that are essential for vertebrate Hh signaling: the membrane protein Dispatched (Disp) and a member of the Scube family of secreted proteins that cooperate to dramatically enhance the secretion and solubility of the cholesterol-modified Hh ligand [31,39].

The Hedgehog (Hh) signaling pathway relies on the primary cilium to regulate tissue patterning and homeostasis, where ciliary localization and trafficking of Hh components lead to pathway activation and regulation. Recent studies reveal specific roles of discrete ciliary regulators, components, and structures in controlling the movement and signaling of Hh components. Active Hh signaling is associated with increased levels of Hh components along the primary cilium or in a ciliary subdomain. On ligand binding to its membrane receptor Ptch1, a dramatic reduction in Ptch1 expression ensues concomitant with an increase of ciliary Smo levels. Hence release of Hh-bound Ptch1 from the cilium allows for Smo entry through dynamic movements of Ptch1 and Smo that occur even in the absence of active Hh signaling (Fig. 3.1) [31,39].

Downstream signaling of the Hedgehog pathway relies on Hh ligands binding to the integral-membrane protein Hh receptor, Patched (Ptch). There are two distinct homologs of the Ptch gene (Ptch1, Ptch2) in vertebrates that are differentially expressed during development. Ptch1$^{-/-}$ is embryonically lethal in mice. In the absence of Hh, Ptch catalytically represses the seven Smoothened (Smo) transmembrane proteins and may involve oxysterols. The subsequent binding of Hh to Ptch antagonizes its repressor function. In vertebrates, transcription of Hh target genes is controlled

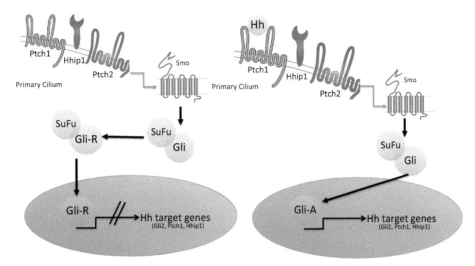

FIGURE 3.1   Hedgehog signaling pathway in mammalian cells. (A) In the absence of *Hh* ligand, Ptch1 inhibits SMO allowing the GLI processing complex containing SUFU to generate transcriptional repressors (*Gli-R*) within the primary cilium. (B) *Hh* ligand binding to *Ptch1* de-represses *Smo* and generates activated GLI factors (*Gli-A*) that induce the expression of Hh target genes.

by Gli1–3 transcription factors [31,39]. Gli1 and Gli2 primarily act as transcriptional activators, whereas Gli3 is the principal transcriptional repressor. However, Gli2 and Gli3 have been shown to possess both activator and repressor functions. In the absence of Hh, the full-length Gli (Gli-FL) transcription factors are cleaved to their repressor forms through phosphorylation cascades that cause retention of Gli-FL proteins in the cytosol. This leads to the ubiquitylation, cleavage, and degradation of the C-terminal peptides, generating the repressor forms of the proteins (Gli- R). Gli-R proteins then localize to the nucleus and repress target gene expression. Upon Hh binding of the Ptch receptor, hyperphosphorylation and activation of Smo ensue before the disassembly of the microtubule-binding Sufu–Gli–FL complex occurs. Smo mediates the disassembly of the Sufu–Gli–FL complex, thus allowing the Gli-FL proteins to localize to the nucleus and activate transcription. Histone deacetylase 6 (HDAC6) appears essential for both full Hh pathway activation and complete repression of basal Hh target gene expression through its impact on Gli2 mRNA and GLI3 protein expression [31,39].

Aside from the traditional Hh signaling pathway, other nonconventional pathways, termed noncanonical Hh signaling pathways, have been described [39]. As such, Hh pathway activation can be triggered by many other intracellular signals. These pathways include: (1) signaling that is independent of Gli-mediated transcription; (2) interactions between Hh signaling proteins and components of other molecular pathways, such as TGF-β, KRAS–MAPK/ERK, PI3K–AKT, IGF, TNF-α induced mTOR/S6K1 activation, and inactivation of hSNF5 (a regulator of chromatin remodeling, also known as SMARCB1); (3) unconventional interactions between Hh signaling proteins. These noncanonical signals are largely attributed to various tumor-associated

signaling pathways integrating with Hh signaling, in part by influencing the activity of GLI transcription factors. Determining the role of these noncanonical pathways, and the molecular crosstalk between them, is an important consideration for the ongoing development of Hh-therapeutics.

NOTCH SIGNALING

Since it was first identified a century ago in *Drosophila melanogaster*, Notch signaling has been extensively characterized as a hugely important regulator of cell fate in a variety of organisms and tissues [40]. The Notch signaling pathway plays a critical role in embryonic development, self-renewal of stem cells, and carcinogenesis [41]. Aberrant Notch signaling has been linked to a wide variety of diseases, and can either suppress or promote disease phenotypes, depending on the cell type and the context [38,40].

Mammals express four transmembrane Notch receptors (Notch-1, Notch-2, Notch-3, and Notch-4) and five canonical transmembrane ligands (Delta-like [DLL] 1, DLL 3, DLL 4, Jagged1, and Jagged2) that combine in a cell-to-cell manner to transduce Notch signaling. Delta and Jagged ligands share many similarities but differ because Delta's smaller extracellular domains can mediate Notch activation in *trans* (from cell to cell) and Notch inhibition in *cis* (on the same cell). The affinity of the ligands for Notch receptors is governed by glycosylation through the addition of sugars by fucosyltransferase and Fringe family *N*-acetyl-glucosamine-transferases [40].

On binding, Notch receptors undergo three proteolytic cleavages. Notch precursor proteins are cleaved (S1) by a furin-like convertase to produce the mature Notch receptor, which is a heterodimer consisting of Notch extracellular (NEC) and Notch transmembrane (N™) subunits. A second cleavage (S2) by a disintegrin and metalloproteinase domain containing protein 10 or 17 (ADAM10 or ADAM17) occurs upon ligand–receptor engagement and NEC dissociation from N™. This cleavage releases a short extracellular peptide and generates a short-lived intermediate that is cleaved again (S3) by the γ-secretase complex. The S3 cleavage releases the intracellular portion of Notch (NICD). NICD translocates to the nucleus and binds to the CBF-1-suppressor of hairless/Lag1 [(CSL) also known as RBP-jκ], a constitutive transcriptional repressor, displacing corepressors and recruiting coactivators, such as mastermind-like (MAML) proteins, homologous to Drosophila mastermind, to form a Notch–CSL–MAML complex that recruits multiple transcriptional regulators forming the "Notch transcriptional complex" (NTC) to drive Notch target gene expression including the hairy/enhancer of split (HES) family and hairy/enhancer-of-split related with YRPW motif-like protein (Hey) family of basic helix–loop–helix transcription factors (Fig. 3.2; [38,40,41].

VASCULAR TARGETS FOR CHEMOTHERAPY—ANGIOGENESIS

A common feature of all solid tumors is their ability to elicit the formation of new blood vessels through the processes of angiogenesis to support tumor growth and favor metastatic dissemination [42]. Angiogenesis, initially described as the formation of new blood vessels from pre-existing ones, is regulated by activator and inhibitor molecules with numerous different proteins identified to date in either category [15,43]. Vascular endothelial growth factor (VEGF) and epidermal growth factor (EGF) are considered the most important angiogenic stimuli [44] and these lead to

preferential differentiation of specific endothelial cells into so-called "tip cells," which start to migrate and exist at the leading front of growing vessels. Once endothelial cells have transformed into vascular tubes, mesenchyme-derived mural cells (MCs), referred to as pericytes/vascular smooth muscle cells (PC/vSMCs), are recruited to the outer layer of the neovasculature [45].

Several important properties of tumor angiogenesis present as potential targets for cancer therapy, which include: (1) endothelial cell migration/tip cell formation, (2) structural abnormalities of tumor vessels, (3) hypoxia, (4) lymphangiogenesis, (5) elevated interstitial fluid pressure, (6) poor perfusion, (7) disrupted circadian rhythms, (8) tumor-promoting inflammation, (9) tumor-promoting fibroblasts, and (10) tumor-cell metabolism/acidosis [43].

During tumor angiogenesis, ECs receive continuous signals to sprout and develop, generating vessels that are structurally and functionally abnormal. An emerging mechanism playing a central role in shaping the tumor vasculature is the endothelial-vesicular network that regulates trafficking/export and degradation of key signaling proteins and membrane receptors, including the VEGF receptor-2/3 and members of the Notch pathway. The VEGF receptor (VEGFR)-3 (for lymphatic endothelial cells), VEGFR-1 and–2 (for vascular endothelial cells), PDGF-BB, and the Notch ligand, delta-like ligand-4 (Dll4) have all been shown to contribute to the endothelial tip cell phenotype [44,46]. Normally, ECs located behind the tip cell, the so-called "stalk cells," express VEGFR-1 and Notch-1 and -4 to maintain a quiescent state, maturation of the vascular wall, lumen formation, and perfusion [47]. However, unlike the quiescent phenotype normally associated with a healthy vasculature, this process becomes disrupted in cancer, culminating in excessive

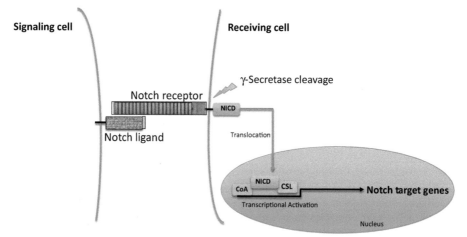

FIGURE 3.2 **Notch signaling pathway in mammalian cells.** In the absence of Notch ligands (Jagged, Delta), the CBF-1-Suppressor of Hairless/Lag1 (*CSL*; also known as RBP-jκ) acts a constitutive transcriptional repressor to inhibit Notch target gene expression. On ligand binding to the Notch receptor, *NICD* translocates to the nucleus and binds to the CBF-1-Suppressor of Hairless/Lag1 (*CSL*), displacing corepressors and recruiting coactivators (*CoA*), such as Mastermind-like (MAML) proteins to form a Notch–CSL–CoA complex that recruits multiple transcriptional regulators to drive Notch target gene expression including the Hairy/Enhancer of Split (HES) family and Hairy/enhancer-of-split related with YRPW motif-like protein (Hey) family of basic helix–loop–helix transcription factors.

tip-cell formation and migration of vascular ECs [48]. As a result, tumor neovasculature displays key structural and functional abnormalities that include leakiness, poor coverage by vascular supportive cells including pericytes and vSMCs, growth and remodeling, high tortuosity and lack of arterial or venous identity, and chaotic blood flow, all leading to overall poor functionality and perfusion [49].

As tumor angiogenesis is a complex process involving discrete interactions between tumor cells, ECs, phagocytes, and their secreted factors which may act as promoters or inhibitors of angiogenesis, many signaling pathways are involved but Notch signaling has emerged as the most notable pathway [43,46,50]. Upon VEGF binding to VEGFR2 in the tip cells, activated VEGFR2 induces the transcription of the Notch ligand DLL4. Expression of DLL4 on the tip cells induces the activating cleavage of NICD the in the stalk cells and the Notch target genes hairy/enhancer of split-1 (HES1) and hairy/enhancer-of-split related with YRPW motif 1 (HEY1). In the tumor context, specific inhibition of the Notch signaling pathway also results in hyperactive sprouting and reduced vessel function, resulting in overall reduced tumor growth [50]. Increasingly it is also clear that Notch signaling promotes the growth of tumor cells through the maintenance of CSCs [51].

It is also apparent that the type of tumor and the tissue from which it is derived dictate the overall response to Notch, as different tumors and tumor subtypes express different Notch receptors and ligands [52]. The level of post-translational modifications of the Notch receptor, in particular glycosylation, in addition to the degree of noncanonical Notch signaling and Notch interactions with Wnt and Hh pathways in different cell types, dictate the overall effect of Notch [53]. This diversity is important as targeting Notch has the potential to affect multiple cell types within a tumor or vascular lesion from resident stem cells, to immune cells, vascular endothelial cells, and tumor cells. Notch's oncogenic capacity is controlled in a coordinated manner with several known oncogenes [54], including TGF-β, WNT/β-catenin, IL-6, and NF-κB, as well as by the Notch pathway itself. One of the Notch ligands, Jagged1 (JAG1), is overexpressed in many cancer types, and plays an important role in several aspects of tumor biology [41]. In addition, JAG1 can indirectly affect cancer through regulation of the tumor neovasculature and immune cell infiltration [40]. Notch ligand, Delta-like 4 (Dll4) also plays a key role in tumor angiogenesis [48]. DLL4 expressed by endothelial tip cells suppresses the tip phenotype in neighboring stalk cells, thus maintaining a sufficient number of endothelial cells for vascular integrity and adequate tissue perfusion. In some models, JAG1 has been proven to have the opposite effect in that it promotes endothelial cell proliferation and sprouting, and inhibits DLL4-induced Notch signaling in endothelial cells. Thus, JAG1 deletion inhibits sprouting angiogenesis, and JAG1 overexpression opposes DLL4 to

promote sprouting [55,56]. More recent data suggest that Dll4 blocks endothelial activation through Notch1 signaling but also induces Jagged1 expression. Jagged1 then blocks Dll4 signaling through Notch1, allowing endothelial activation by VEGF and endothelial cell growth. Jagged1 also initiates maturation of the newly formed vessels, possibly by binding and activating endothelial Notch4. Importantly, mice administered with a Notch4 agonistic antibody mimicked the MC phenotype of endothelial Jag1 overexpressing mutants without affecting angiogenic growth, which is thought to be Notch1 dependent. Collectively, endothelial Jagged1 is likely to operate downstream of Dll4/Notch1 signaling to activate Notch4 and regulate vascular maturation. Thus, Jagged1 not only counteracts Dll4/Notch in the endothelium but also generates a balance between angiogenic growth and maturation processes in vivo [57].

VEGF-A is secreted by tumor cells, inflammatory cells, and other cell types and binds the VEGFR2 receptor (or VEGFR2/VEGFR3 heterodimer) on the tip cells of endothelial vessel sprouts [43,58]. Monoclonal antibodies targeting the VEGFR2 or VEGFR3 receptor inhibit tumor angiogenesis and block tumor growth in mice, supporting its key putative role [59]. VEGFR2/3 activates several downstream signaling pathways, including the ERK kinase and Akt cascades, resulting in increased endothelial cell migration. VEGF-A also binds to neuropilin (NRP1), which interacts with VEGFR2 and potentiates its function. Importantly, VEGFR2 activation in the tip cells promotes the transcription of the Notch ligand DLL4, which activates Notch in the stalk cells, where it promotes vessel stability. In the stalk cells, angiopoetin-2 (ANG-2) can contribute to endothelial cell proliferation by inhibiting its receptor TEK tyrosine kinase (TIE2). However, in the established vasculature ANG-1 binds and activates TIE2, thereby stabilizing the vessels and inhibiting angiogenesis [58].

VASCULAR TARGETS FOR CHEMOTHERAPY—VASCULOGENIC MIMICRY

Another important facet of tumor neovascularization has been the discovery that tumor cells themselves assemble to form vascular channels, independent of ECs [60,61]. Such tumor cell-mediated vascular formation lacking ECs is referred to as vasculogenic mimicry (VM). VM is a new tumor vascular paradigm, independent of angiogenesis, that describes the specific ability of aggressive CSCs to form vessel-like networks that provide adequate blood supply for tumor growth [62]. VM is also associated with tumor invasion, metastasis, and poor cancer patient prognosis [62]. Generally, VM characteristics can be summarized as follows: (1) positive periodic acid-Schiff (PAS) and negative CD31 staining; (2) the channel is lined by tumor cells rather than endothelial cells; (3) the expression of a multipotent, stem cell-like phenotype; (4) extracellular matrix remodeling; and (v) VM has connection with the tumor microcirculation system, providing blood for tumor growth.

These vessel-like networks typically develop from differentiation of bone-marrow-derived CD34+-hematopoietic stem cells. Other cell types can also participate, including endothelial progenitor cells (EPCs) and CSC-differentiated vascular cells [60,63,64]. This differentiation of tumor stem-like cells to ECs is responsible for the maintenance of the pathological characteristics of the tumor microenvironment [43]. Although the individual contributions of subpopulations of stem cells (i.e., CD133+ and CD133− for glioblastoma vascularization) into VM are still controversial [65], a significant population (~20%) of CSCs derived from patients are capable of transdifferentiation into pericytes and SMCs that participate in both VM and angiogenesis. Moreover, VEGFR2 gene knockdown or treatment with a VEGFR2 kinase inhibitor (SU1498) impedes this transdifferentiation and subsequent VM in xenograft models and in cultured cells, an effect that is independent of VEGF, unlike CSC transdifferentiation to ECs, which is VEGF dependent [66].

Bone-marrow-derived EPCs are also an important mediator of the angiogenic response through the production of paracrine factors and their incorporation into the lumen of tumor neovasculature. Importantly, EPC depletion leads to a delayed tumor angiogenic response and impaired tumor growth and spread [67]. Dicer-regulated miRNAs are small noncoding RNAs (18–23 bp in size) generated by the consecutive activity of 2 RNAseIII enzymes, Drosha and Dicer that regulate gene activity by sequence-specific binding to mRNA, triggering either translational repression or RNA degradation. They are key factors involved in normal cell function, embryological development, and stem-cell biology [68], so it is not surprising that EPC functionality is tightly regulated by specific microRNAs (miRNAs). Although the role of metastasis-linked miRNAs has been controversial, there is a strong link between miR-10b, the epithelial-to-mesenchymal transition (EMT) and tumorigenesis [69]. Moreover, specific miRNAs, miR-10b and miR-196b have both been implicated in angiogenesis in vitro [70] and their contribution to tumor angiogenesis using Dicer-floxed mice and EPCs traced with an Id1 proximal promoter-LV reporter has recently been reported in vivo to show for the first time that Dicer is required for EPC-mediated tumor angiogenesis [64].

VASCULAR TARGETS FOR CHEMOTHERAPY—MICROVESICULAR TRAFFICKING

Although tumor angiogenesis is a tightly regulated process involving a number of angiogenic factors, a further mechanism of cell-to-cell communication for the modulation

of the tumor angiogenic process has been proposed [71]. Nonapoptotic membrane vesicles that include exosomes and microvesicles are released in the nanosize range and contain critical components of the cell of origin. These vesicles transfer bioactive lipids, proteins, and nucleic acids from one cell to another, and thereby induce changes in the phenotype and functions of the recipient cells [71,72]. Tumor cells, inflammatory cells, and stem/progenitor cells have all been shown to release these vesicles with angiogenic like-properties suggesting that they may act under different physiological and pathological conditions [73].

Endocytosis and vesicle trafficking mechanisms also play a pivotal role in EC activation and in regulating the extent of Notch signaling in ECs [74]. Notch signals not only from the plasma membrane but also from the endosomes and lysosomes, after both ligand-dependent and -independent Notch activation [75]. This endocytotic process for both Notch receptor or its ligand after binding generates the physical forces necessary to dissociate and activate the receptor [74]. Importantly, EC-specific depletion of Notch1 compromises vessel normalization [74]. ECs can also secrete and capture exosomes, facilitating communication within the endothelium and other cell types. Although endothelial-derived exosomes may contain proteins with a proangiogenic potential, EC-derived exosomes also incorporate DLL4 and transfer it to neighboring ECs, modulating filopodia, and sprout formation through Notch signaling activation in the recipient ECs [76].

Similar evidence for a putative role for Notch and the mechanisms of action of these exosomal vesicles in vascular homeostasis and in the angiogenic processes occurring in tumors, inflammation and tissue regeneration has been purported [74]. Numerous drugs and biological agents have recently been developed to interfere with tumor angiogenesis, including anti-human EGF receptor 2 agents, VEGF inhibitors, and tyrosine kinase inhibitors (TKIs). These angiogenesis inhibitors typically work by blocking the activity of growth factors secreted by the tumor that initiate the formation of new blood vessels or signaling pathways in endothelial cells that are targets for the secreted growth factors. These targeted therapies are all important components of current treatment strategies [43].

VASCULAR TARGETS FOR CHEMOTHERAPY—VESSEL MATURATION

The recruitment of mural cells (MCs), namely pericytes and vSMCs, is essential to the maturation of newly formed vessels [77]. Sonic hedgehog (SHh) was originally implicated in the formation of larger and more muscularized vessels. More recently autocrine production of SHh by MCs has been shown to be a downstream effector of PDGF-BB for MC migration and recruitment in neovessels (Fig. 3.3) [77].

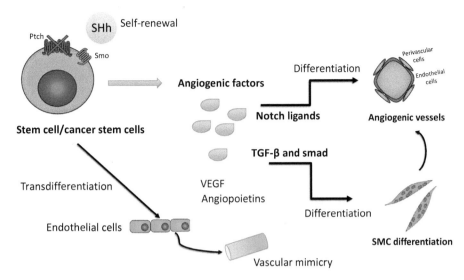

FIGURE 3.3 **Hedgehog and notch promote angiogenesis:** Stem cells can be activated by SHh and activation of its pathways to produce cytokines and growth factors that promote angiogenesis including VEGF-A and Notch ligands and vascular mimicry (VM).

HEDGEHOG AND CANCER BIOLOGY

Self-renewal and cell-fate determination of resident stem cells is controlled by both cell-autonomous (intrinsic) and non-cell-autonomous (extrinsic) pathways during the regenerative process [78]. The dysfunctional regulation of these pathways, resulting in stem cell expansion, is a key initiating event in both carcinogenesis and vascular disease progression.

The Hedgehog (Hh) pathway is an established regulator of fundamental processes in vertebrate embryonic develop-ment including stem-cell maintenance, cell differentiation, tissue polarity, and cell proliferation [39]. Constitutive acti-vation of the Hh pathway leading to tumorigenesis has been widely reported for basal-cell carcinomas (BCCs) [79] and medulloblastoma [80]. A variety of other human cancers, including brain, gastrointestinal, lung, breast, and prostate cancers, also demonstrate inappropriate activation of this pathway [14].

In general, the tumor microenvironment resembles that of a stem-cell niche (Fig. 3.4), comprised of noncancer support cells, such as immature myeloid cells, cancer-associated

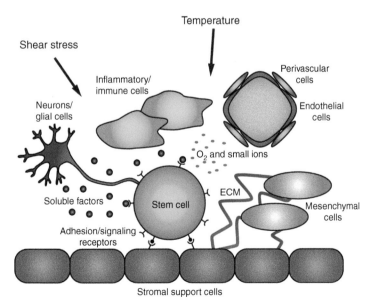

FIGURE 3.4 **The stem cell niche.** The stem cell niche is composed of multiple niche support cells, such as stromal and mesenchymal cells, that provide stimuli to a small subpopulation of stem cells. The stem cells are responsive to cellular and acellular regulatory components within the niche. These regu-lator components control the fate of the stem cells, be it proliferation, self-renewal, differentiation, fate, programmed cell death, retention, or migration.

fibroblasts, and neural cells, with neighboring tumor cells and a subpopulation of CSCs [18,39]. These CSCs are responsible for the ability of cancers to renew, reoccur, and metastasize. Not surprisingly, given the vast range of cellular responses it elicits and its roles in stem cell regulation, the Hh signaling pathway has been implicated in the etiology of many cancers through numerous mechanisms where it promotes cell growth and survival, angiogenesis, metastasis, chemoresistance, and CSCs self-renewal, fuelling the basic requirements for all cancerous growth [18].

Aberrant Hh pathway activation has been identified in several human cancers [81]. These include loss of function Ptch1 mutations in Gorlin's syndrome, gain of function Smo mutations in BCCs and the upregulation of Gli1 in glioblastomas (Fig. 3.5) [79]. Mutations resulting in an increase in Hh ligands within the tumor microenvironment have also been described [82]. In cancers of colon, prostate, and small-cell lung cancer, there is an increase in Hh autocrine/juxtacrine signaling where tumor cells both produce and respond to Hh proteins [83]. Upregulation of Hh paracrine signaling has been determined in certain tumor microenvironments. Stromal cells in B-cell

lymphomas and multiple myelomas produce Hh ligands to stimulate growth of tumor cells, whereas tumor cells in pancreatic and colon cancers have been reported to produce Hh ligands to stimulate infiltrating stromal cells to produce signaling factor required for tumor growth [84]. In some cases, Hh signaling may also be upregulated due to other signaling cascades. In breast cancer, the PI3K/AKT pathway is upregulated and protects members of the Hh signaling cascade from degradation, leading to constituent activation of the Hh pathway [83].

Many Hh target genes regulate proliferation, apoptosis, and cell-cycle advancement. The Hh pathway has been found to be highly active in diffuse large B-cell lymphomas (DLBCL), resulting in their upregulated cell growth and survival [85]. Cell-cycle arrest is seen in these cells after Hh inhibition with cyclopamine due to downregulation of the B-cell Lymphoma 2 (Bcl-2) protein. Inhibition of Gli transcription factors resulted in decreased expression of the cell-cycle control and proproliferation proteins Cyclin-D1 and Cyclin D2; Cyclin E1 and p53 in brain tumor medulloblastoma; embryonal carcinoma stem cells from teratocarcinomas; and colon cancer cells [86–88].

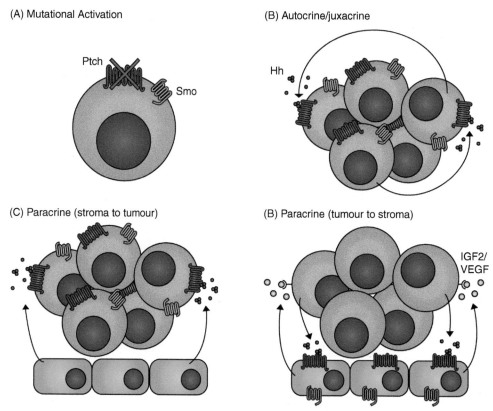

FIGURE 3.5 Proposed models of Hh signaling in cancer. (A) Mutational activations within the signaling cascade can result in nonligand mediated signaling. Loss-of-function *Ptch* mutations have been described in Gorlin's syndrome, whereas gain of function *Smo* mutations have been reported in BCC cells. (B) Ligand-mediated autocrine/juxacrine signaling occurs in some colon cancers where the tumor cells both produce and respond to *Hh* proteins. (C) Ligand-mediated paracrine signaling where stromal cells provide the tumor cells with sufficient Hh ligands has been reported in B-cell lymphomas and multiple myelomas. (D) Ligand-mediated paracrine signaling where the tumor cells stimulate Hh-responsive stromal cells to produce the required factors to maintain the tumor microenvironment occurs in pancreatic and colon cancer.

Hh signaling has also been implicated in the metastasis of many tumors, such as pancreatic, breast, and colon cancers and medulloblastomas [89]. Hh acts upstream of angiogenic factors, such as VEGF and the angiopoietins, and has been found to promote hematogenous metastasis in some cancers [90,91]. Pancreatic ductal adenocarcinoma (PDAC) cells upregulate the expression of angiogenic factors in proangiogenic progenitor cells in the bone marrow and promote their migration through modulation of the Hh pathway. Treatment of PDAC xenografts in mice with cyclopamine results in a significant decrease in tumor vasculature [90,91]. Additionally, overstimulation of colorectal cancer xenografts in mice with SHh upregulates angiogenesis when compared to control tumors [90]. Increased expression of Gli1 upregulates osteopontin, a secreted growth factor involved in chemotaxis in breast and pancreatic cancer cells, which promotes their metastasis to bone marrow. Moreover, osteopontin increases osteoclast differentiation and enhances tumor osteolysis [92]. It appears that SHh promotes metastasis in breast cancers primarily by upregulating cysteine-rich angiogenic inducer 61, CD24, matrix metalloproteinase-2 (MMP-2), and MMP-9 [93].

In addition to the secretion of chemattractants, Hh pathway promotes metastasis by promoting epithelial-mesenchymal transition (EMT), a process that produces highly motile and invasive cells [94]. EMT in pancreatic cancer cells is activated via noncanonical activation of the Hh pathway and is substantially inhibited in cells treated with cyclopamine. Hh mediates this by promoting the expression of Snail and Twist, which results in the downregulation of the adhesion protein, E-cadherin [95]. Expression of Snail and Twist in human mammary epithelial cells from nonadherent mammary cancer cell clusters in culture (mammospheres) induced EMT and produced stem-cell-like cells that were similar to mammary stem cells and were more prolific and invasive than untreated human mammary epithelial cells [96].

One of the most notable aspects of Hh signaling in cancer is its maintenance of CSCs [84]. The Gli1 transcription factor was first isolated and found to be upregulated in glioma CSCs. Smo RNA interference and cyclopamine administration of glioma stem-cell cultures (gliomaspheres) attenuates Gli1 and Ptch1 expression, leading to a reduction in proliferation and self-renewal, whereas stimulation of the Hh pathway with SHh results in increased growth and number of gliomaspheres [97]. The same effects can be seen in leukemic stem cells [98]. Loss-of-function Smo mutations reduce the tumor-forming properties of Bcr–Abl, a fusion oncogene associated with chronic myelogenous leukemia [99]. Additionally, cyclopamine decreases self-renewal and induces apoptosis of leukemic progenitor forms in vitro [100]. SHh also stimulates multiple myeloma CSC self-renewal in vitro, a response that is attenuated after cyclopamine treatment [98]. Recently, compelling evidence suggests that Hedgehog (Hh) signaling mediates the trans-

duction of signals between stromal and lymphoma cells. The gain of cell-autonomous activation of the Hh pathway seen in lymphomas may represent a survival and/or proliferative advantage for the lymphoma cells and suggest, at least to some degree, stromal independence [101].

HEDGEHOG INHIBITORS IN CANCER THERAPY

Given the activity of Hh signaling in a wide range of cancers, the development of Hh inhibitors as novel anticancer therapies has gained a lot of interest (Fig. 3.6). Cyclopamine was the first compound discovered to antagonize the Hh pathway and, as already described, has been used in various studies to downregulate Hh-mediated metastasis, angiogenesis and chemoresistance in cancer cells. Currently, a number of drugs targeting the Hh pathway are in clinical trials and Vismodegib, a Smo antagonist developed by Genentech, is approved by the US FDA for the treatment of locally advanced and metastatic BCC [102]. Phase-II clinical-trial results demonstrated that the occurrence and size of tumors were significantly reduced in Vismodegib treated BCC patients when compared to subjects on placebo. Only 20% of patients were removed from the study due to adverse side effects. During phase I, Vismodegib also showed therapeutic effects in medulloblastoma patients; however, one subject with metastatic medulloblastoma relapsed and became resistant due to an Smo mutation that prevented Vismodegib binding. Additionally, an NCI-sponsored phase-II study of a FOLFOX chemotherapy regimen with or without Vismodegib has started to recruit colorectal cancer patients [103]. Other Smo antagonists have shown promising results in clinical trials, such as LY2940680, which has been shown to inhibit growth of cancer cells that are resistant to Vismodegib, and IPI-926, another drug that has been developed for the treatment of BCC and shows therapeutic effects in patients with chondrosarcoma bone cancer [104]. A combination of therapies that include Hh inhibitors has also proven efficacious [81].

Collectively, an essential role for Hedgehog in human cancer has been established. Hh signaling has been targeted predominantly using smoothened (SMO) inhibitors. Unfortunately, resistance has also been observed in BCC patients [105] with a critical role of the RAS–MAPK (mitogen-activated protein kinase) pathway in mediating both drug resistance and tumor evolution of SHh pathway-dependent tumors. Therefore, the use of Hh inhibitors targeting the signaling cascade downstream of SMO may represent a more promising strategy. Moreover, in addition to the classical canonical pathway for Hh activation, noncanonical activation of the GLI transcription factors by multiple important signaling pathways (e.g., MAPK, PI3K, TGFβ) has also been described, highlighting the importance of targeting the transcription factors GLI1/2. The most promising agent in this

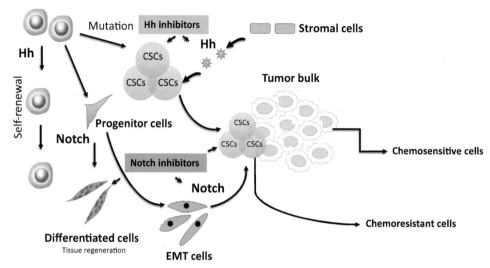

FIGURE 3.6 CSCs, Hh, and Notch signaling pathway; Hh signaling in CSCs. CSCs respond to the Hh ligand, secreted by adjacent stromal cells, tumor cells, or the CSCs themselves, to maintain a "stemness" signature. CSCs are resistant to conventional chemotherapeutics, surviving treatment before expanding and deriving the heterogeneous tumor bulk population, resulting in disease relapse. Recent data indicates that the Notch signaling pathway also plays an important role in the development and progression of many cancers. Emerging evidence suggests that activation of the Notch signaling pathway is mechanistically associated with molecular characteristics of CSCs through EMT. Moreover, CSCs are known to be highly drug-resistant, suggesting that targeted inactivation of Notch and Hedgehog signaling would be useful for overcoming drug resistance and the elimination of CSCs.

context is probably the GLI1/2 inhibitor GANT61 which has been investigated preclinically in numerous tumor types in the last few years. GANT61 appears to be highly effective against human cancer cells and in xenograft mouse models, targeting almost all of the classical hallmarks of cancer and could hence represent a promising treatment option for human cancer [104,106]. In addition, noncanonical signaling, independent of transcriptional changes mediated by the Gli family of transcription factors, has also been reported [107].

Hh-mediated chemoresistance is prevalent in ovarian, pancreatic, prostate, glioma, myeloid leukemic, B-cell lymphoma, and hepatocellular carcinoma cancer cells, and research is on-going to determine the exact mechanisms of drug resistance involved [105–107]. Hh signaling also conferred chemotolerance in esophageal adenocarcinoma, prostate carcinoma, and metastatic squamous cell carcinoma cancer cells via two major adenosine triphosphate-binding cassette (ABC) transporters, ABCB1 and ABCG2 [106]. SHh stimulation showed upregulation of both ABCB1 and ABCG2 and, thus, caused resistance to the chemotherapeutic agents, Taxol, MTX, and VP-16 in the cancer cells in vitro. Survival assays with cyclopamine or RNA interference showed a decrease in SHh-stimulated cancer cell survival; however, these cells still demonstrated enhanced drug resistance when compared to cancer cells that were not treated with SHh, indicating other mechanisms of Hh-mediated chemoresistance. Additionally, more recent studies have demonstrated that Hh signaling directly upregulates ABCB1 in myeloid leukemic cells and ABCG2 in pancreatic stem and DLBCL cells [108].

The therapeutic targeting of Hedgehog (Hh) signaling almost exclusively focuses on receptor or downstream SMO-dependent/independent antagonism; however, Hedgehog's biosynthesis also represents a unique and potentially "druggable" target of this oncogenic signaling pathway. The possibility of generating drugs that target a key biosynthetic step called cholesterolysis, also called cholesteroylation, that generates cholesterol-modified Hh ligand via autoprocessing of a Hedgehog precursor protein has received some attention. Posttranslational modification by cholesterol appears to be restricted to proteins in the Hedgehog family and may offer new therapeutic advantage [109].

HEDGEHOG AND VASCULAR BIOLOGY

The formation of a hierarchical vascular network is essential for both normal development and for the production of new functional vasculature in the adult. The molecular mechanisms that orchestrate the differentiation of vascular endothelial cells into arterial and venous cell fates for regenerative medicine has been widely examined and has presented clues about similar mechanisms required for directed formation and remodeling of vessels in a myriad of pathological settings, such as in arteriosclerosis, atherosclerosis, and diabetes, following myocardial infarction [110]. Studies in several model organisms, such as mouse, zebrafish, and chick, have revealed a number of key signaling pathways that are required for the establishment and maintenance of arterial and venous fates. These include Hh, VEGF,

TGF-β, Wnt, and Notch signaling pathways and a number of transcription factor families including Notch-regulated transcription factors (e.g., HEY and HES), SOX factors, forkhead factors, β-catenin, ETS factors, and COUP-TFII [111]. In particular, Hh proteins play a pivotal role and, as prototypical morphogens, regulate epithelial/mesenchymal interactions of limbs, vascular, lung, gut, hair follicles, and bone during development [39]. Several studies establish Hh as pivotal to pattern specific events in early blood vascular development through VEGF- and Notch-dependent and -independent mechanisms [112].

The involvement of SHh in postnatal neovascularization has been confirmed in addition to that which occurs during embryologic development [113,114]. Exogenous administration of SHh induces angiogenesis and accelerates repair of the ischemic myocardium and skeletal muscle, significantly accelerates wound healing by inducing arteriogenesis [115], and restores nerve function in diabetic neuropathy by promoting angiogenesis [114]. The presence of Hh receptors on cultured EPCs but not mature endothelial cells suggests that SHh might preferentially modulate human EPCs and CD34+ cells [116]. Indeed, recent studies confirm that SHh therapies promotes angiogenesis in ischemic skeletal muscle [117] and increases angiogenesis in ischemic myocardium following myocardial infarction [118]. Moreover, SHh signaling promotes CD34+ cell function and increases differentiation into the vascular lineages [116].

Over the last decade, an intimate and functional association between various stem cells and the vasculature has emerged that contributes to tissue homeostasis and repair [23]. In particular, undifferentiated CD34$^-$, CD105$^+$, and VEGF receptor 2 (Flk1)$^+$ mesenchymal stem-cell (MSC) populations have been successfully isolated from human fetal aorta [119,120]. Treatment of these cells with inductive stimuli in vitro (VEGF, PDGF-BB, or osteogenic/adipogenic induction media) gave rise to EC and SMC, respectively, and they also exhibited high angiogenic potential in vivo [119,120]. Similarly, adult human aorta contains CD34$^+$ and c-kit$^+$ progenitor stem cells within the media and adventitia that are capable of transition to EC and SMC phenotypes on inductive stimulation [121].

The potential of using MSCs and vascular progenitor cells for therapeutic regenerative medicine purposes has been widely reported [122], yet several recent studies have also described the putative role of vascular stem cells in controlling vessel maintenance and regeneration which may be critical to the pathogenesis of several vascular proliferative diseases conditions [123,124]. Adventitial Sca1$^+$ progenitor stem cells contribute to atherosclerotic lesions in vein grafts [125], whereas medial Sox10/Sox17/S100β positive multipotent vascular stem cells are responsible for the accumulation of SMCs within arteriosclerotic vessels [23]. Lineage tracing studies that map differentiated SMCs using *Myh11–Cre–LoxP* transgenic animals are in disagreement about the origin of the accumulated SMCs [23,126,127]. Cell fate mapping studies that specifically track stem cells using *Nestin-Cre* and *Wnt1–Cre* mice clearly demonstrate that the accumulated SMCs within the intima of arteriosclerotic vessels and following artery/vein grafting are also derived from a neural stem-cell background [128,129].

The adventitia surrounds the medial layer of blood vessels. It is a hub of activity with complex and dynamic interactions between many different players including leukocytes, microvessels, nerves, and lymphatics [26]. It also houses resident vascular stem cells whose formation and maintenance depend, in part, on Hh signaling [130,131]. These Hh responsive AdvSca1$^+$ stem cells have been characterized in mice and are shown to be pivotal to atherosclerotic lesions in vein grafts [125] and the remodeling of the vessel wall during arteriosclerosis [128]. Indeed, AdvSca1$^+$ progenitor cells with SMC lineage potential migrate to the neointima in vein graft models and contribute to ≈30% of intimal SMCs in atherosclerotic lesions from ApoE-deficient mice [125]. Moreover, during transplant arteriosclerosis, adventitial tissues labeled as transplanted in rat aortic allografts revealed that the adventitia was the major source of intimal cells [132], whereas cell-fate mapping demonstrated a neural background for these cells following carotid artery and vein grafting using Wnt1–Cre mice [129]. Importantly, selective perivascular knockdown of the Hh receptor, Ptch1, in arteriosclerotic vessels attenuated the intimal medial thickening associated with this disease [133]. The importance of Hedgehog signaling within adventitial sites is further validated by the appearance of stromal tumors arising from the adventitia of blood vessels that originated from AdvSca1 progenitor cells using a transgenic mouse model of pancreatic cancer [134].

Finally, the chemotherapeutic drug Sirolimus, also known as rapamycin, is a widely prescribed treatment for in-stent restenosis using drug-eluting stents and it stimulates adventitial progenitor stem cells grown on scaffolds to migrate in a CXCR4-dependent manner to form neointimal lesion-like accumulations of SMCs [30]. In addition, sirolimus stimulated differentiation of AdvSca1 progenitor cells into SMCs but not endothelial cells in vitro [30].

NOTCH SIGNALING AND TUMOR BIOLOGY

There is now a widespread acceptance that many forms of cancer contain cells that exhibit stem-like characteristics of self-renewal that drive tumorigenesis. Moreover, CSCs may contribute to metastasis as their relative resistance to chemotherapy and radiotherapy may contribute to a relapse [22].

Notch signaling is known to play an important role in normal stem-cell function and is thought to become dysfunctional during neoplasia (Fig. 3.6). Dysfunctional Notch ligands, Notch receptors, and downstream Notch targets have been reported in several tumors, including cervical, head and neck, endometrial, renal, lung, pancreatic, ovarian, prostate, esophageal, oral, hepatocellular, and gastric carcinomas; osteosarcoma mesothelioma; melanoma; gliomas; and medulloblastomas [51]. Notch is also dysfunctional in some hematological malignancies other than T-ALL. These include Hodgkin lymphomas, anaplastic large-cell non-Hodgkin lymphomas, some acute myeloid leukemias (AMLs), B-cell chronic lymphoid leukemias (B-CLLs), and multiple myeloma (MM) [41]. In most instances, it is exaggerated Notch activation that is responsible for the neoplasia but is some cases, like in squamous epithelia, it is the loss of Notch stimuli that can result in cancer [135].

It is now well recognized that cancer progression not only requires dysfunctional signaling pathways and accumulated genetic alterations in cancer cells but also relies on the support from tumor microenvironment [101]. As with Hh signaling, the tumor microenvironment is critical to the overall repercussions of the oncogenic transformation. In this context, Notch signaling regulates both the formation of CSCs and the acquisition of the EMT phenotype, which are both also associated with drug resistance [136]. Indeed, an epithelial gene signature is strongly associated with the responsiveness to EGF receptor inhibition with erlotinib in lung cancer cells and with gefitinib and cetuximab for squamous cell carcinoma [137,138]. EMT also promotes chemoresistance to paclitaxel, vincristine, and oxaliplatin and EMT has been associated with resistance gemcitabine-resistant pancreatic cancer, oxaliplatin-resistant colorectal cancer, lapatinib-resistant breast cancer, and paclitaxel-resistant ovarian carcinoma [41].

Notch activation also promotes endothelial mesenchymal stem cell (MSC) transition (EndoMT) that leads to decreased endothelial markers (vascular endothelial-cadherin, tyrosine kinase with immunoglobulin-like and EGF-like domain [Tie]1, Tie2, platelet-endothelial cell adhesion molecule-1, and endothelial nitric oxide synthase) and upregulation of mesenchymal markers (α-SMA, fibronectin, and platelet-derived growth factor receptors) [139]. Notch interacts with several factors notably TGF-β, Snail, Slug [140] either directly or by stabilizing these factors for downstream signaling critical to EMT [136]. EMT signatures in prostate cancer are characterized by increased expression of Notch-1, Sox2, Nanog, Oct4, and Lin28B and a close association between Notch and Hedgehog in controlling CSCs [141]. Notch1 levels are also highly expressed in bone metastases in these patient cohorts suggesting a putative role for Notch driven EMT in prostate cancer [142].

Bone is frequently targeted for metastasis and is known to be hypoxic. This hypoxic microenvironment is believed to promote self-renewal of hematopoietic stem cells, and Notch, which is activated by hypoxia, can induce EMT during tumor progression [143]. Dysfunctional Notch signaling is associated with both the mobilization and spread of primary tumor cells to distant locations and Notch-driven EMT and mesenchymal–epithelial transition play important roles during tumor invasion, metastasis, and therapeutic resistance. The paradigm of EMT inducing a CSC phenotype that provides a mechanistic basis for metastasis, chemoresistance, tumor dormancy, and delayed recurrence is attractive [51]. Notch signaling, much like Hedgehog, is one of a few putative signaling pathways that control the generation and self-renewal of CSCs, at least in part through EMT. Exaggerated expression of Jagged1 is associated with increased incidence of triple-negative breast cancer (TNBC) bone metastasis, and tumor cells that overexpress Jagged1 generate severe osteolytic lesions [144]. Notch-1 also mediates the induction of Tregs by MSCs and therefore promotes tumorigenesis by dampening antitumor immune responses [145].

NOTCH INHIBITORS

Several classes of Notch inhibitors have been developed that include monoclonal antibodies against Notch receptors or ligands; decoys (soluble forms of the extracellular domain of Notch receptor or Notch ligands); blocking peptides; gamma-secretase inhibitors (GSIs) or natural compounds [41]. GSIs are the most widely studied and are less specific than biologics, but have the greater potential of favorable biodistribution and pan-Notch inhibition. In EGF receptor 2 (Her2)/Neu positive BT474 xenografts, the combination of two chemically different GSIs with trastuzumab dramatically inhibited tumor recurrence, producing complete cures in most animals treated with one drug and all animals treated with another [146]. Since GSIs given as single agents prevented tumor regression with no significant effect on tumor volume, the most likely reason is their effect on CSC fate. Despite this, an enormous therapeutic opportunity still exists for modulators of Notch signaling as this pathway is essential for EMT and CSC maintenance, angiogenesis, and, in many cases, proliferation and survival of cancer cells [51]. Non-GSI strategies to target Notch signaling, including stapled peptides, decoys, monoclonal antibodies to Notch ligands or receptors, or inhibitors of downstream mediators may also prove useful in some indications.

NOTCH SIGNALING AND VASCULAR BIOLOGY

Notch signaling in the cardiovascular system is important not only during human embryonic development but also during vascular repair of injury and vascular pathogenesis. Notch promotes SMC differentiation marker-gene expression, but its effects appear context-dependent in that Notch is capable of initially promoting a contractile phenotype in SMC before the onset of a negative feedback loop to antagonize the effect [147]. Overexpression of the active intracellular domain (NICD) in 10T1/2 or human SMC cells stimulated SMC differentiation marker-gene expression, and RBP-Jκ as shown to interact with the SM α-actin promoter. Endothelial-specific deletion of Jagged1 resulted in embryonic lethality and severe defects in vascular SMC investment of vessels. In addition, neural crest cell-specific expression of a dominant negative MAML that inhibits all Notch family members disrupted aortic arch development and reduced SMC differentiation. The decrease in artery maturation observed in Notch3 deficient mice and the requirement for Notch3 in EC-dependent MC differentiation provides additional evidence that Notch activation is important for vascular SMC identity. A mutation in Notch3 is causal for cerebral autosomal dominant arteriopathy with subcortical infarcts and leukoencephaly (CADASIL), a neurovascular disorder associated with SMC abnormalities [147].

Studies have demonstrated that expression of NICD inhibited SMC differentiation and this effect was due, in part, to upregulation of the canonical Notch target genes of the Hey family of Notch target genes which have been shown to inhibit SMC differentiation by interfering with SRF/myocardin binding to CArG elements and by directly inhibiting the function of the NICD/RBP–Jκ complex [38,148]. Both Notch1 and 3 receptors, and Notch target genes Hey1 and Hey2, are upregulated in arteriosclerotic vessels, whereas inhibition of Notch1 and Hey2 in vivo causes reduced-injury-induced vessel remodeling, confirming a putative role for Notch signaling in promoting intimal hyperplasia within rodent models [149,150]. Expression of soluble Jag-1, which acts as an inhibitor of Notch signaling, is also sufficient to reduce balloon induced-injury and neointimal lesion formation of rat carotid arteries [151]. Similar changes in Notch signaling have been reported in human lesions [152].

CHEMOTHERAPY AND VASCULAR DISEASE

The cardiovascular side effects that arise from chemotherapy are considerable. Some chemotherapy agents cause the heart muscle to weaken soon after chemotherapy begins. Angiogenesis inhibitors that suppress new blood vessel formation cause hypertension and may increase the risk of blood clots and heart failure [153]. Hormonal therapies can cause stroke, heart attacks, and blood clots. Other agents can trigger low blood flow to the heart (ischemia), heart attack, arrhythmias, or inflammation of the sac (pericardium) around the heart. The severity of such toxicity depends on many factors including (1) molecular site of action, (2) the immediate and cumulative dose, (3) the method of administration, (4) the presence of any underlying cardiac condition, and (5) the demographics of the patient [153].

The most relevant cardiotoxic effect is following treatment with anthracyclines that can lead to heart failure [154]. It is broadly classified into three categories: (1) acute, (2) early onset chronic progressive cardiomyopathy, and (3) late onset chronic progressive cardiomyopathy. They differ in time of onset, clinical characteristics, associated risk factors, and molecular mechanisms, but generally involve oxidative stress and apoptosis. Oxidative stress, ion dysfunction, and alterations of the cardiac-specific gene expression collectively cooperate at inducing cardiomyopathy. Early detection combines 2D-echocardiography and/or radionuclide angiography and recent methods, such as tissue Doppler imaging, strain rate echocardiography, and sampling of serial troponin and/or NT-proBNP levels. Dexrazoxane has proven effective in the prevention of dose-related toxicity in children and adults [155]. The oxidative stress leads to cardiac myocyte death as well as activation of the so-called "fetal gene program" that is a feature of many forms of heart failure [154]. Moreover, because cardiomyocytes lack free radical-detoxifying enzymes (catalase or superoxide dismutase), free radicals eventually destroy the mitochondria. This drives a cellular stress response that activates a host of kinase pathways including mitogen/stress-activated protein kinase (MAPKs and SAPKs) linking anthracyclines to the apoptotic pathway [154].

High doses of the alkylating drugs cyclophosphamide and ifosfamide may also result in a reversible heart failure and in life-threatening arrhythmias. Myocardial ischemia induced by the antimetabolites 5-fluorouracil and capecitabine impacts the prognosis of patients with prior CAD. Severe arrhythmias may also complicate administration of microtubule inhibitors [156]. Anthracycline-induced apoptosis appears to involve a mitochondrial pathway, in particular Bax, cytochrome c, and caspase-3 activity [154]. Cytochrome c is released by anthracyclines from the mitochondria and interacts with Apaf-1 and pro-caspase-9 to generate caspase-9, which activates caspase-3 to induce apoptosis [154].

Targeted therapies with the antibody-based tyrosine kinases (TK) inhibitors trastuzumab and, to a lesser extent, alemtuzumab induce heart failure or asymptomatic LV dysfunction in 1–4% and 10%, respectively. Cetuximab and rituximab induce hypotension, whereas bevacizumab may promote severe hypertension and venous thromboembolism. Small molecule TK inhibitors may also elicit LV dysfunction in only few patients treated with imatinib mesylate, but in a substantially higher proportion of those receiving the multitargeted TK inhibitor sunitinib or the recently approved drugs erlotinib, lapatinib, and dasatinib. The target effect of these inhibitors is caused by a target promoting both cancer cell growth and cardiomyocyte function. The off-target effect, instead, occurs when an inhibitor causes an inhibition of a "bystander" target (i.e., a target not essential to kill cancer cells but involved in cardiomyocyte survival) [157]. In contrast to the toxic effects of anthracyclines on cardiac myocytes, which are dose-dependent, irreversible ultrastructural changes, trastuzumab-associated cardiac dysfunction are thought to be idiosyncratic and at least partially reversible since no structural damage has been detected by myocardial biopsies of patients. Under normal circumstances, recovery is complete following withdrawal or cessation of the treatment [157].

It is thought that disruption of the human EGF receptor 2 (HER2) signaling underlies the mechanism of action of these inhibitors within the heart. HER2 is involved in cardiomyocyte development and survival [158]. Neuregulin 1 (NRG1) is produced by cardiac endothelial cells, binds the human EGF receptor 4 (HER4, also known as ERBB4) on cardiomyocytes and promotes heterodimerization with HER2, leading to activation of various downstream intracellular signaling pathways: ERK–MAPK, phosphatidylinositol 3-kinase P13K-Akt pathways and Src–FAK (focal adhesion kinase). This HER2 upregulation occurred within 3 weeks of antracycline therapy, but not in heart failure unrelated to anthracycline treatment, suggesting that the higher incidence of cardiotoxicity in patients on concurrent treatment may be HER2 dependent [157].

One novel mechanism proposed for some targeted molecular chemotherapy-induced cardiotoxicity is the inadvertent interruption in the homeostasis of cardiac stem cells, thereby depleting the resident cardiac stem cell pool. As a result, the heart loses the capability of regeneration and repair and demonstrates features of cardiotoxicity. This hypothesis is supported by several lines of emerging evidence: the high incidence of cardiotoxicity in pediatric cancer patients who still have more cardiac stem cells in the myocardium; the rescue of anthracycline cardiomyopathy by injection of cardiac stem cells; and the adverse cardiotoxicity induced by inhibitors of oncogenic kinases or pathways which target cardiac stem cells besides cancer cells, and the demonstration of depletion of cardiac stem cells after anthracyclines [159]. This may promote our growing appreciation that cardiac stem cells represent new targets of chemotherapy that contribute to cardiotoxicity and open up novel strategies for the preservation or expansion of the cardiac stem-cells pool to overcome cardiotoxicity associated with chemotherapy.

Recent analysis suggests that TKIs initiate a novel cascade of events traversing through MSCs to leukemic cells, leading to resistance. Specifically, MSCs exposed to TKIs acquired a new functional status with the expression of genes encoding for chemo-attractants, adhesion molecules, and pro-survival growth factors, and this priming enabled leukemic cells to form clusters underneath the MSCs. This cluster formation was associated with the protection of ALL cells from therapy as leukemic cells switched from BCR-ABL signaling to IL-7R/Janus kinase signaling to survive in the MSC milieu. These findings illustrate a novel pathway in the evolution of TKI resistance and may contribute in part to the cardiotoxic effects of TKIs [158]. Finally, a lot of interest has recently focused on whether β-blockers, statins, and/or angiotensin-converting enzyme (ACE)-inhibitors might have therapeutic and/or preventative effects in cancer patients that exhibit any cardiotoxic effects of these drugs [159].

CONCLUSIONS

The developmental regulatory pathways of Notch and Hedgehog are key contributors to both tumor angiogenesis and resident vascular, and nonvascular stem-cell fate that underlies the pathogenesis of many cancers and vascular proliferative disease. The commonalities in signaling pathways for both diseases, and the putative role of stem cells in their etiology suggest that therapies targeting these pathways in cancer may well affect their beneficial role in vascular regenerative biology and vascular homeostasis and thereby contribute to the associated cardiotoxic effects of many forms of chemotherapy.

REFERENCES

[1] Hanahan D, Weinberg RA. Hallmarks of cancer: the next generation. Cell 2011;144:646–74.

[2] Li D, de Glas NA, Hurria A. Cancer and aging: general principles, biology, and geriatric assessment. Clin Geriatr Med 2016;32:1–15.

[3] Uryga AK, Bennett MR. Ageing induced vascular smooth muscle cell senescence in atherosclerosis. J Physiol (Lond) 2015;594:2115–24.

[4] van Kruijsdijk RCM, van der Graaf Y, Peeters PHM, Visseren FLJ. Second manifestations of ARTerial disease (SMART) study group. Cancer risk in patients with manifest vascular disease: effects of smoking, obesity, and metabolic syndrome. Cancer Epidemiol Biomarkers Prev 2013;22:1267–77.

[5] Canavese M, Santo L, Raje N. Cyclin dependent kinases in cancer: potential for therapeutic intervention. Cancer Biol Ther 2012;13:451–7.

[6] Fuster JJ, Fernández P, González-Navarro H, Silvestre C, Nabah YNA, Andrés V. Control of cell proliferation in atherosclerosis: insights from animal models and human studies. Cardiovasc Res 2010;86:254–64.

[7] McEver RP. Selectins: initiators of leucocyte adhesion and signalling at the vascular wall. Cardiovasc Res. 2015;107:331–9.

[8] Blandin A-F, Renner G, Lehmann M, Lelong-Rebel I, Martin S, Dontenwill M. β1 Integrins as therapeutic targets to disrupt hallmarks of cancer. Front Pharmacol 2015;6:279.

[9] MacKay CE, Knock GA. Control of vascular smooth muscle function by Src-family kinases and reactive oxygen species in health and disease. J Physiol (Lond) 2015;593:3815–28.

[10] Bhattacharyya S, Tumour Saha J. Oxidative stress and host T cell response: cementing the dominance. Scand J Immunol 2015;82:477–88.

[11] Pinilla-Ibarz J, Sweet K, Emole J, Fradley M. Long-term BCR-ABL1 tyrosine kinase inhibitor therapy in chronic myeloid leukemia. Anticancer Res 2015;35:6355–64.

[12] Goumans M-J, Valdimarsdottir G, Itoh S, Rosendahl A, Sideras P, Dijke ten P. Balancing the activation state of the endothelium via two distinct TGF-beta type I receptors. EMBO J 2002;21:1743–53.

[13] Lee YC, Michael M, Zalcberg JR. An overview of experimental and investigational multikinase inhibitors for the treatment of metastatic colorectal cancer. Expert Opin Investig Drugs 2015;24:1307–20.

[14] Olsen CL, Hsu P-P, Glienke J, Rubanyi GM, Brooks AR. Hedgehog-interacting protein is highly expressed in endothelial cells but down-regulated during angiogenesis and in several human tumors. BMC Cancer 2004;4:43. Available from: http://www.biomedcentral.com/1471-2407/4/43.

[15] Jomrich G, Schoppmann SF. Targeting HER 2 and angiogenesis in gastric cancer. Expert Rev Anticancer Ther 2016;16(1):111–22.

[16] Courboulin A, Ranchoux B, Cohen-Kaminsky S, Perros F, Bonnet S. MicroRNA networks in pulmonary arterial hypertension: share mechanisms with cancer? Curr Opin Oncol 2016;28:72–82.

[17] Sekijima T, Tanabe A, Maruoka R, Fujishiro N, Yu S, Fujiwara S, Yuguchi H, Yamashita Y, Terai Y, Ohmichi M. Impact of platinum-based chemotherapy on the progression of atherosclerosis. Climacteric 2011;14:31–40.

[18] Vermeulen L, Sprick MR, Kemper K, Stassi G, Medema JP. Cancer stem cells—old concepts, new insights. Cell Death Differ 2008;15:947–58.

[19] Tomasetti C, Vogelstein B. Cancer etiology. Variation in cancer risk among tissues can be explained by the number of stem cell divisions. Science 2015;347:78–81.

[20] Metcalfe C, de Sauvage FJ. Hedgehog fights back: mechanisms of acquired resistance against Smoothened antagonists. Cancer Res 2011;71:5057–61.

[21] Queiroz KC, Ruela-de-Sousa RR, Fuhler GM, Aberson HL, Ferreira CV, Peppelenbosch MP, Spek CA. Hedgehog signaling maintains chemoresistance in myeloid leukemic cells. Oncogene 2010;29:6314–22.

[22] Steg AD, Bevis KS, Katre AA, Ziebarth A, Dobbin ZC, Alvarez RD, Zhang K, Conner M, Landen CN. Stem cell pathways contribute to clinical chemoresistance in ovarian cancer. Clin Cancer Res 2012;18:869–81.

[23] Tang Z, Wang A, Yuan F, Yan Z, Liu B, Chu JS, Helms JA, Li S. Differentiation of multipotent vascular stem cells contributes to vascular diseases. Nat Commun 2012;3:875.

[24] Alexander MR, Owens GK. Epigenetic control of smooth muscle cell differentiation and phenotypic switching in vascular development and disease. Annu Rev Physiol 2012;74:13–40.

[25] Lao KH, Zeng L, Xu Q. Endothelial and smooth muscle cell transformation in atherosclerosis. Curr Opin Lipidol 2015;26:449–56.

[26] Majesky MW. Adventitia and perivascular cells. Arterioscler Thromb Vasc Biol 2015;35:e31–5.

[27] Rostama B, Peterson SM, Vary CPH, Liaw L. Notch signal integration in the vasculature during remodeling. Vascul Pharmacol 2014;63:97–104.

[28] Caliceti C, Nigro P, Rizzo P, Ferrari R. ROS, Notch, and Wnt signaling pathways: crosstalk between three major regulators of cardiovascular biology. Biomed Res Int 2014;2014:318714–8.

[29] Petrova R, Joyner AL. Roles for Hedgehog signaling in adult organ homeostasis and repair. Development 2014;141:3445–57.

[30] Wong MM, Winkler B, Karamariti E, Wang X, Yu B, Simpson R, Chen T, Margariti A, Xu Q. Sirolimus stimulates vascular stem/progenitor cell migration and differentiation into smooth muscle cells via epidermal growth factor receptor/extracellular signal-regulated kinase/β-catenin signaling pathway. Arterioscler Thromb Vasc Biol 2013;33:2397–406.

[31] Mooney CJ, Hakimjavadi R, Fitzpatrick E, Kennedy E, Walls D, Morrow D, Redmond EM, Cahill PA. Hedgehog and resident vascular stem cell fate. Stem Cells Int 2015;2015:468428.

[32] Kamiya K, Ozasa K, Akiba S, Niwa O, Kodama K, Takamura N, Zaharieva EK, Kimura Y, Wakeford R. Long-term effects of radiation exposure on health. Lancet 2015;386:469–78.

[33] Grover S, Lou PW, Bradbrook C, Cheong K, Kotasek D, Leong DP, Koczwara B, Selvanayagam JB. Early and late changes in markers of aortic stiffness with breast cancer therapy. Intern Med J 2015;45:140–7.

[34] Wu Y-T, Chen C-Y, Lai W-T, Kuo C-C, Huang Y-B. Increasing risks of ischemic stroke in oral cancer patients treated with radiotherapy or chemotherapy: a nationwide cohort study. Int J Neurosci 2015;125:808–16.

[35] Harding JL, Sooriyakumaran M, Anstey KJ, Adams R, Balkau B, Brennan-Olsen S, Briffa T, Davis TME, Davis WA, Dobson A, Giles GG, Grant J, Huxley R, Knuiman M, Luszcz M, Mitchell P, Pasco JA, Reid CM, Simmons D, Simons LA, Taylor AW, Tonkin A, Woodward M, Shaw JE, Magliano DJ. Hypertension, antihypertensive treatment and cancer incidence and mortality: a pooled collaborative analysis of 12 Australian and New Zealand cohorts. J Hypertens 2016;34:149–55.

[36] Vatanen A, Sarkola T, Ojala TH, Turanlahti M, Jahnukainen T, Saarinen-Pihkala UM, Jahnukainen K. Radiotherapy-related arterial intima thickening and plaque formation in childhood cancer survivors detected with very-high resolution ultrasound during young adulthood. Pediatr Blood Cancer 2015;62:2000–6.

[37] Takebe N, Miele L, Harris PJ, Jeong W, Bando H, Kahn M, Yang SX, Ivy SP. Targeting Notch, Hedgehog, and Wnt pathways in cancer stem cells: clinical update. Nat Rev Clin Oncol 2015;12:445–64.

[38] Morrow D, Guha S, Sweeney C, Birney Y, Walshe T, O'Brien C, Walls D, Redmond EM, Cahill PA. Notch and vascular smooth muscle cell phenotype. Circ Res 2008;103:1370–82.

[39] Briscoe J, Thérond PP. The mechanisms of Hedgehog signalling and its roles in development and disease. Nat Rev Mol Cell Biol 2013;14:416–29.

[40] D'Souza B, Miyamoto A, Weinmaster G. The many facets of Notch ligands. Oncogene 2008;27:5148–67.

[41] Takebe N, Nguyen D, Yang SX. Targeting notch signaling pathway in cancer: clinical development advances and challenges. Pharmacol Ther 2014;141:140–9.

[42] Folkman J. Tumor angiogenesis: therapeutic implications. N Engl J Med 1971;285:1182–6.

[43] Wang Z, Dabrosin C, Yin X, Fuster MM, Arreola A, Rathmell WK, Generali D, Nagaraju GP, El-Rayes B, Ribatti D, Chen YC, Honoki K, Fujii H, Georgakilas AG, Nowsheen S, Amedei A, Niccolai E, Amin A, Ashraf SS, Helferich B, Yang X, Guha G, Bhakta D, Ciriolo MR, Aquilano K, Chen S, Halicka D, Mohammed SI, Azmi AS, Bilsland A, Keith WN, Jensen LD. Broad targeting of angiogenesis for cancer prevention and therapy. Semin Cancer Biol 2015;35 Suppl:S224–43.

[44] Ferrara N. VEGF as a therapeutic target in cancer. Oncology 2005;69(Suppl 3):11–6.

[45] Armulik A, Genové G, Betsholtz C. Pericytes: developmental, physiological, and pathological perspectives, problems, and promises. Dev Cell 2011;21:193–215.

[46] Hellström M, Phng L-K, Hofmann JJ, Wallgard E, Coultas L, Lindblom P, Alva J, Nilsson A-K, Karlsson L, Gaiano N, Yoon K, Rossant J, Iruela-Arispe ML, Kalén M, Gerhardt H, Betsholtz C. Dll4 signalling through Notch1 regulates formation of tip cells during angiogenesis. Nature 2007;445:776–80.

[47] Jakobsson L, Franco CA, Bentley K, Collins RT, Ponsioen B, Aspalter IM, Rosewell I, Busse M, Thurston G, Medvinsky A, Schulte-Merker S, Gerhardt H. Endothelial cells dynamically compete for the tip cell position during angiogenic sprouting. Nat Cell Biol 2010;12:943–53.

[48] Ridgway J, Zhang G, Wu Y, Stawicki S, Liang W-C, Chanthery Y, Kowalski J, Watts RJ, Callahan C, Kasman I, Singh M, Chien M, Tan C, Hongo J-AS, de Sauvage F, Plowman G, Yan M. Inhibition of Dll4 signalling inhibits tumour growth by deregulating angiogenesis. Nature 2006;444:1083–7.

[49] Hida K, Maishi N, Sakurai Y, Hida Y, Harashima H. Heterogeneity of tumor endothelial cells and drug delivery. Adv Drug Deliv Rev 2016;99:140–7.

[50] Hoey T, Yen W-C, Axelrod F, Basi J, Donigian L, Dylla S, Fitch-Bruhns M, Lazetic S, Park I-K, Sato A, Satyal S, Wang X, Clarke MF, Lewicki J, Gurney A. DLL4 blockade inhibits tumor growth and reduces tumor-initiating cell frequency. Cell Stem Cell 2009;5:168–77.

[51] Yuan X, Wu H, Xu H, Xiong H, Chu Q, Yu S, Wu GS, Wu K. Notch signaling: an emerging therapeutic target for cancer treatment. Cancer Lett 2015;369:20–7.

[52] Takebe N, Warren RQ, Ivy SP. Breast cancer growth and metastasis: interplay between cancer stem cells, embryonic signaling pathways and epithelial-to-mesenchymal transition. Breast Cancer Res 2011;13:211.

[53] Takeuchi H, Haltiwanger RS. Significance of glycosylation in Notch signaling. Biochem Biophys Res Commun 2014;453:235–42.

[54] Dominguez M. Oncogenic programmes and Notch activity: an 'organized crime'? Semin Cell Dev Biol 2014;28:78–85.

[55] Bhadada SV, Goyal BR, Patel MM. Angiogenic targets for potential disorders. Fundam Clin Pharmacol 2011;25:29–47.

[56] Benedito R, Roca C, Sörensen I, Adams S, Gossler A, Fruttiger M, Adams RH. The notch ligands Dll4 and Jagged1 have opposing effects on angiogenesis. Cell 2009;137:1124–35.

[57] Pedrosa A-R, Trindade A, Fernandes A-C, Carvalho C, Gigante J, Tavares AT, Diéguez-Hurtado R, Yagita H, Adams RH, Duarte A. Endothelial Jagged1 antagonizes Dll4 regulation of endothelial branching and promotes vascular maturation downstream of Dll4/Notch1. Arterioscler Thromb Vasc Biol 2015;35:1134–46.

[58] Carmeliet P, Jain RK. Principles and mechanisms of vessel normalization for cancer and other angiogenic diseases. Nat Rev Drug Discov 2011;10:417–27.

[59] Witte L, Hicklin DJ, Zhu Z, Pytowski B, Kotanides H, Rockwell P, Böhlen P. Monoclonal antibodies targeting the VEGF receptor-2 (Flk1/KDR) as an anti-angiogenic therapeutic strategy. Cancer Metastasis Rev 1998;17:155–61.

[60] Wang R, Chadalavada K, Wilshire J, Kowalik U, Hovinga KE, Geber A, Fligelman B, Leversha M, Brennan C, Tabar V. Glioblastoma stem-like cells give rise to tumour endothelium. Nature 2010;468:829–33.

[61] Dong J, Zhao Y, Huang Q, Fei X, Diao Y, Shen Y, Xiao H, Zhang T, Lan Q, Gu X. Glioma stem/progenitor cells contribute to neovascularization via transdifferentiation. Stem Cell Rev 2011;7:141–52.

[62] Qiao L, Liang N, Zhang J, Xie J, Liu F, Xu D, Yu X, Tian Y. Advanced research on vasculogenic mimicry in cancer. J Cell Mol Med 2015;19:315–26.

[63] Shao R, Taylor SL, Oh DS, Schwartz LM. Vascular heterogeneity and targeting: the role of YKL-40 in glioblastoma vascularization. Oncotarget 2015;6:40507–18.

[64] Plummer PN, Freeman R, Taft RJ, Vider J, Sax M, Umer BA, Gao D, Johns C, Mattick JS, Wilton SD, Ferro V, McMillan NAJ, Swarbrick A, Mittal V, Mellick AS. MicroRNAs regulate tumor angiogenesis modulated by endothelial progenitor cells. Cancer Res 2013;73:341–52.

[65] Chiao M-T, Yang Y-C, Cheng W-Y, Shen C-C, Ko J-L. CD133+ glioblastoma stem-like cells induce vascular mimicry in vivo. Curr Neurovasc Res 2011;8:210–9.

[66] Yao X, Ping Y, Liu Y, Chen K, Yoshimura T, Liu M, Gong W, Chen C, Niu Q, Guo D, Zhang X, Wang JM, Bian X. Vascular endothelial growth factor receptor 2 (VEGFR-2) plays a key role in vasculogenic mimicry formation, neovascularization and tumor initiation by Glioma stem-like cells. PLoS One 2013;8:e57188.

[67] Gao D, Nolan DJ, Mellick AS, Bambino K, McDonnell K, Mittal V. Endothelial progenitor cells control the angiogenic switch in mouse lung metastasis. Science 2008;319:195–8.

[68] O'Connell RM, Rao DS, Chaudhuri AA, Baltimore D. Physiological and pathological roles for microRNAs in the immune system. Nat Rev Immunol 2010;10:111–22.

[69] Ma L, Teruya-Feldstein J, Weinberg RA. Tumour invasion and metastasis initiated by microRNA-10b in breast cancer. Nature 2007;449:682–8.

[70] Suárez Y, Fernández-Hernando C, Pober JS, Sessa WC. Dicer dependent microRNAs regulate gene expression and functions in human endothelial cells. Circ Res 2007;100:1164–73.

[71] Kahlert C, Kalluri R. Exosomes in tumor microenvironment influence cancer progression and metastasis. J Mol Med 2013;91:431–7.

[72] Bruno S, Collino F, Iavello A, Camussi G. Effects of mesenchymal stromal cell-derived extracellular vesicles on tumor growth. Front Immunol 2014;5:382.

[73] Pap E, Pállinger E, Falus A. The role of membrane vesicles in tumorigenesis. Crit Rev Oncol Hematol 2011;79:213–23.

[74] Maes H, Olmeda D, Soengas MS, Agostinis P. Vesicular trafficking mechanisms in endothelial cells as modulators of the tumor vasculature and targets of antiangiogenic therapies. FEBS J 2015;283:25–38.

[75] Zheng L, Saunders CA, Sorensen EB, Waxmonsky NC, Conner SD. Notch signaling from the endosome requires a conserved dileucine motif. Mol Biol Cell 2013;24:297–307.

[76] Sheldon H, Heikamp E, Turley H, Dragovic R, Thomas P, Oon CE, Leek R, Edelmann M, Kessler B, Sainson RCA, Sargent I, Li J-L, Harris AL. New mechanism for Notch signaling to endothelium at a distance by Delta-like 4 incorporation into exosomes. Blood 2010;116:2385–94.

[77] Liebner S, Liebner S. Sonic hedgehog causes mural cells to jump "n" run. Blood 2014;123:2285–6.

[78] Jones DL, Rando TA. Emerging models and paradigms for stem cell ageing. Nat Cell Biol 2011;13:506–12.

[79] Cirrone F, Harris CS. Vismodegib and the hedgehog pathway: a new treatment for basal cell carcinoma. Clin Ther 2012;34:2039–50.

[80] Rudin CM, Hann CL, Laterra J, Yauch RL, Callahan CA, Fu L, Holcomb T, Stinson J, Gould SE, Coleman B, LoRusso PM, Hoff Von DD, de Sauvage FJ, Low JA. Treatment of medulloblastoma with hedgehog pathway inhibitor GDC-0449. N Engl J Med 2009;361:1173–8.

[81] Brechbiel J, Miller-Moslin K, Adjei AA. Crosstalk between hedgehog and other signaling pathways as a basis for combination therapies in cancer. Cancer Treat Rev 2014;40:750–9.

[82] Gomes DC, Jamra SA, Leal LF, Colli LM, Campanini ML, Oliveira RS, Martinelli CE, Elias PCL, Moreira AC, Machado HR, Saggioro F, Neder L, Castro M, Antonini SR. Sonic Hedgehog pathway is up-regulated in adamantinomatous craniopharyngiomas. Eur J Endocrinol 2015;172:603–8.

[83] Ramaswamy B, Lu Y, Teng KY, Nuovo G, Li X, Shapiro CL, Majumder S. Hedgehog signaling is a novel therapeutic target in tamoxifen-resistant breast cancer aberrantly activated by PI3K/AKT pathway. Cancer Res 2012;72:5048–59.

[84] Merchant AA, Matsui W. Targeting hedgehog—a cancer stem cell pathway. Clin Cancer Res 2010;16:3130–40.

[85] Kim JE, Singh RR, Cho-Vega JH, Drakos E, Davuluri Y, Khokhar FA, Fayad L, Medeiros LJ, Vega F. Sonic hedgehog signaling proteins and ATP-binding cassette G2 are aberrantly expressed in diffuse large B-cell lymphoma. Mod Pathol 2009;22:1312–20.

[86] Oliver TG, Grasfeder LL, Carroll AL, Kaiser C, Gillingham CL, Lin SM, Wickramasinghe R, Scott MP, Wechsler-Reya RJ. Transcriptional profiling of the Sonic hedgehog response: a critical role for N-myc in proliferation of neuronal precursors. Proc Natl Acad Sci 2003;100:7331–6.

[87] Vestergaard J, Lind-Thomsen A, Pedersen MW, Jarmer HO, Bak M, Hasholt L, Tommerup N, Tümer Z, Larsen LA. GLI1 is involved in cell cycle regulation and proliferation of NT2 embryonal carcinoma stem cells. DNA Cell Biol 2008;27:251–6.

[88] Kang HN, Oh SC, Kim JS, Yoo YA. Abrogation of Gli3 expression suppresses the growth of colon cancer cells via activation of p53. Exp Cell Res 2012;318:539–49.

[89] Katoh Y, Katoh M. Hedgehog target genes: mechanisms of carcinogenesis induced by aberrant hedgehog signaling activation. Curr Mol Med 2009;9:873–86.

[90] Nakamura K, Sasajima J, Mizukami Y, Sugiyama Y, Yamazaki M, Fujii R, Kawamoto T, Koizumi K, Sato K, Fujiya M, Sasaki K, Tanno S, Okumura T, Shimizu N, Kawabe J-I, Karasaki H, Kono T, Ii M, Bardeesy N, Chung DC, Kohgo Y. Hedgehog promotes neovascularization in pancreatic cancers by regulating Ang-1 and IGF-1 expression in bone-marrow derived pro-angiogenic cells. PLoS One 2010;5:e8824.

[91] Chen W, Tang T, Eastham-Anderson J, Dunlap D, Alicke B, Nannini M, Gould S, Yauch R, Modrusan Z, DuPree KJ, Darbonne WC, Plowman G, de Sauvage FJ, Callahan CA. Canonical hedgehog signaling augments tumor angiogenesis by induction of VEGF-A in stromal perivascular cells. Proc Natl Acad Sci 2011;108:9589–94.

[92] Das S, Harris LG, Metge BJ, Liu S, Riker AI, Samant RS, Shevde LA. The hedgehog pathway transcription factor GLI1 promotes malignant behavior of cancer cells by up-regulating osteopontin. J Biol Chem 2009;284:22888–97.

[93] Harris LG, Pannell LK, Singh S, Samant RS, Shevde LA. Increased vascularity and spontaneous metastasis of breast cancer by hedgehog signaling mediated upregulation of cyr61. Oncogene 2011;31:3370–80.

[94] Li X, Ma Q, Xu Q, Liu H, Lei J, Duan W, Bhat K, Wang F, Wu E, Wang Z. SDF-1/CXCR4 signaling induces pancreatic cancer cell invasion and epithelial-mesenchymal transition in vitro through non-canonical activation of Hedgehog pathway. Cancer Lett 2012;322:169–76.

[95] Omenetti A, Porrello A, Jung Y, Yang L, Popov Y, Choi SS, Witek RP, Alpini G, Venter J, Vandongen HM, Syn W-K, Baroni GS, Benedetti A, Schuppan D, Diehl AM. Hedgehog signaling regulates epithelial-mesenchymal transition during biliary fibrosis in rodents and humans. J Clin Invest 2008;118:3331–42.

[96] Mani SA, Guo W, Liao M-J, Eaton EN, Ayyanan A, Zhou AY, Brooks M, Reinhard F, Zhang CC, Shipitsin M, Campbell LL, Polyak K, Brisken C, Yang J, Weinberg RA. The epithelial-mesenchymal transition generates cells with properties of stem cells. Cell 2008;133:704–15.

[97] Clement V, Sanchez P, de Tribolet N, Radovanovic I, Ruiz i Altaba A. HEDGEHOG-GLI1 signaling regulates human glioma growth, cancer stem cell self-renewal, and tumorigenicity. Curr Biol 2007;17:165–72.

[98] Zhao C, Chen A, Jamieson CH, Fereshteh M, Abrahamsson A, Blum J, Kwon HY, Kim J, Chute JP, Rizzieri D, Munchhof M, VanArsdale T, Beachy PA, Reya T. Hedgehog signalling is essential for maintenance of cancer stem cells in myeloid leukaemia. Nature 2009;458:776–9.

[99] Dierks C, Beigi R, Guo G-R, Zirlik K, Stegert MR, Manley P, Trussell C, Schmitt-Graeff A, Landwerlin K, Veelken H, Warmuth M.

[100] Bar EE, Chaudhry A, Lin A, Fan X, Schreck K, Matsui W, Piccirillo S, Vescovi AL, DiMeco F, Olivi A, Eberhart CG. Cyclopamine-mediated hedgehog pathway inhibition depletes stem-like cancer cells in glioblastoma. Stem Cells 2007;25:2524–33.

[101] Blonska M, Agarwal NK, Vega F. Shaping of the tumor microenvironment: stromal cells and vessels. Semin Cancer Biol 2015;34: 3–13.

[102] Xin M. Hedgehog inhibitors: a patent review (2013–present). Expert Opin Ther Pat 2015;25:549–65.

[103] Berlin J, Bendell JC, Hart LL, Firdaus I, Gore I, Hermann RC, Mulcahy MF, Zalupski MM, Mackey HM, Yauch RL, Graham RA, Bray GL, Low JA. A randomized phase II trial of vismodegib versus placebo with FOLFOX or FOLFIRI and bevacizumab in patients with previously untreated metastatic colorectal cancer. Clin Cancer Res 2013;19:258–67.

[104] Ruch JM, Kim EJ. Hedgehog signaling pathway and cancer therapeutics: progress to date. Drugs 2013;73:613–23.

[105] Zhao X, Ponomaryov T, Ornell KJ, Zhou P, Dabral SK, Pak E, Li W, Atwood SX, Whitson RJ, Chang ALS, Li J, Oro AE, Chan JA, Kelleher JF, Segal RA. RAS/MAPK activation drives resistance to Smo inhibition, metastasis, and tumor evolution in Shh pathway–dependent tumors. Cancer Res 2015;75:3623–35.

[106] Sims-Mourtada J, Izzo JG, Ajani J, Chao KSC. Sonic Hedgehog promotes multiple drug resistance by regulation of drug transport. Oncogene 2007;26:5674–9.

[107] Brennan D, Chen X, Cheng L, Mahoney M, Riobo NA. Noncanonical hedgehog signaling. Vitam Horm 2012;88:55–72.

[108] Singh S, Chitkara D, Mehrazin R, Behrman SW, Wake RW, Mahato RI. Chemoresistance in prostate cancer cells is regulated by miRNAs and Hedgehog pathway. PLoS One 2012;7:e40021.

[109] Callahan BP, Wang C. Hedgehog cholesterolysis: specialized gatekeeper to oncogenic signaling. Cancers (Basel) 2015;7:2037–53.

[110] Cristofaro B, Emanueli C. Possible novel targets for therapeutic angiogenesis. Curr Opin Pharmacol 2009;9:102–8.

[111] Swift MR, Weinstein BM. Arterial-venous specification during development. Circ Res 2009;104:576–88.

[112] Coultas L, Nieuwenhuis E, Anderson GA, Cabezas J, Nagy A, Henkelman RM, Hui CC, Rossant J. Hedgehog regulates distinct vascular patterning events through VEGF-dependent and -independent mechanisms. Blood 2010;116:653–60.

[113] Pola R, Ling LE, Silver M, Corbley MJ, Kearney M, Blake Pepinsky R, Shapiro R, Taylor FR, Baker DP, Asahara T, Isner JM. The morphogen Sonic hedgehog is an indirect angiogenic agent upregulating two families of angiogenic growth factors. Nat Med 2001;7:706–11.

[114] Kusano KF, Allendoerfer KL, Munger W, Pola R, Bosch-Marce M, Kirchmair R, Yoon Y-S, Curry C, Silver M, Kearney M, Asahara T, Losordo DW. Sonic hedgehog induces arteriogenesis in diabetic vasa nervorum and restores function in diabetic neuropathy. Arterioscler Thromb Vasc Biol 2004;24:2102–7.

[115] Asai J, Takenaka H, Kusano KF, Ii M, Luedemann C, Curry C, Eaton E, Iwakura A, Tsutsumi Y, Hamada H, Kishimoto S, Thorne T, Kishore R, Losordo DW. Topical sonic hedgehog gene therapy accelerates wound healing in diabetes by enhancing endothelial progenitor cell-mediated microvascular remodeling. Circulation 2006;113:2413–24.

[116] Kanaya K, Masaaki I, Okazaki T, Nakamura T, Horii-Komatsu M, Alev C, Akimaru H, Kawamoto A, Akashi H, Tanaka H, Asahi M,

Expansion of Bcr-Abl-positive leukemic stem cells is dependent on hedgehog pathway activation. Cancer Cell 2008;14:238–49.

Asahara T. Sonic Hedgehog signaling regulates vascular differentiation and function in human CD34 positive cells: vasculogenic CD34(+) cells with Sonic Hedgehog. Stem Cell Res 2015;14: 165–76.

[117] Palladino M, Gatto I, Neri V, Stigliano E, Smith RC, Pola E, Straino S, Gaetani E, Capogrossi M, Leone G, Hlatky L, Pola R. Combined therapy with sonic hedgehog gene transfer and bone marrow-derived endothelial progenitor cells enhances angiogenesis and myogenesis in the ischemic skeletal muscle. J Vasc Res 2012;49:425–31.

[118] Mackie AR, Klyachko E, Thorne T, Schultz KM, Millay M, Ito A, Kamide CE, Liu T, Gupta R, Sahoo S, Misener S, Kishore R, Losordo DW. Sonic hedgehog-modified human CD34+ cells preserve cardiac function after acute myocardial infarction. Circ Res 2012;111:312–21.

[119] Invernici G, Emanueli C, Madeddu P, Cristini S, Gadau S, Benetti A, Ciusani E, Stassi G, Siragusa M, Nicosia R, Peschle C, Fascio U, Colombo A, Rizzuti T, Parati E, Alessandri G. Human fetal aorta contains vascular progenitor cells capable of inducing vasculogenesis, angiogenesis, and myogenesis in vitro and in a murine model of peripheral ischemia. Am J Pathol 2007;170:1879–92.

[120] Fang B, Li Y, Song Y, Li N. Isolation and characterization of multipotent progenitor cells from the human fetal aorta wall. Exp Biol Med (Maywood). 2010;235:130–8.

[121] Pacilli A, Pasquinelli G. Vascular wall resident progenitor cells: a review. Exp Cell Res 2009;315:901–14.

[122] Dar A, Domev H, Ben-Yosef O, Tzukerman M, Zeevi-Levin N, Novak A, Germanguz I, Amit M, Itskovitz-Eldor J. Multipotent vasculogenic pericytes from human pluripotent stem cells promote recovery of murine ischemic limb. Circulation 2012;125:87–99.

[123] Orlandi A. The contribution of resident vascular stem cells to arterial pathology. Int J Stem Cells 2015;8:9–17.

[124] Psaltis PJ, Simari RD. Vascular wall progenitor cells in health and disease. Circ Res 2015;116:1392–412.

[125] Chen Y, Wong MM, Campagnolo P, Simpson R, Winkler B, Margariti A, Hu Y, Xu Q. Adventitial stem cells in vein grafts display multilineage potential that contributes to neointimal formation. Arterioscler Thromb Vasc Biol 2013;33:1844–51.

[126] Herring BP, Hoggatt AM, Burlak C, Offermanns S. Previously differentiated medial vascular smooth muscle cells contribute to neointima formation following vascular injury. Vasc Cell 2014;6:21.

[127] Nemenoff RA, Horita H, Ostriker AC, Furgeson SB, Simpson PA, VanPutten V, Crossno J, Offermanns S, Weiser-Evans MCM. SDF-1α induction in mature smooth muscle cells by inactivation of PTEN is a critical mediator of exacerbated injury-induced neointima formation. Arterioscler Thromb Vasc Biol 2011;31:1300–8.

[128] Wan M, Li C, Zhen G, Jiao K, He W, Jia X, Wang W, Shi C, Xing Q, Chen Y-F, Jan De Beur S, Yu B, Cao X. Injury-activated transforming growth factor β controls mobilization of mesenchymal stem cells for tissue remodeling. Stem Cells 2012;30:2498–511.

[129] Liang M, Liang A, Wang Y, Jiang J, Cheng J. Smooth muscle cells from the anastomosed artery are the major precursors for neointima formation in both artery and vein grafts. Basic Res Cardiol 2014;109:431.

[130] Morrow D, Cullen JP, Liu W, Guha S, Sweeney C, Birney YA, Collins N, Walls D, Redmond EM, Cahill PA. Sonic Hedgehog induces Notch target gene expression in vascular smooth muscle cells via VEGF-A. Arterioscler Thromb Vasc Biol 2009;29:1112–8.

[131] Passman JN, Dong XR, Wu S-P, Maguire CT, Hogan KA, Bautch VL, Majesky MW. A sonic hedgehog signaling domain in the arterial adventitia supports resident Sca1+ smooth muscle progenitor cells. Proc Natl Acad Sci USA 2008;105:9349–54.

[132] Grudzinska MK, Kurzejamska E, Bojakowski K, Soin J, Lehmann MH, Reinecke H, Murry CE, Soderberg-Naucler C, Religa P. Monocyte chemoattractant protein 1-mediated migration of mesenchymal stem cells is a source of intimal hyperplasia. Arterioscler Thromb Vasc Biol 2013;33:1271–9.

[133] Redmond EM, Hamm K, Cullen JP, Hatch E, Cahill PA, Morrow D. Inhibition of patched-1 prevents injury-induced neointimal hyperplasia. Arterioscler Thromb Vasc Biol 2013;33:1960–4.

[134] Tian H, Callahan CA, DuPree KJ, Darbonne WC, Ahn CP, Scales SJ, de Sauvage FJ. Hedgehog signaling is restricted to the stromal compartment during pancreatic carcinogenesis. Proc Natl Acad Sci USA 2009;106:4254–9.

[135] Olivieri F, Recchioni R, Marcheselli F, Abbatecola AM, Santini G, Borghetti G, Antonicelli R, Procopio AD. Cellular senescence in cardiovascular diseases: potential age-related mechanisms and implications for treatment. Curr Pharm Des 2013;19:1710–9.

[136] Fender AW, Nutter JM, Fitzgerald TL, Bertrand FE, Sigounas G. Notch-1 promotes stemness and epithelial to mesenchymal transition in colorectal cancer. J Cell Biochem 2015;116:2517–27.

[137] Xie M, Zhang L, He C-S, Xu F, Liu J-L, Hu Z-H, Zhao L-P, Tian Y. Activation of Notch-1 enhances epithelial-mesenchymal transition in gefitinib-acquired resistant lung cancer cells. J Cell Biochem 2012;113:1501–13.

[138] Byers LA, Diao L, Wang J, Saintigny P, Girard L, Peyton M, Shen L, Fan Y, Giri U, Tumula PK, Nilsson MB, Gudikote J, Tran H, Cardnell RJG, Bearss DJ, Warner SL, Foulks JM, Kanner SB, Gandhi V, Krett N, Rosen ST, Kim ES, Herbst RS, Blumenschein GR, Lee JJ, Lippman SM, Ang KK, Mills GB, Hong WK, Weinstein JN, Wistuba II, Coombes KR, Minna JD, Heymach JV. An epithelial-mesenchymal transition gene signature predicts resistance to EGFR and PI3K inhibitors and identifies Axl as a therapeutic target for overcoming EGFR inhibitor resistance. Clin Cancer Res 2013;19:279–90.

[139] Liu J, Dong F, Jeong J, Masuda T, Lobe CG. Constitutively active Notch1 signaling promotes endothelial-mesenchymal transition in a conditional transgenic mouse model. Int J Mol Med 2014;34:669–76.

[140] Chen X, Xiao W, Liu X, Zeng M, Luo L, Wu M, Ye S, Liu Y. Blockade of Jagged/Notch pathway abrogates transforming growth factor β2-induced epithelial-mesenchymal transition in human retinal pigment epithelium cells. Curr Mol Med 2014;14:523–34.

[141] Suzman DL, Antonarakis ES. Clinical implications of hedgehog pathway signaling in prostate cancer. Cancers (Basel) 2015;7:1983–93.

[142] Jadaan DY, Jadaan MM, McCabe JP. Cellular plasticity in prostate cancer bone metastasis. Prostate Cancer 2015;2015:651580.

[143] Xing F, Okuda H, Watabe M, Kobayashi A, Pai SK, Liu W, Pandey PR, Fukuda K, Hirota S, Sugai T, Wakabayshi G, Koeda K, Kashiwaba M, Suzuki K, Chiba T, Endo M, Mo Y-Y, Watabe K. Hypoxia-induced Jagged2 promotes breast cancer metastasis and self-renewal of cancer stem-like cells. Oncogene 2011;30:4075–86.

[144] Zanotti S, Canalis E. Notch regulation of bone development and remodeling and related skeletal disorders. Calcif Tissue Int 2012;90:69–75.

[145] Ikemoto T, Sugimoto K, Shimada M, Utsunomiya T, Morine Y, Imura S, Arakawa Y, Kanamoto M, Iwahashi S-I, Saito Y, Yamada S. Clinical role of Notch signaling pathway in intraductal papillary mucinous neoplasm of the pancreas. J Gastroenterol Hepatol 2015;30:217–22.

[146] Pandya K, Meeke K, Clementz AG, Rogowski A, Roberts J, Miele L, Albain KS, Osipo C. Targeting both Notch and ErbB-2 signalling

pathways is required for prevention of ErbB-2-positive tumour recurrence. Br J Cancer 2011;105:796–806.

[147] Boucher J, Gridley T, Liaw L. Molecular pathways of notch signaling in vascular smooth muscle cells. Front Physiol 2012;3:81.

[148] Doi H, Iso T, Shiba Y, Sato H, Yamazaki M, Oyama Y, Akiyama H, Tanaka T, Tomita T, Arai M, Takahashi M, Ikeda U, Kurabayashi M. Notch signaling regulates the differentiation of bone marrow-derived cells into smooth muscle-like cells during arterial lesion formation. Biochem Biophys Res Commun 2009;381:654–9.

[149] Zhang B, Pu WT. Notching up vascular regeneration. Cell Res 2014;24:777–8.

[150] Redmond EM, Liu W, Hamm K, Hatch E, Cahill PA, Morrow D. Perivascular delivery of Notch 1 siRNA inhibits injury-induced arterial remodeling. PLoS One 2014;9:e84122.

[151] Caolo V, Schulten HM, Zhuang ZW, Murakami M, Wagenaar A, Verbruggen S, Molin DGM, Post MJ. Soluble Jagged-1 inhibits neointima formation by attenuating Notch-Herp2 signaling. Arterioscler Thromb Vasc Biol 2011;31:1059–65.

[152] Liu Z-J, Tan Y, Beecham GW, Seo DM, Tian R, Li Y, Vazquez-Padron RI, Pericak-Vance M, Vance JM, Goldschmidt-Clermont PJ, Livingstone AS, Velazquez OC. Notch activation induces endothelial cell senescence and pro-inflammatory response: implication of Notch signaling in atherosclerosis. Atherosclerosis 2012;225:296–303.

[153] Yeh ETH, Tong AT, Lenihan DJ, Yusuf SW, Swafford J, Champion C, Durand J-B, Gibbs H, Zafarmand AA, Ewer MS. Cardiovascular complications of cancer therapy: diagnosis, pathogenesis, and management. Circulation 2004;109:3122–31.

[154] Chen B, Peng X, Pentassuglia L, Lim CC, Sawyer DB. Molecular and cellular mechanisms of anthracycline cardiotoxicity. Cardiovasc Toxicol 2007;7:114–21.

[155] Ewer MS, Hoff Von DD, Benjamin RS. A historical perspective of anthracycline cardiotoxicity. Heart Fail Clin 2011;7:363–72.

[156] de Azambuja E, Ameye L, Diaz M, Vandenbossche S, Aftimos P, Hernández SB, Shih-Li C, Delhaye F, Focan C, Cornez N, Vindevoghel A, Beauduin M, Lemort M, Paesmans M, Suter T, Piccart-Gebhart M. Cardiac assessment of early breast cancer patients 18 years after treatment with cyclophosphamide-, methotrexate-, fluorouracil- or epirubicin-based chemotherapy. Eur J Cancer 2015;51:2517–24.

[157] Raschi E, Vasina V, Ursino MG, Boriani G, Martoni A, De Ponti F. Anticancer drugs and cardiotoxicity: insights and perspectives in the era of targeted therapy. Pharmacol Ther 2010;125:196–218.

[158] Negro A, Brar BK, Lee K-F. Essential roles of Her2/erbB2 in cardiac development and function. Recent Prog Horm Res 2004;59:1–12.

[159] Huang C, Zhang X, Ramil JM, Rikka S, Kim L, Lee Y, Gude NA, Thistlethwaite PA, Sussman MA, Gottlieb RA, Gustafsson AB. Juvenile exposure to anthracyclines impairs cardiac progenitor cell function and vascularization resulting in greater susceptibility to stress-induced myocardial injury in adult mice. Circulation 2010;121:675–83.

Chapter 4

Molecular Mechanisms of Anthracycline-Induced Cardiotoxicity

R. Moudgil and E.T.H. Yeh

Department of Cardiology, The University of Texas, MD Anderson Cancer Center, Houston, TX, United States

An upsurge of research was seen in mid-20th century, primarily geared toward identifying newer antibiotics. In the process, anthracyclines were isolated as new antiinfectious agent with effective tumor cytotoxic activity. Since then there has been an explosion of basic science/clinical investigations and currently anthracyclines are extensively used in various chemotherapy regimen. Today they form an indispensable part of chemotherapy for breast cancer, soft tissue sarcomas, non-Hodgkin's lymphomas, acute lymphoblastic, myeloblastic, and myelogenous leukemias [1–4]. However, the success of anthracyclines has been marred by the cardiotoxicities. The anthracycline-mediated cardiotoxicity has been subdivided into three categories; acute, subacute, and late cardiac damage [4,5].

Acute morbidity occurs during or shortly after the drug infusion and includes arrhythmias (supraventricular tachycardia, ventricular ectopy) accompanied, in some patients, by heart failure and pericarditis–myocarditis syndrome [8,9]. The subacute cardiac toxicity occurs within few weeks, clinically resembles myocarditis with edema and thickening of the left ventricular walls, and is associated with diastolic dysfunction and increased mortality [10]. In contrast to the late anthracycline-mediated cardiotoxicity, improvement in left ventricular function has been noted to occur in these subacute patients [6–8]. Furthermore, the mechanism responsible for the acute toxicity may involve an inflammatory response, which differs from the generally accepted cause of the chronic anthracycline cardiotoxicity [5,7]. Clinically, the most significant effect of anthracyclines is the late cardiac damage leading to left ventricular dysfunction and congestive heart failure, which will be the main focus of this chapter [5,7]. The dogma of the anthracycline-mediated cardiotoxicty is of the fact that each temporal event has its own mechanisms; therefore, they differ in outcomes [9].

Over the last years, the significance of the cardiac toxicity mediated by the anticancer treatment has increased markedly because of improved oncological patient survivorship, and the introduction of new anticancer drugs with unique toxicities. The awareness regarding chemotherapy-mediated cardiotoxicity, specifically anthracycline has grown and currently the American College of Cardiology and American Heart Association guidelines state that patients receiving chemotherapy may be considered a Stage A heart failure group (defined as those with increased risk of developing cardiac dysfunction) [10]. Therefore, it is apt to discuss the current development in this field. To that end, the focus of this chapter will be to highlight some of the historical and clinical perspectives with identification of the risk factors of anthracycline therapy as it pertains to cardiotoxicity. The main idea will be to address the current dogma in molecular mechanisms. At the end of this chapter, the current strategies employed to limit anthracycline mediated cardiotoxicity will be discussed.

HISTORICAL AND CLINICAL PERSPECTIVES

The family of anthracycline drugs originated in the 1950s with the identification of daunorubicin from the soil bacterium *Streptomyces peucetius* [11]. In the 1960s, daunorubicin was found to be quite effective in treating leukemias and lymphomas [12]. The same decade also saw isolation of a derivative of daunorubicin, 14-hydroxydaunomycin or adriamycin [later to be renamed Doxorubicin (DOX)], which had more efficacy as an antitumor agent than its predecessor [13,14]. Since these initial investigations of this class of antitumor agents, anthracycline chemotherapeutic agents has been used in treatment of various solid organ tumors and hematologic malignancies [13]. Subsequently, several newer anthracycline have been developed, including epirubicin (a semisynthetic epimer of DOX), with particular activity in breast, stomach, and urinary tract carcinoma [15]. Furthermore, idarubicin (a chemical analog of daunorubicin) was developed with improved efficacy against acute myelogenous leukemia [16]. Valrubicin, a semisynthetic analog of DOX, is administered directly into the bladder to treat bladder cancer [17] as its systemic toxicity precludes its use intravenously [18]. In addition, mitoxantrone, although not an anthracycline, shares many features with them (including cardiotoxicity) and is used for the treatment of breast or prostate cancer, acute myeloid leukemia, and non-Hodgkin's lymphoma [19]. Needless to say, introduction of anthracyclines into clinical practice has been one of the major successes of modern oncology.

Although DOX has become one of the most effective chemotherapeutic agents, it was noted early on that its use was complicated by the development of heart failure [20]. In a retrospective analysis of over 4000 patients receiving DOX performed by Von Hoff et al. [21], 2.2% of the patients developed clinical signs and symptoms of congestive heart failure. Because the study was based on clinician-identified signs and symptoms of congestive heart failure, incorporation of subclinical left-ventricular dysfunction would result in higher incidence of the cardiovascular disease in DOX patients, as acknowledged by the authors themselves [21]. This study went on to conclude that the prevalence of heart failure markedly increased with a cumulative dose of 550 mg/m^2 of DOX [21], which is now recognized as one of the greatest determinants in the development of anthracycline mediated heart failure [22].

Moreover, data from three trials (two in breast and one in non-small-cell lung cancer) conducted between 1988 and 1992 in which cardiotoxicity was prospectively assessed showed that the rate of conventional DOX-related CHF was 5% at a cumulative dose of 400 mg/m^2, 16% at a dose of 500 mg/m^2, and 26% at a dose of 550 mg/m^2 [22]. Furthermore, subclinical events occurred in about 30% of the patients, even at doses of 180–240 mg/m^2 [23], about 13 years after the treatment. Interestingly, histopathologic changes can be seen in endomyocardial biopsy specimens from patients who have received as little as 240 mg/m^2 of DOX [24]. These findings suggest that there is no safe dose of anthracyclines. Even doses as low as 100 mg/m^2 have been associated with reduced cardiac function [24,25]. However, individual susceptibility to cardiomyopathy is highly unpredictable. For instance, early studies suggested that some patients had no significant cardiac complications despite exposure to doses as high as 1000 mg/m^2 [21]. On the other hand, 25% of women who received six cycles of cyclophosphamide, epirubicin, and 5-fluorouracil developed an asymptomatic decline of 10% or more in left ventricular ejection fraction (LVEF) after 5 years [26]. Thus, cardiotoxicity can be expected at any dose of DOX; and the incidence is higher with cumulative dose, specific regimens involving combination chemotherapies, and longer cancer survivorship.

This is especially concerning as the age of newly diagnosed cancer patients is rising. Of all newly diagnosed cancers, 70% will be in patients older than 65 years [27]. Kendal [28] recently assessed the complex interaction between age, comorbidity, and cancer site on the chances of death among more than 780 000 people registered on the Surveillance, Epidemiology and End Results (SEER) database after a cancer diagnosis in the period 1984–1993. The median age at diagnosis was 67 years. Among those with breast cancer who attained an age of 75 years or older during follow-up, the cumulative probability of dying from a comorbid condition far outweighed risk of death from their tumor [28]. Thus, chemotherapy-mediated cardiotoxicity will be more prevalent.

Perhaps the most affected patients are the childhood cancer survivors. In the USA, the 5-year survival rate for childhood cancer is now roughly 80%, a substantial improvement from the 58% documented in the mid-1970s [29]. The relative risk reduction in mortality has been roughly 66%, owing to advances in treatment over the last 40 years [29]. However, long-term morbidity and mortality is still present due to chemotherapies administered for initial oncological disease [30–32]. This longitudinal risk is manifested, after cancer recurrence and secondary malignancies, with cardiovascular-related disease [32,33]. The yearly mortality rate from cardiac causes gradually increases until it exceeds that of recurrence at 30 year [33]. Survivors are eightfold more likely than the general population to die from cardiovascular-related disease [34]. Furthermore, 13% of all excess deaths beyond 45 years of survival have been attributed to cardiac causes [35]. Survivors are also 9 times as likely to have had a cerebrovascular event, 10 times as likely to have coronary heart disease, and 15 times as likely to have heart failure during the first 30 years after cancer diagnosis compared to their siblings without cancer [30]. Although these effects could be result of increased prevalence of the metabolic syndrome, including a high body mass index, obesity, insulin resistance, hypertension, and dyslipidemia, in the childhood leukemia survivors [30,36]. Studies of childhood leukemia survivors have also shown that these increased risks can persist at least up to 45 years after treatment [37].

In an observational hospital-based cohort of 1362 childhood cancer survivors beyond 5 years, van der Pal [38] analyzed the incidence and risk factors for symptomatic cardiac events. There were 50 cardiac events, including 27 cases of CHF in 42 survivors, mean age 27 years. They calculated the 30-year cause-specific cumulative incidence of cardiac events in three groups, such as anthracycline plus irradiation 12.6%, anthracycline alone 7.3%, and irradiation alone 4.0% [38]. In a recent study of over 100 childhood leukemia survivors, almost two-thirds (66.7%) of adult patients were classified as low cardiorespiratory fitness compared with only 26.3% of adult non-cancer participants [39]. By the age of 45 years, the incidence of absolute risk of coronary artery disease, heart failure, valvular disease, and arrhythmia among survivors is 4.4, 4.5, 1.4, and 0.9%, respectively, when compared to their siblings [40]. Thus, the cumulative long-term burden and the lost years due to anthracycline toxicities is a major concern in pediatric population.

RISK FACTORS

As noted previously, the greatest risk factor for anthracycline-induced cardiotoxicity is the cumulative dose. Various studies have corroborated this evidence and now there is clear dose–response relationship of heart failure with anthracycline doses [24,41]. Although it is well established with higher DOX dosing, pathological damage still occurs at low dose though clinical manifestation can take up to three to four decades [24,25,37]. Thus, cumulative anthracycline dose was the most consistently reported as an accurate and robust predictor of cardiotoxicity.

In addition to the cumulative dose, other risk factors have been identified that increase the risk of anthracycline-induced cardiotoxicity, including old age [28], hypertension [21], concomitant treatment with cyclophosphamide [42], trastuzumab [43], and/or paclitaxel [44]. Of particular interest is the interaction between anthracyclines, such as DOX, and trastuzumab, as they form the bases for adjuvant therapy in breast cancer patients.

More recently, other risk factors have been isolated. Exposure to 250 mg/m^2 or more of anthracyclines and radiation dose of more than 1200 cGy to the heart increased the relative hazard of congestive heart failure by two- to sixfold as compared to nonirradiated survivors, thus making a radiation therapy as a risk factor [34]. SEER database analysis also highlighted prior heart disease as a major risk factor [45]. African-American ethnicity, diabetes, very high or very low body weight, or severe comorbidities, are some of the newly identified risk factors [45,46].

The risk factors for cardiotoxicity in children are somewhat different. A higher cumulative dose of anthracycline is still the predominant risk factors, with higher dose of radiation and African-American ethnicity as common risk factors between young and old. However, risk factors, such as younger age at diagnosis [22,47], female sex [48], and trisomy 21 [48] are unique to the pediatric population.

The identification of high-risk patients is important as they should be offered preventive means to reduce the risk of cardiotoxicity or intensive noninvasive monitoring (e.g., tissue Doppler imaging echocardiography, and/or MRI) to enable early recognition of cardiotoxicity and therefore therapeutic adjustments. However, it is also associated with cost as delay in administration of chemotherapy due to cardiotoxicity can have dire consequences on oncological outcomes. This has been especially highlighted in recent meta-analysis which showed that overall survival decreased by 15% for every 4-week delay in initiation of adjuvant chemotherapy. The results are also consistent across disease free survival analysis [49]. Thus, a critical balance hangs in the decision-making process of whether the chemotherapy should be continued in the face of cardiotoxicity or stopped due to potential major adverse cardiovascular events. Therefore, identification of risk factors is key in modulating therapy and providing an effective surveillance.

MOLECULAR MECHANISMS OF DOX MEDIATED CARDIOTOXICITY

Reactive Oxygen Species Production

Enzymatic Reaction

NAD(P)H-oxidoreductases family, including cytochrome P450 enzymes, mitochondrial NADH dehydrogenase [complex I of the electron transport chain (ETC)], and xanthine dehydrogenase, can catalyze the one-electron transfer from NAD(P)H to the quinone moiety to the tetra-cycle ring C of DOX, resulting in the formation of a semiquinone radical [50,51]. Its unpaired electron can be donated to oxygen forming superoxide radicals (O^{2-}), thereby regenerating its parental quinone and reducing molecular oxygen to a superoxide radical (O^{2-}), in a process termed as redox cycling [52]. The dismutation of O^{2-} to hydrogen peroxide (H_2O_2) is catalyzed by superoxide dismutase or may occur spontaneously [50,52]. H_2O_2 is a relatively stable and low-toxicity molecule, and under physiological conditions is eliminated by catalase or glutathione peroxidase. However, H_2O_2 and O^{2-} may generate highly reactive and toxic hydroxyl radicals (OH). This takes place during the Haber–Weiss reaction, catalyzed by transition metals—especially iron [53]. Alternatively, the semiquinone can oxidize and deglycosylate to generate a 7-deoxyaglycone and another O^{2-} [53]. The deoxyaglycone is particularly active, being strongly lipophilic, to penetrate and intercalate with lipids, in particular cardiolipin, of the mitochondrial membranes [1]. It can generate O^{2-} and H_2O_2 through a futile cycle catalyzed by NADH dehydrogenase of the ETC [1].

Initial studies in anthracycline-mediated oxygen radical production looked at the direct concentrations of downstream effector and proved that indeed these chemotherapies produce ROS [54,55]. Later the role of these enzymes in the O^{2-} production and thereby development of DOX cardiomyopathy was based on the evidence murine knock out models, such as Nox2/NAD(P)H oxidase-deficient mice which showed preserved LVEF, stroke volume, and numerous other indices of cardiac contractility compared with the wild-type mice, both treated with DOX (4 mg/kg at 0, 7, and 14 days) [56]. Additionally, the pathological changes associated with DOX, such as cardiomyocyte apoptosis, interstitial fibrosis, and myocardial atrophy were abrogated [56].

Antioxidant interventions in large animals (pig, dogs, etc.) exposed to a chronic DOX regimen have been much less successful than interventions in smaller animals—mostly murine models [1,57]. This was subsequently extended to human studies which were negative, as many findings were contradictory to the outcomes described from acute anthracycline cardiotoxicity models. This includes equivocal findings on cardioprotection between untreated or treated group (such as vitamin E [58,59], N-acetylcysteine [60], and amifostin [61,62]). Berthiaume et al. [58] found suppression of DOX-induced oxidative stress through dietary supplementation of vitamin E, but the treatment had no effect on the cardiac parameters. In addition, although significant protection was conferred by two flavonoid derivatives [63,64] (mono-HER and frederine), further experiments showed that cardioprotective effects were not sustained in longer follow-up. Although vitamin C has been suggested to decrease the mortality rate induced by both acute and subchronic DOX treatment, cardioprotective effects have been evaluated against repeated anthracycline treatment only in a very low DOX cumulative dose (2 mg/kg) [65]. Overall, the pathophysiological implication of this pathway in clinical setting remains elusive.

DOX–Fe Complexes

DOX binds to iron (Fe) both in the ferric (Fe^{3+}) and ferrous (Fe^{2+}) forms, generating DOX:Fe complexes (1:1, 2:1,3:1) [66,67]. In the presence of a reducing system (NADH cytochrome P450 reductase or thiols, such as cysteine or glutathione), the anthracycline-Fe^{3+} complex is reduced to anthracycline-Fe^{2+}, which can react with O_2 to form O^{2-}, which in turn dismutates to H_2O_2 and/or produces OH via Haber–Weiss reaction. In the absence of reducing systems, anthracycline Fe^{3+} can gain an electron by an intramolecular redox reaction, forming a free radical anthracycline—Fe^{2+}; which upon exposure to O_2, yields O^{2-} and anthracycline Fe^{2+} [50]. Alternatively, excess amount of H_2O_2, under physiological conditions, is enzymatically eliminated by the concerted actions of catalase and glutathione peroxidase. Cardiomyocytes possess low levels of catalase, which is less efficient than glutathione peroxidase at low H_2O_2 concentrations [68]. Therefore, cytosolic glutathione peroxidase, due to its low Km for H_2O_2, is preferentially involved in the detoxification of this peroxide. DOX can selectively inhibit the cardiac forms of glutathione peroxidase (both the cytosolic and the mitochondrial isoforms), and thereby resulting in net production of H_2O_2. Furthermore, apart from the ROS, cardiac exposure to anthracyclines may be also connected with the deregulation of the nitric oxide network [69]. Overproduction of ROS and NO yields reactive nitrogen species, particularly the powerful oxidant—peroxynitrite [69].

In the early 1980s, Myers et. al. [70] have shown formation of anthracycline–Fe complexes and resulting oxidative damage of biomembranes in vitro; a damage which was immune to classical ROS scavengers. Later on, augmentation of anthracycline cardiotoxicity by iron has been demonstrated in isolated rat cardiomyocytes, where prior iron loading resulted in marked lactate dehydrogenase release and changes in cell contractility [71] with DOX exposure. Intravenous iron loading resulted in severe weight loss and a twofold increase in the rate of mortality in DOX treated mice [72]. In both studies, the unfavorable effects of iron on DOX cardiotoxicity could be eliminated by the iron chelator deferoxamine.

Panjrath et al. [73] showed a substantial increase in DOX cardiotoxicity by dietary iron loading, concluding that body iron stores as well as iron bioavailability in tissue may be important independent predictors of susceptibility to DOX cardiotoxicity. Similarly, Hfe-deficient mice (a model of human hereditary hemochromatosis, a disorder resulting in body iron overload) exhibited significantly greater sensitivity to DOX-induced cardiotoxicity. Increased mortality after chronic DOX treatment was observed in both Hfe$^{-/-}$ and Hfe$^{+/-}$ mice compared with wild-type animals. DOX-treated Hfe$^{-/-}$ mice had a higher degree of mitochondrial damage and iron deposits in the heart than did the wild-type mice [74].

In the first in vivo studies, Herman et al. [75] have shown that razoxane pretreatment (100 mg/kg) can partially decrease the mortality rate and ameliorate certain signs of acute cardiovascular toxicity induced by sublethal daunorubicin doses (50 and 25 mg/kg) in Syrian golden hamsters [76]. With recognition of clinical importance of chronic anthracycline cardiotoxicity, the interest has been shifted toward the animal models receiving repeated cycles of clinically relevant individual anthracycline doses. With an accumulating body of evidence, it has become firmly established that dexrazoxane (DEX) is able to effectively protect the heart and cardiomyocytes from chronic anthracycline cardiotoxicity in various animal models, including rabbits, dogs, mice, normotensive, and spontaneously hypertensive rats, guinea pigs, and pigs, which was later extended to human subjects [31,77–80]. Initially, the cardioprotective effect of DEX was attributed to its iron chelating properties. ADR-925, a DEX hydrolysis product, can chelate free intracellular iron as well as displace Fe3 + from its complex with DOX; these effects have been long accepted as responsible for cardioprotection [81]. Furthermore, it has been demonstrated that in iron-overload conditions, the anthracycline-induced cardiotoxicity is markedly increased [72]. Taken together, this provided a strong rationale for studies of anthracycline cardiotoxicity prevention with iron chelators. However, other potent iron chelators failed to show a cardioprotective response.

Deferoxamine [also desferrioxamine (DFO)] is a well-established hexadentate-chelating agent long used to remove excess iron from the body. In iron overload, it acts by binding free iron in the bloodstream and enhances its elimination in the urine [82]. Voest et al. [83] showed that at the concentration of 200 μM DFO was the most effective protectant of the six various chelators tested, including

DEX. However, with slight increase of DFO concentration to 500 µM, its protective effects completely disappeared. Herman et al. [84] have reported a failure of DFO to achieve a meaningful cardioprotection and reduction of DOX-induced death. Another iron chelator, deferiprone, is an orally effective α-ketohydroxypyridine iron chelator, effective as a monotherapy or in combination with DFO [82]. In a clinically relevant and DEX-validated model of chronic anthracycline-induced cardiotoxicity in rabbits, deferiprone showed no alleviation in either anthracycline-induced oxidative stress or the LV cardiac damage and CHF, as assessed by both echocardiography and LV catheterization [85]. Deferiprone was administered orally in two doses of 10 and 50 mg/kg, 45 min before each DAU injection (3 mg/kg i.v.), and the higher deferiprone dose (50 mg/kg, well tolerated when administered alone) actually led to earlier animal deaths [86]. Similar results have been published for other iron chelators, such as deferasirox [87], aroylhydrazones (at higher doses) [88,89], and di-2-pyridylketone 4,4-dimethyl-3-thiosemicarbazone (Dp44mT) [90]. In essence, iron chelators were unsuccessful in alleviating anthracycline-mediated cardiotoxicity.

DOX/DNA/Top-II Beta Ternary Complex

It has been well-studied that one of the mechanisms of DOX induced tumor-cytotoxic effect is mediated by topoisomerase II alpha inhibition [91]. Toposiomerase II alpha (Top2A) is an enzyme that regulates the overwinding or underwinding of DNA during DNA repair process [92]. They play an important role in regulating cellular processes, such as replication, transcription, and chromosomal segregation by altering DNA topology [92]. On the other hand, topoisomerase II beta (Top2B) serves the same function in quiescent cells. Since they share catalytic mechanisms and have a high degree of amino acid similarity (~70% identity at the amino acid level) [93]; we embarked on a project to study the role of Top2B in murine cardiac cells treated with DOX. We successfully demonstrated that [94]: (1) in rats, the molecular phenotype of acute and chronic DOX cardiomyopathy is characterized by the formation of a ternary DNA–Top2B–DOX cleavage complex, that triggers double-strand breaks in the DNA; (2) the acute stage is characterized by upregulation of the apoptotic pathway signaling, specifically *Apaf-1, Bax, Mdm-2,* and *Fas*. Under chronic condition, (3) the genes implicated in mitochondrial dysfunction and oxidative phosphorylation were diminished by downregulation of peroxisome proliferator activated receptor gamma, coactivator 1 alpha (*Ppargc-1a*), and beta (*Ppargc-1b*) [94]. This resulted in (4) downregulation of key components of the ETC, such as *Ndufa3, Sdha,* and *Atp5a1,* culminating with (5) ultrastructural mitochondrial damage with vacuolization [94]. The mitochondria were also (6) dysfunctional as measured by oxygen consumption

and changes in mitochondrial membrane potential. The end result was (7) an increase in end systolic and end-diastolic volumes with decrease in ejection fraction (EF) [94]. The formation of the ternary complex is also responsible for the production of most (70%) DOX-induced ROS. Therefore the oxidative stress is preferentially a result of the DOX-induced DNA damage and of the consequent changes in the transcriptome rather than of the redox-cycling of DOX. Transgenic mice with cardiomyocyte-specific deletion of Top2B were indeed protected from the acute and progressive or chronic DOX-induced heart failure, and did not exhibit the severe cardiomyopathic phenotype of the wild-type mice. Therefore, Top2B is required to initiate the entire phenotypic cascade of DOX-induced cardiomyopathy [94]. Other studies also identified the activation of the p53 pathway to DNA-damage and the consequent apoptosis and mitochondrial dysfunction in cultured cardiomyocytes treated with DOX [95,96]. (Fig. 4.1).

Furthermore, it is well known that two genes, PPAR coactivator1-alpha and 1-beta (Ppargc-1a and Ppargc-1b), nuclear genes coding for the transcription coactivators peroxisome proliferator-activated receptor gamma coactivator 1 (PGC-1)alpha and PGC-1beta, respectively, are expressed in the heart as essential coactivators in the activity of PPAR gamma, nuclear respiratory factor-1, and estrogen-related receptor alpha [97,98]. PGC-1alpha and PGC-1beta are master regulators of mitochondrial biogenesis, including genes controlling mtDNA replication, the expression of oxidative phosphorylation enzymes (OXPHOS) and the β oxidation of fatty acids, and are therefore essential regulators of the ATP production [97,98]. These two genes were downregulated by 50% in rat and mouse hearts treated with DOX (25 mg/kg for 72 h) [94], whereas, after a single injection of DOX (15 mg/kg), the expression of PGC-1alpha, as well as the myocardial levels of its mRNA were severely decreased [99]. Therefore, DOX interferes with the expression of nuclear-encoded mitochondrial genes and causes defective mitochondrial DNA replication, DNA depletion, decreased ETC/OXPHOS function and increased mitochondrial protein oxidation, and apoptosis prior to left ventricular dilation and decreased EF. These findings, according to some authors, are in line with the oxidative hypothesis of DOX cardiotoxicity [94,99].

The corroborating evidence of topoisomerase II beta mechanism is provided by the use of DEX. In vivo DEX has shown significant protection against DOX-induced cardiotoxicity in numerous preclinical models, such as mouse, rat, hamster, rabbit, and dog [61,77,100,101]. In addition, the cardioprotective effects were evident in both acute and chronic models of DOX-induced cardiomyopathy [90,102]. These findings were extended to human subjects in various clinical trials also [31,77–80]. It appears that DEX can block ATP hydrolysis and inhibit the reopening of the ATPase domain, thereby trapping the topoisomerase

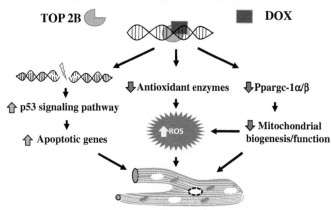

Myofibrillar disarray and vacuolization

FIGURE 4.1 **Schematic representation of DOX/DNA/ Top II beta ternary complex.** Activation of the ternary complex results in activation of three primary signaling pathways. DNA double-stranded break increases p53 signaling resulting in increased apoptotic gene expression. Furthermore, there is increased production of reactive oxygen species (*ROS*) via decreased superoxide dismutase (SOD) and other antioxidant enzymes resulting in ultrastructural damage. Additionally, there is a downregulation of peroxisome-proliferation-activated receptor gamma coactivator-1 alpha and beta (*Ppargc-1 α/β*) which results in mitochondrial biogenesis and dysfunction. Cumulatively, these pathways culminate into myofibrillar disarray and vacuolization. Please note red mitochondria denotes mitochondrial dysfunction and damage.

complex on DNA and blocking enzyme turnover [103], which may be its predominant mechanism. Therefore, making the topoisomerase II beta catalytic site unavailable for DOX activity thereby providing cardioprotection. Although DEX also has been regarded as a potent iron chelator, other compounds in the same family with same chelation properties have failed to provide any degree of cardioprotection, as mentioned previously. In addition, a recent study looking at DEX effects also provides proof that DEX amelioration of anthracycline-mediated cardiotoxicity is primarily through its actions on topoisomerase II beta [104]. In the end the cardioprotection conferred by DEX is due to its unique effect on topoisomerase II beta. Thus, topoisomerase provides a unifying mechanism of DOX mediated cardiotoxicity.

STRATEGIES TO LIMIT ANTHRACYCLINE TOXICITIES

Opting Out of Using Anthracyclines for Chemotherapy

Anthracycline forms an integral part of many chemotherapy regimens and therefore, they have been used in various hematological and solid tumor malignancies. Studies have been done to substitute anthracyclines with other chemotherapeutic combinations, however, the results have been less successful.

One of the largest, single randomized trials comparing anthracycline-based chemotherapy with cyclophosphamide, methotrexate, fluorouracil (CMF; where fluorouracil is 5-FU) was the Southwest Oncology Group (SWOG)/Intergroup trial (INT 0102) [105]. In this study, 4400 women with node-negative breast cancer were stratified into high- or low-risk groups according to tumor size (≥2 cm as high risk) or hormone-receptor-negative (high risk). The object of the study was to determine whether the cyclophosphamide, DOX (Adriamycin), 5-FU (CAF) is superior to CMF. All high-risk women were randomized to receive CAF or

classical oral CMF chemotherapy for six cycles, with or without tamoxifen for 5 years; low-risk patients did not receive adjuvant treatment. Recurrence rates were 15% in the CAF group and 18% in the CMF arm (13% and 15%, respectively, with the addition of tamoxifen). Estimated 5-year overall survival in CAF-treated patients was 92%, compared with 90% in the CMF group. The investigators concluded that CAF is slightly superior to CMF, with the risk of increased but manageable acute toxicity [105].

The National Cancer Institute of Canada (NCIC) MA.5 trial randomized 710 premenopausal women with node-positive breast cancer to receive oral CMF or CEF (cyclophosphamide, 75 mg/m² orally on days 1–14; epirubicin, 60 mg/m² IV on days 1 and 8; and 5-FU, 500 mg/m² IV on days 1 and 8) for six cycles or oral CMF (cyclophosphamide, 100 mg/m² orally on days 1–14; methotrexate, 40 mg/m² IV on days 1 and 8; and 5-FU, 600 mg/m² IV on days 1 and 8 [106]. The NCIC MA.5 trial reported a significantly better 5-year disease-free survival of 63% in the CEF group versus 53% in the CMF group (relative risk reduction = 29%). Overall survival at 5 years in the CEF group was 77%, compared to 70% with CMF (relative risk reduction = 19%) [106]. An update of this trial showed that patients who received CEF adjuvant chemotherapy continued to have an improved survival at 10-year follow-up with a 10-year disease-free survival rate of 52% for patients who received CEF compared to 45% for CMF patients, and the 10-year overall survival was 62% and 58% for CEF and CMF patients, respectively [107]. Overall, anthracycline-based therapy proved to be more beneficial over the short-term and long-term disease for survival rate and overall mortality. Addition of anthracycline therapy to the existing CMF regimen in a European trial showed epirubicin (ECMF) curbs mortality, as a significantly higher number of deaths on treatment were noted in the CMF group compared to the ECMF group (13 vs. 4 patients). The relapse-free survival rate was significantly better in the ECMF group—83% versus 77%—with a 31% reduction in recurrence. Overall survival was also significantly better in the ECMF group compared to the CMF group (88% vs. 82.7%). In summary, sequential ECMF significantly prolongs relapse-free survival and overall survival compared to CMF adjuvant chemotherapy. [108] A more recent study demonstrated that capecitabine, considered a less aggressive regimen, leads to almost twice the rate of disease recurrence and death when compared with standard chemotherapy with either CMF or cyclophosphamide plus DOX in women aged 65 years and older with early breast cancer [109].

Thus, anthracycline-containing combination chemotherapy reduces cumulative 10-year breast cancer mortality by an absolute 4.6% when compared with nonanthracycline-based regimens [110] and therefore is a conventional part of chemotherapy regimen in breast cancer. Similar results have been found in other hematological and solid organ malignancies [111]. However, anthracycline does not form the basis of numerous cancer regimens (such as chronic myelogenous leukemia, renal cell carcinoma, etc.), due to tumor resistance and toxicity; therefore, more studies are warranted to identify suitable alternatives to anthracycline in individual oncological diseases.

Substituting DOX With Other Anthracycline

Over the past five decades, more than 2000 modified anthracycline chemical structures have been synthesized and tested. The main effort was to reduce cardiotoxicity while retaining their unique cytostatic/cytotoxic effectiveness. Although several anthracycline derivatives have been evaluated in clinical trials, only epirubicin [108] and idarubicin [112] received approval for clinical use. Unfortunately, clinical trials have not confirmed lower cardiotoxicity of idarubicin as compared to DOX [112]. Similar results have been found with epirubicin also.

40-Epidoxorubicin, or epirubicin, is an analog of DOX with equivalent efficacy and less cardiotoxicity on a milligram to milligram comparison [113–115]. In a prospective randomized comparison of DOX and epirubicinin patients with breast cancer, epirubicin was associated with a longer median duration of response at 11.9 months compared to 7.1 months with DOX [116]. The cumulative doses at which CHF occurred was $1134 \, mg/m^2$ with epirubicin compared to $492 \, mg/m^2$ with DOX [116]. In a meta-analysis of 13 studies comparing DOX with epirubicin, the majority of which included women with advanced or metastatic breast cancer, epirubicin was associated with a significantly decreased risk of clinical cardiotoxicity, subclinical cardiotoxicity, and any cardiac event compared to DOX [117]. Epirubicin-induced cardiotoxicity is also dose- dependent, and the Food and Drug Administration recommends a maximum cumulative dose of $900 \, mg/m^2$ [118]. However, in an analysis of 1097 patients, the safe maximum cumulative dosage was found to be lower when risk factors, such as age, radiation, and underlying cardiac risk factors were taken into consideration [119]. In addition a critical analysis by Cochrane Database has identified no difference in cardiotoxicity between epirubicin and DOX at equipotent doses [120].

In the Nordic Group's randomized trial, 455 untreated patients with aggressive non-Hodgkin's lymphoma (NHL) aged 60–86 years were randomized to CHOP or a similar regimen in which the $50 \, g/m^2$ DOX was replaced by $10 \, mg/m^2$ mitoxantrone (CNOP) [121]. CHOP was significantly superior to CNOP in time to treatment failure and overall survival. The similar study conducted earlier by Sonneveld et al. [122] found that randomization to CNOP resulted in a poorer outcome than with CHOP chemotherapy (at 3 years, 42% of CHOP and 26% of CNOP patients were alive). In a randomized study to test a regimen devised specifically for use in elderly patients (70 years and older) with intermediate- and high-grade NHL, VP-16 plus mitoxantrone and prednimustine achieved significantly poorer progression free and overall survival than CHOP [123]. Therefore, CHOP is still considered the gold standard of treatment. Numerous other trials have reached a similar conclusion where DOX fared better than a less toxic replacement drug [120,124].

Continuous Infusion

Replacing bolus administration with slow infusions does not significantly affect anthracycline area under the curve (AUC) but diminishes anthracycline peak level and anthracycline accumulation in the heart [1]. As such, various trials were carried out with anthracycline infusion. Recently, a Cochrane review was published which looked at the current available data in this field [125]. They identified seven RCTs addressing different anthracycline infusion durations. The meta-analysis showed a statistically significant lower rate of clinical heart failure with an infusion duration of 6 h or longer as compared to a shorter infusion duration (relative risk (RR) = 0.27; 95% confidence interval (CI) 0.09–0.81; 5 studies; 557 patients) in adult solid tumor population. As far as the peak DOX dose was concerned, two RCTs addressing less than 60 mg/m(2) versus 60 mg/m(2) or more, one RCT addressing a liposomal DOX peak dose of 25 mg/m(2) versus 50 mg/m(2) and one RCT addressing an epirubicin peak dose of 83 mg/m(2) versus 110 mg/m(2) [125]. In none of the studies a significant difference in the occurrence of clinical heart failure was identified. Thus, anthracycline infusion duration of 6 h or longer reduces the risk of clinical heart failure and subclinical cardiac damage to some extent [125]. However, the review was only performed in an adult population with solid tumors.

In the pediatric population, the results of infusion of anthracycline have been disappointing. A randomized trial in children with high-risk ALL found that continuous infusion offered no additional cardiac protection over bolus administration in a median follow-up of 8 years postdiagnosis [126]. A follow-up at 10 years also revealed no incremental therapeutic efficacy with infusion [127]. This is further supported by other studies that also looked at cardiovascular outcomes in patients after 5–7 years of treatment [128,129]. However, despite a lack of evidence for cardioprotection, anthracycline administration by continuous infusion is still incorporated into pediatric treatment protocols for cardioprotection [127].

PEGylated Liposomal DOX

PEGylated liposomal DOX comprises an aqueous core of DOX hydrochloride encapsulated in liposomes with a protective hydrophilic outer coating of surface-bound methoxypolyethylene glycol [130,131]. Delivery of DOX in a PEGylated liposomal form decreases the circulating concentrations of free DOX and results in selective uptake of the agent in tumor cells.

In preclinical studies, PEGylated liposomal DOX demonstrated antitumor activity in several animal models of colon, breast, ovarian, lung, and other types of cancer, markedly inhibiting tumor growth rates and improving survival rate [132]. Furthermore, in a mouse mammary carcinoma (MC2) model, PEGylated liposomal DOX displayed efficacy against both high- and low-growth fraction tumor variants, MC2A and MC2B [133]. Thus, PEGylated liposomal DOX proved to be effective in animal studies [132]. In addition, in three randomized [134–136], open-label, multicenter trials, monotherapy with PEGylated liposomal DOX was as effective as DOX or capecitabine in the first-line treatment of metastatic breast cancer, and as effective as vinorelbine or combination mitomycin plus vinblastine in taxane-refractory metastatic breast cancer. PEGylated liposomal DOX alone was as effective as topotecan or gemcitabine alone in patients with progressive ovarian cancer resistant or refractory to platinum- or paclitaxel-based therapy, as per three randomized multicenter trials [137–139].

Although effective antitumor activity led to the development and sustainability of PEGylated liposomal DOX, the reduced cardiotoxic effect also provides benefit. The risk of symptomatic cardiotoxicity with PEGylated liposomal DOX appears low. In several studies there was no evidence of symptomatic cardiotoxicity when PEGylated liposomal DOX was administered as monotherapy or as part of combination therapy, irrespective of patients' prior exposure to anthracyclines, including high cumulative doses [134,140,141]. In the pivotal trial in patients with metastatic breast cancer, PEGylated liposomal DOX 50 mg/m^2 every 4 weeks was associated with a significantly ($p < 0.001$) lower risk of LVEF-defined cardiotoxicity than DOX 60 mg/m^2 every 3 weeks (HR 3.16; 95% CI 1.58, 6.31); this effect

was observed irrespective of cardiovascular risk factors, including age greater than 65 years and prior anthracycline exposure [134]. Ten of 254 recipients of PEGylated liposomal DOX (median cumulative anthracycline dose 293 mg/m^2) developed LVEF-defined cardiotoxicity compared with 48 of 255 recipients of conventional DOX (median cumulative anthracycline dose 361 mg/m^2). Of the patients that experienced cardiotoxicity, none in the PEGylated liposomal DOX group and 10 in the DOX group developed signs or symptoms of congestive heart failure [134]. Furthermore, high cumulative doses of PEGylated liposomal DOX were associated with a low risk of clinically significant cardiac dysfunction in patients with malignancies [140,141]. In a pooled analysis of patients with solid tumors ($n = 418$), the incidence of clinically significant cardiac dysfunction was low in PEGylated liposomal DOX 50 mg/m^2 recipients (lifetime cumulative anthracycline doses up to 1532 mg/m^2) [142]. Thirteen (15%) of 88 patients who received a cumulative anthracycline dose of more than 400 mg/m^2 had at least one clinically significant change in LVEF; however, only one patient discontinued treatment because of clinical symptoms of congestive heart failure. In a subset of eight patients who received cumulative anthracycline doses of 509–1680 mg/m^2, endomyocardial biopsies demonstrated mild or no cardiotoxicity (Billingham cardiotoxicity scores of grades 0–1.5) [142].

PEGylated liposomal DOX exhibited a relatively favorable cardiac safety profile compared with conventional DOX and other available chemotherapy agents. The most common treatment-related adverse events included myelosuppression, palmar–plantar erythrodysesthesia, and stomatitis, although these are manageable with appropriate supportive measures [142]. Thus, PEGylated liposomal DOX is a useful option in the treatment of various malignancies, including metastatic breast cancer, ovarian cancer, multiple myeloma, and AIDS-related Kaposi's sarcoma [143]. However, the cost associated with administering the drug has prevented its widespread adoption as conventional anthracycline therapy [144].

Dexrazoxane

DEX (ICRF-187, ADR-529) and the corresponding racemic mixture—razoxane (ICRF-159, ADR-159)—belong to bisdioxopiperazine agents originally developed by Creighton et al. [145] as potential anticancer agents. The authors aimed to find cell-permeable EDTA prodrugs that could target biometals of vital importance within the cancer cells [145]. However, anticancer effects of DEX and razoxane have been later attributed to TOP2 inhibition [146,147]. Razoxane has passed through extensive preclinical development as an anticancer drug. DEX and other bisdioxiopiperazines (ICRF- 159, ICRF-193, and IRCF-194) have shown cytotoxicity in leukemic cells and cause DNA damage and apoptosis in various hematological cell lines at clinically achievable (4–5 μM) concentrations [81,145]. DEX has some clinical anticancer activity as a single agent. Work reviewed by Kovacevic et al. [148] has shown that DEX can induce DNA double-strand breaks as measured by the formation of the phosphorylated forms of the histone H2AX [termed serine 139 phosphorylated histone H2A (c-H2AX)] in cancer cells. Although it was being developed as anticancer agent, using H9c2 myoblasts and fibroblasts from TOP2b knockout mice, Lyu et al. [149] have suggested that the parent compound DEX may be protective through inhibition of anthracycline-induced and TOP2b-mediated DNA damage, thus opening a window of DEX as a protective agent in anthracycline induced cardiotoxicity.

More evidence of support emerged when DEX was shown to be cardioprotective in DOX treated population. Cardioprotective effects of DEX against anthracycline-induced cardiotoxicity have been unanimously demonstrated in numerous clinical trials and in both adults and children [79,80,150–153]. Importantly, significant cardioprotection has been achieved in various chemotherapy regimens, using different DEX-to-anthracycline ratios and different types of anthracyclines in clinical use. Cardioprotective potential of DEX has been evaluated by clinical examination (incidence of cardiac events and symptoms of CHF), using cardiac function examinations (echocardiography or radionuclide ventriculography), by analysis of biochemical markers (e.g., plasma concentrations of cardiac troponins), and/or endomyocardial biopsy. Today, DEX has passed all the stages of preclinical and clinical research and has been finally approved in Europe and the United States for cardioprotection in patients treated with anthracyclines (Cardioxane and Zinecard) with several generic preparations recently available (Procard and Cardynax). More recently, DEX has also been approved for treatment of accidental extravasation of anthracyclines (Savene). Thus, dexrazoxane's role as protective agent against anthracycline induced cardiotoxicity has been firmly established.

Concern for potential interference of DEX with anticancer effects of anthracycline has arisen from one phase-III trial [80], in which a significant difference in objective response was reported (47% vs. 61%, respectively, $n = 293$, $p = 0.019$). Although high response in the placebo group was quite unusual, and no other endpoints (including survival or time to progression) were affected in either of these studies, DEX was suspected for negative effect on tumor response [80]. This study has been extensively analyzed with a conclusion that DEX cannot be blamed for reduction in tumor response [154]. No significant effect on any oncological parameter has been found ever since, and most importantly, careful metaanalyses of all randomized clinical trials have found no evidence for this hypothesis [155,156]. However, the outcome of this study was reflected in recommendations for DEX use given by various oncological societies.

The American Society of Clinical Oncology, Chemotherapy, and Radiotherapy Expert Panel maintained caution and recommended using DEX only in very limited conditions (e.g., patients who have received more than 300 mg/m^2 for metastatic breast cancer and who may benefit from continued DOX treatment) [157]. Since this was an isolated study and overwhelming evidence exists against this assertion, the time has come to revisit this cautionary note.

Another controversial issue about DEX pertains to an increased risk of second malignancies. This was observed in survivors of Hodgkin lymphoma who had received DOX in combination with etoposide. By having considered that both DOX and etoposide as well as DEX inhibited topoisomerase IIα, albeit by different mechanisms and with different efficacies, it was postulated that combining the three drugs could exceed a threshold above which topoisomerase inhibitors caused genetic instability in normal tissues [158]. This report led the European Medicine Agency to conclude that DEX should not be used in children due to the risk of second malignancies. Two studies of survivors of childhood acute lymphoblastic leukemia reached the opposite conclusion and did not detect an increased risk of second malignancies from DEX [159,160]. Thus, risk:benefit analysis supports a wider clinical usage of DEX with the possible exception of conditions in which patients received etoposide or etoposide-anthracycline combinations. In essence, cautionary considerations should be limited to select groups. Despite these isolated studies, DEX is a bona fide cardioprotective agent against anthracycline-induced toxicity and as such should be used as a part of most anthracycline-based chemotherapy regimens.

CONCLUSIONS

Anthracycline is heralded as an old drug with unwavering antitumor efficacy. Its application has been widespread and forms an integral part of the therapeutic armamentarium. However, widespread use has been accompanied by its cardiotoxicity. Understanding and delineating the mechanism is the first step in ameliorating the side effects of anthracyclines, and therefore we should be vigorous in our pursuit. Although the mechanisms are becoming apparent, present use of various strategies to limit cardiotoxic effects are clearly warranted to prevent cardiopathological squeal. The risk:benefit ratio of various strategies and/or medications to abrogate cardiotoxicity have to be critically analyzed to ensure that recommendations follow a sound empirical burden of data, especially in the context of dexrazoane. This is very important especially in pediatric population as well as in adults who are increasing in number from cancer survivorship as combating cancer should not expose them to increased cardiovascular risk and/or events. In the end, more research is warranted to address this issue.

REFERENCES

[1] Minotti G, Menna P, Salvatorelli E, Cairo G, Gianni L. Anthracyclines: molecular advances and pharmacologic developments in antitumor activity and cardiotoxicity. Pharmacol Rev 2004; 56:185–229.

[2] Ewer MS, Ewer SM. Cardiotoxicity of anticancer treatments: what the cardiologist needs to know. Nat Rev Cardiol 2010;7:564–75.

[3] Eschenhagen T, Force T, Ewer MS, et al. Cardiovascular side effects of cancer therapies: a position statement from the Heart Failure Association of the European Society of Cardiology. Eur J Heart Fail 2011;13:1–10.

[4] Yeh ET, Bickford CL. Cardiovascular complications of cancer therapy: incidence, pathogenesis, diagnosis, and management. J Am Coll Cardiol 2009;53:2231–47.

[5] Slordal L, Spigset O. Heart failure induced by non-cardiac drugs. Drug Saf 2006;29:567–86.

[6] Bristow MR, Thompson PD, Martin RP, Mason JW, Billingham ME, Harrison DC. Early anthracycline cardiotoxicity. Am J Med 1978;65:823–32.

[7] Dazzi H, Kaufmann K, Follath F. Anthracycline-induced acute cardiotoxicity in adults treated for leukaemia. Analysis of the clinicopathological aspects of documented acute anthracycline-induced cardiotoxicity in patients treated for acute leukaemia at the University Hospital of Zurich, Switzerland, between 1990 and 1996. Ann Oncol 2001;12:963–6.

[8] Hayek ER, Speakman E, Rehmus E. Acute doxorubicin cardiotoxicity. N Engl J Med 2005;352:2456–7.

[9] Bristow MR, Mason JW, Billingham ME, Daniels JR. Doxorubicin cardiomyopathy: evaluation by phonocardiography, endomyocardial biopsy, and cardiac catheterization. Ann Intern Med 1978;88:168–75.

[10] Lenihan DJ. Progression of heart failure from AHA/ACC stage A to stage B or even C: can we all agree we should try to prevent this from happening? J Am Coll Cardiol 2012;60:2513–4.

[11] Di MA, Cassinelli G, Arcamone F. The discovery of daunorubicin. Cancer Treat Rep 1981;65(Suppl. 4):3–8.

[12] Tan C, Tasaka H, Yu KP, Murphy ML, Karnofsky DA. Daunomycin, an antitumor antibiotic, in the treatment of neoplastic disease. Clinical evaluation with special reference to childhood leukemia. Cancer 1967;20:333–53.

[13] Arcamone F, Cassinelli G, Fantini G, et al. Adriamycin, 14- hydroxydaunomycin, a new antitumor antibiotic from *S. peucetius* var. caesius. Biotechnol Bioeng 1969;11:1101–10.

[14] Di MA, Gaetani M, Scarpinato B. Adriamycin (NSC-123,127): a new antibiotic with antitumor activity. Cancer Chemother Rep 1969;53:33–7.

[15] Bonfante V, Bonadonna G, Villani F, Martini A. Preliminary clinical experience with 4-epidoxorubicin in advanced human neoplasia. Recent Results Cancer Res 1980;74:192–9.

[16] Bonfante V, Ferrari L, Villani F, Bonadonna G. Phase I study of 4-demethoxydaunorubicin. Invest New Drugs 1983;1:161–8.

[17] Vecchi A, Spreafico F, Sironi M, Cairo M, Garattini S. The immunodepressive and hematotoxic activities of *N*-trifluoro-acetyladriamycin-14-valerate. Eur J Cancer 1980;16:1289–96.

[18] Greenberg RE, Bahnson RR, Wood D, et al. Initial report on intravesical administration of *N*-trifluoroacetyladriamycin-14-valerate (AD 32) to patients with refractory superficial transitional cell carcinoma of the urinary bladder. Urology 1997;49:471–5.

[19] Powles TJ. Evolving clinical strategies: innovative approaches to the use of mitoxantrone—introduction. Eur J Cancer Care (Engl) 1997;6:1–3.

[20] Lefrak EA, Pitha J, Rosenheim S, Gottlieb JA. A clinicopathologic analysis of adriamycin cardiotoxicity. Cancer 1973;32:302–14.

[21] Von Hoff DD, Layard MW, Basa P, et al. Risk factors for doxorubicin-induced congestive heart failure. Ann Intern Med 1979;91: 710–7.

[22] Swain SM, Whaley FS, Ewer MS. Congestive heart failure in patients treated with doxorubicin: a retrospective analysis of three trials. Cancer 2003;97:2869–79.

[23] Vandecruys E, Mondelaers V, De Wolf D, Benoit Y, Suys B. Late cardiotoxicity after low dose of anthracycline therapy for acute lymphoblastic leukemia in childhood. J Cancer Surviv 2012;6: 95–101.

[24] Nysom K, Holm K, Lipsitz SR, et al. Relationship between cumulative anthracycline dose and late cardiotoxicity in childhood acute lymphoblastic leukemia. J Clin Oncol 1998;16:545–50.

[25] van der Pal HJ, van Dalen EC, Hauptmann M, et al. Cardiac function in 5-year survivors of childhood cancer: a long-term follow-up study. Arch Intern Med 2010;170:1247–55.

[26] Chapman JA, Meng D, Shepherd L, et al. Competing causes of death from a randomized trial of extended adjuvant endocrine therapy for breast cancer. J Natl Cancer Inst 2008;100:252–60.

[27] Balducci L, Extermann M. Cancer and aging. An evolving panorama. Hematol Oncol Clin North Am 2000;14:1–16.

[28] Kendal WS. Dying with cancer: the influence of age, comorbidity, and cancer site. Cancer 2008;112:1354–62.

[29] American Cancer Society. Facts and Figures 2015; 2015.

[30] Oeffinger KC, Mertens AC, Sklar CA, et al. Chronic health conditions in adult survivors of childhood cancer. N Engl J Med 2006;355:1572–82.

[31] Lipshultz SE, Colan SD, Gelber RD, Perez-Atayde AR, Sallan SE, Sanders SP. Late cardiac effects of doxorubicin therapy for acute lymphoblastic leukemia in childhood. N Engl J Med 1991;324: 808–15.

[32] Tukenova M, Guibout C, Oberlin O, et al. Role of cancer treatment in long-term overall and cardiovascular mortality after childhood cancer. J Clin Oncol 2010;28:1308–15.

[33] Mertens AC, Liu Q, Neglia JP, et al. Cause-specific late mortality among 5-year survivors of childhood cancer: the Childhood Cancer Survivor Study. J Natl Cancer Inst 2008;100:1368–79.

[34] Mulrooney DA, Yeazel MW, Kawashima T, et al. Cardiac outcomes in a cohort of adult survivors of childhood and adolescent cancer: retrospective analysis of the Childhood Cancer Survivor Study cohort. BMJ 2009;339. b4606.

[35] Reulen RC, Winter DL, Frobisher C, et al. Long-term cause-specific mortality among survivors of childhood cancer. JAMA 2010;304:172–9.

[36] Gurney JG, Ness KK, Sibley SD, et al. Metabolic syndrome and growth hormone deficiency in adult survivors of childhood acute lymphoblastic leukemia. Cancer 2006;107:1303–12.

[37] Moller TR, Garwicz S, Barlow L, et al. Decreasing late mortality among five-year survivors of cancer in childhood and adolescence: a population-based study in the Nordic countries. J Clin Oncol 2001;19:3173–81.

[38] van der Pal HJ, van Dalen EC, van Delden E, et al. High risk of symptomatic cardiac events in childhood cancer survivors. J Clin Oncol 2012;30:1429–37.

[39] Tonorezos ES, Snell PG, Moskowitz CS, et al. Reduced cardiorespiratory fitness in adult survivors of childhood acute lymphoblastic leukemia. Pediatr Blood Cancer 2013;60:1358–64.

[40] Armstrong GT, Oeffinger KC, Chen Y, et al. Modifiable risk factors and major cardiac events among adult survivors of childhood cancer. J Clin Oncol 2013;31:3673–80.

[41] Lipshultz SE, Adams MJ. Cardiotoxicity after childhood cancer: beginning with the end in mind. J Clin Oncol 2010;28:1276–81.

[42] Gottdiener JS, Appelbaum FR, Ferrans VJ, Deisseroth A, Ziegler J. Cardiotoxicity associated with high-dose cyclophosphamide therapy. Arch Intern Med 1981;141:758–63.

[43] Seidman A, Hudis C, Pierri MK, et al. Cardiac dysfunction in the trastuzumab clinical trials experience. J Clin Oncol 2002;20:1215–21.

[44] Gianni L, Munzone E, Capri G, et al. Paclitaxel by 3-hour infusion in combination with bolus doxorubicin in women with untreated metastatic breast cancer: high antitumor efficacy and cardiac effects in a dose-finding and sequence-finding study. J Clin Oncol 1995;13:2688–99.

[45] Pinder MC, Duan Z, Goodwin JS, Hortobagyi GN, Giordano SH. Congestive heart failure in older women treated with adjuvant anthracycline chemotherapy for breast cancer. J Clin Oncol 2007;25:3808–15.

[46] Lotrionte M, Biondi-Zoccai G, Abbate A, et al. Review and meta-analysis of incidence and clinical predictors of anthracycline cardiotoxicity. Am J Cardiol 2013;112:1980–4.

[47] Lipshultz SE, Lipsitz SR, Sallan SE, et al. Chronic progressive cardiac dysfunction years after doxorubicin therapy for childhood acute lymphoblastic leukemia. J Clin Oncol 2005;23:2629–36.

[48] Krischer JP, Epstein S, Cuthbertson DD, Goorin AM, Epstein ML, Lipshultz SE. Clinical cardiotoxicity following anthracycline treatment for childhood cancer: the Pediatric Oncology Group experience. J Clin Oncol 1997;15:1544–52.

[49] Yu KD, Huang S, Zhang JX, Liu GY, Shao ZM. Association between delayed initiation of adjuvant CMF or anthracycline-based chemotherapy and survival in breast cancer: a systematic review and meta-analysis. BMC Cancer 2013;13:240.

[50] Simunek T, Sterba M, Popelova O, Adamcova M, Hrdina R, Gersl V. Anthracycline-induced cardiotoxicity: overview of studies examining the roles of oxidative stress and free cellular iron. Pharmacol Rep 2009;61:154–71.

[51] Muller I, Niethammer D, Bruchelt G. Anthracycline-derived chemotherapeutics in apoptosis and free radical cytotoxicity (Review). Int J Mol Med 1998;1:491–4.

[52] Chen S, Deng PS, Bailey JM, Swiderek KM. A two-domain structure for the two subunits of NAD(P)H:quinone acceptor oxidoreductase. Protein Sci 1994;3:51–7.

[53] Sterba M, Popelova O, Vavrova A, et al. Oxidative stress, redox signaling, and metal chelation in anthracycline cardiotoxicity and pharmacological cardioprotection. Antioxid Redox Signal 2013;18:899–929.

[54] Davies KJ, Doroshow JH, Hochstein P. Mitochondrial NADH dehydrogenase-catalyzed oxygen radical production by adriamycin, and the relative inactivity of 5-iminodaunorubicin. FEBS Lett 1983;153:227–30.

[55] Doroshow JH, Davies KJ. Comparative cardiac oxygen radical metabolism by anthracycline antibiotics, mitoxantrone, bisantrene, 4'-(9-acridinylamino)-methanesulfon-m-anisidide, and neocarzinostatin. Biochem Pharmacol 1983;32:2935–9.

[56] Zhao Y, McLaughlin D, Robinson E, et al. Nox2 NADPH oxidase promotes pathologic cardiac remodeling associated with Doxorubicin chemotherapy. Cancer Res 2010;70:9287–97.

[57] Menna P, Paz OG, Chello M, Covino E, Salvatorelli E, Minotti G. Anthracycline cardiotoxicity. Expert Opin Drug Saf 2012;11:S21–36.

[58] Berthiaume JM, Oliveira PJ, Fariss MW, Wallace KB. Dietary vitamin E decreases doxorubicin-induced oxidative stress without preventing mitochondrial dysfunction. Cardiovasc Toxicol 2005;5:257–67.

[59] Breed JG, Zimmerman AN, Dormans JA, Pinedo HM. Failure of the antioxidant vitamin E to protect against adriamycin-induced cardiotoxicity in the rabbit. Cancer Res 1980;40:2033–8.

[60] Herman EH, Ferrans VJ, Myers CE, Van Vleet JF. Comparison of the effectiveness of (+/-)-1,2-bis(3,5-dioxopiperazinyl-1-yl)propane (ICRF-187) and N-acetylcysteine in preventing chronic doxorubicin cardiotoxicity in beagles. Cancer Res 1985;45:276–2781.

[61] Herman EH, Zhang J, Chadwick DP, Ferrans VJ. Comparison of the protective effects of amifostine and dexrazoxane against the toxicity of doxorubicin in spontaneously hypertensive rats. Cancer Chemother Pharmacol 2000;45:329–34.

[62] Rigatos SK, Stathopoulos GP, Dontas I, et al. Investigation of doxorubicin tissue toxicity: does amifostine provide chemoprotection? An experimental study. Anticancer Res 2002;22:129–34.

[63] van Acker FA, Boven E, Kramer K, Haenen GR, Bast A, van der Vijgh WJ. Frederine, a new and promising protector against doxorubicin-induced cardiotoxicity. Clin Cancer Res 2001;7:1378–13784.

[64] van Acker SA, Kramer K, Grimbergen JA, van den Berg DJ, van der Vijgh WJ, Bast A. Monohydroxyethylrutoside as protector against chronic doxorubicin-induced cardiotoxicity. Br J Pharmacol 1995;115:1260–4.

[65] Fujita K, Shinpo K, Yamada K, et al. Reduction of adriamycin toxicity by ascorbate in mice and guinea pigs. Cancer Res 1982;42:309–16.

[66] Olson RD, Mushlin PS. Doxorubicin cardiotoxicity: analysis of prevailing hypotheses. FASEB J 1990;4:3076–86.

[67] Xu X, Persson HL, Richardson DR. Molecular pharmacology of the interaction of anthracyclines with iron. Mol Pharmacol 2005;68:261–71.

[68] Kalyanaraman B, Joseph J, Kalivendi S, Wang S, Konorev E, Kotamraju S. Doxorubicin-induced apoptosis: implications in cardiotoxicity. Mol Cell Biochem 2002;234-235:119–24.

[69] Fogli S, Nieri P, Breschi MC. The role of nitric oxide in anthracycline toxicity and prospects for pharmacologic prevention of cardiac damage. FASEB J 2004;18:664–75.

[70] Myers CE, Gianni L, Simone CB, Klecker R, Greene R. Oxidative destruction of erythrocyte ghost membranes catalyzed by the doxorubicin-iron complex. Biochemistry 1982;21:1707–12.

[71] Hershko C, Link G, Tzahor M, et al. Anthracycline toxicity is potentiated by iron and inhibited by deferoxamine: studies in rat heart cells in culture. J Lab Clin Med 1993;122:245–51.

[72] Link G, Tirosh R, Pinson A, Hershko C. Role of iron in the potentiation of anthracycline cardiotoxicity: identification of heart cell mitochondria as a major site of iron-anthracycline interaction. J Lab Clin Med 1996;127:272–8.

[73] Panjrath GS, Patel V, Valdiviezo CI, Narula N, Narula J, Jain D. Potentiation of Doxorubicin cardiotoxicity by iron loading in a rodent model. J Am Coll Cardiol 2007;49:2457–64.

[74] Miranda CJ, Makui H, Soares RJ, et al. Hfe deficiency increases susceptibility to cardiotoxicity and exacerbates changes in iron metabolism induced by doxorubicin. Blood 2003;102:2574–80.

[75] Herman E, Ardalan B, Bier C, Waravdekar V, Krop S. Reduction of daunorubicin lethality and myocardial cellular alterations by pretreatment with ICRF-187 in Syrian golden hamsters. Cancer Treat Rep 1979;63:89–92.

[76] Herman EH, Mhatre RM, Chadwick DP. Modification of some of the toxic effects of daunomycin (NSC-82,151) by pretreatment with the antineoplastic agent ICRF 159 (NSC-129,943). Toxicol Appl Pharmacol 1974;27:517–26.

[77] Herman EH, Ferrans VJ. Preclinical animal models of cardiac protection from anthracycline-induced cardiotoxicity. Semin Oncol 1998;25:15–21.

[78] Imondi AR. Preclinical models of cardiac protection and testing for effects of dexrazoxane on doxorubicin antitumor effects. Semin Oncol 1998;25:22–30.

[79] Marty M, Espie M, Llombart A, et al. Multicenter randomized phase III study of the cardioprotective effect of dexrazoxane (Cardioxane) in advanced/metastatic breast cancer patients treated with anthracycline-based chemotherapy. Ann Oncol 2006;17: 614–22.

[80] Swain SM, Whaley FS, Gerber MC, et al. Cardioprotection with dexrazoxane for doxorubicin-containing therapy in advanced breast cancer. J Clin Oncol 1997;15:1318–32.

[81] Hasinoff BB, Hellmann K, Herman EH, Ferrans VJ. Chemical, biological and clinical aspects of dexrazoxane and other bisdioxopiperazines. Curr Med Chem 1998;5:1–28.

[82] Kalinowski DS, Richardson DR. The evolution of iron chelators for the treatment of iron overload disease and cancer. Pharmacol Rev 2005;57:547–83.

[83] Voest EE, van Acker SA, van der Vijgh WJ, van Asbeck BS, Bast A. Comparison of different iron chelators as protective agents against acute doxorubicin-induced cardiotoxicity. J Mol Cell Cardiol 1994;26:1179–85.

[84] Herman EH, Zhang J, Ferrans VJ. Comparison of the protective effects of desferrioxamine and ICRF-187 against doxorubicin-induced toxicity in spontaneously hypertensive rats. Cancer Chemother Pharmacol 1994;35:93–100.

[85] Simunek T, Klimtova I, Kaplanova J, et al. Rabbit model for in vivo study of anthracycline-induced heart failure and for the evaluation of protective agents. Eur J Heart Fail 2004;6:377–87.

[86] Popelova O, Sterba M, Simunek T, et al. Deferiprone does not protect against chronic anthracycline cardiotoxicity in vivo. J Pharmacol Exp Ther 2008;326:259–69.

[87] Hasinoff BB, Patel D, Wu X. The oral iron chelator ICL670A (deferasirox) does not protect myocytes against doxorubicin. Free Radic Biol Med 2003;35:1469–79.

[88] Sterba M, Popelova O, Simunek T, et al. Iron chelation-afforded cardioprotection against chronic anthracycline cardiotoxicity: a study of salicylaldehyde isonicotinoyl hydrazone (SIH). Toxicology 2007;235:150–66.

[89] Simunek T, Sterba M, Popelova O, et al. Pyridoxal isonicotinoyl hydrazone (PIH) and its analogs as protectants against anthracycline-induced cardiotoxicity. Hemoglobin 2008;32:207–15.

[90] Rao VA, Zhang J, Klein SR, et al. The iron chelator Dp44mT inhibits the proliferation of cancer cells but fails to protect from doxorubicin-induced cardiotoxicity in spontaneously hypertensive rats. Cancer Chemother Pharmacol 2011;68:1125–34.

[91] Bodley A, Liu LF, Israel M, et al. DNA topoisomerase II-mediated interaction of doxorubicin and daunorubicin congeners with DNA. Cancer Res 1989;49:5969–78.

[92] Schoeffler AJ, Berger JM. DNA topoisomerases: harnessing and constraining energy to govern chromosome topology. Q Rev Biophys 2008;41:41–101.

[93] Corbett KD, Berger JM. Structure of the topoisomerase VI-B subunit: implications for type II topoisomerase mechanism and evolution. EMBO J 2003;22:151–63.

[94] Zhang S, Liu X, Bawa-Khalfe T, et al. Identification of the molecular basis of doxorubicin-induced cardiotoxicity. Nat Med 2012;18:1639–42.

[95] L'Ecuyer T, Sanjeev S, Thomas R, et al. DNA damage is an early event in doxorubicin-induced cardiac myocyte death. Am J Physiol Heart Circ Physiol 2006;291:H1273–80.

[96] Liu J, Mao W, Ding B, Liang CS. ERKs/p53 signal transduction pathway is involved in doxorubicin-induced apoptosis in H9c2 cells and cardiomyocytes. Am J Physiol Heart Circ Physiol 2008;295:H1956–65.

[97] Kelly DP, Scarpulla RC. Transcriptional regulatory circuits controlling mitochondrial biogenesis and function. Genes Dev 2004;18:357–68.

[98] Leone TC, Kelly DP. Transcriptional control of cardiac fuel metabolism and mitochondrial function. Cold Spring Harb Symp Quant Biol 2011;76:175–82.

[99] Suliman HB, Carraway MS, Ali AS, Reynolds CM, Welty-Wolf KE, Piantadosi CA. The CO/HO system reverses inhibition of mitochondrial biogenesis and prevents murine doxorubicin cardiomyopathy. J Clin Invest 2007;117:3730–41.

[100] Hasinoff BB, Herman EH. Dexrazoxane: how it works in cardiac and tumor cells. Is it a prodrug or is it a drug? Cardiovasc Toxicol 2007;7:140–4.

[101] Herman EH, el-Hage A, Ferrans VJ. Protective effect of ICRF-187 on doxorubicin-induced cardiac and renal toxicity in spontaneously hypertensive (SHR) and normotensive (WKY) rats. Toxicol Appl Pharmacol 1988;92:42–53.

[102] Herman EH, Ferrans VJ. Timing of treatment with ICRF-187 and its effect on chronic doxorubicin cardiotoxicity. Cancer Chemother Pharmacol 1993;32:445–9.

[103] Nitiss JL. Targeting DNA topoisomerase II in cancer chemotherapy. Nat Rev Cancer 2009;9:338–50.

[104] Vavrova A, Jansova H, Mackova E, et al. Catalytic inhibitors of topoisomerase II differently modulate the toxicity of anthracyclines in cardiac and cancer cells. PLoS One 2013;8:e76676.

[105] Hutchins LF, Green SJ, Ravdin PM, et al. Randomized, controlled trial of cyclophosphamide, methotrexate, and fluorouracil versus cyclophosphamide, doxorubicin, and fluorouracil with and without tamoxifen for high-risk, node-negative breast cancer: treatment results of Intergroup Protocol INT-0102. J Clin Oncol 2005;23: 8313–21.

[106] Levine MN, Bramwell VH, Pritchard KI, et al. Randomized trial of intensive cyclophosphamide, epirubicin, and fluorouracil chemotherapy compared with cyclophosphamide, methotrexate, and fluorouracil in premenopausal women with node-positive breast cancer. National Cancer Institute of Canada Clinical Trials Group. J Clin Oncol 1998;16:2651–8.

[107] Levine MN, Pritchard KI, Bramwell VH, et al. Randomized trial comparing cyclophosphamide, epirubicin, and fluorouracil with cyclophosphamide, methotrexate, and fluorouracil in premenopausal

women with node-positive breast cancer: update of National Cancer Institute of Canada Clinical Trials Group Trial MA5. J Clin Oncol 2005;23:5166–70.

[108] Poole CJ, Earl HM, Hiller L, et al. Epirubicin and cyclophosphamide, methotrexate, and fluorouracil as adjuvant therapy for early breast cancer. N Engl J Med 2006;355:1851–62.

[109] Muss HB, Berry DA, Cirrincione CT, et al. Adjuvant chemotherapy in older women with early-stage breast cancer. N Engl J Med 2009;360:2055–65.

[110] Early Breast Cancer Trialists' Collaborative G, Peto R, Davies C, et al. Comparisons between different polychemotherapy regimens for early breast cancer: meta-analyses of long-term outcome among 100,000 women in 123 randomised trials. Lancet 2012;379:432–44.

[111] Hortobagyi GN. Anthracyclines in the treatment of cancer. An overview. Drugs 1997;54(Suppl. 4):1–7.

[112] Li X, Xu S, Tan Y, Chen J. The effects of idarubicin versus other anthracyclines for induction therapy of patients with newly diagnosed leukaemia. Cochrane Database Syst Rev 2015;6. CD010432.

[113] Brambilla C, Rossi A, Bonfante V, et al. Phase II study of doxorubicin versus epirubicin in advanced breast cancer. Cancer Treat Rep 1986;70:261–6.

[114] Jain KK, Casper ES, Geller NL, et al. A prospective randomized comparison of epirubicin and doxorubicin in patients with advanced breast cancer. J Clin Oncol 1985;3:818–26.

[115] Kaklamani VG, Gradishar WJ. Epirubicin versus doxorubicin: which is the anthracycline of choice for the treatment of breast cancer? Clin Breast Cancer 2003;4(Suppl. 1):S26–33.

[116] Blanco JG, Sun CL, Landier W, et al. Anthracycline-related cardiomyopathy after childhood cancer: role of polymorphisms in carbonyl reductase genes--a report from the Children's Oncology Group. J Clin Oncol 2012;30:1415–21.

[117] Smith LA, Cornelius VR, Plummer CJ, et al. Cardiotoxicity of anthracycline agents for the treatment of cancer: systematic review and meta-analysis of randomised controlled trials. BMC Cancer 2010;10:337.

[118] Ryberg M, Nielsen D, Skovsgaard T, Hansen J, Jensen BV, Dombernowsky P. Epirubicin cardiotoxicity: an analysis of 469 patients with metastatic breast cancer. J Clin Oncol 1998;16:3502–8.

[119] Ryberg M, Nielsen D, Cortese G, Nielsen G, Skovsgaard T, Andersen PK. New insight into epirubicin cardiac toxicity: competing risks analysis of 1097 breast cancer patients. J Natl Cancer Inst 2008;100:1058–67.

[120] van Dalen EC, Michiels EM, Caron HN, Kremer LC. Different anthracycline derivates for reducing cardiotoxicity in cancer patients. Cochrane Database Syst Rev 2010;5. CD005006.

[121] Osby E, Hagberg H, Kvaloy S, et al. CHOP is superior to CNOP in elderly patients with aggressive lymphoma while outcome is unaffected by filgrastim treatment: results of a Nordic Lymphoma Group randomized trial. Blood 2003;101:3840–8.

[122] Sonneveld P, de Ridder M, van der Lelie H, et al. Comparison of doxorubicin and mitoxantrone in the treatment of elderly patients with advanced diffuse non-Hodgkin's lymphoma using CHOP versus CNOP chemotherapy. J Clin Oncol 1995;13:2530–9.

[123] Tirelli U, Errante D, Van Glabbeke M, et al. CHOP is the standard regimen in patients > or = 70 years of age with intermediate-grade and high-grade non-Hodgkin's lymphoma: results of a randomized study of the European Organization for Research and Treatment of Cancer Lymphoma Cooperative Study Group. J Clin Oncol 1998;16:27–34.

[124] Hohloch K, Zwick C, Ziepert M, et al. Significant dose Escalation of Idarubicin in the treatment of aggressive Non- Hodgkin Lymphoma leads to increased hematotoxicity without improvement in efficacy in comparison to standard CHOEP-14: 9-year follow up results of the CIVEP trial of the DSHNHL. Springerplus 2014;3:5.

[125] van Dalen EC, van der Pal HJ, Caron HN, Kremer LC. Different dosage schedules for reducing cardiotoxicity in cancer patients receiving anthracycline chemotherapy. Cochrane Database Syst Rev 2009;4. CD005008.

[126] Lipshultz SE, Miller TL, Lipsitz SR, et al. Continuous versus bolus infusion of doxorubicin in children with ALL: long-term cardiac outcomes. Pediatrics 2012;130:1003–11.

[127] Lipshultz SE, Cochran TR, Franco VI, Miller TL. Treatment-related cardiotoxicity in survivors of childhood cancer. Nat Rev Clin Oncol 2013;10:697–710.

[128] Gupta M, Steinherz PG, Cheung NK, Steinherz L. Late cardiotoxicity after bolus versus infusion anthracycline therapy for childhood cancers. Med Pediatr Oncol 2003;40:343–7.

[129] Levitt GA, Dorup I, Sorensen K, Sullivan I. Does anthracycline administration by infusion in children affect late cardiotoxicity? Br J Haematol 2004;124:463–8.

[130] Pignata S, Scambia G, Ferrandina G, et al. Carboplatin plus paclitaxel versus carboplatin plus pegylated liposomal doxorubicin as first-line treatment for patients with ovarian cancer: the MITO-2 randomized phase III trial. J Clin Oncol 2011;29:3628–35.

[131] Sharpe M, Easthope SE, Keating GM, Lamb HM. Polyethylene glycol-liposomal doxorubicin: a review of its use in the management of solid and haematological malignancies and AIDS-related Kaposi's sarcoma. Drugs 2002;62:2089–126.

[132] Vail DM, Amantea MA, Colbern GT, Martin FJ, Hilger RA, Working PK. Pegylated liposomal doxorubicin: proof of principle using preclinical animal models and pharmacokinetic studies. Semin Oncol 2004;31:16–35.

[133] Vaage J, Donovan D, Mayhew E, Uster P, Woodle M. Therapy of mouse mammary carcinomas with vincristine and doxorubicin encapsulated in sterically stabilized liposomes. Int J Cancer 1993;54:959–64.

[134] O'Brien ME, Wigler N, Inbar M, et al. Reduced cardiotoxicity and comparable efficacy in a phase III trial of pegylated liposomal doxorubicin HCl (CAELYX/Doxil) versus conventional doxorubicin for first-line treatment of metastatic breast cancer. Ann Oncol 2004;15:440–9.

[135] Al-Batran SE, Guntner M, Pauligk C, et al. Anthracycline rechallenge using pegylated liposomal doxorubicin in patients with metastatic breast cancer: a pooled analysis using individual data from four prospective trials. Br J Cancer 2010;103:1518–23.

[136] Keller AM, Mennel RG, Georgoulias VA, et al. Randomized phase III trial of pegylated liposomal doxorubicin versus vinorelbine or mitomycin C plus vinblastine in women with taxane-refractory advanced breast cancer. J Clin Oncol 2004;22:3893–901.

[137] Gordon AN, Fleagle JT, Guthrie D, Parkin DE, Gore ME, Lacave AJ. Recurrent epithelial ovarian carcinoma: a randomized phase III study of pegylated liposomal doxorubicin versus topotecan. J Clin Oncol 2001;19:3312–22.

[138] Mutch DG, Orlando M, Goss T, et al. Randomized phase III trial of gemcitabine compared with pegylated liposomal doxorubicin in patients with platinum-resistant ovarian cancer. J Clin Oncol 2007;25:2811–8.

[139] Pujade-Lauraine E, Wagner U, Aavall-Lundqvist E, et al. Pegylated liposomal Doxorubicin and Carboplatin compared with Paclitaxel and Carboplatin for patients with platinum-sensitive ovarian cancer in late relapse. J Clin Oncol 2010;28:3323–9.

[140] Kesterson JP, Odunsi K, Lele S. High cumulative doses of pegylated liposomal doxorubicin are not associated with cardiac toxicity in patients with gynecologic malignancies. Chemotherapy 2010;56:108–11.

[141] Yildirim Y, Gultekin E, Avci ME, Inal MM, Yunus S, Tinar S. Cardiac safety profile of pegylated liposomal doxorubicin reaching or exceeding lifetime cumulative doses of 550 mg/m2 in patients with recurrent ovarian and peritoneal cancer. Int J Gynecol Cancer 2008;18:223–7.

[142] Agency EM. Caelyx (doxorubicin hydrochloride in a pegylated. liposomal formulation); 2011. Avialble from:

[143] Duggan ST, Keating GM. Pegylated liposomal doxorubicin: a review of its use in metastatic breast cancer, ovarian cancer, multiple myeloma and AIDS-related Kaposi's sarcoma. Drugs 2011;71:2531–58.

[144] Smith DH, Adams JR, Johnston SR, Gordon A, Drummond MF, Bennett CL. A comparative economic analysis of pegylated liposomal doxorubicin versus topotecan in ovarian cancer in the USA and the UK. Ann Oncol 2002;13:1590–7.

[145] Creighton AM, Birnie GD. The effect of bisdioxopiperazines on the synthesis of deoxyribonucleic acid, ribonucleic acid and protein in growing mouse-embryo fibroblasts. Biochem J 1969;114:58P.

[146] Classen S, Olland S, Berger JM. Structure of the topoisomerase II ATPase region and its mechanism of inhibition by the chemotherapeutic agent ICRF-187. Proc Natl Acad Sci USA 2003;100: 10629–34.

[147] Tanabe K, Ikegami Y, Ishida R, Andoh T. Inhibition of topoisomerase II by antitumor agents bis(2,6-dioxopiperazine) derivatives. Cancer Res 1991;51:4903–8.

[148] Kovacevic Z, Kalinowski DS, Lovejoy DB, Quach P, Wong J, Richardson DR. Iron chelators: development of novel compounds with high and selective anti-tumour activity. Curr Drug Deliv 2010;7(3):194–207.

[149] Lyu YL, Kerrigan JE, Lin CP, et al. Topoisomerase IIbeta mediated DNA double-strand breaks: implications in doxorubicin cardiotoxicity and prevention by dexrazoxane. Cancer Res 2007; 67:8839–46.

[150] Lipshultz SE, Rifai N, Dalton VM, et al. The effect of dexrazoxane on myocardial injury in doxorubicin-treated children with acute lymphoblastic leukemia. N Engl J Med 2004;351:145–53.

[151] Lipshultz SE, Scully RE, Lipsitz SR, et al. Assessment of dexrazoxane as a cardioprotectant in doxorubicin-treated children with high-risk acute lymphoblastic leukaemia: long-term follow-up of a prospective, randomised, multicentre trial. Lancet Oncol 2010;11:950–61.

[152] Speyer JL, Green MD, Zeleniuch-Jacquotte A, et al. ICRF-187 permits longer treatment with doxorubicin in women with breast cancer. J Clin Oncol 1992;10:117–27.

[153] Yu Y, Kalinowski DS, Kovacevic Z, et al. Thiosemicarbazones from the old to new: iron chelators that are more than just ribonucleotide reductase inhibitors. J Med Chem 2009;52:5271–94.

[154] Swain SM, Vici P. The current and future role of dexrazoxane as a cardioprotectant in anthracycline treatment: expert panel review. J Cancer Res Clin Oncol 2004;130:1–7.

[155] Seymour L, Bramwell V, Moran LA. Use of dexrazoxane as a cardioprotectant in patients receiving doxorubicin or epirubicin chemotherapy for the treatment of cancer. The Provincial Systemic Treatment Disease Site Group. Cancer Prev Control 1999;3:145–59.

[156] van Dalen EC, Caron HN, Dickinson HO, Kremer LC. Cardioprotective interventions for cancer patients receiving anthracyclines. Cochrane Database Syst Rev 2008;6. CD003917.

[157] Schuchter LM, Hensley ML, Meropol NJ, Winer EP. American Society of Clinical Oncology C, Radiotherapy Expert P. 2002 update of recommendations for the use of chemotherapy and radiotherapy protectants: clinical practice guidelines of the American Society of Clinical Oncology. J Clin Oncol 2002;20:2895–903.

[158] Tebbi CK, London WB, Friedman D, et al. Dexrazoxane-associated risk for acute myeloid leukemia/myelodysplastic syndrome and other secondary malignancies in pediatric Hodgkin's disease. J Clin Oncol 2007;25:493–500.

[159] Salzer WL, Devidas M, Carroll WL, et al. Long-term results of the pediatric oncology group studies for childhood acute lymphoblastic leukemia 1984-2001: a report from the children's oncology group. Leukemia 2010;24:355–70.

[160] Vrooman LM, Neuberg DS, Stevenson KE, et al. The low incidence of secondary acute myelogenous leukaemia in children and adolescents treated with dexrazoxane for acute lymphoblastic leukaemia: a report from the Dana-Farber Cancer Institute ALL Consortium. Eur J Cancer 2011;47:1373–9.

Chapter 5

Cardiotoxic Effects of Anti-VEGFR Tyrosine Kinase Inhibitors

E. Bronte*, A. Galvano*, G. Novo** and A. Russo*

*Department of Surgical, Oncological and Oral Sciences, Section of Medical Oncology, University of Palermo, Palermo, Italy; **Department of Internal Medicine and Cardiovascular Disease, University of Palermo, Palermo, Italy

INTRODUCTION

The bloodstream is essential to deliver oxygen and nutrients to the tissues and remove catabolites through endothelial cells of vessels. New vessels are important for the growth and development of tissues. Experiments conducted since the mid-1950s revealed that tumors stimulated endothelial cells to become highly active from a resting state. As in physiological settings, the formation of new vessels is fundamental for growth of the tissue or tumor. Angiogenesis is driven by the tumor in a sort of mutualistic relationship. This evidence led to Judah Folkman's idea of blocking the process of vascularization, which he called "antiangiogenesis" in order to limit tumor growth. This opened up a new research field [1–6]. Over the years, control of the angiogenic process has become an important therapeutic target. Antiangiogenic therapy supports the action of old therapies, such as chemotherapy and radiotherapy, and in some cases exceeds their limits. Two main types of molecules have been developed. These are monoclonal antibodies (such as bevacizumab and ramucirumab) and tyrosine kinase inhibitors (TKIs) (such as sorafenib, sunitinib, regorafenib, etc.). Another molecule has been developed acting as VEGF-trap. It is aflibercept [7–13].

In this chapter we will discuss about the biology of VEGF and its pathway, and will also focus on how TKIs act in cells and how they lead to cardiotoxic side effects.

ANGIOGENESIS: A TWO-EDGED SWORD

Development of new blood vessels from pre-existing blood vessels is called angiogenesis and is a normal physiologic process, particularly during the development of the embryo and fetus, and in adults during the ovarian cycle and in wound healing. Angiogenesis is the product of the balance between proangiogenic factors and antiangiogenic factors.

Proangiogenic factors promote angiogenesis and comprise two categories: classical and nonclassical factors. Classical factors are vascular endothelial growth factor (VEGF), platelet-derived growth factor (PDGF), hepatocyte growth factor (HGF), angiopoietins (Ang), insulin-like growth factors (IGFs), fibroblast growth factors (FGFs), which are basicFGF (bFGF also called FGF-2) and acidicFGF (aFGF also called FGF-1), tumor necrosis factor (TNF), interleukins (ILs), in particular IL-6 and IL-8, transforming growth factor-α (TGF-α) and TGF-β. Nonclassical factors are stem-cell factor (SCF), tryptase and chymase. Antiangiogenic factors inhibit angiogenesis and comprise two categories: matrix-derived and non-matrix-derived factors. Matrix-derived factors are arresten, canstatin, endorepellin, endostatin, thrombospondins (TSPs): TSP-1 and TSP-2, tumstatin. Non-matrix-derived factors are interferons (INFs), interleukins (ILs, e.g. IL-4 and IL-12), angiostatin, chondromodulin I, tissue inhibitors of matrix metalloproteinases (TIMPs), soluble Fms-like tyrosine kinase 1 (sFlt-1), platelet factor-4, troponin I, and vasostatin (Fig. 5.1) [14–29].

Conditions such as blood-vessel constriction or obstruction, or systemic hypoxia (e.g., due to lung disease or high altitude) stimulate production of proangiogenic factors which attempt to compensate for the deficit through the production of new blood vessels. Hypoxia-inducible factor-1 (HIF-1), in the cytosol, is the key regulator of oxygen homeostasis. HIF-1 is constituted by two subunits α and β. HIF-1β is an aryl hydrocarbon nuclear receptor translocator (ARNT). The two subunits α and β possess basic helix–loop–helix (bHLH) and PER–ARNT–SIM homology (PAS) domains in their amino-terminal half, which are required for heterodimerization. The subunits α and β are part of a transcription factor family. In normoxic conditions HIF-1α is hydroxylated by prolyl hydroxylase enzymes (PHDs) on proline residues in the position 402 and 564, which are located within

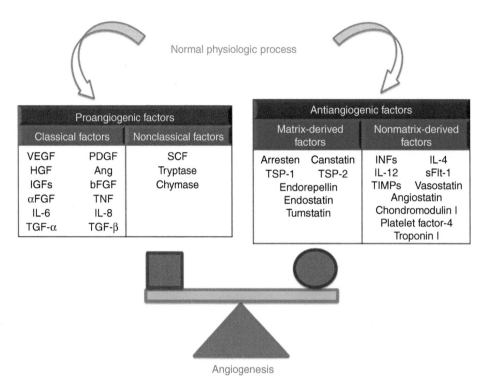

FIGURE 5.1 The angiogenic process is the result of the equilibrium between proangiogenic factors and antiangiogenic factors.

ODDD (O_2-dependent degradation domain). This hydroxylation determines the interaction with the von Hippel–Lindau (VHL) E3 ligase complex which results in ubiquitination of HIF-1α, leading to its proteasomal degradation. On the other hand, in hypoxic conditions there is a reduction in the quantity of substrates and coactivators of hydroxylation, such as O_2, Fe(II), and 2-oxoglutarate resulting in a decrease of HIF-1α hydroxylation and its accumulation in the cytosol. HIF-1α is then translocated to the nucleus, where HIF-1β is constitutively present. The interaction of coactivators, such as CBP/p300, with the two domains C-TAD and N-TAD on the C-terminus of the protein HIF-1α, helps the dimer HIF-1α/β for DNA binding on hypoxia response elements (HREs) and for the subsequent transcriptional activation. HREs are located within O_2-regulated genes. The transcription of target genes by HIF-1 includes angiogenic and hematopoietic growth factors, glycolytic enzymes, and glucose transporters. Among them, there is, for example, erythropoietin (EPO), which is necessary for red-blood-cell production. The production of erythrocytes increases the transport of oxygen to tissues so as to reach O_2 homeostasis. Other transcriptional products are endothelin-1 (ET-1), glucose transporter 1 and 3, IGF-II, nitric oxide synthase 2 (NOS2), VEGF and VEGF receptor FLT-1. HIF-α is a member of a family which also includes HIF-2α, also known as EPAS (endothelial PAS protein), and HIF-3α, also called IPAS (inhibitory PAS). HIF-2α is present in endothelium, lung, and cartilage. HIF-3α acts as a dominant negative inhibitor of HIF-1α DNA binding [30–34].

The transcription of target genes by HIF-1 leads to the production of several molecules, importantly including VEGF. The increased production of VEGF and other proangiogenic factors stimulate the creation of new vessels. VEGF isoforms interact with their receptors, VEGFRs, which are tyrosine kinases present on endothelial cell membranes. The interaction of VEGF with VEGFR activates an intracellular signal transduction pathway promoting survival, proliferation, and migration of the endothelial cells and tube formation. Angiogenesis consists of multiple processes: (1) endothelial cell division. Under the stimulus of proangiogenic factors endothelial cells become highly active. They have a significant mitotic index and develop the capability to migrate and disrupt the extracellular matrix (including tight junctions and gap junctions). (2) Pre-existing basement membrane rupture. (3) Endothelial cell migration. Endothelial cells invade the perivascular tissue, where they further proliferate. (4) New basement membrane development. (5) Tube formation. (6) Pericyte recruitment.

At first the growing tumor is in balance with blood supply and all cells receive sufficient nutrients and oxygen. However, as the tumor grows, it outstrips the blood supply needed for continued growth. The hypoxic tumor cells produce proangiogenic factors (e.g., VEGF) in excess of ambient antiangiogenic factors, so angiogenesis is triggered. These cells also interact by autocrine and paracrine pathways. The excessive cell growth and production of growth factors produce an uncontrolled angiogenesis, which result in a chaotic microvascular bed with ineffective blood flow and regions of hypoxia. A vicious cycle is created that facilitates tumor growth and metastasis [35–42].

VASCULAR ENDOTHELIAL GROWTH FACTOR AND VEGFR SIGNALING PATHWAY

VEGF family members include VEGF-A, VEGF-B, VEGF-C, VEGF-D, and placental growth factor (PlGF). Among them, the most important one is VEGF-A, which has at least six splice variants ($VEGF_{121}$, $VEGF_{145}$, $VEGF_{165}$, $VEGF_{183}$, $VEGF_{189}$, and $VEGF_{206}$). The most common isoform contains 165 amino acid residues ($VEGF_{165}$). Each of these growth factor isoforms interacts with VEGF receptors on endothelial cells to activate them and to start the angiogenic process. VEGFRs are a family of homodimeric tyrosine kinase receptors that include VEGFR1, VEGFR2, and VEGFR3. VEGFR1 and VEGFR2 are involved in vascular angiogenesis and VEGFR1 can transphosphorylate VEGFR2. Besides, between these two, VEGFR2 has a major part in angiogenesis. VEGFR3 features lymphangiogenesis and it does not interact with VEGF-A. When VEGF is secreted, it binds to VEGFR, triggering homodimerization and autophosphorylation, thus allowing the activation of several cytoplasmic signaling molecules. There are two main signaling cascade pathways, which start from VEGF/VEGFR interaction: the RAS–RAF–MEK–ERK pathway and phosphatidylinositol-3-kinase (PI3K)/PTEN/Akt pathway. These signaling pathways lead to the transcription of genes involved in proliferation and survival of pre-existing endothelial cells. The first pathway is called the MAPK cascade. It starts from RAS, which is part of the protein family of small GTPases. RAS isoforms are KRAS, NRAS, and HRAS. When activated, RAS changes its state from the inactive form with GDP bound to the active form which binds GTP. There is a conformational switch, which facilitates its binding to RAF, the first kinase of the pathway. RAF is a serine/threonine kinase, with three isoforms [ARAF, BRAF, and CRAF (this last one also called Raf-1)]. Activated RAS recruits RAF to the membrane and activates it. RAF in turn phosphorylates and stimulates the kinase MEK, which activates the kinase ERK through phosphorylation. Lastly ERK phosphorylates several molecules, which include other kinases and transcription factors. This sequential activation of molecules starts various cellular phenomena linked to cell-cycle progression, cell proliferation or differentiation, protein translation and evasion from cell death related to the intensity and time duration of the signal.

The second pathway is the PI3K/PTEN/Akt pathway, which induces cell growth and survival. PI3K is the starting point of the cascade. It is possible to distinguish three classes of PI3Ks in correlation with structure and function, of which class IA is the main class involved in cancer. Class IA PI3Ks are initiated through receptor tyrosine kinases (RTKs) by growth factors (such as VEGF). Class IA PI3Ks are heterodimers composed of two parts: a regulatory subunit, p85, and a catalytic subunit, p110. When the p85 regulatory subunit interacts with the phosphotyrosine residues on RTKs or adaptors or activated Ras, it releases p110 to the plasma membrane where it phosphorylates phosphatidylinositol 4,5-bisphosphate (PI [4,5] P2) on the 3′OH position, generating PI(3,4,5)P3. PIP3 attracts phosphoinositide-dependent kinase 1(PDK1) and Akt, so that PDK1 phosphorylates Akt at threonine 308, thereby activating it. Activated Akt moves from cell membrane to cytoplasm to phosphorylate intracellular substrates but it also moves to the nucleus. It activates various regulators involved in transcription, such as CREB, E2F, and nuclear factor κB (NF-κB). Normally NF-κB is constitutively inhibited in the cytoplasm by IκB (inhibitory κ B protein kinase). When NF-κB is activated, it translocates to the nucleus where it stimulates the expression of several target genes governing cell proliferation, invasion, and inflammation. Thus, Akt has a part in survival, invasion, metastasis, cell cycle progression, migration, senescence, drug resistance, and DNA damage repair. Akt favors cell survival through the phosphorylation and inhibition of proapoptotic Bcl-2 family members and Mdm2, involved in p53-mediated apoptosis. Akt also inhibits the tuberous sclerosis complex-2 (TSC2) gene product tuberin by phosphorylating it. Tuberin is normally bound to hamartin, which is the product of TSC1. Tuberin is a GTPase-activating protein and consequently it is an inhibitor of the Ras-like small G protein Rheb. When TSC2 is phosphorylated, Rheb is activated which in turn activates the mammalian target of rapamycin (mTOR)—containing protein complex mTORC1. This activated complex on one hand triggers the p70 ribosomal S6 kinase (S6K1), whereas on the other hand inhibits the elongation-initiation factor 4E binding protein-1 (4E-BP1) through phosphorylation. These events lead to increased protein synthesis resulting in cell growth. The S6K through a feedback mechanism limits PI3K activation. It also inhibits the adaptor protein insulin receptor substrate 1, which is involved in insulin and IGF-1-mediated PI3K activation. Another mTOR complex mTORC2, phosphorylates Akt on serine 473 [43–50].

MECHANISMS OF ACTION OF TYROSINE KINASE INHIBITORS TARGETING VEGFR

The study of the VEGF/VEGFR pathway revealed the central role of this pathway in angiogenesis and led to the development of various drugs designed to inhibit it. The present-day armamentarium includes antibodies targeting VEGF and/or VEGFRs, soluble VEGF receptors, or receptor hybrids. Additionally there are TKIs that selectively target one or more than one VEGFR. TKIs have been developed to target not only VEGF receptors but also other targets, not only earning the name of "multikinase" inhibitors but also giving rise

TABLE 5.1 Molecular Targets of Anti-VEGFR Tyrosine Kinase Inhibitors

Drug	Molecular Target												
	VEGFR-1	VEGFR-2	VEGFR-3	PDGFRα	PDGFRβ	c-KIT	FLT3	CSF1R	RET	Raf-1	BRAF	TIE2	FGFR1
Sunitinib	✓	✓	✓	✓	✓	✓	✓	✓	✓				
Sorafenib		✓	✓	✓	✓	✓	✓			✓	✓		
Regorafenib	✓	✓	✓		✓	✓			✓	✓	✓	✓	✓
Axitinib	✓	✓	✓										
Nintedanib	✓	✓	✓	✓	✓		✓		✓				✓
Vandetanib	✓	✓	✓		✓				✓				
Pazopanib	✓	✓	✓	✓	✓	✓							✓
Vatalanib	✓	✓	✓	✓		✓							
Cediranib	✓	✓	✓	✓	✓	✓							✓
Cabozantinib	✓	✓	✓			✓	✓		✓			✓	
Lenvatinib	✓	✓	✓	✓		✓			✓				✓
Linifanib	✓	✓	✓	✓	✓								
Telatinib		✓	✓		✓								
Brivanib	✓	✓	✓										✓
Foretinib	✓	✓	✓	✓	✓	✓	✓					✓	
Motesanib	✓	✓	✓	✓	✓	✓							
Lucitanib	✓	✓	✓	✓	✓								✓
Fruquintinib	✓	✓	✓										
Tivozanib	✓	✓	✓										
Apatinib		✓											

to off-target toxicity (Table 5.1). For example, regorafenib and sorafenib also inhibit RAF-1, B-RAF, PDGF receptor-β (PDGFRβ), and c-KIT. In particular, drugs targeting both VEGFRs and PDGFRs carry out inhibition on two fronts, blocking VEGFR on endothelial cells and PDGFR on pericytes as well as on VEGFRs expressed in tumor cells. TKIs affect not only tumor vasculature but also normal vasculature, which explains the cardiovascular toxicity evinced by this class of drugs. Acting on tumor vasculature they limit tumor growth and metastasis. TKIs mainly inhibit the tyrosine kinase activity of the receptor thus blocking the transmission of the signal after the interaction between VEGF and its receptor VEGFR. VEGF signaling promotes several cell functions, including cell survival and migration. Blockade of the receptor suppresses tumor cell survival, migration, and invasion [49,51,52].

CARDIOTOXIC EFFECTS BY ANTIANGIOGENIC DRUGS

TKIs act both on tumor and normal cells, thus leading to side effects including hypertension, renal vascular injury, and heart failure (HF). The cardiovascular side effects involve HF, hypertension, coronary artery vasospasm, and acute coronary syndrome, QT interval prolongation, asymptomatic or less commonly, symptomatic reduction of left ventricular ejection fraction (LVEF), and acute myocardial infarction (MI). It is possible to differentiate two types of toxicity, on-target toxicity, and off-target toxicity. In the first one, the toxicity is target related, which means that the kinase inhibited by the TKI carries out a crucial role in heart or vasculature. This cannot be overcome by developing more specific inhibitory molecules. Off-target toxicity is due to the fact that TKIs are multikinase inhibitors limited in their selectivity. Thus if the drug inhibits a kinase that is unrelated to tumor cytotoxicity but plays a role in cardiovascular function, off-target toxicity would develop. An example of off-target toxicity is the inhibition of AMPK (AMP-activated protein kinase) by sunitinib, an inhibitor of VEGFRs, PDGFRs, and c-KIT. AMPK has an important role in the metabolic homeostasis of the heart through regulation of energy stress. It is activated if the level of energy is decreased in the cardiomyocyte resulting in an increase in AMP levels. After activation, AMPK inhibits the energy-consuming pathways such as protein and fatty acid synthesis, and it stimulates the production of energy by activating fatty acid oxidation and glycolysis. The inhibition by sunitinib has opposite effects because the energy consuming pathways are not suppressed and activation of energy-generating pathways is limited. This state of energy depletion paves the way to the activation of apoptosis (including mitochondrial membrane depolarization and cytochrome c release). Studies have demonstrated that there is myocardial cell loss by this drug which may be due to AMPK inhibition as well as loss of survival signals through VEGFR, PDGFR, and c-KIT [49,53–55].

The most frequent cardiovascular complication is hypertension, which is tightly linked to VEGF/VEGFR pathway inhibition. Indeed the increase in blood pressure is closely related to the treatment scheme, with hypertension occurring during cycles of drug administration and regressing between cycles. The interaction between VEGF and VEGFR2 activates the receptor, signaling through Src, PI3K, and phospholipase C (PLC), resulting in conversion of PIP2 to PIP3 by PI3K. PIP3 and PD1K activate Akt which in turn induces endothelial nitric oxide synthase (eNOS) to produce nitric oxide (NO). The activated enzyme PLC otherwise converts PIP2 to inositol trisphosphate (IP3) and diacylglycerol. IP3 is a second messenger which promotes Ca^{2+} influx into the cell, which also contributes to stimulate eNOS activity to produce NO. The latter activates guanylyl cyclase, increasing cGMP which leads to vasodilation, limits platelet aggregation, and suppressed growth of smooth muscle cells. Thus when TKIs inhibit signal transduction the final effect is a remarkable reduction in NO synthesis, resulting in vasoconstriction (thus hypertension) and endothelial dysfunction (microvascular impairment). These considerations are confirmed by the evidence that reduced VEGF-A production contributes to HF due in part to modified microvascular growth and reduced capillary density. Normally, VEGF helps to mitigate hypertension, but anti-VEGF therapy compromises this effect. Uncontrolled hypertension contributes to left ventricular hypertrophy; pathologic cardiac remodeling is characterized by cardiomyocyte hypertrophy that is not matched by an increase in capillary density. Studies in animal models indeed demonstrated an impairment in microvascular density, thinned ventricular walls, and lowered contractile function after deletion of the VEGF gene. These conditions favor the evolution from myocardial hypertrophy to HF, even though there are also other factors such as impaired calcium homeostasis in cardiomyocytes, interstitial fibrosis, and changes in energy metabolism. It has to be noted that the reduction in NO production not only determines vasoconstriction and endothelial dysfunction but also alters renal sodium handling, which supports in the long term the persistence of hypertension and renovascular injury.

Studies revealed that sunitinib plays a role in regulating ET-1 levels in blood. The increment in ET-1 quantity indicates that ET pathway is important in TKI-induced hypertension development. The VEGF/VEGFR interruption alters the equilibrium between NO and ET-1, facilitating vasoconstriction. ET-1 induces vasoconstriction through nicotinamide adenine dinucleotide phosphate (NADPH) oxidase and the production of reactive oxygen radicals. Vasoconstriction facilitates hypertension. Another concurrent factor in maintaining hypertension in the long term is thyroid dysfunction. It has been reported that TKIs can cause hypothyroidism detected by a rise in TSH levels. Regardless of the etiology of the hypertension, it is important to control it with antihypertensives [49,56].

PDGF is an important glycoprotein that acts as a growth factor in various cell types. Among these cell types are smooth muscle cells, stromal cells, cardiomyocytes, and endothelial cells. The two PDGF receptors (α and β) are present in cells that have an oncogenic potential, contributing to the growth of gastrointestinal stromal tumor (GIST), glioblastoma, and chronic myelomonocytic leukemia. A study by Edelberg et al. revealed that PDGF mediates the interaction between cardiomyocytes and endothelial cells nearby. This interaction sustains angiogenesis and endothelial function, an interaction that is impaired in aged heart tissue. Deletion of the gene for PDGFRβ in cardiomyocytes results in impaired adjustment to afterload stress accompanied by a decrease in cardiac capillary density and consequently local tissue hypoxia. These processes contribute to pathologic remodeling characterized by ventricular hypertrophy and chamber dilation culminating in HF. Thus HF is the result of two combined effects. On the one hand the impairment in the production of NO causes hypertension, which is responsible for afterload stress of the heart. On the other hand the suppression of PDGFRβ limits the normal capacity to adapt to afterload stress. A recent study of sunitinib showed that the drug reduces the number of pericytes in the coronary microcirculation, thereby altering coronary microvasculature and further contributing to local tissue hypoxia, which underlies cardiac dysfunction [49,57,58].

Another important cardiovascular adverse event due to TKIs is thromboembolism. The interaction of VEGF with VEGFR activates the MAPK pathway and upregulates the prosurvival factor Bcl-2 in endothelial cells. The related protein Bcl-x_L, is an antiapoptotic factor that upregulates VEGF-A production in endothelial cells and in platelets and contributes to microvascular stability. VEGF-A/VEGFR2 also regulates the expression of proteins of the intercellular junctional complexes. VEGF-A modifies the endothelial cell through the increase of vascular permeability, upregulation of urokinase, tissue plasminogen activator, and the vascular-cell-adhesion molecule (VCAM). The three major isoforms of VEGF-A are present in megakaryocytes and platelets and are released during thrombin stimulation. Platelet activating factor (PAF), which is a proinflammatory molecule, stimulates the expression of VEGF-A by endothelial cells. VEGF released by cells activates VEGFR2 via autocrine and paracrine signaling. The paracrine pathway

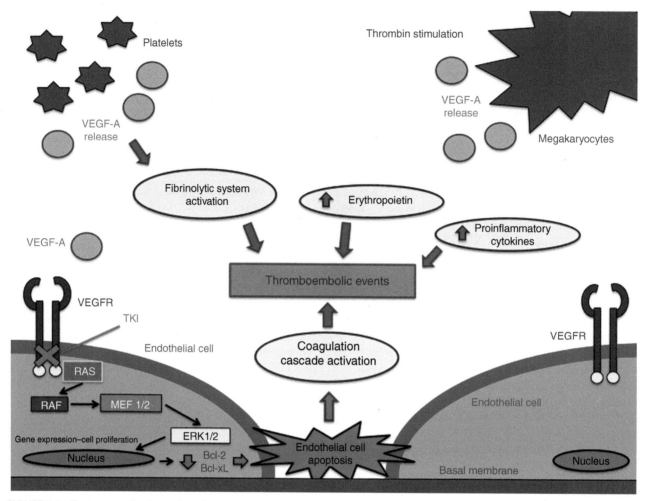

FIGURE 5.2 **Factors contributing to thromboembolism during TKI therapy.**

supports vascular permeability in abnormal conditions such as inflammation, and is therefore crucial for angiogenesis in cancer and inflammation. The VEGFR blockage during TKI therapy lowers Bcl-x_L and Bcl-2 levels, leading to apoptosis. Endothelial cell apoptosis exposes the subendothelial basement membrane, activating the coagulation cascade and paving the way for thromboembolic events. Furthermore, platelets release VEGF, which activates the fibrinolytic system, further contributing to thromboembolic events. VEGF is not only implicated in the production of NO by the endothelium but also in the production of PGI2, the reduction of which contributes to thrombosis, having an antiplatelet activity. The suppression of VEGF activity determines a consequential inversely proportional increase of EPO, which is responsible for the increase in hematocrit and blood viscosity, further contributing to the prothrombotic state. Elevated levels of proinflammatory cytokines also expose the patient to a higher risk of thrombosis (Fig. 5.2). Finally, the tumor itself contributes to the prothrombotic state through the release of procoagulant factors in response to TKI therapy [49,59].

ANTI-VEGFR TYROSINE KINASE INHIBITORS

Sunitinib

Sunitinib is a small orally administered multitarget inhibitor of tyrosine kinase receptors that carries out its anticancer activity on different targets that regulate angiogenesis, survival, and cell proliferation including VEGFRs 1-3, PDGFRα and PDGFRβ, c-KIT, FMS-like tyrosine kinase-3 (FLT3), CFS-1 receptor (CSF1R), and the product of the human RET gene (RET).

At present sunitinib is used for the treatment of various neoplasms such as unresectable GIST [60,61] and unresectable or metastatic well-differentiated pancreatic neuroendocrine tumors [57]. In all these trials sunitinib demonstrated a cardiotoxicity profile peculiar enough to be further evaluated. Although sunitinib is a generally well-tolerated medication, hypertension is the most common side effect with a grade >2 hypertension risk ratio (RR) of 23 compared to placebo, as shown by a meta-analysis of approximately 5000 patients. Rini et al. further demonstrated that this adverse event required a dose adjustment or the addition of a drug in 6.8% of cases and that sunitinib is associated with a higher incidence of left ventricular dysfunction than other TKIs. Cardiac involvement was confirmed by an observational study in which Schmidinger et al. reported an increased incidence of cardiac event defined as elevated cardiac enzymes, symptomatic arrhythmia requiring treatment, new left ventricular dysfunction, or acute coronary syndrome in one third of patients treated with sunitinib. In another observational study, Schmidinger et al. reported that patients with advanced renal cancer receiving chemotherapy with sunitinib or sorafenib developed a higher incidence of cardiovascular events and, in particular, 40.5% of them registered ECG rhythm changes including conduction disturbances, axis change, QRS amplitude changes, ST segment depression, and elevation, T wave changes and QT prolongation; 18% of these were symptomatic, with clinical symptoms such as angina, dyspnea, and dizziness. Subsequently, many of these patients developed reduced LVEF, regional contractile dysfunctions, relaxation disturbances greater than grade 1, and pericardial effusion. In the GIST setting, researchers have documented an increased incidence of cardiovascular events. Chu et al. reported in patients with GIST previously treated with imatinib, that sunitinib treatment caused cardiac events in 11% of patients, with reductions in LVEF $\geq$15%, and increased blood pressure > G2 in 17% of patients. The authors also noted that many of the patients treated with sunitinib or sorafenib exhibited in an increase of cardiac biomarkers such as creatine kinase myocardial band (CK-MB; 54.5% vs. 78.6%) and troponins (54.5% vs. 21.4%) [56–58,60–64].

Sorafenib

Sorafenib is an orally administered multitarget small molecule inhibitor of tyrosine and serine/threonine kinases including VEGFR2 VEGFR3, PDGFRα and PDGFRβ, c-KIT, FLT3, v-raf-1 murine leukemia viral oncogene homolog 1 (RAF1) including BRAF kinases. This molecule is currently approved for the treatment of various cancers and in particular advanced hepatocellular carcinoma Child-Pugh Class A or B and advanced renal-cell carcinoma (RCC).

Sorafenib was evaluated by Llovet et al. in a phase-III randomized controlled trial in which it was compared against placebo in two cohorts of patients with advanced HCC never treated with chemotherapy. Sorafenib showed a significant benefit in terms of overall survival and a good profile of cardiovascular tolerability (fatigue >G2 4% vs. 3%; blood pressure >G2 2% vs. 1%). Cardiac ischemia or infarction occurred in 3% versus 1% of patients. Cardiac events were also reported in another phase-III randomized trial by Cheng et al. in which the incidence of heart attack

or cardiac ischemia occurring during treatment was 2.7% in sorafenib-treated patients and 1.3% in the placebo-treated group.

In another randomized controlled phase-III trial sorafenib was compared with placebo for the treatment of previously treated metastatic RCC demonstrating a significant benefit in terms of overall survival. The increased incidence of cardiovascular toxicity (fatigue >G2 14% vs. 5%; blood pressure >G2 4% vs. 0%) was similar to that recorded in the expanded access cohort of 2504 patients (blood pressure >G2 5%). Subsequent retrospective analysis showed that the increase in pressure was predictive of tumor response to treatment with sorafenib. Escudier et al. reported 22 events of myocardial ischemia (4.9% vs. 1.4%) and CHF (1.7% vs. 0.7%) among patients treated with sorafenib versus placebo. They also attributed an increase of the QT/QTc interval with consequent alteration of ventricular repolarization to sorafenib. In conclusion, sorafenib is a well-tolerated drug with a cardiotoxicity profile associated with higher incidence of hypertension (usually well controlled with a standard antihypertensive therapy), cardiac ischemia and infarction, with a higher risk for thromboembolic events (RR 3.03) as showed by a meta-analysis of more than 10,000 patients [65–69].

Regorafenib

Regorafenib is an oral multikinase inhibitor with a triple mechanism of action against targets involved in the regulation of angiogenesis, cell proliferation, and tumor stroma, including VEGFR1-3, TIE2, FGFR1 and PDGFRβ, c-KIT, and RET, along with the intracellular signaling kinases c-RAF/RAF-1, and its BRAF V600E mutant. Regorafenib is currently indicated for the treatment of refractory advanced colorectal cancer and advanced GIST resistant to imatinib and sunitinib chemotherapies. Like the other TKIs, regorafenib has a cardiotoxic profile. A recent meta-analysis assessed the risk of hypertension in patients taking regorafenib and reported a RR of hypertension >G2 of 8.39 and an incidence of hypertension >G2 of 12.5%. The authors point out that the overall incidence of hypertension differs significantly on the basis of the type of pathology (56.1% among patients with GIST, 49.0% among patients with RCC, 27.8% among patients with metastatic colorectal cancer, and 36.1% among patients with hepatocellular carcinoma). The incidence was highest with GIST and lowest with RCC, but it was clinically manageable with treatment interruption or dose reduction. Of note, in the randomized controlled phase-III GRID trial, authors reported one patient with cardiac arrest. Regorafenib was also studied in metastatic colorectal cancer in two large phase-III randomized controlled trial, the CORRECT trial and the CONCUR trial (the first on a western population and the second on an Asian population). Hypertension >G2 was reported in 7%

and 11%, whereas fatigue >G2 was reported in 9% and 3%, respectively. Furthermore, in the CONCUR study, 1 patient had an atrial fibrillation, 1 patient had mesenteric ischemia, and 1 patient had dyspnea, whereas in the CORRECT trial, authors reported all-grade dyspnea in 6% and nosebleeds in 7% of patients [70–72].

Axitinib

Axitinib is a third-generation selective inhibitor of VEGF receptors 1–3 and is indicated for the treatment of patients with advanced renal cancer after failure of prior treatment with sunitinib or a cytokine. Axitinib also has a cardiovascular toxicity profile revealed by the various trials in which it was evaluated. Axitinib is associated with a significant increase in cases of hypertension, as demonstrated by a recent meta-analysis of Abdel-Rahman where the subgroup of patients treated with Axitinib had a RR of hypertension (all grades) of 2.63; this value is not significantly different from the other drugs studied in this analysis (sunitinib RR 3.48; cediranib RR 2.26). In contrast, treatment with sunitinib significantly increased the risk of bleeding (sunitinib RR 2.80 vs. axitinib RR 1.02 vs. cediranib RR 1.11) and venous thromboembolism (sunitinib RR 2.05 vs. axitinib RR 0.53 vs. cediranib RR 0.51). There was no subgroup analysis of arterial hypertension >G2 but this information can be extrapolated from the analysis of outcomes of individual trials reported in the meta-analysis (axitinib 15.5% vs. 5.5% in controls). No information on high-grade left-ventricular dysfunction was reported. The cardiovascular profile of axitinib was also investigated in another meta-analysis by Qi et al. which included trials involving various tumors (metastatic RCC, metastatic melanoma, metastatic breast cancer, advanced non-small-cell lung cancer (NSCLC), pancreatic cancer, and all histological subtypes of advanced thyroid cancer), although the majority of cases were renal and pancreatic advanced neoplasms. The reported incidence of all grades hypertension was 40.1% (RR 3.00), whereas the incidence of hypertension >G2 was 13.1% (RR 1.71) and was associated with treatment interruption or reduction of the dose of the drug. Furthermore, the increase in the incidence of all grades of hypertension was greater in patients with renal neoplasms (57.6%) compared to other neoplasms (28.4%), which was also the case for hypertension >G2 (28.4% vs. 7.2%). Finally in a recent analysis of the phase-III AXIS published by Rini et al. in which axitinib was compared with sorafenib, the authors reported an incidence of 40% for hypertension of all degrees and 16% for hypertension >G2 (trial not blinded); the causes for drug discontinuation were fatigue (1%; 4) and transient ischemic attack (<1%; 3). Further analysis also revealed a relationship between diastolic blood pressure > or equal to 90 mmHg and tumor response: thus hypertension may not only predict efficacy of treatment with

axitinib but also suggests that antitumor effect and cardiovascular toxicity may be inseparable [73–76].

Nintedanib

Nintedanib is a novel oral selective TKI against all subtypes of VEGF, FGF and PDGFRα and β, together with RET and FLT3. Nintedanib is usually very well tolerated, with a favorable cardiovascular safety profile tested in various neoplastic diseases including RCC, HCC, ovarian/endometrial cancer, lung cancer, breast cancer, prostate cancer, gliomas, and colorectal cancer. In a phase-II trial in advanced renal neoplasms, Eisen et al. reported that nintedanib, unlike other TKI molecules, does not give rise to QTc interval prolongations. Furthermore, cardiovascular adverse events were not encountered. Nintedanib has been studied as a single agent and in association with chemotherapeutic regimens, with the best results in the treatment of advanced lung and ovarian cancers. Nintedanib was investigated in the LUME-Lung 1 phase-III, randomized, double-blind trial, which compared nintedanib plus docetaxel versus docetaxel plus placebo in patients with locally advanced/metastatic non-small-cell lung cancer after failure of first-line therapy. The most common adverse events in patients in the experimental arm included diarrhea responsive to supportive care and reversible elevation of liver enzymes managed with dose reduction. Furthermore, the only reported cardiac adverse event was hypertension <G2 in 15.4% of the patients. Recently du Bois et al. reported their experience in patients suffering from advanced ovarian cancer and treated upfront with a standard first-line chemotherapy regimen containing carboplatin and paclitaxel plus nintedanib or placebo. In this randomized phase-III trial the most common adverse events were gastrointestinal too; in particular, diarrhea >G2 had an incidence of almost 22% in nintedanib arm versus 2% in the placebo arm. Drug-related adverse events leading to death occurred in three patients in the nintedanib group but none of these was correlated to cardiovascular events (diarrhea, kidney failure, and peritonitis) [77,78].

Vandetanib

Vandetanib is another oral small molecule TKI with multitarget action against receptors including VEGFR1, VEGFR2, VEGFR3, EGFR, RET, PDGFRβ. This drug has been approved for the treatment of advanced medullary thyroid cancer and has also been studied in the treatment of advanced NSCLC. This drug has a cardiotoxic profile like the other TKIs and has been the subject of several meta-analyses. Zang et al. analyzed alterations of the QTc interval in patients with neoplasms and treated with vandetanib and observed a 3.7% incidence of high-grade prolonged QTc interval in patients with nonthyroid cancers and 12.0% in patients with medullary thyroid cancer. A subsequent meta-analysis of W-X Qi et al. included 11 trials and more than 3000 patients with advanced NSCLC and advanced thyroid cancer; they reported an increased incidence of hypertension >G2 in patients with lung cancer (7.6%, RR 10.22) and thyroid cancer (8.8%), but incidence was lower in patients with other neoplasms (3.4%). This suggests that incidence of hypertension may be significantly influenced by the type of neoplasia. This suggests that all patients receiving vandetanib should be monitored for hypertension, and in cases of severe or persistent hypertension despite the initiation of antihypertensive treatment, dose reduction or interruption may be necessary. The risk of developing high blood pressure in patients with advanced NSCLC was also the subject of a recent meta-analysis performed by Y. Liu et al., in which the authors showed that vandetanib compared to control was responsible for a significant increase in the risk of hypertension (RR 5.58) and prolongation of QTc interval (RR 7.90). Cardiovascular toxicity may be underestimated in the first-line treatment due to the small amount of data from only two studies; further studies are needed to define the risk of patients in this setting [79–81].

Pazopanib

Pazopanib is another multitarget oral TKI that exerts its action against VEGFR1, VEGFR2, VEGFR3, PDGFRα and β, FGFR1, FGFR3, c-KIT, LCK, and macrophage colony-stimulating factor-1 receptor. It is currently available for treatment of patients with advanced renal cancer and soft-tissue sarcomas, although it has also been studied in advanced epithelial ovarian cancer.

Like the other TKIs, pazopanib has a particular cardiovascular toxicity profile that has been evaluated in detail by WX Qi et al. in a meta-analysis of the major studies, which showed that pazopanib significantly increased the risk of high blood pressure >G2 (RR 2.87) with an incidence of 6.8% among patients with advanced RCC and 6.2% among other malignancies without statistically significant differences between the groups; it was associated with an increase in morbidity and interruption of chemotherapic treatment. Pazopanib is also responsible for abnormal ventricular repolarization. AM Pick et al. in their review recommended a close monitoring of ECG and cardiac enzymes in patients with existing heart disorders or QT prolongation, due to an increased incidence of torsades de pointes (less than 2%); they recommended avoiding other drugs with direct action on the same cardiac phase. The same authors point out that Pazopanib is also associated with thromboembolic events with an incidence of MI and cerebrovascular accidents of about 3% versus 0% in placebo group. These data were similar to those of another study about ovarian cancers in which CN Sternberg et al. reported an increased incidence of cardiovascular events (MI/ischemia 2%, cerebrovascular

accident <1%, and transient ischemic attack <1% compared with the none reported in the placebo arm). In treatment of advanced soft tissue sarcomas (PALETTE trial), pazopanib was associated with increased incidence of fatigue (fatigue >G2 13%) and hypertension (>G2 7%) with a significant reduction in LVEF compared with placebo (5% vs. 3%) [82–84].

Vatalanib

Vatalanib is a small molecule TKI that interferes with the ATP-binding site of VEGFR1-3, with an inhibitory action also against c-KIT and PDGFRα. The safety profile of vatalanib has been evaluated in several malignancies although larger studies were performed in the treatment of metastatic colorectal cancer and in advanced NSCLC. In colorectal cancer, vatalanib was evaluated in two randomized phase-III trials. In the CONFIRM 1 study, previously untreated metastatic colorectal cancer patients were randomly assigned to receive FOLFOX chemotherapic regimen plus valatanib or placebo. The authors reported a significant increase in cardiovascular toxicity >G2 among patients assigned to the experimental treatment compared to placebo (hypertension 23.0% vs. 6.8%, pulmonary embolism 5.7% vs. 1.7%, with no significant difference in venous thromboembolism incidence (5.2% vs. 3.5%). In the study CONFIRM 2, patients with advanced colorectal neoplasm whose disease had recurred or progressed during or within 6 months of treatment with irinotecan in combination with fluoropyrimidine were randomly assigned to a FOLFOX chemotherapic regimen plus vatalanib or placebo. The cardiac toxicity profile reported by the authors was very similar to that reported in the CONFIRM 1 trial and in particular they noted an increase in >G2 hypertension (21.8% vs. 6.0%) and fatigue (14.7% vs. 7.4%). In vatalanib arm, there was also a higher incidence of deep vein thrombosis, pulmonary embolism, and thromboembolic events. Vatalanib was evaluated in an uncontrolled phase-II trial in patients with NSCLC (stage IIIB or IV) who had disease progression on a first-line platinum-containing or chemoradiotherapy regimen. They reported an incidence of hypertension >G2 of 12%, fatigue >G2 of 2% and pulmonary embolism >G2 of 6%; two patients died from causes probably related to the treatment (pulmonary hemorrhage) [85–87].

Cediranib

Cediranib is an indole–ether quinazoline molecule and a potent small TKI, orally taken. It is a pan-VEGF receptor TKI (VEGFR-1, VEGFR-2, VEGFR-3), with greater selectivity for VEGFR-2; it also inhibits PDGFRs (PDGFRα, PDGFRβ) and c-KIT. Studies revealed that this molecule has an IC_{50} of <0.001 μM for VEGFR2, <0.003 μM for VEGFR3, <0.002 μM for c-KIT, <0.005 μM for PDGFRβ,

<0.036 µM for PDGFRα, and <0.026 µM for FGFR-1. It has been studied in patients with recurrent glioblastoma that failed standard therapy, in epithelial ovarian cancer combined with platinum-based chemotherapy, in advanced biliary tract cancer, in NSCLC, in colon cancer, breast cancer, metastatic renal cancer, and hormone-refractory prostate cancer. Hypertension and fatigue are the main side effects reported. The Recentin in Glioblastoma Alone and With Lomustine (REGAL) study is a randomized, phase-III, placebo-controlled, partially blinded study evaluating the efficacy of cediranib in monotherapy or in combination with lomustine versus lomustine alone in 325 patients with recurrent glioblastoma who previously received radiation and temozolomide. They were assigned 2:2:1 to receive cediranib (30 mg) in monotherapy, cediranib (20 mg) plus lomustine (110 mg/m^2), or lomustine (110 mg/m^2) plus placebo. Among grade 3 and 4 adverse events the authors noted hypertension and pulmonary embolism. Hypertension was present in 18 patients (14.1%) receiving cediranib alone, but occurred in only 8 patients (6.5%) receiving cediranib plus lomustine. No G > 2 hypertension was encountered in the group placebo plus lomustine. Pulmonary embolism occurred in four patients (3.1%) with cediranib, in six patients (4.9%) receiving cediranib plus lomustine, and in four patients (6.3%) in the group receiving placebo plus lomustine. Unfortunately the study did not satisfy the primary end point of demonstrating a benefit in progression-free survival for either cediranib-containing arm versus lomustine, even though preclinical studies suggested synergistic activity of anti-VEGF therapy in combination with radiation. For this reason cediranib has been studied in combination with chemoradiotherapy in a phase-II trial. A randomized, open-label, phase-II study recruited 90 women with measurable platinum-sensitive, relapsed, high-grade serous or endometrioid ovarian, fallopian tube, or primary peritoneal cancer, and women with deleterious germline BRCA1/2 mutations. They were divided in two groups: 46 women received olaparib 400 mg twice daily, whereas 44 received the combination of cediranib 30 mg daily and olaparib 200 mg twice daily. The most common G > 2 side effects were fatigue, diarrhea, and hypertension. Incidence of these adverse events was higher in the cediranib plus olaparib group, confirming the phase-I findings. No hypertension was observed in the olaparib group. In the cediranib plus olaparib group, hypertension of varying severity was encountered: G1, two patients (5%), G1-2, fifteen patients (34%), G3, seventeen patients (39%), and G4, one patient (2%). Fatigue of grade 2–3 was increased about twofold in the group cediranib plus olaparib in comparison with the olaparib group (54% vs. 26%). Another phase-II study evaluated the use of cediranib in this group of cancers. Of 23 women who received the drug at a dose of 45 mg, 10 patients (43%) had grade-1–2 hypertension, 8 patients (35%) had grade 3, whereas 2 patients (9%) had grade-4

hypertension. Eleven patients (48%) had grade-1–2 fatigue and seven patients (30%) had grade-3 fatigue. Two patients (9%) had grade-1–2 chest pain and two patients (9%) had grade-4 myocardial ischemia. In the same study 51 patients were treated with cediranib at the dose of 30 mg, among them 22 patients (43%) had grade-1–2 hypertension, 14 patients (27%) had grade-3 hypertension, whereas no grade-4 hypertension was reported. Fatigue (grade 1–2) was reported in 26 patients (51%) and grade 3 in 10 patients (20%). Three patients (6%) had grade-1–2 chest pain. Different results were reported in a placebo-controlled, randomized, double-blind phase-II trial of patients with metastatic carcinoma or who developed metastatic disease or local pelvic recurrence after radical treatment. Sixty-nine patients received carboplatin AUC of 5 plus paclitaxel 175 mg/m^2 by infusion every 3 weeks for a maximum of six cycles with cediranib 20 mg or placebo orally once daily until disease progression. Among the 34 patients receiving standard chemotherapy plus cediranib grade-1/2 hypertension was present in 19 patients (59%); no grade 3 or 4 was reported. Dyspnea grade 1/2 was present in 4 patients (13%), whereas no grade 3 or 4 was noted. Fatigue grade 1/2 was present in 26 patients (81%), grade 3 in 4 patients (13%), with no grade 4 fatigue. A randomized, double-blind, placebo-controlled phase-III trial (ICON 6, NCT00532194) compared cediranib versus placebo in combination with carboplatin and paclitaxel in platinum-sensitive recurrent ovarian cancer patients. In this study 456 women were randomly assigned to receive standard therapy with carboplatin and paclitaxel plus placebo followed by placebo as maintenance therapy, or carboplatin and paclitaxel plus cediranib 20 mg/day followed by placebo as maintenance therapy or cediranib 20 mg/day as maintenance therapy. In this study grade-3 hypertension was encountered in 4 patients (7%). A recent multicenter, placebo-controlled, randomized phase II trial of 124 patients with histologically confirmed or cytologically confirmed advanced biliary tract cancer were treated with first-line cisplatin and gemcitabine chemotherapy (25 mg/m^2 cisplatin and 1000 mg/m^2 gemcitabine, on days 1 and 8 every 21 days, for up to eight cycles) with either 20 mg cediranib or placebo once a day until disease progression. Cediranib was received by 62 patients. Grade-1/2 fatigue was seen in 36 patients (58%) and grade-3/4 fatigue in 16 patients (26%) in the cediranib group. Grade-1/2 hypertension was present in 19 patients (31%), while grade 3/4 was present in 23 (37%). Fifteen patients (24%) had grade-1/2 dyspnea, whereas only one patient (2%) had grade-3/4 dyspnea. MI grade 3/4 occurred in one patient (2%). Unfortunately, cediranib did not enhance the progression-free survival of these patients. Ongoing phase-III trials are studying cediranib for the first-line treatment of metastatic colorectal cancer (mCRC). These are HORIZON II and HORIZON III. The HORIZON II trial compares chemotherapy (FOLFOX or XELOX) with cediranib or placebo in patients with metastatic colorectal cancer, while the HORIZON III compares mFOLFOX6 (modified 5-fluorouracil [5-FU]/leucovorin/oxaliplatin) in combination with cediranib versus mFOLFOX6 in combination with bevacizumab. An open-labeled, single-agent, phase-II study evaluated the development of hypertension and proteinuria in 46 patients with recurrent epithelial ovarian carcinoma receiving cediranib. The authors reported a rapid onset of hypertension: by the third day of drug administration, 67% patients developed hypertension, 73% by day 7, and 87% by the end of the study. Grade-3 hypertension developed in 43% of patients, and 24% developed grade 3 fatigue [88–100].

Cabozantinib

Cabozantinib is a TKI approved for the treatment of patients with progressive, metastatic medullary thyroid cancer (mMTC). It has been also studied in advanced prostate cancer and advanced RCC. Studies revealed that it inhibits the activity of multiple kinases including RET, MET, VEGFR-1, -2 and -3, KIT, TRKB, FLT-3, AXL, and TIE-2. Elisei et al. conducted a double-blind, phase-III trial in which they compared cabozantinib (140 mg per day) to placebo in a 2:1 ratio in 330 patients with documented radiographic progression of mMTC. Among these patients, 219 were treated with cabozantinib. Common cardiovascular side effects in cabozantinib-treated patients included fatigue, hypertension, asthenia, and dyspnea. All grades fatigue was present in 86 patients (40.7%), with grade 3–4 in 20 patients (9.3%). All grades hypertension was present in 70 patients (32.7%), with grade 3–4 in 18 (8.4%). All grades asthenia was present in 45 patients (21%), with grade 3–4 in 12 (5.6%). All grades dyspnea was reported in 29 patients (13.6%), whereas grade 3–4 dyspnea occurred in 5 patients (2.3%). Severe adverse events were more frequent in cabozantinib-treated patients (214 patients). These included pulmonary embolism in 5 patients (2.3% vs. 0% in placebo group) and hypertension in 5 patients (2.3% vs 0%). Among the grade-5 adverse events which occurred within 30 days of last dose of cabozantinib, treatment-related events included respiratory failure, sudden death, and cardiopulmonary failure (total three patients). Cabozantinib (140 mg per day) in this study achieved a statistically significant enhancement of progression-free survival in these patients. In a phase-II study by Smith et al., 144 patients with chemotherapy-pretreated metastatic castration-resistant prostate cancer (mCRPC) received open-label cabozantinib; 93 patients received a daily dose of 100 mg, whereas the other 51 patients received 40 mg daily until tumor progression or intolerable toxicity. Cardiovascular side effects reported in the study were dose-related fatigue, dyspnea, hypertension, and pulmonary embolism. In the 100-mg cabozantinib cohort 77 patients (83%) had all grades fatigue, of which 25 patients (27%) presented grade 3–4 fatigue. All grades dyspnea was

present in 30 patients (32%), of which 6 patients (6%) had grade 3–4 dyspnea. All grades hypertension was present in 23 patients (25%), of which 14 patients (15%) had grade 3–4 hypertension. In the 40-mg cabozantinib cohort 32 patients (63%) had all grades fatigue, of which 7 patients (14%) suffered grade 3–4 fatigue. All grades dyspnea was present in 13 patients (25%), of which one patient (2%) had grade 3–4 dyspnea. All grades hypertension was present in 10 patients (20%), of which 6 patients (12%) had grade 3–4 hypertension. Incidence of grade 3–4 pulmonary embolism was 8% in the 100-mg cohort, versus 18% in the 40-mg cohort. The study found that the drug exhibited significant clinical activity in mCRPC. Cabozantinib has also been studied in a randomized, open-label, phase-III trial, the METEOR trial, comparing the efficacy of cabozantinib to everolimus, in 658 patients with RCC and disease progression after VEGFR-targeted therapy. Patients received cabozantinib 60 mg daily (330 patients) or everolimus 10 mg daily. The cardiovascular side effects were fatigue, hypertension, asthenia, dyspnea and peripheral edema. All grades fatigue was present in 186 patients (56%), grade 3–4 fatigue was present in 30 (9%). All grades hypertension developed in 122 patients (37%), with grade 3–4 hypertension in 49 (15%). All grades asthenia occurred in 62 patients (19%), with grade 3–4 asthenia in 14 (4%). All grades dyspnea was present in 62 patients (19%), with grade 3–4 in 10 (3%). All grades peripheral edema was present in 31 patients (9%), with no grade 3 or 4. The study revealed longer progression-free survival in the cabozantinib group than in the everolimus group. Other studies showed that there was a higher incidence of thrombotic events using the drug in comparison with placebo. Venous thromboembolism showed an incidence of 6% versus 3% and arterial thromboembolism 2% versus 0%. The studies in patients with mMTC evaluated the effect of this drug on QTc interval. There was a mild increase in QTcF of 10–15 ms after four weeks of treatment, but none of the patients had a QTcF > 500 ms [101–104].

Lenvatinib

Lenvatinib, another TKI, inhibits mainly VEGFR1 (FLT1), VEGFR2 (KDR), and VEGFR3 (FLT4), but it also inhibits other kinases including FGF receptors FGFR1, 2, 3, and 4, PDGFRα, KIT, and RET. It has been approved for the treatment of patients with locally recurrent or metastatic, progressive, radioactive iodine-refractory differentiated thyroid cancer. It has also been studied in advanced hepatocellular carcinoma and metastatic RCC.

The SELECT trial, a randomized, double-blind, multicenter phase-III study, evaluated 612 patients with progressive thyroid cancer refractory to iodine-131 treatment, of which 392 were randomized to receive lenvatinib at a dose of 24 mg per day in 28-day cycles (261 patients) or placebo (131 patients). The authors observed all grades hypertension in 67.8% patients, with grade 3–4 hypertension in 41.8%. All grades fatigue or asthenia was present in 59%, with grade 3–4 in 9.2%. All grades peripheral edema occurred in 11.1%, grade 3–4 in 0.4%. All grades pulmonary embolism was present in 2.7%, with grade 3–4 in 2.7%. This study showed improvements with lenvatinib compared to placebo in progression-free survival and tumor response rate, although patients who received lenvatinib had more side effects. Recently Schlumberger et al. conducted a phase-II multicenter, open-label, single-arm trial in patients with medullary thyroid carcinoma. Lenvatinib was administered to 59 patients once a day at a starting dose of 24 mg in 28-day treatment cycles for eight cycles in the absence of disease progression, uncontrolled toxicities, or death. They reported all grades fatigue in 31 patients (53%), with grade 3–4 in 3 (5%). All grades hypertension was present in 30 patients (51%), of which 4 (7%) had grade 3–4. All grades dyspnea occurred in 16 patients (27%), of which one patient (2%) had grade 3–4. One patient (2%) interrupted treatment due to hypertension. Among serious adverse events that occurred in 51% of patients, pulmonary embolism occurred in 3.4%. Motzer et al. studied this drug in a randomized, phase-II, open-label, multicenter trial in advanced or metastatic clear-cell RCC, enrolling patients to receive lenvatinib plus everolimus or single-agent lenvatinib or single-agent everolimus. The treatment was taken once a day in 28-day continuous cycles. Patients received the single-agent therapy with lenvatinib 24 mg daily (two capsules of 10 mg and one capsule of 4 mg). Single-agent lenvatinib was received by 52 patients. Of these, 22 (42%) had grade 1–2 fatigue or asthenia, whereas 4 patients (8%) had grade-3 fatigue or asthenia; no grade 4 was reported. Grade 1–2 hypertension was present in 16 patients (31%), whereas 9 patients (17%) had grade-3 hypertension; no grade 4 was registered. Peripheral edema was present only grade 1–2 in eight patients (15%). Grade 1–2 dyspnea was experienced by 10 patients (19%); only one patient had grade-3 dyspnea (2%), and no patient developed grade-4 dyspnea. One patient receiving single-agent lenvatinib had a fatal MI [105–109].

Linifanib

Linifanib is another oral TKI drug. Its activity is selective for the VEGF and platelet-PDGF receptors, thereby blocking two of the most important signaling pathways involved in tumor progression. The activity and efficacy of linifanib has been studied in many tumors (NSCLC, renal cancer, hepatocellular cancer, colorectal cancer, and breast cancer). The major results were achieved in the field of advanced NSCLC. A prospective randomized phase-II study evaluated linifanib at two different doses (7.5 and 12.5 mg) versus placebo in combination with carboplatin and paclitaxel. The addition of linifanib significantly improved progression free survival (PFS) [5.2 months for placebo vs. 10.2 months

(7.5 mg dose) or 8.3 months (12.5 mg dose)]. Both treatment arms containing linifanib authors reported an increased incidence of adverse events, the most common of which included diarrhea (27.7%), anemia (14.3%), and high blood pressure (4.3%); thrombocytopenia was the most frequent cause of treatment interruption and/or reduction of the associated chemotherapy regimen. The tolerability profile of linifanib was already investigated in previous phase-I studies. In particular, Chiu YL et al. conducted a careful study of linifanib's effects on cardiac ventricular repolarization. Although the study was small (24 patients, in a crossover design), they concluded that linifanib, unlike other TKI, does not cause an increased risk of QTc prolongation at the highest concentration for the maximum tolerated dose of the drug [110,111].

Telatinib

Telatinib is an orally active small molecule TKI with activity toward VEGFR2-3 and PDGFRβ. The activity of this molecule has been assessed in several kinds of cancer. Mross et al. published a multicenter phase-I study in which 29 heavily pretreated patients with advanced colorectal cancer were treated with telatinib at 600 up to 1500 mg twice daily showing that the molecule had a substantial effect on tumor shrinkage and also showed a favorable safety profile. High blood pressure was the most common adverse event (all grades, 36%, grade 3, 28%) but was clinically manageable with appropriate antihypertensive therapy, although in three patients it was necessary to reduce the dose, interrupt treatment, or discontinue treatment. Authors also observed fatigue (2% grade 1–2 in non-continuous dosing schedule, and 7% in the continuous dosing schedule) and diarrhea as specific toxicities requiring dose reduction or interruption of treatment. At the time of this writing, results of phase-II trials have not been published. One phase-II trial will evaluate telatinib in combination with chemotherapy in patients with advanced gastric cancer (NCT00952497) [112].

Brivanib

Much scientific evidence has also shown that among the factors responsible for angiogenesis, a key role belongs to the FGF. For this reason, new molecules were synthesized with the ability to selectively block VEGF and FGF simultaneously with the intent to overcome drug resistance to VEGF pathway inhibitors.

Brivanib is an oral dual inhibitor of the growth signals from the activation of VEGFR and FGFR that demonstrated a tenacious antitumor and antiangiogenic activity. This drug has been tested in several cancers including colorectal cancer, hepatocellular cancer, renal cell cancer, and NSCLC. A phase-I study demonstrated high activity of brivanib in solid tumors; the main toxicities of the drug at the maximum tolerated dose (800 mg continuous, intermittent 800 mg, and 400 mg bid) consisted of nausea, diarrhea, fatigue (15–25% G3-4), dizziness, hypertension (15-25% G3-4), headache and anorexia; cardiac ventricular repolarization changes were not reported. Two randomized phase-III studies evaluated brivanib at 800 mg orally daily in advanced hepatocellular carcinoma. The study BRISK-FL is a noninferiority study that compared brivanib with the standard sorafenib in patients with advanced hepatocellular carcinoma without prior chemotherapy. The study BRISK-PS evaluated patients who progressed on/after or were intolerant to sorafenib that were randomly assigned (2:1) to receive brivanib 800 mg orally once per day plus best supportive care (BSC) or placebo plus BSC. Both studies failed to demonstrate any benefit in terms of overall survival and also reported a characteristic dose-dependent increase in the incidence of toxicities with brivanib (BRISK-FL fatigue >G2 14.5%; blood pressure >G2 13.3%—BRISK-PS fatigue >G2 13%; blood pressure >G2 16%) which were responsible for a decrease in performance status in patients assigned to brivanib. The authors of both studies report deaths that were considered possibly related to treatment in the experimental arm not clearly attributed to cardiovascular function abnormalities. Finally another randomized phase-III study investigated the efficacy of brivanib in combination with cetuximab (anti EGFR moAb) compared to single-agent cetuximab plus placebo in patients with chemotherapy-refractory advanced colorectal cancer. Authors did not demonstrate any significant benefit in terms of survival global but only in terms of progression free survival at the cost of a significant increase in related toxicity (fatigue >G2 25%; blood pressure >G2 11%; dyspnea >G2 8%) and a more rapid deterioration of patient performance status, terminating further experimental trials with this drug [113–117].

Foretinib

Foretinib is an oral multikinase inhibitor targeting MET, RON, AXL, Tie-2, VEGFR, c-KIT, Flt-3, and PDGFR signaling pathways.

Foretinib activity was evaluated in several preliminary studies where it was found to be particularly active against gastric and renal cancer. In particular MA Shah et al. studied Foretinib in a phase-II trial in which the drug was administered on an intermittent or daily schedule in a single cohort of unselected previously treated patients with advanced or metastatic gastric cancer. Although neither mode of drug administration caused significant toxicity, including the cardiovascular profile (fatigue >G2 4.2% and 3.8%; blood pressure >G2 6.3% and 15.4%), foretinib as a single agent did not show significant effect on tumor regression except for patients carrying a MET gene amplification. In another phase-II study, TK Choueiri et al. evaluated the activity of

foretinib with the same intermittent or daily schedules in 74 patients with locally advanced, bilateral multifocal, or metastatic sporadic papillary RCC or known hereditary papillary RCC, and observed appreciable antitumor activity (overall response rate 13.5%), especially in the subgroup of patients carrying a germline mutation of the MET gene. Drug treatment was also associated with significant cardiovascular toxicity for both intermittent and daily regimens (blood pressure >G2 35.1% and 68%; fatigue >G2 5.4% and 8.0%; proteinuria >G2 5% and 5%). They also reported nine events of nonfatal pulmonary embolism of which three were only recognized at the time of disease progression [118,119].

Motesanib

Motesanib is an angiogenesis inhibitor that targets VEGFR1-3 and also exerts direct antitumor activity by acting as an antagonist PDGFR and c-KIT. Its chemical structure and mechanism of action make motesanib a very promising molecule against tumor-mediated angiogenesis. Motesanib has been evaluated in several phase-I and -II and preclinical trials, but in large phase-III randomized trials, it has not shown significant benefits on major clinical endpoints of overall survival or progression-free survival. In the phase-III randomized controlled MONET-1 study, GV Scagliotti et al. did not detect any improvement in overall survival and minimal cardiotoxicity comparing motesanib to placebo when used in combination with carboplatin and paclitaxel in patients with lung cancer, squamous cell non-small-cell stage IV. However, a preplanned analysis of an Asian subgroup conducted by Kubota et al. found encouraging results in terms of objective response rate, progression-free survival, and overall survival, providing a strong rationale for the phase-III randomized controlled MONET-A study among Asian patients in Japan, South Korea, Taiwan, and Hong Kong. This trial of 401 patients with Stage IV or recurrent nonsquamous NSCLC randomized patients in a 1:1 ratio to paclitaxel and carboplatin plus either placebo or motesanib. Although Motesanib exhibited no significant difference in cardiovascular toxicity >G2 between motesanib and placebo, the drug failed to demonstrate efficacy in terms of objective response rate, progression-free survival, and overall survival [120,121].

Lucitanib

Lucitanib is a newer oral FGFR1-2, VEGFR1-3, and PGFRα-β inhibitor, although preclinical proteomics analyses suggest it may exert its antitumor activity through additional unidentified targets. Lucitanib assessment in the clinical setting is still at a very preliminary stage. It has been tested in a single phase-I/IIa trial on solid tumors, showing promising results in terms of effectiveness (complete + partial response 26–50% depending on tumor subgroup) with a maximum tolerated dose of 15 mg/day. Cardiovascular toxicity was frequently enountered including hypertension (all grades 91%; >G2 57.9%) requiring antihypertensive medication, dose reduction, or discontinuation, as well as asthenia (42%) and proteinuria (57%). Based on the preliminary findings of efficacy, lucitanib will be investigated in further trials (NCT02202746, NCT02053636) [122,123].

Fruquintinib

Fruquintinib is another recently-developed oral TKI which exerts its antitumor activity through the selective blocking of VEGFR1-3. Fruquintinib is still at an early stage in clinical trials. In a phase-Ib trial fruquintinib has shown good efficacy with a sufficient safety profile when used at 5 mg once daily dose in cycles of 3 weeks on and 1 week off in patients with previously treated advanced colorectal cancer. The most significant toxicities were hand–foot syndrome (HFS), hoarseness, proteinuria, hypertension, and fatigue (no incidence data are reported). Further studies are ongoing (NCT02415023, NCT02691299, NCT02314819) [124].

Tivozanib

Tivozanib is an oral TKI that selectively inhibits the signal transduction pathway activated by VEGFR1-3 receptors. Preclinical studies of tivozanib demonstrated activity on xenograft models of RCC and have justified its extensive testing in this clinical setting. Phase-I studies of Tivozanib at a dose of 1.5 mg/day for 4 weeks on and 2 weeks off reported promising clinical responses with side effects of arterial hypertension, fatigue, and headache. On the basis of these data, tivozanib was evaluated in a discontinuation phase-II randomized trial in patients with advanced RCC; the most common severe adverse event (G3-4) was hypertension (12%), and elevation of GGT (16%). Subsequently, tivozanib was evaluated in a large confirmatory phase-III randomized, controlled trial (TIVO-1) in which tivozanib 1.5 mg/day for 3 weeks on and 1 week off was compared with sorafenib 400 mg/day in patients with advanced RCC not previously treated with VEGF or mTOR inhibitors. Tivozanib study showed particular cardiovascular toxicity characterized by blood pressure >G2 in 27% (vs. 18% on the sorafenib arm) and from fatigue >G2 5% (vs. 4% with sorafenib). Hypertension was the leading cardiovascular cause dose reduction (2% vs. 4%). In tivozanib arm it should be noted that many deaths were associated with cardiovascular complications (two deaths resulted from myocardial infarction, two from cardiac failure, and one each from hypertension, dyspnea, cerebrovascular accident, aortic aneurysm rupture, coronary arteriosclerosis artery, cardiac arrest, apnea, pulmonary embolism), and for these reasons, in addition to the negative trend shown in median overall survival (28.8 vs. 29.3 months) and to the poor US study accrual (only 3%) the FDA denied permission to register this drug for this indication [125–127].

Apatinib

Apatinib is another oral TKI that acts by selective inhibition of VEGFR-2 signal transduction. The first studies that evaluated the antitumor activity in solid tumors demonstrated safety of apatinib at a dose of 500 mg/day. Experimentation with apatinib has been mainly in the field of gastric and breast cancer. X. Hu et al. evaluated apatinib in previously treated advanced non triple-negative breast neoplasm. The apatinib cardiovascular profile was very similar to that of other TKIs, with hypertension >G2 in 21.1%, with almost half of the patients requiring dose reduction. A similar experience was encountered in the triple negative patients at the same dose, with hypertension >G2 in 11.9% of patients in combination with fatigue >G2 in 3.4%. In this study, authors also reported one symptomatic pericardial effusion and one uncontrolled atrial fibrillation thought to be treatment related. Apatinib has shown promise in the treatment of advanced gastric cancer, where two schedules of administration were evaluated (850 mg daily vs. 425 mg twice daily) in a randomized controlled phase-II study in heavily pretreated patients. The cardiotoxicity profile was characterized by high blood pressure >G2 and fatigue >G2 similar in the two groups (8% vs. 11%; 2% vs. 2%), but showing a better overall safety profile when used in the schedule 425 mg twice daily [128–130].

CONCLUSIONS

The goal of this chapter is to provide to the reader a quick and useful guide regarding the use of TKIs in oncology with a focus on cardiovascular toxicity. To do this we have tried to collect all the data available in the literature, although some of the agents in this drug class are still at an early stage of experimentation. The TKIs exert their anticancer activity by inhibiting signal transduction of ligands and their receptors regulating tumor proliferation, its relationship with the microenvironment and particularly with angiogenesis. The angiogenesis mechanisms involve several key molecules such as VEGF and the corresponding receptor (VEGFR), whose action is crucial for the development and spread of solid tumors. It was amply demonstrated by preclinical studies that angiogenesis increases the metastatic potential of various malignancies such as hepatocellular carcinoma. The main TKIs studied in the antineoplastic field are sunitinib, sorafenib, regorafenib, axitinib, and pazopanib. They have proven to be effective in the treatment of various cancers such as colorectal, kidney, and liver. The management of adverse events related to the drug is crucial to increase the overall survival of patients maintaining a good quality of life. Surely, among the most important side effects, also in consideration of the aforementioned mechanism of action, there are those of the cardiovascular type, which require dose reductions and/or discontinuation of treatment, thereby limiting their efficacy. The risk for a cardiovascular event is related to the underlying cardiovascular risk of the patient. Patients with pre-existing chronic disease such as hypertension, diabetes, renal disease, or previous cardiovascular event are considered at highest risk, so proactive management of these conditions is warranted before administering a TKI. As revealed by the pivotal clinical trials, the occurrence of a G3 type event, however rare, must necessarily result in a temporary interruption of the treatment and/or a reduction of 50% of the dose of the drug on the basis of individual tolerance. Among the main events reported in the trials include high blood pressure, the incidence of which is significantly different depending on the type of cancer (RCC vs. non-RCC 25.9% versus 20.4%, RR 1.27, 95% CI: 1.13-1:43, p <0.001), although patients with RCC may have higher blood pressure at the outset. For Sunitinib, RR was 8.20 for patients with RCC (95% CI: 4.70 to 14:29), and only 1.42 for patients with GIST (95% CI: 0.81 to 4.2). This may be related to the higher levels of VEGF found in patients with clear cell RCC due to loss of function in Von Hippel-Lindau (VHL), or more likely because of the increased rate of nephrectomies, with reduction of nephrons and glomerular filtration rate in patients with RCC responsible for a reduced urinary excretion of the drug and perhaps also impaired sodium clearance. The use of TKIs is responsible in turn for cardiac and renal damage. It was reported that high blood pressure was associated with reduction of left ventricular function during treatment with sunitinib in patients with RCC, although the mechanism is still unclear, and although it was not possible to exclude direct cardiotoxicity of the drug. Some authors postulate that ventricular dysfunction may depend on the direct action of the VEGF pathway causing an alteration of the vascular architecture responsible for a lower microvascular density and diminished production of NO. The treatment schedule influences the risk of developing high blood pressure. In particular, H. Zhu et al. showed in a meta-analysis that the continuous administration of TKIs has an increased risk of higher blood pressure than the intermittent schedule (RR 1:32, 95% CI: 1.18–1.48, $P < 0.001$), probably due to the unremitting action of the drug on the vasculature. With regard to kidney damage, it has been shown that this may arise from cardiovascular abnormalities. The TKIs can contribute to renal injury through hypertension as well as direct effects on VEGFR signaling in the renal tubules and glomeruli. While arterial hypertension is one of the most common challenges managing patients receiving TKIs, hypertension has also been recognized as a predictor of tumor response, suggesting that antitumor effects and cardiovascular side effects may be inseparable.

Management of patients receiving TKIs should nevertheless provide for close blood pressure monitoring and appropriate medical management of hypertension. Treatments may include the use of angiotensin converting enzyme (ACE) inhibitors or angiotension-II receptor blockers (ARBs) that have demonstrated antiangiogenic effects in xenograft models. Nondihydropyridine calcium channel blockers that induce secretion of VEGF should be avoided in preference to the dihydropyridines (amlodipine, nifedipine). Despite these suggestions, the best therapeutic approach is not fully established, and is further complicated by interactions between TKIs and antihypertensive agents, necessitating further studies. Some authors suggest avoiding drugs that interfere with the CYP3A4 because of the potential increase in TKI effect. Blood pressure control can also include diuretics, alpha blockers, and beta blockers, although most data are from studies using bevacizumab. The limits of interpretation of data about hypertension are numerous. First, many trials reported hypertension as values >150/100 mmHg or an increase of 20 mmHg rather than values >140/90 mmHg, and no randomized controlled trials were designed with the aim to standardize this measurement. In addition, baseline blood pressure was not always reported, although such information is essential in nephrectomized patients may already have secondary hypertension.

Cardiovascular toxicity should not, however, limit the use of these drugs, as they have demonstrated great utility in the treatment of some cancers such as RCC, which until recently had few or no medical treatment options. Several authors, having noted the correlation between high blood pressure (>140/90 mmHg) and tumor response, have suggested hypertension may predict efficacy and might be helpful in selecting subgroups of patients most likely to benefit from the therapy. Because of the increased risk of cardiovascular complications including end-stage heart disease in these patients, there is great interest in early detection of cardiovascular toxicity. Recently K.A. Bordun et al. recreated hypertension in mice treated with bevacizumab or sunitinib and showed that the echocardiographic assessment by tissue velocity imaging (TVI) could detect early LV systolic dysfunction before the appearance of abnormalities in conventional echocardiographic indices. Of course, much more needs to be done in the development of these techniques but these encouraging findings suggest that this approach may help to prevent more severe cardiovascular events [56,57,60,62,131–144].

REFERENCES

[1] Claesson-Welsh L. Blood vessels as targets in tumor therapy. Ups J Med Sci 2012;117(2):178–86.

[2] WOOD S Jr. Pathogenesis of metastasis formation observed in vivo in the rabbit ear chamber. AMA Arch Pathol 1958;66(4):550–68.

[3] Greenblatt M, Shubi P. Tumor angiogenesis: transfilter diffusion studies in the hamster by the transparent chamber technique. J Natl Cancer Inst 1968;41(1):111–24.

[4] Ehrmann RL, Knoth M. Choriocarcinoma. Transfilter stimulation of vasoproliferation in the hamster cheek pouch. Studied by light and electron microscopy. J Natl Cancer Inst 1968;41(6):1329–41.

[5] Folkman J. Tumor angiogenesis: therapeutic implications. N Engl J Med 1971;285(21):1182–6.

[6] Tannock IF. The relation between cell proliferation and the vascular system in a transplanted mouse mammary tumor. Br J Cancer 1968;22(2):258–73.

[7] Schlaeppi JM, Wood JM. Targeting vascular endothelial growth factor (VEGF) for anti-tumor therapy, by anti-VEGF neutralizing monoclonal antibodies or by VEGF receptor tyrosine-kinase inhibitors. Cancer Metastasis Rev 1999;18(4):473–81.

[8] Manley PW, Bold G, Brüggen J, Fendrich G, Furet P, Mestan J, Schnell C, Stolz B, Meyer T, Meyhack B, Stark W, Strauss A, Wood J. Advances in the structural biology, design and clinical development of VEGF-R kinase inhibitors for the treatment of angiogenesis. Biochim Biophys Acta. 2004;1697(1–2):17–27.

[9] Yang JC, Haworth L, Sherry RM, Hwu P, Schwartzentruber DJ, Topalian SL, Steinberg SM, Chen HX, Rosenberg SA. A randomized trial of bevacizumab, an anti-vascular endothelial growth factor antibody, for metastatic renal cancer. N Engl J Med 2003;349(5):427–34.

[10] Miller KD, Chap LI, Holmes FA, Cobleigh MA, Marcom PK, Fehrenbacher L, Dickler M, Overmoyer BA, Reimann JD, Sing AP, Langmuir V, Rugo HS. Randomized phase III trial of capecitabine compared with bevacizumab plus capecitabine in patients with previously treated metastatic breast cancer. J Clin Oncol 2005;23(4):792–9.

[11] Geng L, Donnelly E, McMahon G, Lin PC, Sierra-Rivera E, Oshinka H, Hallahan DE. Inhibition of vascular endothelial growth factor receptor signaling leads to reversal of tumor resistance to radiotherapy. Cancer Res 2001;61(6):2413–9.

[12] Ferrara N. Vascular endothelial growth factor as a target for anticancer therapy. Oncologist 2004;9 Suppl 1:2–10.

[13] Zhao Y, Adjei AA. Targeting angiogenesis in cancer therapy: moving beyond vascular endothelial growth factor. Oncologist 2015;20(6):660–73.

[14] Folkman J. Angiogenesis: an organizing principle for drug discovery? Nat Rev Drug Discov 2007;6(4):273–86.

[15] Marek-Trzonkowska N, Kwieczy ska A, Reiwer-Gostomska M, Koli ski T, Molisz A, Siebert J. Arterial hypertension is characterized by imbalance of pro-angiogenic versus anti-angiogenic factors. PLoS One 2015;10(5).

[16] Fràter-Schröder M, Risau W, Hallmann R, Gautschi P, Böhlen P. Tumor necrosis factor type alpha, a potent inhibitor of endothelial cell growth in vitro, is angiogenic in vivo. Proc Natl Acad Sci USA 1987;84(15):5277–81.

[17] Marech I, Leporini C, Ammendola M, Porcelli M, Gadaleta CD, Russo E, De Sarro G, Ranieri G. Classical and non-classical proangiogenic factors as a target of antiangiogenic therapy in tumor microenvironment. Cancer Lett 2015;. pii: S0304-3835(15)00483-8.

[18] Herbst RS, Hong D, Chap L, Kurzrock R, Jackson E, Silverman JM, Rasmussen E, Sun YN, Zhong D, Hwang YC, Evelhoch JL, Oliner JD, Le N, Rosen LS. Safety, pharmacokinetics, and antitumor activity of AMG 386, a selective angiopoietin inhibitor, in adult patients with advanced solid tumors. J Clin Oncol 2009;27(21):3557–65.

[19] Seghezzi G, Patel S, Ren CJ, Gualandris A, Pintucci G, Robbins ES, Shapiro RL, Galloway AC, Rifkin DB, Mignatti P. Fibroblast growth factor-2 (FGF-2) induces vascular endothelial growth factor (VEGF) expression in the endothelial cells of forming capillaries: an autocrine mechanism contributing to angiogenesis. J Cell Biol 1998;141(7):1659–73.

[20] Nyberg P, Xie L, Kalluri R. Endogenous inhibitors of angiogenesis. Cancer Res 2005;65(10):3967–79.

[21] Ständker L, Schrader M, Kanse SM, Jürgens M, Forssmann WG, Preissner KT. Isolation and characterization of the circulating form of human endostatin. FEBS Lett 1997;420(2–3):129–33.

[22] Good DJ, Polverini PJ, Rastinejad F, Le Beau MM, Lemons RS, Frazier WA, Bouck NP. A tumor suppressor-dependent inhibitor of angiogenesis is immunologically and functionally indistinguishable from a fragment of thrombospondin. Proc Natl Acad Sci USA 1990;87(17):6624–8.

[23] Lingen MW, Polverini PJ, Bouck NP. Retinoic acid and interferon alpha act synergistically as antiangiogenic and antitumor agents against human head and neck squamous cell carcinoma. Cancer Res 1998;58(23):5551–8.

[24] Volpert OV, Fong T, Koch AE, Peterson JD, Waltenbaugh C, Tepper RI, Bouck NP. Inhibition of angiogenesis by interleukin 4. J Exp Med. 1998;188(6):1039–46.

[25] Voest EE, Kenyon BM, O'Reilly MS, Truitt G, D'Amato RJ, Folkman J. Inhibition of angiogenesis in vivo by interleukin 12. J Natl Cancer Inst 1995;87(8):581–6.

[26] Cornelius LA, Nehring LC, Harding E, Bolanowski M, Welgus HG, Kobayashi DK, Pierce RA, Shapiro SD. Matrix metalloproteinases generate angiostatin: effects on neovascularization. J Immunol 1998;161(12):6845–52.

[27] Hagedorn M, Zilberberg L, Wilting J, Canron X, Carrabba G, Giussani C, Pluderi M, Bello L, Bikfalvi A. Domain swapping in a COOH-terminal fragment of platelet factor 4 generates potent angiogenesis inhibitors. Cancer Res 2002;62(23):6884–90.

[28] Moses MA, Wiederschain D, Wu I, Fernandez CA, Ghazizadeh V, Lane WS, Flynn E, Sytkowski A, Tao T, Langer R. Troponin I is present in human cartilage and inhibits angiogenesis. Proc Natl Acad Sci USA 1999;96(6):2645–50.

[29] Pike SE, Yao L, Jones KD, Cherney B, Appella E, Sakaguchi K, Nakhasi H, Teruya-Feldstein J, Wirth P, Gupta G, Tosato G. Vasostatin, a calreticulin fragment, inhibits angiogenesis and suppresses tumor growth. J Exp Med 1998;188(12):2349–56.

[30] Wang GL, Jiang BH, Rue EA, Semenza GL. Hypoxia-inducible factor 1 is a basic-helix-loop-helix-PAS heterodimer regulated by cellular O_2 tension. Proc Natl Acad Sci USA 1995;92(12):5510–4.

[31] Wang GL, Semenza GL. Purification and characterization of hypoxia-inducible factor 1. J Biol Chem 1995;270(3):1230–7.

[32] Jiang BH, Semenza GL, Bauer C, Marti HH. Hypoxia-inducible factor 1 levels vary exponentially over a physiologically relevant range of O_2 tension. Am J Physiol 1996;271(4 Pt 1).

[33] Semenza GL. HIF-1: mediator of physiological and pathophysiological responses to hypoxia. J Appl Physiol (1985) 2000;88(4):1474–80.

[34] Galdeano C, Gadd MS, Soares P, Scaffidi S, Van Molle I, Birced I, Hewitt S, Dias DM, Ciulli A. Structure-guided design and optimization of small molecules targeting the protein-protein interaction between the von Hippel-Lindau (VHL) E3 ubiquitin ligase and the hypoxia inducible factor (HIF) alpha subunit with in vitro nanomolar affinities. J Med Chem 2014;57(20):8657–63.

[35] Karamysheva AF. Mechanisms of angiogenesis. Biochemistry (Mosc) 2008;73(7):751–62.

[36] Dvorak HF. Angiogenesis: update 2005. J Thromb Haemost 2005;3(8): 1835–42.

[37] Sun JF, Phung T, Shiojima I, Felske T, Upalakalin JN, Feng D, Kornaga T, Dor T, Dvorak AM, Walsh K, Benjamin LE. Microvascular patterning is controlled by fine-tuning the Akt signal. Proc Natl Acad Sci USA 2005;102(1):128–33.

[38] Zeng H, Dvorak HF, Mukhopadhyay D. Vascular permeability factor (VPF)/vascular endothelial growth factor (VEGF) peceptor-1 down-modulates VPF/VEGF receptor-2-mediated endothelial cell proliferation, but not migration, through phosphatidylinosit 3-kinase-dependent pathways. J Biol Chem 2001;276(29):26969–79.

[39] Ucuzian AA, Gassman AA, East AT, Greisler HP. Molecular mediators of angiogenesis. J Burn Care Res 2010;31(1):158–75.

[40] Armulik A, Abramsson A, Betsholtz C. Endothelial/pericyte interactions. Circ Res 2005;97(6):512–23.

[41] Folkman J, Haudenschild C. Angiogenesis in vitro. Nature 1980;288(5791):551–6.

[42] Wakui S, Furusato M, Ohshige H, Ushigome S. Endothelial-pericyte interdigitations in rat subcutaneous disc implanted angiogenesis. Microvasc Res 1993;46(1):19–27.

[43] Ferrara N, Gerber HP, LeCouter J. The biology of VEGF and its receptors. Nat Med 2003;9(6):669–76.

[44] Cross MJ, Dixelius J, Matsumoto T, Claesson-Welsh L. VEGF-receptor signal transduction. Trends Biochem Sci 2003;28(9):488–94.

[45] Ferrara N, Kerbel RS. Angiogenesis as a therapeutic target. Nature 2005;438(7070):967–74.

[46] Ellis LM, Hicklin DJ. VEGF-targeted therapy: mechanisms of antitumor activity. Nat Rev Cancer 2008;8(8):579–91.

[47] Lee SH, Jeong D, Han YS, Baek MJ. Pivotal role of vascular endothelial growth factor pathway in tumor angiogenesis. Ann Surg Treat Res 2015;89(1):1–8.

[48] Caraglia M, Santini D, Bronte G, Rizzo S, Sortino G, Rini GB, Di Fede G, Russo A. Predicting efficacy and toxicity in the era of targeted therapy: focus on anti-EGFR and anti-VEGF molecules. Curr Drug Metab 2011;12(10):944–55.

[49] Bronte G, Bronte E, Novo G, Pernice G, Lo Vullo F, Musso E, Bronte F, Gulotta E, Rizzo S, Rolfo C, Silvestris N, Bazan V, Novo S, Russo A. Conquests and perspectives of cardio-oncology in the field of tumor angiogenesis-targeting tyrosine kinase inhibitor-based therapy. Expert Opin Drug Saf 2015;14(2):253–67.

[50] Courtney KD, Corcoran RB, Engelman JA. The PI3K pathway as drug target in human cancer. J Clin Oncol. 2010;28(6):1075–83.

[51] Ellis LM, Hicklin DJ. VEGF-targeted therapy: mechanisms of antitumor activity. Nat Rev Cancer 2008;8(8):579–91.

[52] Bronte E, Bronte G, Novo G, Bronte F, Bavetta MG, Lo Re G, Brancatelli G, Bazan V, Natoli C, Novo S, Russo A. What links BRAF to the heart function? New insights from the cardiotoxicity of BRAF inhibitors in cancer treatment. Oncotarget 2015;6(34):35589–601.

[53] Kerkela R, Woulfe KC, Durand JB, Vagnozzi R, Kramer D, Chu TF, Beahm C, Chen MH, Force T. Sunitinib-induced cardiotoxicity is mediated by off-target inhibition of AMP-activated protein kinase. Clin Transl Sci 2009;2(1):15–25.

[54] Greineder CF, Kohnstamm S, Ky B. Heart failure associated with sunitinib: lessons learned from animal models. Curr Hypertens Rep 2011;13(6):436–41.

[55] Kappers MH, van Esch JH, Sleijfer S, Danser AH, van den Meiracker AH. Cardiovascular and renal toxicity during angiogenesis inhibition: clinical and mechanistic aspects. J Hypertens 2009;27(12):2297–309.

[56] Motzer RJ, Hutson TE, Tomczak P, Michaelson MD, Bukowski RM, Rixe O, Oudard S, Negrier S, Szczylik C, Kim ST, Chen I, Bycott PW, Baum CM, Figlin RA. Sunitinib versus interferon alfa in metastatic renal-cell carcinoma. N Engl J Med 2007;356(2):115–24.

[57] Raymond E, Dahan L, Raoul JL, Bang YJ, Borbath I, Lombard-Bohas C, Valle J, Metrakos P, Smith D, Vinik A, Chen JS, Hörsch D, Hammel P, Wiedenmann B, Van Cutsem E, Patyna S, Lu DR, Blanckmeister C, Chao R, Ruszniewski P. Sunitinib malate for the treatment of pancreatic neuroendocrine tumors. N Engl J Med 2011;364(6):501–13.

[58] Rini BI, Cohen DP, Lu DR, Chen I, Hariharan S, Gore ME, Figlin RA, Baum MS, Motzer RJ. Hypertension as a biomarker of efficacy in patients with metastatic renal cell carcinoma treated with sunitinib. J Natl Cancer Inst 2011;103(9):763–73.

[59] Greineder CF, Kohnstamm S, Ky B. Heart failure associated with sunitinib: lessons learned from animal models. Curr Hypertens Rep 2011;13(6):436–41.

[60] Chu TF, Rupnick MA, Kerkela R, Dallabrida SM, Zurakowski D, Nguyen L, Woulfe K, Pravda E, Cassiola F, Desai J, George S, Morgan JA, Harris DM, Ismail NS, Chen JH, Schoen FJ, Van den Abbeele AD, Demetri GD, Force T, Chen MH. Cardiotoxicity associated with tyrosine kinase inhibitor sunitinib. Lancet 2007;370(9604):2011–9.

[61] Llovet JM, Ricci S, Mazzaferro V, Hilgard P, Gane E, Blanc JF, de Oliveira AC, Santoro A, Raoul JL, Forner A, Schwartz M, Porta C, Zeuzem S, Bolondi L, Greten TF, Galle PR, Seitz JF, Borbath I, Häussinger D, Giannaris T, Shan M, Moscovici M, Voliotis D, Bruix J, Investigators Study SHARP, Group. Sorafenib in advanced hepatocellular carcinoma. N Engl J Med 2008;359(4):378–90.

[62] Demetri GD, van Oosterom AT, Garrett CR, Blackstein ME, Shah MH, Verweij J, McArthur G, Judson IR, Heinrich MC, Morgan JA, Desai J, Fletcher CD, George S, Bello CL, Huang X, Baum CM, Casali PG. Efficacy and safety of sunitinib in patients with advanced gastrointestinal stromal tumor after failure of imatinib: a randomised controlled trial. Lancet 2006;368(9544):1329–38.

[63] Gupta R, Maitland ML. Sunitinib, hypertension, and heart failure: a model for kinase inhibitor-mediated cardiotoxicity. Curr Hypertens Rep 2011;13(6):430–5.

[64] Schmidinger M, Zielinski CC, Vogl UM, Bojic A, Bojic M, Schukro C, Ruhsam M, Hejna M, Schmidinger H. Cardiac toxicity of sunitinib and sorafenib in patients with metastatic renal cell carcinoma. J Clin Oncol 2008;26(32):5204–12.

[65] Cheng AL, Kang YK, Chen Z, Tsao CJ, Qin S, Kim JS, Luo R, Feng J, Ye S, Yang TS, Xu J, Sun Y, Liang H, Liu J, Wang J, Tak WY, Pan H, Burock K, Zou J, Voliotis D, Guan Z. Efficacy and safety of sorafenib in patients in the Asia-Pacific region with advanced hepatocellular carcinoma: a phase III randomised, double-blind, placebo-controlled trial. Lancet Oncol 2009;10(1):25–34.

[66] Escudier B, Eisen T, Stadler WM, Szczylik C, Oudard S, Staehler M, Negrier S, Chevreau C, Desai AA, Rolland F, Demkow T, Hutson TE, Gore M, Anderson S, Hofilena G, Shan M, Pena C, Lathia C, Bukowski RM. Sorafenib for treatment ofrenal cell carcinoma: Final efficacy and safety results of the phase III treatment approaches in renal cancer global evaluation trial. J Clin Oncol 2009;27(20):3312–8.

[67] Stadler WM, Figlin RA, McDermott DF, Dutcher JP, Knox JJ, Miller WH Jr, Hainsworth JD, Henderson CA, George JR, Hajdenberg J, Kindwall-Keller TL, Ernstoff MS, Drabkin HA, Curti BD, Chu L, Ryan CW, Hotte SJ, Xia C, Cupit L, Bukowski RM, Study ARCCS, Investigators. Safety and efficacy results of the advanced renal cell carcinoma sorafenib expanded access program in North America. Cancer 2010;116(5):1272–80.

[68] Choueiri TK, Schutz FA, Je Y, Rosenberg JE, Bellmunt J. Risk of arterial thromboembolic events with sunitinib and sorafenib: a systematic review and meta-analysis of clinical trials. J Clin Oncol 2010;28(13):2280–5.

[69] Wang Z, Xu J, Nie W, Huang G, Tang J, Guan X. Risk of hypertension with regorafenib in cancer patients: a systematic review and meta-analysis. Eur J Clin Pharmacol 2014;70(2):225–31.

[70] Demetri GD, Reichardt P, Kang YK, Blay JY, Rutkowski P, Gelderblom H, Hohenberger P, Leahy M, von Mehren M, Joensuu H, Badalamenti G, Blackstein M, Le Cesne A, Schöffski P, Maki RG, Bauer S, Nguyen BB, Xu J, Nishida T, Chung J, Kappeler C, Kuss I, Laurent D, Casali PG, GRID study investigators. Efficacy and safety of regorafenib for advanced gastrointestinal stromal tumors after failure of imatinib and sunitinib (GRID): an international, multicentre, randomised, placebo-controlled, phase 3 trial. Lancet 2013;381(9863):295–302.

[71] Li J, Qin S, Xu R, Yau TC, Ma B, Pan H, Xu J, Bai Y, Chi Y, Wang L, Yeh KH, Bi F, Cheng Y, Le AT, Lin JK, Liu T, Ma D, Kappeler C, Kalmus J, Kim TW, CONCUR Investigators. Regorafenib plus best supportive care versus placebo plus best supportive care in Asian patients with previously treated metastatic colorectal cancer (CONCUR): a randomised, double-blind, placebo-controlled, phase 3 trial. Lancet Oncol 2015;16(6):619–29.

[72] Abdel-Rahman O, Fouad M. Risk of cardiovascular toxicities in patients with solid tumors treated with sunitinib, axitinib, cediranib or regorafenib: an updated systematic review and comparative meta-analysis. Crit Rev Oncol Hematol 2014;92(3):194–207.

[73] Qi WX, He AN, Shen Z, Yao Y. Incidence and risk of hypertension with a novel multi-targeted kinase inhibitor axitinib in cancer patients: a systematic review and meta-analysis. Br J Clin Pharmacol 2013;76(3):348–57.

[74] Rini BI, Quinn DI, Baum M, Wood LS, Tarazi J, Rosbrook B, Arruda LS, Cisar L, Roberts WG, Kim S, Motzer RJ. Hypertension among patients with renal cell carcinoma receiving axitinib or sorafenib: analysis from the randomized phase III AXIS trial. Target Oncol 2015;10(1):45–53.

[75] Rini BI, Schiller JH, Fruehauf JP, Cohen EE, Tarazi JC, Rosbrook B, Bair AH, Ricart AD, Olszanski AJ, Letrent KJ, Kim S, Rixe O. Diastolic blood pressure as a biomarker of axitinib efficacy in solid tumors. Clin Cancer Res D 2011;17(11):3841–9.

[76] Eisen T, Shparyk Y, Macleod N, Jones R, Wallenstein G, Temple G, Khder Y, Dallinger C, Studeny M, Loembe AB, Bondarenko I. Effect of small angiokinase inhibitor nintedanib (BIBF 1120) on QT interval in patients with previously untreated, advanced renal cell cancer in an open-label, phase II study. Invest New Drugs 2013;31(5):1283–93.

[77] du Bois A, Kristensen G, Ray-Coquard I, Reuss A, Pignata S, Colombo N, Denison U, Vergote I, Del Campo JM, Ottevanger P, Heubner M, Minarik T, Sevin E, de Gregorio N, Bidzi ski M, Pfisterer J, Malander S, Hilpert F, Mirza MR, Scambia G, Meier W, Nicoletto MO, Bjørge L, Lortholary A, Sailer MO, Merger M, Harter P. AGO Study Group led Gynecologic Cancer Intergroup (GCIG)/European Network of Gynaecologic Oncology Trials Groups (ENGOT) Intergroup Consortium. Standard first-line chemotherapy with or without nintedanib for advanced ovarian cancer (AGO-OVAR 12): a randomised, double-blind, placebo-controlled phase 3 trial. Lancet Oncol 2016;17(1):78–89.

[78] Zang J, Wu S, Tang L, Xu X, Bai J, Ding C, Chang Y, Yue L, Kang E, He J. Incidence and risk of QTc interval prolongation among cancer patients treated with vandetanib: a systematic review and meta-analysis. PLoS One 2012;7(2):e30353.

[79] Qi WX, Shen Z, Lin F, Sun YJ, Min DL, Tang LN, He AN, Yao Y. Incidence and risk of hypertension with vandetanib in cancer patients: a systematic review and meta-analysis of clinical trials. Br J Clin Pharmacol 2013;75(4):919–30.

[80] Liu Y, Liu Y, Fan ZW, Li J, Xu GG. Meta-analysis of the risks of hypertension and QTc prolongation in patients with advanced non-small cell lung cancer who were receiving vandetanib. Eur J Clin Pharmacol 2015;71(5):541–7.

[81] Qi WX, Lin F, Sun YJ, Tang LN, He AN, Yao Y, Shen Z. Incidence and risk of hypertension with pazopanib in patients with cancer: a meta-analysis. Cancer Chemother Pharmacol 2013;71(2):431–9.

[82] Pick AM, Nystrom KK. Pazopanib for the treatment of metastatic renal cell carcinoma. Clin Ther 2012;34(3):511–20.

[83] van der Graaf WT, Blay JY, Chawla SP, Kim DW, Bui-Nguyen B, Casali PG, Schöffski P, Aglietta M, Staddon AP, Beppu Y, Le Cesne A, Gelderblom H, Judson IR, Araki N, Ouali M, Marreaud S, Hodge R, Dewji MR, Coens C, Demetri GD, Fletcher CD, Dei Tos AP, Hohenberger P, Soft Tissue EORTC, Bone Sarcoma Group PALETTE, study group. Pazopanib for metastatic soft-tissue sarcoma (PALETTE): a randomised, double-blind, placebo-controlled phase 3 trial. Lancet 2012;379(9829):1879–86.

[84] Hecht JR, Trarbach T, Hainsworth JD, Major P, Jäger E, Wolff RA, Lloyd-Salvant K, Bodoky G, Pendergrass K, Berg W, Chen BL, Jalava T, Meinhardt G, Laurent D, Lebwohl D, Kerr D. Randomized, placebo-controlled, phase III study of first-line oxaliplatin-based chemotherapy plus PTK787/ZK 222584, an oral vascular endothelial growth factor receptor inhibitor, in patients with metastatic colorectal adenocarcinoma. J Clin Oncol 2011;29(15):1997–2003.

[85] Van Cutsem E, Bajetta E, Valle J, Köhne CH, Hecht JR, Moore M, Germond C, Berg W, Chen BL, Jalava T, Lebwohl D, Meinhardt G, Laurent D, Lin E. Randomized, placebo-controlled, phase III study of oxaliplatin, fluorouracil, and leucovorin with or without PTK787/ZK 222584 in patients with previously treated metastatic colorectal adenocarcinoma. J Clin Oncol 2011;29(15):2004–10.

[86] Gauler TC, Besse B, Mauguen A, Meric JB, Gounant V, Fischer B, Overbeck TR, Krissel H, Laurent D, Tiainen M, Commo F, Soria JC, Eberhardt WE. Phase II trial of PTK787/ZK 222584 (vatalanib) administered orally once-daily or in two divided daily doses as second-line monotherapy in relapsed or progressing patients with stage IIIB/IV non-small-cell lung cancer (NSCLC). Ann Oncol 2012;23(3):678–87.

[87] Norden AD, Drappatz J, Wen PY. Novel anti-angiogenic therapies for malignant gliomas. Lancet Neurol 2008;7(12):1152–60.

[88] Batchelor TT, Sorensen AG, di Tomaso E, Zhang WT, Duda DG, Cohen KS, Kozak KR, Cahill DP, Chen PJ, Zhu M, Ancukiewicz M, Mrugala MM, Plotkin S, Drappatz J, Louis DN, Ivy P, Scadden DT, Benner T, Loeffler JS, Wen PY, Jain RK. AZD2171, a pan-VEGF receptor tyrosine kinase inhibitor, normalizes tumor vasculature and alleviates edema in glioblastoma patients. Cancer Cell 2007;11(1):83–95.

[89] Ruscito I, Gasparri ML, Marchetti C, De Medici C, Bracchi C, Palaia I, Imboden S, Mueller MD, Papadia A, Muzii L, Panici PB. Cediranib in ovarian cancer: state of the art and future perspectives. Tumor Biol 2016;37(3):2833–9.

[90] Robinson ES, Matulonis UA, Ivy P, Berlin ST, Tyburski K, Penson RT, Humphreys BD. Rapid development of hypertension and proteinuria with cediranib, an oral vascular endothelial growth factor receptor inhibitor. Clin J Am Soc Nephrol 2010;5(3):477–83.

[91] Raja FA, Griffin CL, Qian W, Hirte H, Parmar MK, Swart AM, Ledermann JA. Initial toxicity assessment of ICON6: a randomised trial of cediranib plus chemotherapy in platinum-sensitive relapsed ovarian cancer. Br J Cancer 2011;105(7):884–9.

[92] Heckman CA, Holopainen T, Wirzenius M, Keskitalo S, Jeltsch M, Ylä-Herttuala S, Wedge SR, Jürgensmeier JM, Alitalo K. The tyrosine kinase inhibitor cediranib blocks ligand-induced vascular endothelial growth factor receptor-3 activity and lymphangiogenesis. Cancer Res 2008;68(12):4754–62.

[93] Robertson JD, Botwood NA, Rothenberg ML, Schmoll HJ. Phase III trial of FOLFOX plus bevacizumab or cediranib (AZD2171) as first-line treatment of patients with metastatic colorectal cancer: HORIZON III. Clin Colorectal Cancer 2009;8(1):59–60.

[94] Batchelor TT, Mulholland P, Neyns B, Nabors LB, Campone M, Wick A, Mason W, Mikkelsen T, Phuphanich S, Ashby LS, Degroot J, Gattamaneni R, Cher L, Rosenthal M, Payer F, Jürgensmeier JM, Jain RK, Sorensen AG, Xu J, Liu Q, van den Bent M. Phase III randomized trial comparing the efficacy of cediranib as monotherapy, and in combination with lomustine, versus lomustine alone in patients with recurrent glioblastoma. J Clin Oncol 2013;31(26):3212–8.

[95] Liu JF, Barry WT, Birrer M, Lee JM, Buckanovich RJ, Fleming GF, Rimel B, Buss MK, Nattam S, Hurteau J, Luo W, Quy P, Whalen C, Obermayer L, Lee H, Winer EP, Kohn EC, Ivy SP, Matulonis UA. Combination cediranib and olaparib versus olaparib alone for women with recurrent platinum-sensitive ovarian cancer: a randomised phase 2 study. Lancet Oncol 2014;15(11):1207–14.

[96] Richter S, Seah JA, Pond GR, Gan HK, Mackenzie MJ, Hotte SJ, Mukherjee SD, Murray N, Kollmannsberger C, Heng D, Haider MA, Halford R, Ivy SP, Moore MJ, Sridhar SS. Evaluation of second-line and subsequent targeted therapies in metastatic renal cell cancer (mRCC) patients treated with first-line cediranib. Can Urol Assoc J. 2014;8(11-12):398–402.

[97] Hirte H, Lheureux S, Fleming GF, Sugimoto A, Morgan R, Biagi J, Wang L, McGill S, Ivy SP, Oza AM. A phase 2 study of cediranib in recurrent or persistent ovarian, peritoneal or fallopian tube cancer: a trial of the Princess Margaret. Chicago and California Phase II Consortia. Gynecol Oncol 2015;138(1):55–61.

[98] Valle JW, Wasan H, Lopes A, Backen AC, Palmer DH, Morris K, Duggan M, Cunningham D, Anthoney DA, Corrie P, Madhusudan S, Maraveyas A, Ross PJ, Waters JS, Steward WP, Rees C, Beare S, Dive C, Bridgewater JA. Cediranib or placebo in combination with cisplatin and gemcitabine chemotherapy for patients with advanced biliary tract cancer (ABC-03): a randomised phase 2 trial. Lancet Oncol 2015;16(8):967–78.

[99] Jiang Y, Allen D, Kersemans V, Devery AM, Bokobza SM, Smart S, Ryan AJ. Acute vascular response to cediranib treatment in human non-small-cell lung cancer xenografts with different tumor stromal architecture. Lung Cancer 2015;90(2):191–8.

[100] Symonds RP, Gourley C, Davidson S, Carty K, McCartney E, Rai D, Banerjee S, Jackson D, Lord R, McCormack M, Hudson E, Reed N, Flubacher M, Jankowska P, Powell M, Dive C, West CM, Paul J. Cediranib combined with carboplatin and paclitaxel in patients with metastatic or recurrent cervical cancer (CIRCCa): a randomised, double-blind, placebo-controlled phase 2 trial. Lancet Oncol 2015;16(15):1515–24.

[101] Elisei R, Schlumberger MJ, Müller SP, Schöffski P, Brose MS, Shah MH, Licitra L, Jarzab B, Medvedev V, Kreissl MC, Niederle B, Cohen EE, Wirth LJ, Ali H, Hessel C, Yaron Y, Ball D, Nelkin B, Sherman SI. Cabozantinib in progressive medullary thyroid cancer. J Clin Oncol 2013;31(29):3639–46.

[102] Smith DC, Smith MR, Sweeney C, Elfiky AA, Logothetis C, Corn PG, Vogelzang NJ, Small EJ, Harzstark AL, Gordon MS, Vaishampayan UN, Haas NB, Spira AI, Lara PN Jr, Lin CC, Srinivas S, Sella A, Schöffski P, Scheffold C, Weitzman AL, Hussain M. Cabozantinib in patients with advanced prostate cancer: results of a phase II randomized discontinuation trial. J Clin Oncol 2013;31(4):412–9.

[103] Smith MR, Sweeney CJ, Corn PG, Rathkopf DE, Smith DC, Hussain M, George DJ, Higano CS, Harzstark AL, Sartor AO, Vogelzang NJ, Gordon MS, de Bono JS, Haas NB, Logothetis CJ, Elfiky A, Scheffold C, Laird AD, Schimmoller F, Basch EM, Scher HI. Cabozantinib in chemotherapy-pretreated metastatic castration-resistant prostate cancer: results of a phase II nonrandomized expansion study. J Clin Oncol 2014;32(30):3391–9.

[104] Choueiri TK, Escudier B, Powles T, Mainwaring PN, Rini BI, Donskov F, Hammers H, Hutson TE, Lee JL, Peltola K, Roth BJ, Bjarnason GA, Géczi L, Keam B, Maroto P, Heng DY, Schmidinger M, Kantoff PW, Borgman-Hagey A, Hessel C, Scheffold C, Schwab GM, Tannir NM, Motzer RJ, Investigators METEOR. Cabozantinib versus everolimus in advanced renal-cell carcinoma. N Engl J Med 2015;373(19):1814–23.

[105] Schlumberger M, Tahara M, Wirth LJ, Robinson B, Brose MS, Elisei R, Habra MA, Newbold K, Shah MH, Hoff AO, Gianoukakis AG, Kiyota N, Taylor MH, Kim SB, Krzyzanowska MK, Dutcus CE, de las Heras B, Zhu J, Sherman SI. Lenvatinib versus placebo in radioiodine-refractory thyroid cancer. N Engl J Med 2015;372(7):621–30.

[106] Fala L. Lenvima (lenvatinib), a multireceptor tyrosine kinase inhibitor. Approved by the FDA for the treatment of patients with differentiated thyroid cancer. Am Health Drug Benefits 2015;8(Spec Feature):176–9.

[107] Schlumberger M, Jarzab B, Cabanillas ME, Robinson B, Pacini F, Ball DW, McCaffrey J, Newbold K, Allison R, Martins RG, Licitra LF, Shah MH, Bodenner D, Elisei R, Burmeister L, Funahashi Y, Ren M, O'Brien JP, Sherman SI. A phase II trial of the multitargeted tyrosine kinase inhibitor lenvatinib (E7080) in advanced medullary thyroid cancer. Clin Cancer Res 2016;22(1):44–53.

[108] Ikeda M, Okusaka T, Mitsunaga S, Ueno H, Tamai T, Suzuki T, Hayato S, Kadowaki T, Okita K, Kumada H. Safety and pharmacokinetics of lenvatinib in patients with advanced hepatocellular carcinoma. Clin Cancer Res 2016;22(6):1385–94.

[109] Motzer RJ, Hutson TE, Glen H, Michaelson MD, Molina A, Eisen T, Jassem J, Zolnierek J, Maroto JP, Mellado B, Melichar B, Tomasek J, Kremer A, Kim HJ, Wood K, Dutcus C, Larkin J. Lenvatinib, everolimus, and the combination in patients with metastatic renal cell carcinoma: a randomised, phase 2, open-label, multicentre trial. Lancet Oncol 2015;16(15):1473–82.

[110] Ramalingam SS, Shtivelband M, Soo RA, Barrios CH, Makhson A, Segalla JG, Pittman KB, Kolman P, Pereira JR, Srkalovic G, Belani CP, Axelrod R, Owonikoko TK, Qin Q, Qian J, McKeegan EM, Devanarayan V, McKee MD, Ricker JL, Carlson DM, Gorbunova VA. Randomized phase II study of carboplatin and paclitaxel with either linifanib or placebo for advanced nonsquamous non-small-cell lung cancer. J Clin Oncol 2015;33(5):433–41.

[111] Chiu YL, Lorusso P, Hosmane B, Ricker JL, Awni W, Carlson DM. Results of a phase I, open-label, randomized, crossover study evaluating the effects of linifanib on QTc intervals in patients with solid tumors. Cancer Chemother Pharmacol 2014;73(1):213–7.

[112] Mross K, Frost A, Scheulen ME, Krauss J, Strumberg D, Schultheiss B, Fasol U, Büchert M, Krätzschmer J, Delesen H, Rajagopalan P, Christensen O. Phase I study of telatinib (BAY 57-9352): analysis of safety, pharmacokinetics, tumor efficacy, and biomarkers in patients with colorectal cancer. Vasc Cell 2011;3:16.

[113] Bergers G, Hanahan D. Modes of resistance to anti-angiogenic therapy. Nat Rev Cancer 2008;8(8):592–603.

[114] Jonker DJ, Rosen LS, Sawyer MB, de Braud F, Wilding G, Sweeney CJ, Jayson GC, McArthur GA, Rustin G, Goss G, Kantor J, Velasquez L, Syed S, Mokliatchouk O, Feltquate DM, Kollia G, Nuyten DS, Galbraith S. A phase I study to determine the safety, pharmacokinetics and pharmacodynamics of a dual VEGFR and FGFR inhibitor, brivanib, in patients with advanced or metastatic solid tumors. Ann Oncol 2011;22(6):1413–9.

[115] Johnson PJ, Qin S, Park JW, Poon RT, Raoul JL, Philip PA, Hsu CH, Hu TH, Heo J, Xu J, Lu L, Chao Y, Boucher E, Han KH, Paik SW, Robles-Aviña J, Kudo M, Yan L, Sobhonslidsuk A, Komov D, Decaens T, Tak WY, Jeng LB, Liu D, Ezzeddine R, Walters I, Cheng AL. Brivanib versus sorafenib as first-line therapy in patients with unresectable, advanced hepatocellular carcinoma: results from the randomized phase III BRISK-FL study. J Clin Oncol 2013;31(28):3517–24.

[116] Llovet JM, Decaens T, Raoul JL, Boucher E, Kudo M, Chang C, Kang YK, Assenat E, Lim HY, Boige V, Mathurin P, Fartoux L, Lin DY, Bruix J, Poon RT, Sherman M, Blanc JF, Finn RS, Tak WY, Chao Y, Ezzeddine R, Liu D, Walters I, Park JW. Brivanib in patients with advanced hepatocellular carcinoma who were intolerant to sorafenib or for whom sorafenib failed: results from the randomized phase III BRISK-PS study. J Clin Oncol 2013;31(28):3509–16.

[117] Matoori S, Leroux JC. Recent advances in the treatment of hyperammonemia. Adv Drug Deliv Rev 2015;90:55–68.

[118] Shah MA, Wainberg ZA, Catenacci DV, Hochster HS, Ford J, Kunz P, Lee FC, Kallender H, Cecchi F, Rabe DC, Keer H, Martin AM, Liu Y, Gagnon R, Bonate P, Liu L, Gilmer T, Bottaro DP. Phase II study evaluating 2 dosing schedules of oral foretinib (GSK1363089), cMET/VEGFR2 inhibitor, in patients with metastatic gastric cancer. PLoS One 2013;8(3):e54014.

[119] Choueiri TK, Vaishampayan U, Rosenberg JE, Logan TF, Harzstark AL, Bukowski RM, Rini BI, Srinivas S, Stein MN, Adams LM, Ottesen LH, Laubscher KH, Sherman L, McDermott DF, Haas NB, Flaherty KT, Ross R, Eisenberg P, Meltzer PS, Merino MJ, Bottaro DP, Linehan WM, Srinivasan R. Phase II and biomarker study of the dual MET/VEGFR2 inhibitor foretinib in patients with papillary renal cell carcinoma. J Clin Oncol 2013;31(2):181–6.

[120] Scagliotti GV, Vynnychenko I, Park K, Ichinose Y, Kubota K, Blackhall F, Pirker R, Galiulin R, Ciuleanu TE, Sydorenko O, Dediu M, Papai-Szekely Z, Banaclocha NM, McCoy S, Yao B, Hei YJ, Galimi F, Spigel DR. International, randomized, placebo-controlled, double-blind phase III study of motesanib plus carboplatin/paclitaxel in patients with advanced nonsquamous non-small-cell lung cancer: MONET1. J Clin Oncol 2012;30(23):2829–36.

[121] Novello S, Scagliotti GV, Sydorenko O, Vynnychenko I, Volovat C, Schneider CP, Blackhall F, McCoy S, Hei YJ, Spigel DR. Motesanib plus carboplatin/paclitaxel in patients with advanced squamous non-small-cell lung cancer: results from the randomized controlled MONET1 study. J Thorac Oncol 2014;9(8):1154–61.

[122] Soria JC, DeBraud F, Bahleda R, Adamo B, Andre F, Dienstmann R, Delmonte A, Cereda R, Isaacson J, Litten J, Allen A, Dubois F, Saba C, Robert R, D'Incalci M, Zucchetti M, Camboni MG, Tabernero J. Phase I/IIa study evaluating the safety, efficacy, pharmacokinetics, and pharmacodynamics of lucitanib in advanced solid tumors. Ann Oncol 2014;25(11):2244–51.

[123] Colzani M, Noberini R, Romanenghi M, Colella G, Pasi M, Fancelli D, Varasi M, Minucci S, Bonaldi T. Quantitative chemical proteomics identifies novel targets of the anti-cancer multi-kinase inhibitor E-3810. Mol Cell Proteomics 2014;13(6):1495–509.

[124] A Phase Ib Study of VEGFR inhibitor fruquintinib in patients with pre-treated advanced colorectal cancer—ASCO 2014 Presentation Abstracts; Abstract # 3548; 2014.

[125] Nosov DA, Esteves B, Lipatov ON, Lyulko AA, Anischenko AA, Chacko RT, Doval DC, Strahs A, Slichenmyer WJ, Bhargava P. Antitumor activity and safety of tivozanib (AV-951) in a phase II randomized discontinuation trial in patients with renal cell carcinoma. J Clin Oncol 2012;30(14):1678–85.

[126] Eskens FA, de Jonge MJ, Bhargava P, Isoe T, Cotreau MM, Esteves B, Hayashi K, Burger H, Thomeer M, van Doorn L, Verweij J. Biologic and clinical activity of tivozanib (AV-951, KRN-951), a selective inhibitor of VEGF receptor-1, -2, and -3 tyrosine kinases, in a 4-week-on, 2-week-off schedule in patients with advanced solid tumors. Clin Cancer Res 2011;17(22):7156–63.

[127] Motzer RJ, Nosov D, Eisen T, Bondarenko I, Lesovoy V, Lipatov O, Tomczak P, Lyulko O, Alyasova A, Harza M, Kogan M, Alekseev BY, Sternberg CN, Szczylik C, Cella D, Ivanescu C, Krivoshik A, Strahs A, Esteves B, Berkenblit A, Hutson TE. Tivozanib versus sorafenib as initial targeted therapy for patients with metastatic renal cell carcinoma: results from a phase III trial. J Clin Oncol 2013;31(30):3791–9.

[128] Li J, Zhao X, Chen L, Guo H, Lv F, Jia K, Yv K, Wang F, Li C, Qian J, Zheng C, Zuo Y. Safety and pharmacokinetics of novel selective vascular endothelial growth factor receptor-2 inhibitor YN968D1 in patients with advanced malignancies. BMC Cancer 2010;10:529.

[129] Hu X, Zhang J, Xu B, Jiang Z, Ragaz J, Tong Z, Zhang Q, Wang X, Feng J, Pang D, Fan M, Li J, Wang B, Wang Z, Zhang Q, Sun S, Liao C. Multicenter phase II study of apatinib, a novel VEGFR inhibitor in heavily pretreated patients with metastatic triple-negative breast cancer. Int J Cancer 2014;135(8):1961–9.

[130] Li J, Qin S, Xu J, Guo W, Xiong J, Bai Y, Sun G, Yang Y, Wang L, Xu N, Cheng Y, Wang Z, Zheng L, Tao M, Zhu X, Ji D, Liu X, Yu H. Apatinib for chemotherapy-refractory advanced metastatic gastric cancer: results from a randomized, placebo-controlled, parallel-arm, phase II trial. J Clin Oncol 2013;31(26):3219–25.

[131] Abdel-Rahman O, Abdelwahab M, Shaker M, Abdelwahab S, Elbassiony M, Ellithy M. Sorafenib for Egyptian patients with advanced hepatocellular carcinoma; single center experience. J Egypt Natl Canc Inst 2014;26(1):9–13.

[132] Abdel-Rahman O, Abdel-Wahab M, Shaker M, Abdel-Wahab S, Elbassiony M, Ellithy M. Sorafenib versus capecitabine in the management of advanced hepatocellular carcinoma. Med Oncol 2013;30(3):655.

[133] Yoshiji H, Kuriyama S, Yoshii J, Ikenaka Y, Noguchi R, Hicklin DJ, Wu Y, Yanase K, Namisaki T, Kitade M, Yamazaki M, Tsujinoue H, Masaki T, Fukui H. Halting the interaction between vascular endothelial growth factor and its receptors attenuates liver carcinogenesis in mice. Hepatology 2004;39(6):1517–24.

[134] Mayer EL, Dhakil S, Patel T, Sundaram S, Fabian C, Kozloff M, Qamar R, Volterra F, Parmar H, Samant M, Burstein HJ. SABRE-B: an evaluation of paclitaxel and bevacizumab with or without sunitinib as first-line treatment of metastatic breast cancer. Ann Oncol 2010;21(12):2370–6.

[135] Maitland ML, Bakris GL, Black HR, Chen HX, Durand JB, Elliott WJ, Ivy SP, Leier CV, Lindenfeld J, Liu G, Remick SC, Steingart R, Tang WH. Cardiovascular Toxicities Panel, Convened by the Angiogenesis Task Force of the National Cancer Institute Investigational Drug Steering Committee. Initial assessment, surveillance, and management of blood pressure in patients receiving vascular endothelial growth factor signaling pathway inhibitors. J Natl Cancer Inst 2010;102(9):596–604.

[136] Kaplan NM, Opie LH. Controversies in hypertension. Lancet 2006;367(9505):168–76.

[137] Peterson JC, Adler S, Burkart JM, Greene T, Hebert LA, Hunsicker LG, King AJ, Klahr S, Massry SG, Seifter JL. Blood pressure control, proteinuria, and the progression of renal disease. The Modification of Diet in Renal Disease Study. Ann Intern Med 1995;123(10):754–62.

[138] Mourad JJ, des Guetz G, Debbabi H, Levy BI. Blood pressure rise following angiogenesis inhibition by bevacizumab. A crucial role for microcirculation. Ann Oncol 2008;19(5):927–34.

[139] Veronese ML, Mosenkis A, Flaherty KT, Gallagher M, Stevenson JP, Townsend RR, O'Dwyer PJ. Mechanisms of hypertension associated with BAY 43-9006. J Clin Oncol 2006;24(9):1363–9.

[140] Zhu X, Stergiopoulos K, Wu S. Risk of hypertension and renal dysfunction with an angiogenesis inhibitor sunitinib: systematic review and meta-analysis. Acta Oncol 2009;48(1):9–17.

[141] Miura S, Fujino M, Matsuo Y, Tanigawa H, Saku K. Nifedipine-induced vascular endothelial growth factor secretion from coronary smooth muscle cells promotes endothelial tube formation via the kinase insert domain-containing receptor/fetal liver kinase-1/NO pathway. Hypertens Res 2005;28(2):147–53.

[142] Bordun KA, Premecz S, daSilva M, Mandal S, Goyal V, Glavinovic T, Cheung M, Cheung D, White CW, Chaudhary R, Freed DH, Villarraga HR, Herrmann J, Kohli M, Ravandi A, Thliveris J, Pitz M, Singal PK, Mulvagh S, Jassal DS. The utility of cardiac biomarkers and echocardiography for the early detection of bevacizumab-and sunitinib-mediated cardiotoxicity. Am J Physiol Heart Circ Physiol 2015;309(4):H692–701.

[143] Goel HL, Mercurio AM. VEGF targets the tumor cell. Nat Rev Cancer 2013;13(12):871–82.

[144] Naib T, Steingart RM, Chen CL. Sorafenib-associated multivessel coronary artery vasospasm. Herz 2011;36(4):348–51.

Chapter 6

Role of Novel Imaging Techniques in Detection of Chemotoxicity: Cardiac Magnetic Resonance and Radionuclide Imaging

B.K. Tamarappoo, M. Motwani and L.E.J. Thomson
Cedars Sinai Medical Center, Los Angeles, CA, United States

INTRODUCTION

Demand for noninvasive evaluation of patients at risk is predicted to increase as a result of more widespread use of potentially cardiotoxic therapy, and improvement in long-term survival rates for many malignancies. The Cancer Treatment Survivorship Facts and Figures 2014–2015, published by the American Cancer Society reports that in January of 2014 there were approximately 14.5 million survivors of cancer in the United States of America. This number is expected to grow to 19 million by January 2024. There are a broad range of cardiac effects that may result from chemotherapy or radiotherapy. Chemotherapy is the mainstay of cancer treatment and often includes medications, such as anthracyclines, HER2/neu receptor antibodies, and cyclophosphamide, which can result in irreversible (type I) or reversible (type II) chemotherapy-related cardiac dysfunction (CRCD) [1,2]. Most effects of cardiotoxicity can be seen a few months to years after treatment. However, in some cases, cardiotoxic effects may be first detected decades after treatment. Additionally, radiation is used in the treatment of breast cancer, lymphoma, esophageal cancer, and certain types of lung cancer. Radiation, particularly of the chest, may also be associated with damage to the myocardium, coronary arteries, and heart valves that may manifest several decades after treatment. Therefore, the need to diagnose cardiotoxicity before clinical changes become irreversible is important.

Based upon a solid foundation of evidence, guidelines for monitoring for CRCD have emphasized serial measurement of left ventricular ejection fraction (LVEF). Nuclear and magnetic resonance imaging (MRI) approaches are considered to be reliable and reproducible, in addition to being superior to standard two-dimensional (2D) echocardiography for measurement of small changes in LVEF [3]. These approaches allow early detection of subclinical decreases in systolic function, with subsequent guideline-based modification of therapy dose and duration.

However, there is recognition that changes can occur in the cardiovascular system impacting more than left ventricular (LV) systolic function as an early or late consequence of cancer therapy. Noninvasive imaging is an invaluable tool for understanding mechanisms of cardiotoxicity at a molecular level. Novel molecular imaging approaches show promise for earlier detection of myocardial damage, which could impact protocols for use of cardioprotection and future treatment guidelines. This chapter will focus on established and evolving novel applications of radionuclide and magnetic resonance imaging for detection of cardiotoxic effects from cancer therapy. In addition to reviewing use of these imaging modalities for measurement of ventricular volume and ejection fraction (EF), the chapter will address additional techniques that may lead to earlier detection of cardiotoxicity.

CURRENT IMAGING GUIDELINES FOR THE DETECTION OF CARDIOTOXICITY

There has been an increasing recognition of the need for early detection of chemotherapy and radiation induced cardiovascular disease and there are several consensus statements and guidelines that have been put forth by the American Heart Association (AHA), the European Association of Cardiovascular Imaging (EACVI), the American Society of Echocardiography (ASE), and the American Society of Clinical Oncology (ASCO). The ASE recommends the use of LVEF with echocardiography before, during, and after chemotherapy [4,5]. They also acknowledge the high interobserver and intraobserver agreement of LVEF measurements made by radionuclide multiple-gated acquisition (MUGA) scans. Additionally, they recommend that due to the high accuracy of cardiac MRI (CMR) for measuring chamber volumes and LVEF, it may also be used in centers where it is available. The AHA recommends monitoring of cardiac function during anthracycline chemotherapy but does not specify the intervals at which LVEF needs to be measured [6]. For survivors of childhood cancer, the Children's Oncology Group has devised risk-based guidelines for follow-up of late effects [7,8]. The ASCO has also recognized the need for routine monitoring; however, there is no precise guide to the frequency of testing.

RADIONUCLIDE IMAGING

Radionuclide imaging measurement of LV function was first used in the 1970s and remains recognized for its accuracy and reproducibility [9–12]. It is variably referred to as equilibrium radionuclide angiography (ERNA), gated blood pool single-photon emission computed tomography (SPECT) or a MUGA scan. The technique requires labeling of a small volume of the patients own red cells with ~20 mCi (740MBq) 99m-Technetium (Tc), with optimal labeling efficiency achieved using a commercially produced in vitro kit [9–12]. Radiolabeled blood is reinjected and multiplanar imaging performed using cardiac ECG gating and a gamma camera, with the scan taking approximately 20 min to be completed. The calculation of ventricular volumes is based upon the emitted energy (counts-based) within a region of interest (ROI) encompassing the left ventricle. The ROI is used to generate LVEF, regional ejection fraction, and various other functional parameters [12].

This imaging approach has advantages of being independent of geometric assumptions and not limited by body size or implanted devices. Red cell labeling is relatively simple, there is widespread availability, and results obtained are not highly operator dependent [3,11–15]. As a three-dimensional (3D) imaging technique it is superior to standard 2D echocardiography with respect to accuracy and reproducibility of measurements, and correlates well with other 3D tools, such as CMR and 3D echocardiography [3,11,13–15]. Disadvantages include the prerequisite for a <10% rate of premature ventricular contractions (PVCs), the use of ionizing radiation, and lack of any information gained about cardiac structure including valvular function and the pericardium.

Multiple studies have proven the effectiveness of MUGA for identification of asymptomatic decline in LVEF in patients receiving anthracyclines [16,17]. Stopping the culprit cardiotoxic therapy and optimization of medical management with heart failure medications has been shown to result in stabilization or recovery of ventricular function. On the basis of these studies, recommendations for use of MUGA to monitor anthracycline induced cardiotoxicity during treatment were proposed [11,16] (Table 6.1).

There is a large amount of information that can be obtained by MUGA beyond LVEF that is worthy of discussion. The use of tomographic imaging allows the acquisition of a 3D volume of gated blood pool data and this has potential advantages for accurate segmentation of both left and right ventricles and the evaluation of regional wall motion [18–21]. Systolic and diastolic motion can be tracked in detail, with accurate calculation of filling rates and time to peak filling in addition to the ability to measure ventricular synchrony [22] (Fig. 6.1). Studies show that MUGA can be used for early detection of diastolic dysfunction, and this could be applied to evaluation of patients for detection of CRCD [18–21]. Optimization of MUGA evaluation of diastolic filling requires use of a narrow acceptance window for R–R interval variation (i.e., inclusion of data from cardiac cycles with similar length of diastole only).

TABLE 6.1 Guideline for Monitoring LVEF During Treatment With Anthracyclines

LVEF >50% at baseline

1. Measurement at total cumulative dose 250–300 mg/m^2
2. Measurement at 450 mg/m^2
3. Measurement before each dose above 450 mg/m^2
4. Discontinue therapy if LVEF decreases by ≥10% from baseline and LVEF ≤50%

LVEF <50% at baseline

1. Do not treat if LVEF <30%
2. Serial measurement before each dose
3. Discontinue therapy if LVEF decreases by ≥10% from baseline or LVEF ≤30%

Anthracycline dose is expressed in mg per m^2 of body surface area. LVEF, left ventricular ejection fraction.
Source: Data from Schwartz RG, et al. Traditional and novel methods to assess and prevent chemotherapy-related cardiac dysfunction noninvasively. J Nucl Cardiol 2013;20(3):443–64; Schwartz RG, et al. Congestive heart failure and left ventricular dysfunction complicating doxorubicin therapy. Seven-year experience using serial radionuclide angiocardiography. Am J Med 1987;82(6):1109–18.

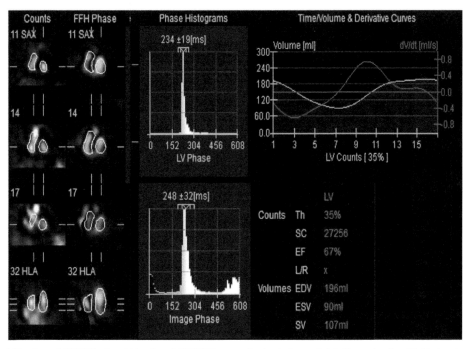

FIGURE 6.1   Gated blood pool SPECT. Gated blood pool SPECT images obtained after radiolabeling red cells with Technetium-99m are automatically segmented and quantified using commercially available software (QBS, quantitative blood pool SPECT, Cedars-Sinai). In addition to calculation of left and right ventricular volumes and ejection fraction, diastolic function metrics can be generated including peak filling rate, mean filling rate over the first third of diastole, and time to peak filling from end systole. Abnormal diastolic relaxation is an early indicator of myocardial dysfunction.

Although standard MUGA is performed at rest, it is possible to combine exercise stress with data acquisition. Sensitivity for detection of subclinical ventricular dysfunction is increased by the use of stress, and studies have demonstrated this with exercise MUGA. This little-used technique requires specialized exercise equipment (supine bicycle) and the patient needs to have sufficient exercise capacity to achieve the necessary workload. MUGA remains recognized as a highly reliable method for early detection of ventricular function decline, with the most frequent indication for this imaging being the evaluation of function prior to, and during chemotherapy. MUGA has been the preferred clinical research tool for serial measurement of LVEF due to the high interobserver agreement and ability to detect small changes in EF [11]. However, for clinical purposes, the estimated dose from ionizing radiation with MUGA of 5–10 mSv is a major contributor to the lack of enthusiasm for routine use compared to echocardiography. Thus echocardiography remains the most widely used noninvasive tool to evaluate cardiac function for clinical purposes, and it is recommended as the test of choice before, during, and after cancer therapy in a recent position paper from the ASE and EACVI (Table 6.2) [5,23]. Clinically, MUGA should be considered for subjects with poor acoustic windows in whom the reliability of echocardiography is diminished. However, it should be noted that the two modalities are not interchangeable and serial evaluations of ventricular function should be performed using the same imaging technique [3,11].

CARDIAC MAGNETIC RESONANCE IMAGING

General Considerations

CMR has become widely available and although considerably more expensive than echocardiography, it has several advantages including providing high-resolution images in any desired plane without restriction to limited acoustic windows, higher accuracy and reproducibility of volumetric measurements, and the unique capacity to characterize tissue composition at the molecular level. Compared to radionuclide imaging and CT, CMR offers versatile cross-sectional imaging without the need for ionizing radiation which is particularly important in patients requiring serial studies. The majority of clinical CMR studies have utilized a 1.5-Tesla (T) field strength magnet with standard commercially available pulse sequences. 3.0 T field strength magnets are becoming more widespread, and have the advantage of increased signal, tempered by increased image artifacts with some cardiac imaging sequences. All standard clinically applicable pulse sequences for evaluation of cardiac structure and function are available from all vendors for both 1.5 and 3 T systems.

A standard clinical CMR scan will require 1 h of imaging time, followed by significant time for postprocessing of images to obtain measurements. A variety of MRI pulse sequences are available for cardiac imaging and the imaging must be tailored to the clinical question.

TABLE 6.2 Comparison of Imaging Techniques Commonly Used for Monitoring Cardiotoxicity

Echocardiography
Readily available and hence most widely used
Uses geometric assumptions for quantification of LVEF and less reliable in dilated ventricles
Gain-dependent edge detection may result in errors
Noncontrast 2D echocardiography has a bias of 0.8% and LOA of −15% to 10% when compared to CMR
Contrast enhanced 2D echocardiography has a bias of 4.6% with LOA of −12.4 to 21.6% when compared to CMR
3D-noncontrast echocardiography exhibits better agreement with CMR than 2D-noncontrast echocardiography
Lower limit of normal using 2D echocardiography: 55% (men and women)
Lower limit of normal using 3D echocardiography: 47–53% (men) and 51–55% (women)
Radionuclide angiography
Reduced resolution and involves radiation compared to echocardiography and CMR
Need for background correction
Errors due to signal from overlapping structures
Lower reproducibility than CMR
Lower limit of normal using radionuclide angiography: 50% (men and women)
Cardiac MRI
Free of geometric assumptions
Greatest reproducibility among the various techniques
Lower limit of normal values using CMR: 55–57% (men) and 54–58% (women)
Expensive and not widely available

CMR, Cardiac MRI; LOA, level of agreement; LVEF, left ventricular ejection fraction.

A standardized approach for CMR for evaluation of suspected CRCD could include a combination of cine imaging, pre- and postcontrast myocardial tissue characterization and possibly specialized sequences to evaluate diastolic relaxation [24–26]. The evaluation of possible metastatic disease involving the heart or central mediastinal vascular structures would be approached differently, as imaging time would be focused toward identification and characterization of tumor tissue. Unlike chest CT, CMR protocols are highly variable depending upon the clinical question, and highly operator dependent for optimization of image quality.

Contraindications to CMR preclude imaging in a small minority of patients. First, implanted electronic devices including but not limited to spinal cord stimulators and infusion pumps are not MR compatible. There is substantial literature evaluating CMR compatibility of implanted surgical devices and this is summarized in a regularly updated reference online resource available at www.mrisafety.com. Noncompatible permanent pacemakers and implanted defibrillators are relative contraindications, with some major centers performing CMR on a case-by-case basis in these patients [27,28]. Although newer generation MR conditional pacemakers and defibrillators are increasingly available, strict adherence to safety protocols and a high-level of expertise is required for both patient safety and to minimize imaging artifact. Claustrophobia can be managed with sedation or anesthesia if CMR must be performed, and is reported to be a significant consideration in <5% of patients [29].

Accurate Quantification of Left Ventricular Ejection Fraction

CMR is one of the most accurate and reproducible tools for quantification of LV volumes and function. As a 3D modality without acoustic window limitation, CMR outperforms standard 2D echocardiography for quantification of LVEF and is a more sensitive tool for early detection of CRCD using serial measurement. CMR has been used as a gold standard among noninvasive imaging tests for assessment of cardiac chamber sizes and function [30,31]. In a study of 117 asymptomatic adults who had received anthracyclines and radiation during childhood, the EF was overestimated and the LV end-systolic and LV end-diastolic volumes were underestimated by 2D transthoracic echocardiography (TTE) compared to CMR [32]. Using CMR-derived LVEF as the gold standard, 3D TTE and 2D TTE misclassified 6 and 11 patients, respectively, as having LVEF ≥ 50%. This study concluded that although echocardiography is more widely available than CMR, and is therefore the most useful screening test, CMR is especially useful for more accurate volumetric quantification in patients with an LVEF of 50–59% by initial screening TTE. In comparing CMR to MUGA, 50 women who were treated with trastuzumab underwent CMR, 2-D TTE, 3-D TTE, and MUGA before initiation, and after 6 and 12 month intervals of treatment. There was a strong correlation between CMR- and MUGA-derived LVEF at all three time points ($r = 0.88, 0.97, 0.87$, respectively) [15].

Practical Considerations for CMR Evaluation of LV Volumes and LVEF

The following technical considerations are highly relevant when discussing accuracy of serial measurement of ventricular volumes and function [30].

Cine imaging is acquired as a stack of 2D images of uniform slice thickness, with a standard interslice gap (frequently 8 mm slice thickness and 2 mm gap) to cover the entire LV from the mitral valve to the apex, and images are in the orientation of the ventricular short axis to allow later standardized segmental description of regional wall motion. Additional long-axis images (ventricular two-chamber and four-chamber views) are usually also acquired, and the total number of cine series for detailed LV volumetric and functional evaluation is 10–15. High temporal and spatial resolution is obtained by the use of cardiac gating, and either respiratory gating or more commonly breath-hold during imaging. Image quality is therefore dependent upon a regular heart rhythm and the ability of the patient to cooperate with breath-holding instructions [25,26].

The postprocessing of images involves use of software to define endocardial and epicardial borders, and is semiautomated with the requirement for the user to make adjustments (Fig. 6.2). Software segmentation tools are less accurate with poor-quality images. A major source of error in measurement of ventricular volumes is related to defining the volume in systole and diastole in the basal short axis,

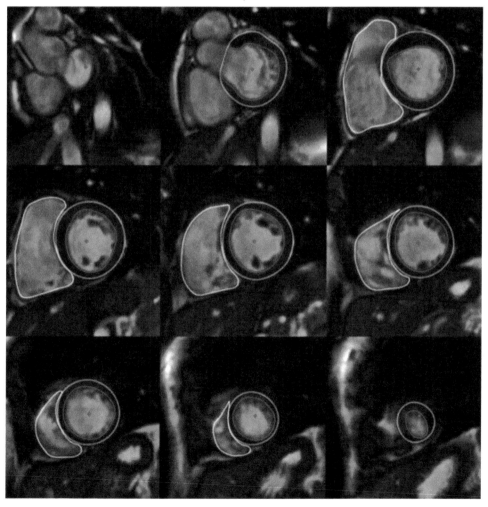

FIGURE 6.2 CMR calculated ventricular volumes. Semiautomatic segmentation of the right and left ventricles involves contours placed at endocardial and epicardial boundaries on a stacked series of cine images. Images are typically acquired in the left ventricular short axis plane, with uniform slice thickness and interslice gap. End diastolic and end systolic volumes, myocardial mass, and ejection fraction are then calculated. Papillary muscles may be included within the ventricular cavity volume or segmented out (and considered as part of myocardial mass); however, consistency is required in whichever approach is chosen.

due to the downward motion of the mitral valve plane during the cardiac cycle. Latest-generation software attempts to minimize this source of error by inclusion of long axis views and mitral annular plane tracking during calculation of ventricular volumes. A second consideration with impact on observed volumes is the segmentation of the papillary muscles and whether papillary muscles are included within the LV cavity volume or added to the myocardial mass measurement. The treatment of the papillary muscle volume needs to be consistent throughout the cardiac cycle and between serial measurements, so as to avoid bias to increase or decrease end systolic volume [25,33].

Serial evaluation of ventricular function should be systematically performed using a standardized cine imaging protocol, the same software for postprocessing and with careful consideration of image datasets side by side to ensure consistency of the above factors.

Recent Advances in CMR Cine Imaging

Hardware and software development leads to an ongoing evolution of imaging sequences, with the motivation of decreased imaging time, improved image quality, and a goal of robust real-time cine 3D volumetric evaluation of the heart. There are ongoing studies of novel approaches to image acquisition and reconstruction, cardiac and respiratory motion correction, and recognition of the need to reduce complexity and time involved with both the acquisition and postprocessing of images.

CMR for Evaluation of Ventricular Strain and Relaxation

The earliest functional changes associated with myocardial insult can be detected by close examination of regional wall motion in terms of both the pattern of systolic contraction and diastolic relaxation. Myocardial stiffness is increased by the presence of either edema or fibrosis, and diastolic relaxation abnormalities are thought to most often precede measurable reduction in systolic function. In many cases of cardiomyopathy, diastolic dysfunction is the predominant finding, and systolic decompensation is observed late in the natural history of disease [34,35]. Heart failure statistics show that 50% of patients with heart failure with preserved ejection fraction (HFpEF).

There are a variety of methods available to measure diastolic function using CMR. At the most basic level, time–volume relation of the LV cavity obtained from a series of breath-hold acquisitions of parallel short-axis planes (Fig. 6.2) or a radial stack of long-axis planes can be used for assessment of LV filling during diastole. The peak filling rate, time to peak filling rate, and atrial filling fraction can be measured [36,37]. This requires high temporal resolution and retrospective gated cine to maximize the accuracy of the time volume curve. This technique has been replaced by the adoption of strain analysis by tissue tagging in CMR [37].

Tagged imaging approaches use the application of a spatially selective saturation pulse to create signal nulling in the myocardium, generally in a pattern of cross hatch or lines that are dark in appearance. The null pattern is applied at end-diastole, and persists throughout the cardiac cycle, during which time images are obtained [38,39]. This allows observation of tag line or grid deformation due to motion. This can be useful for visual evaluation of the relationship between structures, such as inspection of epicardial motion relative to the pericardium. For calculation of strain and relaxation indices, motion of the tag lines can be quantified by assessment of the temporal and spatial changes of image intensity, tag segmentation or a harmonic phase (HARP)–based analysis [40]. To enable acquisition of high-temporal resolution images, parallel imaging techniques, such as simultaneous acquisition of spatial harmonics (SMASH) and sensitivity encoding (SENSE) have been integrated into image acquisition [37,39]. The considerable reduction in scan time results in reduced breath-hold durations, or increased spatial resolution for a given breath-hold duration.

Tagged CMR has been applied to a number of cardiac disease states for both diagnosis of dysfunction and prognostication [39]. In patients with ischemic cardiac disease, myocardial tagging can identify changes in regional function involving the infarcted myocardium versus areas remote from the infarcted myocardium [41]. Dobutamine CMR when combined with myocardial tagging has been shown to detect more angiographically confirmed new wall-motion abnormalities than standard dobutamine CMR [42]. Myocardial tagging also improved the ability to discriminate between patients at risk for major adverse cardiac events (MACE) and those who were likely to remain event-free. Myocardial tagging has also been used to compare the association between regional dysfunction and abnormal myocardial perfusion in hypertrophic cardiomyopathy (HCM) [43]. Although myocardial tagging has not been systematically studied in CRCD, it may offer an opportunity to define early changes in myocardial deformation especially among patients receiving high doses of chemotherapy and the prognostic value of such changes in predicting MACE.

An alternate technique that has been developed to study diastolic function and myocardial deformation is CMR feature tracking (CMR-FT). This is analogous to echocardiographic speckle tracking and allows myocardial deformation to be directly measured from standard steady-state free precession (SSFP) cine images. It involves offline tracking of tissue voxel motion from which longitudinal, circumferential, and radial myocardial deformation can be quantified [44]. In a study of patients with LV dyssynchrony, speckle tracking echocardiography and CMR-FT were shown to provide similar results [45]. In a study of adult patients with a history of Tetralogy of Fallot repair, global circumferential strain showed the highest agreement between speckle tracking echocardiography and CMR-FT, followed by global longitudinal strain [46]. Studies have also shown CMR-FT to serve as reliable marker of myocardial viability and function; with the derived segmental strain measurements showing improvement in myocardial segments with low or no scar burden; but no improvement in those with transmural scar [46,47].

T1 and T2 Weighted Images and Mapping

Basic Principles

CMR uses the body's natural magnetic properties; and for clinical imaging purposes, the hydrogen nucleus (a single proton) is used because of its abundance in water and fat. Within a strong magnetic field, the hydrogen proton's axes align uniformly along the axis of the CMR scanner. When additional radiofrequency energy is added, the magnetic vector is deflected but returns to its resting state when the energy source is turned off. This causes a signal (also a radio wave) to be emitted and this signal is used to create the image.

CMR is unique as an imaging modality in its ability to characterize tissue composition by virtue of the different behaviors of protons in different tissue types when stimulated by radiofrequency pulses within the magnetic field. Multiple transmitted radiofrequency pulses can be used in sequence to emphasize particular tissue characteristic or abnormalities. This occurs because the relaxation of the proton from a higher energy to a lower energy spin state occurs at different rates when the transmitted radiofrequency pulse is switched off. The time it takes for protons to fully relax is measured in two ways. T1 represents longitudinal relaxation and is the time for the magnetic vector in any given region to return to its resting state aligned with the external magnetic field. T2 relaxation is the time needed for the transverse spin to return to its resting state. Protons in different tissues, such as fat and water have different relaxation times and different imaging sequences are used to emphasize or deemphasize particular tissue present in the imaged field. For example, a fat suppression sequence removes signal from adipose tissue, and comparison of images with and without fat suppression will allow evaluation of the adipose content of any structure [48].

T1 and T2 relaxation times have been defined for normal myocardium [49–51]. The normal value depends upon the field strength, age, sex, and the pulse sequence used to acquire the images for calculation of the tissue relaxation rate. T1 and T2 values may vary slightly within different regions of the myocardium, and are influenced by general hydration status and hematocrit. T1 relaxation times also altered dramatically shortened by the addition of gadolinium-based contrast, and normal values have been defined for

myocardium that has been exposed to a standardized dose of contrast [50,51].

A wide range of pathologic processes alter myocardial T1 and T2 values, and the pattern of observed abnormality can be helpful for determining the cause of ventricular dysfunction in newly diagnosed cardiomyopathy. Notably, native (noncontrast) T1 values are significantly increased in the setting of diffuse myocardial fibrosis (due to an expansion in extracellular volume and water content), such as that seen with a chronic cardiomyopathy process or prolonged myocardial insult. Increases in native T1 values are also seen with other processes expanding the ECV, such as myocardial edema or protein deposition (e.g., amyloidosis); while infiltration with other substances, such as lipid or iron causes a reduction in native T1 values [52–56]. Native T2 values increase with myocardial edema and can be observed in acute infarction, acute myocarditis, and following acute ischemic injury [49,50,57].

Imaging performed to emphasize signal from T1 relaxation (T1 weighted imaging) is the basis for "late gadolinium enhancement" or delayed enhancement CMR that has been extensively validated for detection of acute and chronic myocardial infarction. This form of imaging relies upon the presence of normal remote myocardium for optimization of signal differences between normal and abnormal tissue. Nonischemic late enhancement patterns have been described in a variety of cardiomyopathies, and the pattern itself may suggest the underlying cause of cardiac dysfunction in processes, such as myocarditis, HCM, cardiac sarcoid, and cardiac amyloidosis (Fig. 6.3). However, nonischemic cardiomyopathy may not be associated with visually detected abnormality using late gadolinium enhancement, due to the underlying process diffusely involving the myocardium [58].

The development of T1 mapping techniques was in response to the need for a method to detect and quantify diffuse myocardial fibrosis in patients with heart failure, given the hypotheses that diffuse fibrosis was the cause for increased cardiac stiffness and poor clinical outcomes. A prototype T1 mapping sequence was first used in 2008 and it was demonstrated that postcontrast T1 values correlated histologically with fibrosis seen on endomyocardial biopsy, and were reduced in subjects with heart failure compared to controls [59]. Subsequent clinical studies have demonstrated increased values for native T1 mapping in patients with severe aortic stenosis, HCM, and amyloidosis; and reduced native T1 in Anderson–Fabry disease (AFD) [55,58,60,61]. Reduced native T1 is peculiar to AFD and is consequent to increased intracellular storage of glycosphingolipid in myocardium. Thus native T1 values and mapping have a unique ability to differentiate AFD from other causes of left ventricular hypertrophy [55].

T2 mapping was developed and first used in animals and humans in 2009, and has advantages over use of

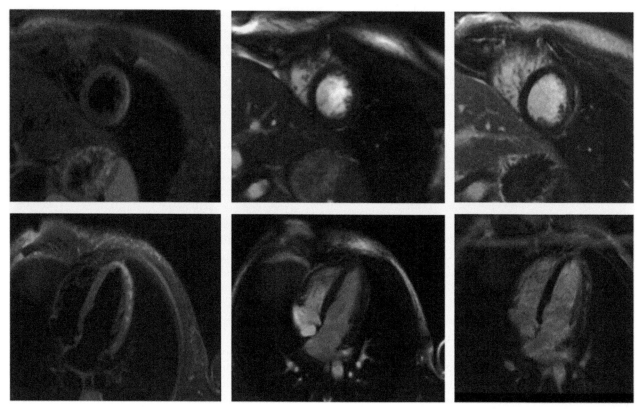

FIGURE 6.3 **CMR tissue characterization in myocarditis.** Images obtained in a patient with acute myocarditis. The left column shows precontrast dark blood T2 weighted images, middle column shows still frame cine images and right column are postcontrast T1 weighted images. There is increased brightness of the left ventricular lateral wall on both the T2 and T1 weighted images, indicating presence of regional myocardial edema and regional scar formation.

standard T2 weighted images in terms of insensitivity to cardiac motion and lack of signal variation seen in standard T2 weighted images [49]. In the setting of cardiac transplantation, it has been suggested that alterations in T2 can be detected using T2 mapping sequences and provide early noninvasive evidence of rejection, with resolution of abnormalities upon treatment [62]. Preliminary small human studies have used T2 weighted imaging sequences to show presence of myocardial edema in patients imaged during or at the end of therapy on the basis of increase in the T2 signal intensity [63].

T1 and T2 Measurement for Evaluation of Cardiotoxicity

In the case of cardiotoxicity from cancer therapy, there is substantial interest in the potential use of T1 and T2 measurement for noninvasive detection of myocardial-tissue abnormalities associated with chemotherapy related cardiotoxicity.

Observations of altered proton relaxation properties of myocardium in animal models of Adriamycin cardiotoxicity date back to the 1980s, with early recognition of native T1 elevation in chronic toxicity, most marked in the setting of overt heart failure, but no observed increase in T2 in this

chronic model [64]. Increase in both native T1 and T2 relaxation times was observed in an animal model evaluating the early effect of low dose Adriamycin, and occurred in association with reduced coronary flow, increased myocardial water content but preserved LV performance [65].

The clinical application of T1 and T2 weighted CMR has been extensively explored for both ischemic and nonischemic cardiomyopathies, and more recently this technique has been included in clinical studies of patients who have received anthracycline-based chemotherapy. A longitudinal assessment of myocardial-tissue characteristics and ventricular function was recently published for a group of adults (86% women) who received cardiotoxic chemotherapy for breast ($n = 51$) or hematologic malignancy ($n = 14$). CMR was performed prior to and at 3 months after initiation of therapy with anthracycline (55%), monoclonal antibody (38%) or an antimicrotubule agent (6%) [66]. There was a decrease in LVEF from $57 \pm 6\%$ to $54 \pm 7\%$ ($P < 0.001$), due to increases in end systolic volume. T2 weighted imaging was analyzable in 52/65 and was assessed by measuring relative signal intensity (ratio of myocardial to skeletal muscle signal) with a percentage of edema calculated as the number of voxels with relative enhancement ≥ 2. Using this approach, there were no appreciable differences at 3 months after chemotherapy initiation. Both native and postcontrast T1 was quantified in a subgroup of 10, and all subjects had late gadolinium enhancement imaging that was evaluated by measuring segmental signal intensity. Focal scarring was not observed in any subject, but the late gadolinium-enhancement image-signal intensity increased significantly at follow-up. In the subgroup who had T1 signal-intensity quantitation, there was no significant change in native or postcontrast T1 values [67].

Extracellular Volume Fraction

Because postcontrast T1 is influenced by a variety of non-pathological factors, such as imaging sequence and field strength, there has been recognition of the value of calculation of ECV as a potentially more reliable indicator of diffuse myocardial fibrosis. Calculation of ECV requires T1 mapping performed before and after contrast, and a known hematocrit value. It is calculated using the formula in Fig. 6.4.

ECV fraction estimation involves direct gadolinium contrast agent-based measurement of the size of the extra-cellular space, reflecting interstitial disease. This measure attempts to dichotomize the myocardium into its cellular (myocardial mass) and extracellular interstitial compartments with estimates expressed as volume fractions or percentages. Alterations in these compartments occur from different physiologic and pathophysiologic biologic processes. Furthermore, interstitial expansion may be reversible and a potential therapeutic target.

The gold standard for evaluation of cellular and extra-cellular volume is endomyocardial biopsy. It has been established, however, that CMR-derived measures of ECV correlate well with histologic collagen volume fraction throughout the whole heart, whereas isolated postcontrast T1 measurement is insufficient for ECV assessment [67].

Human whole heart histological validation was reported in a study that used tissue samples obtained from explanted hearts of six patients undergoing transplantation who had CMR performed at a median interval of 29 days prior to surgery [67]. There was a significant linear relationship between ECV and histologic collagen volume fraction

$$ECV = (1 - \text{hematocrit}) \frac{\left(\dfrac{1}{T1_{\text{myo post}}} - \dfrac{1}{T1_{\text{myo pre}}} \right)}{\left(\dfrac{1}{T1_{\text{blood post}}} - \dfrac{1}{T1_{\text{blood pre}}} \right)}$$

FIGURE 6.4 **Calculation of extracellular volume (ECV) using hematocrit and values for T1 of myocardium (myo) corrected for T1 of blood pool measured prior to and at steady state following administration of gadolinium based contrast.** Factors influencing measured T1 include the MRI system field strength, the sequence used for mapping, and the type of contrast used.

($P < 0.001$), and this relationship was maintained across all ventricular levels, and remained after exclusion of segments with focal scar (defined by presence of late gadolinium enhancement). In the same study 15 male and 15 female normal volunteers aged 32–65 years had variable dose gadolinium CMR for calculation of ECV. Values obtained were different with use of low versus higher dose of contrast when averaged over multiple time points of measurement, and the mean measured ECV increased linearly over time in each group. Additional observations were that ECV varied significantly between myocardial regions, being highest in the septum and lowest in the lateral wall, and that ECV was significantly higher in women than men.

It has been suggested that increase in ECV is a prognostic indicator independent of LVEF. In a CMR study of 793 patients without amyloidosis or HCM being imaged for a variety of indications, ECV was related to all-cause mortality and a composite endpoint of death/cardiac transplant/left ventricular assist device implantation, after adjusting for age, EF, and myocardial infarction size [68]. The same research group additionally reported increased ECV in diabetics compared to nondiabetics, a relationship between increased ECV and CV events in diabetics, and relatively lower ECV in patients receiving medication blocking the renin–angiotensin–aldosterone system [69].

In patients previously exposed to anthracycline therapy this imaging approach has been used to demonstrate presence of diffuse myocardial interstitial fibrosis. A study of asymptomatic long-term childhood cancer survivors aged 22 ± 6 years, who had received cumulative anthracycline dose ≥ 200 mg/m^2, found abnormally elevated ECV in 5/27 subjects [70]. An additional observation in this relatively small study was higher ECV in female compared to male survivors, of uncertain significance in light of aforementioned observations of sex differences in normal volunteers.

A younger group of 30 patients (15 ± 3 year) evaluated by CMR, echocardiography and cardiopulmonary exercise testing at least 2 years after anthracycline treatment had normal LVEF, but peak VO$_2$ 17% lower than age-predicted normal values and this reduction correlated with anthracycline dose ($r = -0.49$, $P = 0.04$). Mean myocardial ECV was comparable to previous studies of young adults ($20.7 \pm 3.6\%$). However ECV correlated with reduced CMR indices of myocardial mass, lower VO$_2$, and higher cumulative dose [71]. It was concluded that ECV may be an early tissue marker of ventricular remodeling in children with normal EF post anthracycline therapy, and related to cumulative dose, exercise capacity, and myocardial wall thinning.

In a study of 21 men and 21 women who received anthracycline-based chemotherapy, the data from CMR was compared to age- and gender-matched controls. Patients were 55 ± 17 years and were imaged a median of 84 months after chemotherapy with cumulative exposure of 282 ± 65 mg/m^2. The overall mean LVEF in this population was $52 \pm 12\%$, and was significantly lower than control group LVEF of $62 \pm 5\%$. In a subset of 14/42 subjects who had pretreatment reduced LVEF, the mean posttreatment LVEF was $38 \pm 8\%$. Mean ECV was elevated in anthracycline-treated patients compared to controls, with an association seen between ECV and left atrial volume and echocardiographic measures of diastolic function [72].

The experience with T1 and T2 mapping and ECV fraction calculation is relatively early, and there is a need to optimize these imaging techniques prior to widespread clinical application. In terms of image acquisition, T1 and T2 parameters are different on the basis of field strength of the magnet, and they are unique to the vendor-specific pulse sequences used. Therefore, the normal range varies according to vendor and pulse sequence type, age, and gender. Image artifact due to physiologic motion or off-resonance effects may also decrease image quality and up to 15% of acquired images may be unsuitable for analysis [70]. Hence there is a need to standardize imaging approaches to facilitate comparisons between different studies. Furthermore, the prognostic significance of changes in T1 and T2 in healthy volunteers and patients are needed in order to gain a comprehensive understanding of patterns in normal health and various pathologic states [73].

CMR Evaluation of Aortic Stiffness

Although myocardial dysfunction leading to development of heart failure is a very important potential consequence of therapy for cancer, it has additionally been recognized that cancer therapies may impact the cardiovascular system more broadly, apparently through generalized vascular insult. Hormonal therapy, such as androgen-deprivation therapy is associated with increased incidence of MI, peripheral arterial disease (PAD), and stroke. Increased risk of PAD [adjusted hazard ratio (HR): 1.16; 95% confidence interval (CI), 1.12–1.21] and venous thromboembolism (adjusted HR: 1.10; 95% CI, 1.04–1.15) was demonstrated in a large-population-based observational study of >180,000 US men $\geq$66 years with prostate cancer followed for median of 5.1 years [74]. Early phase trials of the tyrosine kinase inhibitor sunitinib showed increased mean systolic and diastolic pressure, with 35/75 subjects in a retrospective review developing hypertension [75]. Combination therapy of placlitaxel with bevacizumab versus paclitaxel alone for metastatic breast cancer in a study of 722 patients, reported 14.8% incidence of significant hypertension [76] and significantly more frequent cerebrovascular ischemic events (1.9%) with combination therapy. Anthracyclines have been associated with late subclinical vascular endothelial dysfunction and increased aortic-wall stiffness demonstrated using echocardiographic techniques in a study of 96 long-term survivors of different childhood cancer who were compared with 72 age, weight, and blood pressure matched controls

[77]. Among otherwise healthy individuals, increased aortic stiffness is the most important cause of increasing systolic and pulse pressure in adults over 40. Similar acute changes in aortic stiffness have also been demonstrated in animal and clinical studies of anthracycline cardiotoxicity.

CMR is an excellent tool for evaluation of aortic distensibility and pulse-wave velocity (PWV)—two measures of aortic stiffness. Chaosuwannakit et al. evaluated aortic distensibility in 40 women treated with anthracyclines for breast, or hematologic malignancy and 13 controls with CMR phase-contrast imaging for measurement of PWV. They observed an overall reduction in distensibility and increase in PWV indicating an increase in aortic stiffness [78].

In a recently published study of 29 patients (receiving anthracyclines and trastuzumab for breast cancer) and 12 volunteers, aortic PWV was measured using velocity encoded imaging, in addition to distensibility of the ascending and proximal descending aorta. There were acute changes in PWV and distensibility of the ascending aorta within 4 months of therapy, with persisting reduction in distensibility of the proximal descending aorta at 14 months after therapy in patients receiving chemotherapy, with the greatest change in those receiving anthracyclines alone [79].

CMR for Visualization of Proximal Segments of Coronary Arteries

Invasive coronary angiography or CT coronary angiography are approaches of choice for visualization of the coronary arteries to define the presence and extent of atherosclerotic disease. Both invasive angiography and CT angiography require use of iodinated contrast and expose the patient to a small dose of ionizing radiation. CMR is an alternative validated method for noninvasive visualization of coronary arteries that can be performed without use of contrast (or radiation), and can be used to rule out presence of proximal coronary artery narrowing. This may be particularly helpful for exclusion of proximal coronary stenosis in patients with prior chest radiation therapy.

Coronary magnetic resonance angiography (MRA) is typically performed without the need for contrast agents [80]. The relative signal of the coronary artery, which appears brighter than the surrounding myocardium, is augmented with fat-saturation prepulses, magnetization transfer contrast prepulses, or T2 preparatory pulses [81–83]. Intravenous contrast agents, can be used to improve the contrast-to-noise ratio due to the shortened T1 relaxation time for the intravascular blood pool [84]. The spatial resolution achievable with 3D MRA imaging is typically 0.7–0.8 mm in-plane resolution and 1–3 mm through plane [80,85]. Any improvement in spatial resolution by reducing the field of view is usually offset by a reduction in signal-to-noise ratio and a greater influence of coronary artery motion [85]. Cardiac motion and respiratory motion are key variables that can interfere with optimal visualization of coronary arteries by C and MRA. In order to minimize cardiac motion, images are acquired during mid-diastole. This also provides the ideal imaging opportunity when coronary flow is high. Respiratory motion may be suppressed with the use of breath-holding during image acquisition; however, this depends on the patient's ability to sustain adequate breath-holds particularly when the procedure lasts longer than a few seconds. Navigator echoes are therefore used to track a patient's diaphragmatic motion whereby MRA images are acquired only when the diaphragm is within 3–5 mm of its end-expiratory position [86]. This enables acquisition of a whole heart image without causing patient discomfort. On the other hand, it requires a relatively long duration for image acquisition since image data are collected only when the end-expiratory position of the diaphragm coincides with the period of coronary artery diastasis. A whole heart coronary MRA is acquired over multiple heartbeats and is analogous to coronary CTA. The entire coronary artery tree is imaged in an axially acquired 3D volume and navigator echoes are used for respiratory gating [80]. Acquisition of such a large volumetric data set results in a lower spatial resolution (>1 mm in-plane and through-plane resolution). Data are collected over approximately 100 ms of each cardiac cycle and this may increase the potential for blurring. Nevertheless, the whole-heart coronary MRA approach is widely used for the assessment of coronary arteries [87,88].

An alternate technique for imaging of coronary arteries with CMR uses the steady-state free-precession (SSFP) method. This technique allows acquisition of images with high signal intensity and high contrast between vascular structures and the myocardium without the need for contrast agents [89]. SSFP imaging with free-breathing allows high-quality coronary MRA with superior vessel sharpness compared with standard T2-prepared gradient-echo imaging. To reiterate, the previously described MRA protocols are especially valuable for imaging the proximal portion of the coronary arteries and may be used to exclude presence of ostial or proximal coronary stenosis typical of radiation induced disease [90,91].

EMERGING TECHNIQUES

Iodine-123-MIBG

Alterations in postsynaptic adrenergic efferent neurons in the myocardium have been thought to occur as a compensatory mechanism to offset the upregulation of sympathetic drive that occurs in response to heart failure [92,93]. Iodine-123-meta-iodobenzylguanidine (I-123 MIBG) is an analog of norepinephrine and can be taken up by postsynaptic neurons. It is not metabolized by catechol-O-methyl transferase and is therefore retained, and may serve as a surrogate marker of postsynaptic innervation. Planar gamma camera imaging is used to show distribution of the radiotracer, and quantitative approaches are used to calculate ratio of counts in heart compared to mediastinum, in addition to washout rates of myocardial tracer at baseline compared to 4 h (Fig. 6.5). In patients treated with anthracycline-based

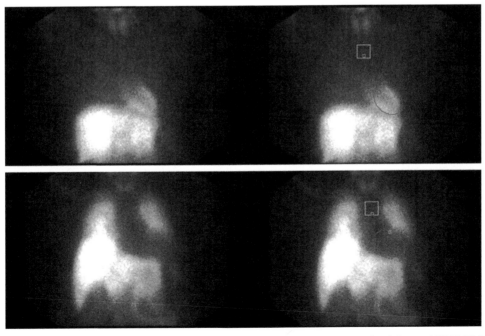

FIGURE 6.5   I-123 MIBG neurohormonal imaging. Planar images showing difference between normal and abnormal I123-MIBG imaging. The top row shows normal tracer uptake in myocardium, with contours around the heart (*red*), and a region in mediastinum (*green*). The bottom row shows abnormally reduced tracer uptake in myocardium relative to mediastinum. Despite the use of thyroid blockade prior to radiopharmaceutical administration there is physiologic uptake in thyroid gland that can be seen in both patients. Lung accumulation of tracer may be increased for a variety of reasons, and may be seen with heart failure.

chemotherapy, I-123 MIBG has been shown to be reduced [93–95]. Furthermore, there may be differences in I-123 MIBG uptake in these patients between the epicardial and endocardial layers suggesting that there may be regional differences in innervation as well as doxorubicin-induced myocardial damage [95].

99mTc-Annexin V

Accelerated apoptosis has been proposed to be one of the mechanisms responsible for myocardial injury caused by doxorubicin [96,97]. Apoptotic cells express phosphatidyl serine residues which serve as a binding site for annexin V. 99mTc-annexin V can therefore serve as a suitable ligand for identification of apoptotic cells in tissues with high apoptotic activity. In animal models of acute and chronic doxorubicin cardiotoxicity, increase in 99mTc-annexin V uptake has been observed. 99mTc-annexin V was also found to be dose dependent and its uptake has been correlated with histopathologic and immunohistochemical evidence of cardiomyocyte apoptosis [97].

Indium-111 Trastuzumab

Direct imaging of the epidermal-growth-factor receptor (EGFR) type 2 which are overexpressed in breast cancer cells is now possible with Indium-111 labeled trastuzumab. This allows visualization of changes in EGFR density in both breast tissue and in the myocardium in response to treatment [98]. The mechanism by which trastuzumab causes myocardial dysfunction is not well known; however, the adverse effects of Her2/neu receptor antibodies administered in combination with anthracycline is well documented. In a study that examined whether myocardial HER2 expression is increased by anthracycline-induced cardiac stress, 10 patients treated with anthracyclines underwent 111-In-trastuzumab scans and compared to a control group of 10 patients with nonanthracycline-related heart failure. Myocardial 111-In-trastuzumab was seen in five asymptomatic anthracycline-treated patients; however, none of 10 heart failure patients showed myocardial uptake [98].

PET–CMR

The emergence of positron emission tomography–CMR (PET–CMR) offers the opportunity to image the myocardium simultaneously with PET, a highly sensitive and quantitative modality that can detect select molecules or metabolites and CMR, which evaluates cardiac anatomy, function, perfusion, and tissue characteristics with excellent spatial and temporal resolution. FDG–PET has been shown to identify inflammation in myocardium far removed from the site of infarction—as defined by region of increase in Gd-DTPA uptake—in a postmyocardial infarction mouse model [99].

More recently, PET–CMR has been used for the assessment of myocardial viability with excellent agreement between FDG uptake imaging by PET and late gadolinium enhancement by CMR [100]. These studies also demonstrated the prognostic value of PET–CMR-based assessment of viability for predicting improvement in regional-wall motion. At this time, PET–CMR has not been specifically applied for the detection of CRCD; however, complementary imaging with PET–CMR may be most valuable in this patient population. We foresee that PET–CMR will greatly improve detection of myocardial damage either through inflammation or apoptosis by the use of novel molecular imaging PET tracers that are being developed in preclinical animal models in combination with MR pulse sequences tailored for identification of inflammation, edema, and fibrosis. This may have significant impact on the early detection of myocardial changes effected by chemotherapy and may improve our understanding of the underlying mechanisms of cardiotoxicity.

CONCLUSIONS

The current approaches used for evaluation of cardiotoxicity including echocardiography, CMR, and serological testing of biomarkers have been limited to relatively small patient populations, most often from single centers in Europe and the United States. One of the most important questions that arise is whether a change in myocardial structure or function that is detected with echocardiography or CMR should prompt a change in treatment including the cessation of potentially curative chemotherapy. Although data from small groups of patients demonstrate the prognostic value of troponin elevation, reduction in global longitudinal strain, or reduction in LVEF in response to chemotherapy, these have not been validated in other large population studies. Furthermore, CMR-based parameters, such as myocardial T1 and T2 have not been studied with respect to their prognostic value in patients who have undergone chemotherapy or radiation. Nevertheless, there has been a great deal of enthusiasm for the use of CMR to detect early myocardial changes in response to chemotherapy and radiation. It therefore becomes very important to understand the long-term prognostic value of myocardial tissue characteristics assessed by CMR before these can be extrapolated to clinical outcomes. Large follow-up studies are therefore needed for patients undergoing cancer treatments and comprehensively studied with these novel imaging parameters over a series of time intervals, in order to give us greater confidence in their prognostic value.

Currently, most patients who undergo chemotherapy with potentially cardiotoxic medications undergo assessment of LV function with either MUGA or echocardiography. In some cases, patients considered to be at high risk for adverse cardiac events may undergo serologic testing of cardiac enzymes. Notably, however, the ASE and the EACVI have recommended the use of CMR for assessment of LV and RV chamber volumes and function especially among patients in whom a cessation of chemotherapy is being considered on the basis of cardiac dysfunction diagnosed by clinical criteria and echocardiographic imaging [5]. Most importantly, these guidelines recommend the use of the same imaging modality especially when monitoring changes in LV function and chamber sizes with sequential imaging tests. For the assessment of subclinical LV dysfunction, the guidelines suggest the use of echocardiography-based strain imaging; however, CMR-based tissue characterization may have an important role to play in detecting subclinical LV dysfunction. This would require a large body of data which examines CMR-based evaluation of edema, inflammation, and fibrosis and its association with the type, dose, and duration of chemotherapy, as well as its relationship with long-term clinical outcomes.

REFERENCES

[1] Suter TM, Ewer MS. Cancer drugs and the heart: importance and management. Eur Heart J 2013;34(15):1102–11.

[2] Curigliano G, et al. Cardiovascular toxicity induced by chemotherapy, targeted agents and radiotherapy: ESMO Clinical Practice Guidelines. Ann Oncol 2012;23(Suppl. 7):vii155–66.

[3] Bellenger NG, et al. Comparison of left ventricular ejection fraction and volumes in heart failure by echocardiography, radionuclide ventriculography and cardiovascular magnetic resonance; are they interchangeable? Eur Heart J 2000;21(16):1387–96.

[4] Lancellotti P, et al. Expert consensus for multi-modality imaging evaluation of cardiovascular complications of radiotherapy in adults: a report from the European Association of Cardiovascular Imaging and the American Society of Echocardiography. J Am Soc Echocardiogr 2013;26(9):1013–32.

[5] Plana JC, et al. Expert consensus for multimodality imaging evaluation of adult patients during and after cancer therapy: a report from the American Society of Echocardiography and the European Association of Cardiovascular Imaging. J Am Soc Echocardiogr 2014;27(9):911–39.

[6] Hunt SA, et al. ACC/AHA 2005 Guideline Update for the Diagnosis and Management of Chronic Heart Failure in the Adult: a report of the American College of Cardiology/American Heart Association Task Force on Practice Guidelines (Writing Committee to Update the 2001 Guidelines for the Evaluation and Management of Heart Failure): developed in collaboration with the American College of Chest Physicians and the International Society for Heart and Lung Transplantation: endorsed by the Heart Rhythm Society. Circulation 2005;112(12):e154–235.

[7] Armenian SH, et al. Recommendations for cardiomyopathy surveillance for survivors of childhood cancer: a report from the International Late Effects of Childhood Cancer Guideline Harmonization Group. Lancet Oncol 2015;16(3):e123–36.

[8] Landier W, et al. Development of risk-based guidelines for pediatric cancer survivors: the Children's Oncology Group Long-Term Follow-Up Guidelines from the Children's Oncology Group Late Effects Committee and Nursing Discipline. J Clin Oncol 2004;22(24):4979–90.

[9] Pavel DG, Zimmer M, Patterson VN. In vivo labeling of red blood cells with 99mTc: a new approach to blood pool visualization. J Nucl Med 1977;18(3):305–8.

[10] Atkins HL, et al. Vascular imaging with 99m Tc-red blood cells. Radiology 1973;106(2):357–60.

[11] de Geus-Oei LF, et al. Scintigraphic techniques for early detection of cancer treatment-induced cardiotoxicity. J Nucl Med 2011;52(4):560–71.

[12] Hesse B, et al. EANM/ESC guidelines for radionuclide imaging of cardiac function. Eur J Nucl Med Mol Imaging 2008;35(4):851–85.

[13] Mitra D, Basu S. Equilibrium radionuclide angiocardiography: its usefulness in current practice and potential future applications. World J Radiol 2012;4(10):421–30.

[14] Skrypniuk JV, et al. UK audit of left ventricular ejection fraction estimation from equilibrium ECG gated blood pool images. Nucl Med Commun 2005;26(3):205–15.

[15] Walker J, et al. Role of three-dimensional echocardiography in breast cancer: comparison with two-dimensional echocardiography, multiple-gated acquisition scans, and cardiac magnetic resonance imaging. J Clin Oncol 2010;28(21):3429–36.

[16] Schwartz RG, Jain D, Storozynsky E. Traditional and novel methods to assess and prevent chemotherapy-related cardiac dysfunction noninvasively. J Nucl Cardiol 2013;20(3):443–64.

[17] Schwartz RG, et al. Congestive heart failure and left ventricular dysfunction complicating doxorubicin therapy. Seven-year experience using serial radionuclide angiocardiography. Am J Med 1987;82(6):1109–18.

[18] Appel JM, et al. Systolic versus diastolic cardiac function variables during epirubicin treatment for breast cancer. Int J Cardiovasc Imaging 2010;26(2):217–23.

[19] Canclini S, et al. Gated blood pool tomography for the evaluation of global and regional left ventricular function in comparison to planar techniques and echocardiography. Ital Heart J 2001;2(1):42–8.

[20] Panjrath GS, Jain D. Monitoring chemotherapy-induced cardiotoxicity: role of cardiac nuclear imaging. J Nucl Cardiol 2006;13(3):415–26.

[21] Reuvekamp EJ, et al. Does diastolic dysfunction precede systolic dysfunction in trastuzumab-induced cardiotoxicity? Assessment with multigated radionuclide angiography (MUGA). J Nucl Cardiol 2015;23(4):824–32.

[22] Seals AA, et al. Comparison of left ventricular diastolic function as determined by nuclear cardiac probe, radionuclide angiography, and contrast cineangiography. J Nucl Med 1986;27(12):1908–15.

[23] Plana JC, et al. Expert consensus for multimodality imaging evaluation of adult patients during and after cancer therapy: a report from the American Society of Echocardiography and the European Association of Cardiovascular Imaging. Eur Heart J Cardiovasc Imaging 2014;15(10):1063–93.

[24] Higgins CB. Which standard has the gold? J Am Coll Cardiol 1992;19(7):1608–9.

[25] Kramer CM, et al. Standardized cardiovascular magnetic resonance imaging (CMR) protocols, society for cardiovascular magnetic resonance: board of trustees task force on standardized protocols. J Cardiovasc Magn Reson 2008;10:35.

[26] Maceira AM, et al. Normalized left ventricular systolic and diastolic function by steady state free precession cardiovascular magnetic resonance. J Cardiovasc Magn Reson 2006;8(3):417–26.

[27] Baikoussis NG, et al. Safety of magnetic resonance imaging in patients with implanted cardiac prostheses and metallic cardiovascular electronic devices. Ann Thorac Surg 2011;91(6):2006–11.

[28] Levine GN, et al. Safety of magnetic resonance imaging in patients with cardiovascular devices: an American Heart Association scientific statement from the Committee on Diagnostic and Interventional Cardiac Catheterization, Council on Clinical Cardiology, and the Council on Cardiovascular Radiology and Intervention: endorsed by the American College of Cardiology Foundation, the North American Society for Cardiac Imaging, and the Society for Cardiovascular Magnetic Resonance. Circulation 2007;116(24):2878–91.

[29] Dewey M, Schink T, Dewey CF. Claustrophobia during magnetic resonance imaging: cohort study in over 55,000 patients. J Magn Reson Imaging 2007;26(5):1322–7.

[30] Hundley WG, et al. ACCF/ACR/AHA/NASCI/SCMR 2010 expert consensus document on cardiovascular magnetic resonance: a report of the American College of Cardiology Foundation Task Force on Expert Consensus Documents. J Am Coll Cardiol 2010;55(23):2614–62.

[31] Constantine G, et al. Role of MRI in clinical cardiology. Lancet 2004;363(9427):2162–71.

[32] Armstrong GT, et al. Screening adult survivors of childhood cancer for cardiomyopathy: comparison of echocardiography and cardiac magnetic resonance imaging. J Clin Oncol 2012;30(23):2876–84.

[33] Sievers B, et al. Impact of papillary muscles in ventricular volume and ejection fraction assessment by cardiovascular magnetic resonance. J Cardiovasc Magn Reson 2004;6(1):9–16.

[34] Owan TE, et al. Trends in prevalence and outcome of heart failure with preserved ejection fraction. N Engl J Med 2006;355(3):251–9.

[35] Yu CM, et al. Progression of systolic abnormalities in patients with "isolated" diastolic heart failure and diastolic dysfunction. Circulation 2002;105(10):1195–201.

[36] Engels G, et al. Evaluation of left ventricular inflow and volume by MR. Magn Reson Imaging 1993;11(7):957–64.

[37] Westenberg JJ. CMR for assessment of diastolic function. Curr Cardiovasc Imaging Rep 2011;4(2):149–58.

[38] Del-Canto I, et al. Characterization of normal regional myocardial function by MRI cardiac tagging. J Magn Reson Imaging 2015;41(1):83–92.

[39] Shehata ML, et al. Myocardial tissue tagging with cardiovascular magnetic resonance. J Cardiovasc Magn Reson 2009;11:55.

[40] Osman NF, et al. Cardiac motion tracking using CINE harmonic phase (HARP) magnetic resonance imaging. Magn Reson Med 1999;42(6):1048–60.

[41] Kramer CM, et al. Regional differences in function within noninfarcted myocardium during left ventricular remodeling. Circulation 1993;88(3):1279–88.

[42] Kuijpers D, et al. Dobutamine cardiovascular magnetic resonance for the detection of myocardial ischemia with the use of myocardial tagging. Circulation 2003;107(12):1592–7.

[43] Soler R, et al. Magnetic resonance imaging of delayed enhancement in hypertrophic cardiomyopathy: relationship with left ventricular perfusion and contractile function. J Comput Assist Tomogr 2006;30(3):412–20.

[44] Schuster A, et al. Cardiovascular magnetic resonance myocardial feature tracking detects quantitative wall motion during dobutamine stress. J Cardiovasc Magn Reson 2011;13:58.

[45] Onishi T, et al. Feature tracking measurement of dyssynchrony from cardiovascular magnetic resonance cine acquisitions: comparison with echocardiographic speckle tracking. J Cardiovasc Magn Reson 2013;15:95.

[46] Padiyath A, et al. Echocardiography and cardiac magnetic resonance-based feature tracking in the assessment of myocardial

mechanics in tetralogy of Fallot: an intermodality comparison. Echocardiography 2013;30(2):203–10.

[47] Schuster A, et al. Cardiovascular magnetic resonance myocardial feature tracking for quantitative viability assessment in ischemic cardiomyopathy. Int J Cardiol 2013;166(2):413–20.

[48] Berger A. Magnetic resonance imaging. BMJ 2002;324(7328):35.

[49] Giri S, et al. T2 quantification for improved detection of myocardial edema. J Cardiovasc Magn Reson 2009;11:56.

[50] Sparrow P, et al. Myocardial T1 mapping for detection of left ventricular myocardial fibrosis in chronic aortic regurgitation: pilot study. AJR Am J Roentgenol 2006;187(6):W630–5.

[51] Messroghli DR, et al. Modified Look-Locker inversion recovery (MOLLI) for high-resolution T1 mapping of the heart. Magn Reson Med 2004;52(1):141–6.

[52] Banypersad SM, et al. Quantification of myocardial extracellular volume fraction in systemic AL amyloidosis: an equilibrium contrast cardiovascular magnetic resonance study. Circ Cardiovasc Imaging 2013;6(1):34–9.

[53] Piechnik SK, et al. Normal variation of magnetic resonance T1 relaxation times in the human population at 1.5 T using ShMOLLI. J Cardiovasc Magn Reson 2013;15:13.

[54] Plymen CM, et al. Diffuse myocardial fibrosis in the systemic right ventricle of patients late after Mustard or Senning surgery: an equilibrium contrast cardiovascular magnetic resonance study. Eur Heart J Cardiovasc Imaging 2013;14(10):963–8.

[55] Sado DM, et al. Identification and assessment of Anderson–Fabry disease by cardiovascular magnetic resonance noncontrast myocardial T1 mapping. Circ Cardiovasc Imaging 2013;6(3):392–8.

[56] White SK, et al. T1 mapping for myocardial extracellular volume measurement by CMR: bolus only versus primed infusion technique. JACC Cardiovasc Imaging 2013;6(9):955–62.

[57] Jellis CL, Kwon DH. Myocardial T1 mapping: modalities and clinical applications. Cardiovasc Diagn Ther 2014;4(2):126–37.

[58] Dass S, et al. Myocardial tissue characterization using magnetic resonance noncontrast t1 mapping in hypertrophic and dilated cardiomyopathy. Circ Cardiovasc Imaging 2012;5(6):726–33.

[59] Iles L, et al. Evaluation of diffuse myocardial fibrosis in heart failure with cardiac magnetic resonance contrast-enhanced T1 mapping. J Am Coll Cardiol 2008;52(19):1574–80.

[60] Bull S, et al. Human non-contrast T1 values and correlation with histology in diffuse fibrosis. Heart 2013;99(13):932–7.

[61] Karamitsos TD, et al. Noncontrast T1 mapping for the diagnosis of cardiac amyloidosis. JACC Cardiovasc Imaging 2013;6(4):488–97.

[62] Usman AA, et al. Cardiac magnetic resonance T2 mapping in the monitoring and follow-up of acute cardiac transplant rejection: a pilot study. Circ Cardiovasc Imaging 2012;5(6):782–90.

[63] Oberholzer K, et al. [Anthracycline-induced cardiotoxicity: cardiac MRI after treatment for childhood cancer]. Rofo 2004;176(9):1245–50.

[64] Thompson RC, et al. Adriamycin cardiotoxicity and proton nuclear magnetic resonance relaxation properties. Am Heart J 1987;113(6):1444–9.

[65] Cottin Y, et al. Early incidence of adriamycin treatment on cardiac parameters in the rat. Can J Physiol Pharmacol 1994;72(2):140–5.

[66] Jordan JH, et al. Longitudinal assessment of concurrent changes in left ventricular ejection fraction and left ventricular myocardial tissue characteristics after administration of cardiotoxic chemotherapies using T1-weighted and T2-weighted cardiovascular magnetic resonance. Circ Cardiovasc Imaging 2014;7(6):872–9.

[67] Miller CA, et al. Comprehensive validation of cardiovascular magnetic resonance techniques for the assessment of myocardial extracellular volume. Circ Cardiovasc Imaging 2013;6(3):373–83.

[68] Wong TC, et al. Association between extracellular matrix expansion quantified by cardiovascular magnetic resonance and short-term mortality. Circulation 2012;126(10):1206–16.

[69] Wong TC, et al. Myocardial extracellular volume fraction quantified by cardiovascular magnetic resonance is increased in diabetes and associated with mortality and incident heart failure admission. Eur Heart J 2014;35(10):657–64.

[70] Toro-Salazar OH, et al. Occult cardiotoxicity in childhood cancer survivors exposed to anthracycline therapy. Circ Cardiovasc Imaging 2013;6(6):873–80.

[71] Tham EB, et al. Diffuse myocardial fibrosis by T1-mapping in children with subclinical anthracycline cardiotoxicity: relationship to exercise capacity, cumulative dose and remodeling. J Cardiovasc Magn Reson 2013;15:48.

[72] Neilan TG, et al. Myocardial extracellular volume by cardiac magnetic resonance imaging in patients treated with anthracycline-based chemotherapy. Am J Cardiol 2013;111(5):717–22.

[73] Lundin J, Ugander M. Clinical utility of cardiac T1- and extracellular volume (ECV) mapping: a brief review. MAGNETOM Flash 2015;1:2.

[74] Hu JC, et al. Androgen-deprivation therapy for nonmetastatic prostate cancer is associated with an increased risk of peripheral arterial disease and venous thromboembolism. Eur Urol 2012;61(6):1119–28.

[75] Chu TF, et al. Cardiotoxicity associated with tyrosine kinase inhibitor sunitinib. Lancet 2007;370(9604):2011–9.

[76] Miller K, et al. Paclitaxel plus bevacizumab versus paclitaxel alone for metastatic breast cancer. N Engl J Med 2007;357(26):2666–76.

[77] Jenei Z, et al. Anthracycline causes impaired vascular endothelial function and aortic stiffness in long term survivors of childhood cancer. Pathol Oncol Res 2013;19(3):375–83.

[78] Chaosuwannakit N, et al. Aortic stiffness increases upon receipt of anthracycline chemotherapy. J Clin Oncol 2010;28(1):166–72.

[79] Grover S, et al. Early and late changes in markers of aortic stiffness with breast cancer therapy. Intern Med J 2015;45(2):140–7.

[80] Bluemke DA, et al. Noninvasive coronary artery imaging: magnetic resonance angiography and multidetector computed tomography angiography: a scientific statement from the american heart association committee on cardiovascular imaging and intervention of the council on cardiovascular radiology and intervention, and the councils on clinical cardiology and cardiovascular disease in the young. Circulation 2008;118(5):586–606.

[81] Li D, et al. Coronary arteries: three-dimensional MR imaging with fat saturation and magnetization transfer contrast. Radiology 1993;187(2):401–6.

[82] Brittain JH, et al. Coronary angiography with magnetization-prepared T2 contrast. Magn Reson Med 1995;33(5):689–96.

[83] Edelman RR, Chien D, Kim D. Fast selective black blood MR imaging. Radiology 1991;181(3):655–60.

[84] Stuber M, et al. Contrast agent-enhanced, free-breathing, three-dimensional coronary magnetic resonance angiography. J Magn Reson Imaging 1999;10(5):790–9.

[85] Spuentrup E, et al. The impact of navigator timing parameters and navigator spatial resolution on 3D coronary magnetic resonance angiography. J Magn Reson Imaging 2001;14(3):311–8.

[86] McConnell MV, et al. Prospective adaptive navigator correction for breath-hold MR coronary angiography. Magn Reson Med 1997;37(1):148–52.

[87] Sakuma H, et al. Assessment of coronary arteries with total study time of less than 30 minutes by using whole-heart coronary MR angiography. Radiology 2005;237(1):316–21.

[88] Piccini D, et al. Respiratory self-navigated postcontrast whole-heart coronary MR angiography: initial experience in patients. Radiology 2014;270(2):378–86.

[89] Deshpande VS, et al. 3D magnetization-prepared true-FISP: a new technique for imaging coronary arteries. Magn Reson Med 2001;46(3):494–502.

[90] McEniery PT, et al. Clinical and angiographic features of coronary artery disease after chest irradiation. Am J Cardiol 1987;60(13):1020–4.

[91] Jaworski C, et al. Cardiac complications of thoracic irradiation. J Am Coll Cardiol 2013;61(23):2319–28.

[92] Matsuo S, et al. Noninvasive identification of myocardial sympathetic and metabolic abnormalities in a patient with restrictive cardiomyopathy–in comparison with perfusion imaging. Ann Nucl Med 2002;16(8):569–72.

[93] Wakasugi S, et al. Myocardial substrate utilization and left ventricular function in adriamycin cardiomyopathy. J Nucl Med 1993;34(9):1529–35.

[94] Jeon TJ, et al. Evaluation of cardiac adrenergic neuronal damage in rats with doxorubicin-induced cardiomyopathy using iodine-131 MIBG autoradiography and PGP 9.5 immunohistochemistry. Eur J Nucl Med 2000;27(6):686–93.

[95] Takano H, et al. Myocardial sympathetic dysinnervation in doxorubicin cardiomyopathy. J Cardiol 1996;27(2):49–55.

[96] Yamanaka S, et al. Amlodipine inhibits doxorubicin-induced apoptosis in neonatal rat cardiac myocytes. J Am Coll Cardiol 2003;41(5):870–8.

[97] Bennink RJ, et al. Annexin V imaging of acute doxorubicin cardiotoxicity (apoptosis) in rats. J Nucl Med 2004;45(5):842–8.

[98] Perik PJ, et al. Indium-111-labeled trastuzumab scintigraphy in patients with human epidermal growth factor receptor 2-positive metastatic breast cancer. J Clin Oncol 2006;24(15):2276–82.

[99] Lee WW, et al. PET/MRI of inflammation in myocardial infarction. J Am Coll Cardiol 2012;59(2):153–63.

[100] Rischpler C, et al. PET/MRI early after myocardial infarction: evaluation of viability with late gadolinium enhancement transmurality vs 18F-FDG uptake. Eur Heart J Cardiovasc Imaging 2015;16(6):661–9.

Chapter 7

Cardiotoxicity Induced by Anticancer Drugs—the Role of Biomarkers

G. Biasillo*, C.M. Cipolla** and D. Cardinale*

*Cardioncology Unit, European Institute of Oncology, IRCCS, Milan, Italy; **Cardiology Division, European Institute of Oncology, IRCCS, Milan, Italy

INTRODUCTION

Modern anticancer therapies lead to a significant improvement in prognosis in oncological patients, However, both conventional and novel anticancer drugs may cause damage to the heart, ultimately affecting patients' survival and quality of life.

In the last decades, both due to the longer expectancy of life and higher knowledge of cardiac toxicity of anticancer drugs, a great amount of studies underlined the importance of chemotherapy-induced cardiotoxicity (CTX) [1–3].

In fact, CTX is one of the most severe complications of cancer treatment and represents an adverse event difficult to manage by the oncologists: even minor cardiac damage may lead to a review of the anticancer therapy, with dose reduction or change in administration schedule. This may impact patient outcome.

The most frequent cardiac complication of CTX is the development of a hypokinetic cardiomyopathy. It usually begins with asymptomatic diastolic or systolic dysfunction and may progress to congestive heart failure (HF), possibly leading to death [4]. Onset time of cardiac toxicity is highly variable. Previously, three types of CTX were described: acute, occurring after a single dose, or a single course of anticancer drugs, with the onset of clinical manifestations within 2 weeks from the end of drug administration; early-onset chronic, developing within 1 year; late-onset chronic, developing years after the end of treatment. However, this classification is based on small, retrospective studies performed in childhood cancer survivor populations [5,6]. Instead, recent findings suggest that drug-induced CTX is a continuum that starts with myocardial cell injury, followed by progressive left ventricular dysfunction (LVD), which if disregarded and not treated, leads to overt HF [7].

The phenomenon of CTX is expected to rise because of the increasing number of patients undergoing anticancer chemotherapy, the improved efficacy of anticancer therapies, and prolonged life expectancy of.

A consistent number of risk factors for CTX have been identified [8]. Some of them are related to the anticancer strategy adopted, such as cumulative dose, use of chemotherapeutic agents in combination resulting in a synergistic toxicity, and prior or concomitant radiation therapy. In particular, radiation therapy may amplify and accelerate the development of cardiovascular injury, inducing endothelial cell damage and compromising coronary artery blood flow [9]. Other risk factors are patient related: age at the time of first therapy administered, preexisting cardiovascular diseases (coronary artery disease, peripheral vascular disease), well-recognized cardiovascular risk factors (hypertension, dyslipidemia, smoking history), and comorbidities (diabetes, obesity, chronic kidney disease). Notably, young patients, with a longer life expectancy, are more exposed to the risk of developing CTX [10]; on the other hand, older age itself is a risk factor, as extensively demonstrated [11].

At present, there is still no single and proper definition of anticancer drug-induced CTX. In fact, the development of any adverse cardiac events, such as acute coronary syndromes, hypertension, arrhythmias, decreased cardiac contractile function, electrocardiographic changes, and thromboembolic events, can be regarded as expressions of CTX.

International cardiologic societies defined CTX as a decline of the left ventricular ejection fraction (LVEF) greater than 10% points with a final LVEF <50% or as a LVEF reduction greater than 15% points with a final LVEF >50% [1]. More recently, expert consensus from the American Society of Echocardiography and the European Association of Cardiovascular Imaging defines CTX as a decline of LVEF greater than 10% points with a final LVEF <53% [12]. This decrease should be confirmed by repeated cardiac imaging.

Although many aspects of CTX need to be better investigated, the severity and the incidence of this phenomenon demand a more accurate prediction of the risk in a preclinical and early clinical stage. This approach would allow the avoidance of restrictions in indications and dose of anticancer agents and drug withdrawal that are recommended when cardiac damage is already clinically evident and moreover to plan closer monitoring.

ANTICANCER DRUGS AND CARDIAC TOXICITY

Several chemotherapeutic agents can induce HF or predispose patients to CTX. Traditional chemotherapeutic agents, such as anthracyclines (ACs), have been known to cause cardiovascular morbidities months or years after administration, and new targeted drugs such as monoclonal antibodies and others, have been recently evaluated (Table 7.1).

AC antibiotics, such as doxorubicin, daunorubicin, and epirubicin, are some of the most effective and widespread chemotherapeutic agents used for the treatment of both hematological and solid malignancies. The therapeutic activity of AC is mediated by their intercalation into the DNA of replicating cells, thereby inhibiting polymerases, and disrupting DNA, RNA, and protein synthesis. The mechanism of AC-induced CTX is not fully understood but it is probably multifactorial. The leading pathway is the increase of reactive oxygen species (ROS) within the cardiac myocyte mitochondria; notably, adult myocytes are more susceptible to ROS because they are terminally differentiated and cannot replace cells damaged during treatment [13,14]. Cardiac damage induced by AC is considered irreversible and

dose dependent. Other authors explored a possible role for topoisomerase 2β in AC-mediated toxicity. In fact, topoisomerase 2β is required for AC to induce DNA double-strand breaks and changes in the transcriptome, leading to mitochondrial dysfunction and generation of ROS. Deleting topoisomerase 2β from cardiomyocytes prevented the development of anthracycline-induced cardiotoxicity in animal models [15]. On the basis of these molecular observations, Vejpongsa et al. hypothesized that topoisomerase 2β could be regarded as a promising molecular target that can be used to design interventions to prevent AC-induced CTX [16,17].

Trastuzumab is a humanized monoclonal antibody directed against the human epidermal growth factor receptor-2 (ErB2, also called EGFR2 or HER2), very effective for the treatment of HER2-positive breast cancer. Evidence from both in vivo and in vitro studies indicate the importance of the HER2 pathway in the heart as well, suggesting that trastuzumab-induced CTX is related to HER2 blockade with subsequent impairment of cell-protective, growth-promoting, antiapoptotic pathways in the myocardium [18].

Trastuzumab enhances the effect of traditional chemotherapy, leading to an increase of the response to the therapy and an improvement in overall survival [19]. On the other hand, its use results in an unexpected risk of CTX, often manifested by an asymptomatic decrease in LVEF. Of interest, different authors have observed that the incidence of cardiac dysfunction increased among patients who received trastuzumab with AC or trastuzumab with paclitaxel [19],

TABLE 7.1 Anticancer Drugs and Cardiovascular Side Effects

Chemotherapeutic Agents	Specific Drug	Indications	CV Side Effects
Anthracycline	Epirubicin	Breast cancer, ovarian cancer, sarcoma	Hypokinetic cardiomyopathy
	Doxorubicin	Breast cancer, lymphoma	
	Daunorubicin	Leukemia	
Pyrimidine analogs	Capecitabine	Breast cancer	Coronary spasm
	5-Fluorouracil	Colorectal cancer	
Alkylating agents	Cyclophosphamide	Breast cancer	Myocarditis
	Cisplatin	Urinary tract cancer	Thrombosis
Antimicrotubule agents	Paclitaxel	Breast cancer, colorectal cancer	Bradycardia
Anti-HER2 agents	Trastuzumab	Breast cancer	Hypokinetic cardiomyopathy
	Lapatinib	Gastric cancer	
Angiogenesis inhibitors	Bevacizumab	Gastric cancer	Hypertension
	Sunitinib	Renal-cell cancer	Thrombosis
	Sorafenib	Hepatocellular cancer	
BCR–ABL inhibitors	Dasatinib	Gastric cancer	QT prolongation and arrhythmias

although it seems that in some cases cardiac dysfunction occurs when trastuzumab is used alone [20].

In contrast to AC-induced CTX, the cardiac injury due to trastuzumab is not related to cumulative dose and is not associated with severe ultrastructural changes on myocardial biopsy; importantly, trastuzumab-induced CTX is often reversible after treatment discontinuation, and can be administered once again, if indicated, after recovery [21]. However, if AC-induced CTX has been reasonably detailed, the features of trastuzumab-induced CTX (the precise pathophysiological mechanism, capacity of recovery, long-term implications, and overall clinical importance) are not fully understood. Some of the uncertainties are due to the fact that HER2-positive breast cancer patients are concomitantly treated with both trastuzumab and AC, making the identification of the effects of each agent from a synergistic interaction between them difficult.

Finally, an increasing number of antiangiogenesis agents are emerging as a therapeutic option for cancer patients. This class of angiogenesis inhibitors are monoclonal antibodies against VEGF receptors (i.e., bevacizumab) and "multitargeted" tyrosine kinase inhibitors (i.e., sunitinib and sorafenib), which block downstream signaling in VEGF and other tumor growth pathways. These agents are associated with adverse cardiovascular events, in particular, the onset of hypertension, thromboembolism, and myocardial ischemia [22]. In fact, they can cause endothelial dysfunction by blocking the capability of endothelial cells to regenerate, decreasing the production of vasodilators, and triggering procoagulant pathways [23].

DETECTION OF CARDIAC TOXICITY

Current Approach

The detection of drug-induced CTX is based, at present, on regular assessment of cardiac function by LVEF measurement using either transthoracic echocardiography (ECHO) or radionuclide multigated acquisition (MUGA) [3,12,24]. However, evidence-based guidelines specifying how often, by what means, or how long cardiac function should be monitored, are lacking. Moreover, this approach has several limitations [1,25]. LVEF assessment has relatively low sensitivity, because no considerable change occurs until significant myocardial damage is present. In fact, cardiac damage is usually detected only after functional impairment has already occurred, precluding any chance of preventing its development. On the other hand, the evidence of a normal LVEF does not exclude the possibility of a late cardiac deterioration given the low predictive value of LVEF assessment, even when serially repeated. Furthermore, measurement of LVEF by ECHO has further limitations: left ventricular geometric assumptions, inadequate visualization of the true left ventricular apex, lack of consideration

of subtle regional wall motion abnormalities, and the inherent variability of measurement. It is also important to consider the load dependency of this measurement. Changes in loading conditions are frequent during chemotherapy and may affect the LVEF value (volume expansion due to the intravenous administration of chemotherapy or volume contraction due to vomiting or diarrhea, changing of arterial pressure values). Moreover, image quality is dependent on the acoustic window, with a high interobserver variability.

Among other imaging modalities, MUGA is only able to detect significant changes in cardiac function, indeed it requires exposure to radioactivity. At present, magnetic resonance imaging represents the gold standard in the evaluation of volume and function of the left ventricle, but it is limited by low availability, high cost, and long processing time. Finally, endomyocardial biopsy is able to provide histological evidence of CTX; at present, it is not used in clinical practice because of its invasiveness and high expertise required [12].

Role of Biomarkers

Over the last decades, the use of cardiac biomarkers has been investigated as a possible new tool aimed at early identification, assessment, and monitoring of drug-induced CTX. It is minimally invasive, economical, repeatable, without direct damage for patients, and without interobserver variability. Most of the existing data regarding use of cardiac biomarkers in an oncological setting refer to troponins, related to cardiomyocyte injury, and natriuretic peptides (NPs), released from the heart in response to volume expansion and increased wall stress.

Early identification of patients who are at risk for drug-induced CTX should be a primary goal to plan and to develop individualized therapeutic strategies and intervention in cancer patients.

Troponin

Troponins constitute a regulatory protein complex composed of three subunits, troponin C (TnC), troponin T (TnT), and troponin I (TnI) (Fig. 7.1). Each unit has a specific function in cell contraction, through mediation of actin–myosin interaction. In particular, TnC binds Ca^{2+} released from the sarcoplasmic reticulum, TnI inhibits the ATPase activity of actomyosin, TnT provides for the binding

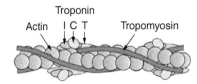

FIGURE 7.1 **Location of cardiac troponin I, cardiac troponin T, and cardiac troponin C.**

of the troponin complex to tropomyosin. TnC is present in all muscle types; on the other hand, three human isoforms have been described for TnT and TnI: one from the cardiac muscle and one from the fast- and the slow-twitch skeletal muscle, respectively. Cardiac troponin is complexed with actin in cardiac myofibrils with an incompletely characterized fraction soluble in the cytoplasm. When an ischemic injury occurs, there is a modification of myocyte membrane integrity, causing rapid depletion of the soluble cytoplasmic pool, followed by larger and more sustained release of troponin into the circulation as the contractile apparatus breaks down.

Cardiac troponins I and T are well-established biomarkers in diagnosis and risk stratification of patients with suspected and proven acute coronary syndromes, according to current guidelines [26]. However, elevation in troponin levels has been observed in other clinical settings, such as left ventricular hypertrophy, HF, acute pulmonary embolism, blunt trauma, sepsis, stroke, renal insufficiency and, more recently, CTX associated with anticancer drugs [27,28].

Studies performed with animal models demonstrated that TnT is released by doxorubicin-damaged myocytes; indeed the serum concentrations of TnT correlated with the dose of drug received as well as the histological degree of myocardial damage [29].

In the clinical setting, a large number of studies performed over the last decades suggest that elevations of cardiac troponin (both TnT and/or TnI) are useful tools in the evaluation of patients receiving potentially cardiotoxic therapy (Table 7.2) [30–50]. Lipshultz first observed an increase in the plasma levels of troponin in about one-third of young patients undergoing chemotherapy, thus suggesting for the first time a possible relationship between myocardial damage and anticancer treatment [30]. In a subsequent study, the same population was followed up for 5 years after the end of treatment; increase in TnT levels occurred during anticancer identified children who would later manifest cardiac abnormalities at ECHO [36].

Similar data were obtained in adult patients. Elevated levels of troponins were founded in patients receiving standard dose of AC, in the days following treatment administration [33,37,38]. In particular, patients with elevated TnT and TnI levels had a significantly greater decrease in LVEF posttreatment than those without elevation [33,37]. TnI has been demonstrated to be a sensitive and specific marker of drug-induced myocardial injury even in patients treated with high-dose AC, able to predict the development of LVD in a very early phase, as well as its severity [31,32]. In fact, in patients showing an increase in TnI, a significant reduction in LVEF after 3 months was observed, and LVEF impairment was still evident at the end of the follow-up; on the other hand patients with normal values of TnI had a transient decrease in LVEF after 3 months, but subsequently recovered to an LVEF greater than 50% (Fig. 7.2) [31]. A larger study performed by the same group confirmed these data: TnI-positive patients had a greater incidence of major adverse cardiac events [35]. In addition, given the very high negative predictive value of the marker, TnI allowed the identification of low-risk patients who will not require further cardiac monitoring, and, on the other hand, the identification of patients at higher risk, requiring closer surveillance.

Recently, the possible role of troponins in the early detection of CTX has also been investigated in patients treated with newer targeted therapies. The role of TnI has been studied in 251 breast cancer patients treated with trastuzumab [41]. It was measured immediately before and immediately after each cycle, and it showed an increase in 14% of the patients. The first TnI increase was observed, in most cases, soon after the first trastuzumab cycle (Fig. 7.3). LVD occurred in 62% of them, and in only 5% of patients with a normal TnI value ($P < 0.001$). HF treatment, including angiotensin-converting enzyme inhibitors (ACEI) and beta-blockers (BB), was promptly initiated, and up-titrated to the maximum-tolerated dose. Patients displaying an increase in TnI during trastuzumab treatment had a threefold lower chance of recovering from cardiac dysfunction and an overall higher incidence of cardiac events, despite optimized HF treatment. These findings suggest that TnI in addition to the early identification of patients at high risk of developing LVD, also allows the identification of patients who will less likely recover from toxicity, possibly distinguishing between reversible and irreversible cardiac injury induced by a sequential treatment with AC and trastuzumab [51].

Further data have also emerged from studies performed in patients with tyrosine-kinase inhibitors. Schmidinger et al. reported an increase in TnT in about 10% of patients with metastatic renal cancer treated with sunitinib or sorafenib, and 90% of them experienced subsequent echocardiographic impairment (decrease in LVEF or regional contraction abnormalities) [40]. Morris showed increased TnI in patients receiving both trastuzumab and lapatinib following AC treatment: of note, the timing of detectable TnI preceded maximum decline in LVEF [42].

Highly Sensitive Troponin

A new generation highly sensitive (HS) troponin assay has been recently developed, which is able to detect very low amounts of troponin. [52] This characteristic is of particular interest in the cardioncological setting. In most patients, in fact, troponin values increases are just slightly above the cut-off.

First studies employing HS-troponin assays were conducted by Sawaya group [43,45]. In particular, they evaluated both HS-troponin and ECHO parameters of myocardial deformation in patients receiving AC, taxanes, and trastuzumab. Global and regional myocardial function by tissue Doppler and strain rate imaging, combined

TABLE 7.2 Clinical Studies Demonstrating Troponins as Predictors of Cardiotoxicity

Study (Year)	Patients (n)	Cancer Type	Drugs	Troponin Type	Cut Off	Timing of Assessment
Lipshultz (1997) [30]	15[a]	ALL	AC	T	0.03 ng/mL	Before CT; 1–3 days after each dose
Cardinale (2000) [31]	201	Various	HD CT	I	0.04 ng/mL	0–12–24–36–72 h after CT
Cardinale (2002) [32]	232	Breast cancer	HD CT	I	0.04 ng/mL	0–12–24–36–72 h after CT
Auner (2002) [33]	30	Hematological	HD Cycl	T	0.03 ng/mL	Before CT; 1–14 days after CT
Sandri (2003) [34]	179	Various	HD CT	I	0.04 ng/mL	0–12–24–36–72 h after CT
Cardinale (2004) [35]	703	Various	HD CT	I	0.04 ng/mL	0–12–24–36–72 h after CT
Lipshultz (2004) [36]	158[a]	ALL	AC	T	0.01 ng/mL	Before CT; daily after induction; 7 days after a CT single dose; end CT
Specchia (2005) [37]	79	Hematological	AC	I	0.15 ng/mL	Before CT; weekly × 4 times
Kilickap (2005) [38]	41	Various	AC	T	0.10 ng/mL	Before CT; 3–5 days after 1st and last dose
Lee (2008) [39]	86	Hematological	AC	I	0.20 ng/mL	Before each dose
Schmidinger (2008) [40]	74	Renal carcinoma	Sunitinib/sorafenib	I	0.03 ng/mL	Before CT; bimonthly during CT
Cardinale (2010) [41]	251	Breast cancer	TRZ	I	0.04 ng/mL	Before and after each cycle
Morris (2011) [42]	95	Breast cancer	AC + taxanes + TRZ/LAP	I	0.30 ng/mL	Every 2 weeks during CT
Sawaya (2011) [43]	43	Breast cancer	AC + taxanes + TRZ	HS-I	0.015 ng/mL	Before CT; after 3 and 6 months during CT
Lipshultz (2010) [44]	205[a]	ALL	AC/AC + dexrazoxane	I/T	Any detectable amount	Before CT; 1–7 days after each dose; end CT
Sawaya (2012) [45]	81	Breast cancer	AC + taxane + TRZ	HS-I	30 pg/mL	Before CT; after 3 and 6 months during CT
Geiger (2012) [46]	50	Various	AC	T	NA	Before CT; after 6 h, 7 days, 3 months
Mornos (2013) [47]	74	Various	AC	HS-T	NA	Before CT; after 6, 12, 24, 52 weeks
Mavinkurve-Groothuis (2013) [48]	60[a]	ALL	AC	HS-T	0.01 ng/mL	Before CT; after 3 and 12 months
Ky (2014) [49]	78	Breast cancer	AC + taxanes + TRZ	HS-I	NA	Before CT; after 3 and 6 months during CT
Putt (2015) [50]	78	Breast cancer	AC + taxanes + TRZ	HS-I	NA	Before CT, after 3, 6, 9, 12, 15 months during CT

AC, Anthracycline-containing chemotherapy; ALL, acute lymphoblastic leukemia; CT, chemotherapy; Cycl, cyclophosphamide; HD, high-dose; HS, ultrasensitive; I, troponin I; LAP, lapatinib; NA, not available; T, troponin T; TRZ, trastuzumab.
[a]Pediatric population.

with HS-troponin I, at baseline, and during chemotherapy were evaluated. Decreases in peak longitudinal strain and increases in HS-TnI concentrations, at the end of the AC treatment, were predictive of subsequent occurrence of LVD. In contrast, other tools, such as changes in LVEF, diastolic function, and N-terminal pro-brain natriuretic peptide (NT-proBNP) evaluated at the same time points, were not predictive of later occurrence of LVD. Notably, elevation in HS-TnI or a decrease in longitudinal strain was associated with higher sensitivity and specificity compared to each parameter alone [45].

More recently, other authors evaluated HS-troponin I as predictor of CTX. In particular they observed, in a similar population of cancer patients treated with AC, taxanes, and

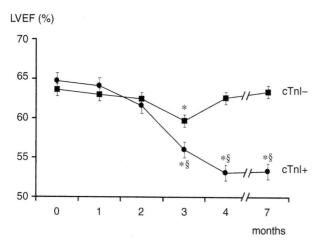

FIGURE 7.2 *LVEF* at baseline and during the 7 months of follow-up of troponin I positive (*cTnI+*) and negative (*cTnI-*) patients. *$P < 0.001$ versus baseline (month 0); $^{\S}P < 0.001$ versus cTnI- group. Data are shown as mean ± 95% CI. *Modified from Cardinale D, et al. Left ventricular dysfunction predicted by early troponin I release after high-dose chemotherapy. J Am Coll Cardiol 2000;36:517–522.*

trastuzumab, that LVD was predicted by a significant rise in HS-Troponin I values compared with baseline [49,50]. Of note in these studies, HS-Troponin I was evaluated in a multiple-biomarker approach.

At present, the only study comparing standard troponin assays and HS-assays in the oncological setting was performed by Salvatici et al [53]. Stocked samples of cancer patients, who were previously monitored during and after chemotherapy through troponin assessment and ECHO evaluation, were retested with an HS-troponin assay. A good correlation between standard and high-sensitivity troponin assays was observed, in agreement with other results obtained in other settings (Fig. 7.4) [53].

Taken all together, these observations pointed out that troponin release may identify subclinical cardiac damage in patients treated with both conventional and newer antineoplastic treatments, possibly representing a final event that is common to different mechanisms underlying the cardiotoxic effect. Indeed, troponin measurement is able to detect CTX very early, and to predict LVD—and associated cardiac events—months before their development, both in patients treated with standard dose and high-dose cardiotoxic drugs, allowing cardiac risk stratification. However, there are still some limitations in the routine employment of troponin in clinical practice. Some studies failed to detect changes in troponin levels during or after anticancer treatments [54,55]. This could be related to different factors: various anticancer protocols employed, varying times of sampling associated with different drug administration schedules, lack of standardization of different assays, cardiac end-points definition and follow-up length [56]. Standardization of routine troponin measurement in the clinical setting to maximize single-time-point assay sensitivity and specificity is needed and should be an important focus for future research.

Natriuretic Peptides

Natriuretic peptides (NPs) are hormones produced by cardiomyocytes and released into circulation in response to wall strain and pressure overload. The more widely investigated members of the NP family are atrial natriuretic peptide (ANP) and brain natriuretic peptide (BNP) and their cosecreted and biologically inactive N-terminal amino acid fragment (NT-proANP and NT-proBNP).

Natriuretic peptides play a pivotal role in the maintenance of cardiovascular homeostasis: in fact they are involved in many physiologic functions including vasodilation,

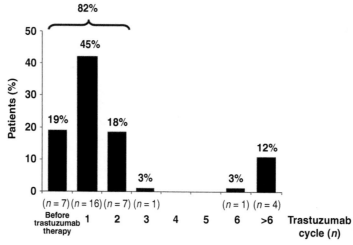

FIGURE 7.3 **Time of the first detection of elevated troponin value.** *Modified from Cardinale D, et al. Trastuzumab-induced cardiotoxicity: clinical and prognostic implications of troponin I evaluation. J Clin Oncol 2010;28:3910–16.*

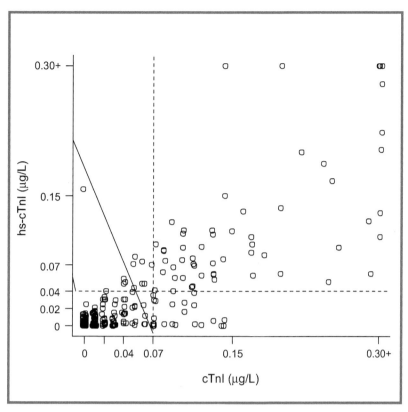

FIGURE 7.4   Correlation between cTnI and cTnI-ultra evaluated at all measurements. Spearman correlation (rho): 0.73. *P* < 0.001. *Modified from Salvatici M, et al. TnI-Ultra assay measurements in cancer patients: comparison with the conventional assay and clinical implication. Scand J Clin Lab Invest 2014;74(5):385–91.*

natriuresis, kaliuresis, inhibition of the renin–angiotensin–aldosterone system and inhibition of sympathetic tone.

BNP and NT-proBNP are gaining acceptance as potentially useful biomarkers in the diagnosis and prognostic stratification of patients with HF [57,58].

In the last decade, great interest has grown about the use of NP in patients with chemotherapy-induced cardiac impairment. Several authors investigated a possible role for BNP and NT-proBNP in particular, in the detection and prediction of CTX. In a very early study performed on 27 patients with hematological malignancy treated with AC, Suzuki observed that persistent elevations of BNP were associated with poor prognosis and reflective of induced diastolic dysfunction, thus suggesting a correlation between NP increase and reduced cardiac tolerance to cardiotoxic agents [59].

After this first report, multiple studies were performed on patients with different malignancies, different ages (both children and adult populations), and different oncologic drugs, and schedules [2,55,60–63]. In most studies persistently elevated levels of posttreatment BNP and/or NT-proBNP correlate with ECHO indexes of myocardial dysfunction [55,63–65]. However, only a few reports indicated NP as strong predictors of LVD after chemotherapy [60,64,65].

In particular, data from Sandri et al [64]. showed that persistently elevated levels of NT-proBNP were able to identify patients who would develop an impairment of both diastolic and systolic function 1 year after high-dose chemotherapy for aggressive malignancies. Three distinct patterns of NT-proBNP concentrations were identified. Of the patients, 31% had no change in NT-proBNP concentrations in the 72 h after therapy; 35% of patients experienced a transient increase with normalization within 72 h. In these two groups, no significant echocardiographic abnormalities were founded during the 1-year follow-up. Conversely, 33% of patients with persistently increased NT-proBNP concentrations at 72 h developed a significant worsening of both diastolic and systolic ECHO indexes. In particular, significant increases in mitral deceleration time, isovolumetric relaxation time and in mitral E/A ratio and significant decrease in LVEF mean value were observed.

Other reports confirmed these findings, showing a close relationship between NP and the development of subclinical myocardial injury due to anticancer drugs [60,63,65]. Some studies, however, found no correlation between NT-proBNP increase and development of cardiac dysfunction in patients receiving AC-based chemotherapy [45,61,62].

The role of NPs in the patients treated with new targeted drugs is less understood. A few studies on small populations, mainly breast cancer patients treated with trastuzumab, have analyzed the information of NP assay in the setting, leading to conflicting results. In fact, although some authors have identified NT-proBNP as a promising tool in the management of the patients treated with new therapy [66,67], others have failed to reveal any predictive role of the NT-proBNP [45,68].

Therefore, although several data are now available, it is not yet possible to draw definite conclusions or indications because of some important limitations affecting the comparison of results coming from different studies. First, most studies were performed on small and heterogeneous populations with different malignancies at various stages and different therapeutic schedules. Furthermore, different laboratory methods were used, with frequently undeclared cutoffs and an extremely broad range of sampling times. Finally, the follow-up duration of the studies was quite variable and the lack of standardized cardiac endpoints were present. New prospective and multi-center studies, including large populations, using well-standardized methods for dosage and with well-defined timing of sampling and cardiologic end-points, are needed to define the appropriate use of NP in this setting.

Newly Proposed Biomarkers

Troponins, BNP, and NT-proBNP are the most studied biomarkers for cardiovascular screening in most clinical settings, including the cardioncological setting, for detection and monitoring of CTX, in cancer patients treated with potentially cardiotoxic drugs, as reported above.

In the last decades, however, an increasing number of circulating biomarkers have aroused researchers' interest in the cardiovascular setting, and more recently even in the cardioncological setting.

Because of the large number of mitochondria in cardiomyocytes and the tight relationship linking oxidative metabolism with myocardial viability, mitochondrial dysfunction is considered as an expression of cardiotoxicity. Therefore, biomarkers related to mitochondrial dysfunction could be studied for monitoring occurrence and extent of cardiac damage; indeed they could be studied in order to prevent mitochondrial cardiotoxic effects of anticancer drugs. Among them, according to current knowledge, cytochrome c, mitochondrial DNA, and oxidized albumin seem to be early and reliable markers of mitochondrial dysfunction [69]. ACs, by generating oxidative stress and alterations in redox status, cause the opening of voltage-dependent channels, leading to mytochondrial membrane permeability changes and the release of proapoptotic proteins from the mitochondria. Cytochrome c is one such protein that can be measured in the circulation as a mitochondrial dysfunction marker, that may anticipate cell necrosis (Fig. 7.5). Preliminary data from an ongoing trial from our institute confirmed that serum cytochrome c may increase during AC-containing chemotherapy (16% of cases, unpublished data) and that its rise temporally precedes the increase of troponin—evidenced in 18% of treated patients. These

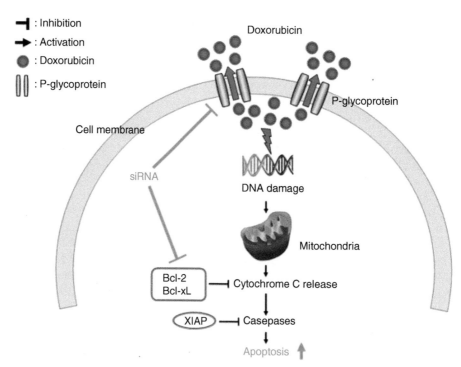

FIGURE 7.5 **Molecular pathway of apoptosis that is triggered by doxorubicin.** Doxorubicin damages DNA; DNA damage induces cytochrome c release in mitochondria which activates caspases, the effectors of apoptosis.

findings suggest that the release of cytochrome c could be a new early marker of CTX, which may precede cell necrosis and the subsequent release of troponin.

Myeloperoxidase (MPO) is an enzyme secreted by polymorphonuclear leucocytes; it has a proatherogenic and pro-oxidant effect and is considered a marker of oxidative stress, causing lipid peroxidation, scavenging of nitric oxide, and inhibition of nitric oxide synthase. In patients with acute coronary syndromes and HF, elevated levels of MPO are predictive of adverse events [70,71]. Notably, MPO seem to provide an additive value to troponin T [70].

In the cardioncological setting, Ky et al. first observed that early changes in MPO levels are associated with subsequent CTX. This result is of particular interest: in fact oxidative stress has been hypothesized to be an important mechanism in AC-mediated CTX. Another important finding is that MPO and TnI used in combination identify a subgroup of patients at increased risk of CTX. Conversely, no association between CTX and other biomarkers, including high-sensitivity C-reactive protein (CRP), NT-proBNP, growth differentiation factor (GDF)-15, placental growth factor (PlGF), soluble VEGF receptor 1 (sFlt-1), and galectin 3 (Gal-3) was found [49].

Subsequently, the same group confirmed that increased levels of MPO are associated with future development of CTX. Interestingly, the study goes beyond previous observations showing an early rise of MPO: in fact, it indicates that increase in MPO throughout the entire course of therapy is significantly associated with development of CTX. Contrary to the previous findings, in this study GDF-15 and PlGF were shown to be associated with CTX: of note, the independence of these markers in the multivariable model suggests additive utility. No association between CRP, NT-proBNP, sFlt-1, and gal-3 and CTX were observed in this study either [50].

Interestingly, in both studies, among molecules shown to be predictive of CTX, each one was modestly predictive by itself, but their combination allowed for a more confident association with subsequent degree of ventricular dysfunction, thus confirming previous observations that a multimarker approach may better stratify the cardiac risk in oncologic patients [45], allowing for preventive strategies.

Heart-type fatty-acid-binding protein (H-FABP) and glycogen phosphorylase BB (GPBB) have been recently evaluated for the early detection of myocardial ischemia. H-FABP is a relatively small cytoplasmic protein for the oxidation of fatty acids and has a good specificity for cardiac muscle. It is rapidly released from the myocardium into the bloodstream in response to an ischemic injury and returns to normal values within 18–30 h. GPBB is a glycogenolytic enzyme providing glucose for the heart muscle tissue. In ischemic tissue, during glycogenolysis, GPBB is released from the sarcoplasmic reticulum into the cytoplasm and then into the circulation through the damaged

cell membrane, returning to normal values within 24–36 h of damage occurrence. In the acute coronary syndrome setting, both markers are regarded as early indicators of cardiac injury due to acute myocardial ischemia [72,73].

The possible roles of H-FABP and GPBB have been investigated in hematological patients receiving AC-based chemotherapy. Whereas El-Ghandour et al. found an association between increased FABP levels and LVEF reduction in patients with cardiac dysfunction [74], Horacek et al. failed to find any association, and reported increases only in GPBB [75]. However, although these markers are highly sensitive and rapidly released after acute myocardial ischemia, they are less specific than troponin for the detection of cardiac damage different from an ischemic insult; further studies on larger number of patients will be needed to better define their potential in the early detection of cardiotoxicity.

PREVENTION OF CARDIAC TOXICITY

Patients undergoing a potentially cardiotoxic treatment are considered to be at increased risk of developing LVD [76]. Existing clinical data suggest that programs aimed at preventing the development of LVD appear strategically more effective than interventions aimed at counteracting an already existing LVD, which can be progressive and irreversible in many cases [1,4].

Accordingly, several preventive strategies to reduce the risk of cardiotoxicity have been proposed. To avoid the development of severe LVD, several preventive measures have been proposed as well. They include limitation of cumulative chemotherapy dose, replacement of bolus administration with slow infusion, use of less cardiotoxic AC analogs, addition of cardioprotectants to the chemotherapeutic regimen, and employment of nutritional supplements.

Cardiotoxicity prevention may be a primary prevention, extended to all patients scheduled for potential cardiotoxic therapy, or could be performed in selected high-risk patients showing preclinical signs of cardiotoxicity,

Primary Prevention

Adding Cardioprotectants to Chemotherapy

Among cardioprotectant agents, dexrazoxane is one of most extensively studied molecules. Some authors observed an association between dexrazoxane administration and reduction of AC-related CTX both in adult patients with different solid tumors and in children with acute lymphoblastic leukemia and Ewing's sarcoma [36,44,77,78]. Still there are some limitations in routine dexrazoxane employment in clinical practice. In fact, according to ASCO guidelines [79], it is recommended as a cardioprotectant agent only in selected patients (metastatic breast cancer patients who have already received more than 300 mg/m^2 of doxorubicin), because of its hypothesized interference with the anticancer efficacy of AC, implication in the occurrence of second malignancies, and myelosuppression. However, metaanalyses of antitumor efficacy and of secondary malignancy occurrences did not find a significant difference between patients who were treated with or without dexrazoxane [77,80].

Other cardioprotective agents such as coenzyme Q10, carnitine, N-acetyl-cysteine, the antioxidant vitamins E and C, erythropoietin, the endothelin-1 receptor antagonist bosentan, the lipid-lowering agent probucol, and statins have been investigated. Preliminary evidence shows that these agents may have cardio-protective effects, but their utility in preventing CTX requires further investigation [14,77].

Adding Cardiovascular Agents to Chemotherapy

The cardioprotective effects of many pharmacologic agents have been demonstrated during cancer therapy. However, most of these findings have been obtained from animal models. In the clinical arena four groups of agents—BB, angiotensin antagonists, statins, and aldosterone antagonists—have proven to be cardioprotective, with similar results in patients treated with ACs or trastuzumab (Table 7.3) [81–91].

Carvedilol has shown antioxidant activity that may result in an effective cardioprotective action against doxorubicin. The first evidence showing cardioprotective effects of BB emerged from an in vitro study [92]. This effect was confirmed in a small randomized study in which prophylactic use of the drug prevented LVD and reduced mortality in a population of AC-treated patients [81].

Different studies conducted over the last decades and performed on animal models have shown that, in rats undergoing short- or long-term administration of doxorubicin, coadministration of ACEI completely prevented the decline in cardiac function, as well as the increase in left ventricular weight induced by doxorubicin [93–96]. Furthermore, other authors demonstrated that doxorubicin cannot induce cardiac injury in angiotensin-II type-I receptor gene knockout

TABLE 7.3 Cardiovascular Drugs Showing a Prophylactic Effect Against Anticancer Drug-Induced Cardiotoxicity

Study (Year)	Study Design/ Follow-Up	N	Cancer Type	Drugs	Intervention	Results
ACEI						
Cardinale (2006) [91]	RCT/12 months	114	Various	HD CT	Enalapril	No LVEF ↓; MACE incidence ↓
ARB						
Nakamae (2005) [88]	RCT/7 days	40	NHL	AC	Valsartan	No LVEDD↑; no BNP, and ANP↑; no QT↑
Cadeddu (2010) [89]	RCT/18 months	49	Various	AC	Telmisartan	No peak strain rate ↓; no interleukin-6 ↑
Heck (2015) [83]	RCT/3–9 months	120	Breast cancer	AC, TRZ	Candesartan	No LVEF↓
Aldosterone antagonists						
Akpek (2015) [90]	RCT/6 months	83	Breast cancer	AC	Spironolactone	No LVEF↓; no TNI and BNP↑
Beta-blockers						
Kalay (2006) [81]	RCT/6 months	50	Various	AC	Carvedilol	No LVEF ↓
Kaya (2012) [87]	RCT/6 months	45	Breast cancer	AC	Nebivolol	No LVEF and NT-proBNP↑
ACEI + beta-blockers						
Bosh (2013) [82]	RCT/6 months	90	Hematological	AC	Enalapril + Carvedilol	No LVEF↓; death↓; HF ↓
Statins						
Acar (2011) [84]	RCT/6 months	40	Hematological	AC	Atorvastatin	No LVEF↓
Seicean (2012) [85]	Retrospective/ 5 years	67	Breast cancer	AC	Statins	HF ↓
Chotenimitkhun (2015) [86]	PO	51	Various	AC	Statin	No LVEF↓

ACEI, Angiotensin-converting enzyme inhibitor; ANP, atrial natriuretic peptide; ARB, angiotensin receptor blocker; BNP, brain natriuretic peptide; HD CT, high-dose chemotherapy; LVEF, left ventricular ejection fraction; LVEDD, left ventricular end-diastolic diameter; HF, heart failure; MACE, major adverse cardiac events; NHL, non-Hodgkin lymphoma; NT-proBNP, N-terminal-pro-brain natriuretic peptide; QT, QT interval; PO, prospective observational; RCT, randomized controlled trial; TNI, troponin I; TRZ, trastuzumab.

mice [97], thus suggesting that angiotensin II could play a key role in the pathogenesis of doxorubicin-induced CTX.

The efficacy of carvedilol, in combination with enalapril, to prevent chemotherapy-induced LVD was explored in the OVERCOME trial [82]. Patients with various hematologic malignancies receiving intensive high-dose chemotherapy were randomized to the intervention group (enalapril plus carvedilol) or the control group (no intervention). LVEF was evaluated before and after chemotherapy administration. After 6 months, no changes in LVEF were observed in the intervention group, but a significant decrease in the control group was present.

The results of the Prevention of Cardiac Dysfunction during Adjuvant Breast Cancer Therapy (PRADA) [83] trial have demonstrated that candesartan—but not metoprolol—concomitantly administered with adjuvant epirubicin-containing chemotherapy, with or without trastuzumab, provides protection against early decline in LV function, assessed with cardiac magnetic resonance.

Statins have been shown to exert antioxidative, antiinflammatory, and other pleiotropic effects. In an animal model it has been demonstrated that pretreatment with fluvastatin blunted anthracycline-induced toxicity, reducing oxidative stress, enhancing expression of the antioxidant enzyme mitochondrial superoxide-dismutase2, and limiting cardiac inflammation [98]. In a small clinical trial of 40 patients with normal LVEF undergoing chemotherapy which included AC, the 6-month LVEF value was unchanged among patients treated with atorvastatin compared with an 8% absolute decrease in controls [84]. In a retrospective observational study, 67 breast cancer patients treated with AC, who had already received statins for alternative indications, uninterrupted statin use was associated with a markedly lower risk for HF and cardiac-related mortality over 2.2 ± 1.7 years of follow-up, compared with 134 propensity-matched controls (HR 0.3, CI 95%.0.1–0.9; $P < 0.03$) [85]. Consistently, Chotenimitkhun et al [86]. more recently found in a prospective observational study that individuals already receiving statin therapy for prevention of cardiovascular disease experienced less deterioration in LVEF at 6 months after AC-containing chemotherapy, than individuals not receiving statins. Prospective randomized control trials are needed to further delineate independent effects of statins on clinical outcomes in oncologic patients.

Role of Biomarkers in Prevention of Cardiac Toxicity

A primary pharmacologic preventive strategy extended to all cancer patients undergoing chemotherapy would have a very high cost–benefit ratio; moreover, patients could be exposed to fewer side effects.

The possibility of identifying patients at high risk of cardiotoxicity by cardiac biomarkers provides a rationale for targeted preventive pharmacological strategies against cardiac dysfunction and its late complications. The therapeutic strategies needed to be implemented in order to reduce the clinical impact of CTX are: (1) use of specific cardiologic treatments during chemotherapy to prevent, or blunt, the rise of biomarkers indicative of myocardial damage; (2) use of cardiologic treatments given only to a selected cancer patient population, in particular to those patients showing an increase in these markers during and after chemotherapy.

Lipshultz et al. selected TnT as a biomarker for monitoring the cardioprotective effect of dexrazoxane in 206 pediatric patients with acute lymphocytic leukemia: dexrazoxane was associated with less frequent TnT elevations compared with a placebo [36]. More recently, in the same population, followed-up for 5 years after treatment, the authors reported that children with at least one increase in TnT during CT showed significant late cardiac abnormalities at echocardiography [44].

The protective effect of nebivolol against AC-induced cardiomyopathy has been demonstrated in a small randomized study [87]. In 27 breast cancer patients receiving nebivolol during AC-therapy, LVEF and NT-proBNP remained unchanged after 6 months from baseline; conversely, in the placebo group a significantly lower LVEF and a higher NT-proBNP value were observed.

The first study evaluating the role of angiotensin II in the AC-induced CTX in humans was conducted by Nakamae et al. These authors showed that, in a randomized trial enrolling a small number of patients free of cardiac diseases, valsartan, an angiotensin-II receptor blocker, administered at the same time as AC-containing chemotherapy, prevented the increase in ANP and BNP, the acute increase in left ventricular diastolic diameter, and the prolongation and in QTc interval [88].

The possible role of another angiotensin-II receptor blocker, telmisartan, in preventing myocardial damage induced by AC was investigated in a randomized study including patients without prior cardiovascular diseases and treated with epirubicin for different kinds of solid cancers. After an 18-month follow-up, patients starting telmisartan a few days before epirubicin showed no significant reduction in myocardial deformation indexes as evaluated by tissue Doppler echocardiography, nor a significant increase in ROS or in interleukin-6, as found in 24 patients receiving epirubicin alone [89,99].

Aldosterone antagonism has very recently been evaluated in a trial including 83 patients randomized to receive spironolactone, or not, and concomitant AC-containing chemotherapy [90]. After 3 weeks of the end of chemotherapy, spironolactone had prevented a decrease in LVEF, blunted the increase in troponin I and NT-proBNP, and also preserved diastolic function.

The usefulness of biomarkers of myocardial damage, and troponin in particular, in selecting patients for prophylactic cardioprotective therapy was investigated in a randomized trial including patients treated with high-dose AC [91]. Among them, 114 patients showed an early increase of TnI: these patients were randomized either to receive enalapril (ACEI group) or not (control group). Treatment with enalapril was started 1 month after chemotherapy and was continued for 1 year. In the ACEI group, LVEF did not change during the follow-up period, whereas, in patients not receiving enalapril, a progressive reduction in LVEF and an increase in ventricle dimensions (both diastolic and systolic) were observed (Table 7.3). Furthermore, patients in the ACEI group had a lower incidence of adverse cardiac events than the other group (Table 7.4).

Similar results were observed in patients treated with developing molecular targeted therapies. In a phase-I trial, Ederhy observed a TnI increase from baseline during treatment with new anti-VEGF monoclonal inhibitors and tyrosine kinase inhibitors in patients with solid metastatic tumors. All patients showing an increase in the marker underwent ECHO, cardiac magnetic resonance, CT scan, and coronary angiography that excluded other possible etiologies of TnI increase. Normalization of TnI values was obtained with BB and aspirin administration. After TnI normalization, all patients were rechallenged with the study drug. No patient experienced any new increase of TnI, and no cardiac events occurred during the following observation period. This study supports previous evidence that troponin may play an important role in the identification of patients at risk for the development of cardiotoxicity who should receive prophylactic treatment, without being excluded from continuing oncologic treatment (Table 7.5) [100].

The International Cardioncology Society (ICOS)-ONE trial is the only randomized study to compare a primary prevention approach with prevention in selected high-risk patients, in patients treated with ACs. The primary objective of the ongoing trial is to assess whether enalapril started concomitantly with AC therapy can prevent cardiotoxicity more effectively than when enalapril is prescribed to selected patients showing an increase in troponin (NCT01968200).

CONCLUSIONS

Anticancer therapy-induced cardiotoxicity still remains a serious problem, strongly affecting both the quality of life and the overall survival of oncologic patients. The most effective approach for minimizing cardiotoxicity is its

TABLE 7.4 Echocardiographic Parameters During the Study Period

		Baseline	Rand.	3 Months	6 Months	12 Months	P Value[a]
EDV (mL)	ACEI-group	101.7 ± 27.4	100.2 ± 26.1	98.1 ± 27.8	97.5 ± 24.5	101.1 ± 26.4	0.045
	Controls	103.2 ± 20.1	103.9 ± 21.0	106.4 ± 21.0	107.1 ± 23.9	104.2 ± 25.6	
ESV (mL)	ACEI-group	38.6 ± 10.8	38.7 ± 10.4	37.3 ± 10.9	37.4 ± 10.3	38.5 ± 11.2	<0.001
	Controls	38.8 ± 10.2	40.5 ± 12.2	49.8 ± 17.6	51.8 ± 16.9	54.4 ± 20.1[†]	
LVEF (%)	ACEI-group	61.9 ± 2.9	61.1 ± 3.2	61.9 ± 3.3	61.6 ± 3.9	62.4 ± 3.5	<0.001
	Controls	62.8 ± 3.4	61.8 ± 4.3	54.2 ± 8.1	51.9 ± 7.9	48.3 ± 9.3[†]	

[a]P value for repeated measures analysis of variance. [†]$P < 0.001$ versus baseline. EDV, end-diastolic volume; ESV, end-systolic volume; LVEF, left ventricular ejection fraction; Rand., randomization.
Source: Modified from Cardinale D, et al. Prevention of high-dose chemotherapy-induced cardiotoxicity in high-risk patients by angiotensin-converting enzyme inhibition. Circulation 2006;114:2474–81.

TABLE 7.5 Cardiac Events in the Study Groups

	Total (n = 114)	ACEI group (n = 56)	Controls (n = 58)	P Value
Sudden death	0 (0%)	0 (0%)	0 (0%)	1.0[a]
Cardiac death	2 (2%)	0 (0%)	2 (3%)	0.49[a]
Acute pulmonary edema	4 (3%)	0 (0%)	4 (7%)	0.07[a]
Heart failure	14 (12%)	0 (0%)	14 (24%)	< 0.001
Arrhythmias requiring treatment	11 (10%)	1 (2%)	10 (17%)	0.01
Cumulative events	31	1	30	< 0.001

[a]By Fisher exact test. ACEI, angiotensin-converting enzyme inhibitor.
Source: Modified from Cardinale D, Colombo A, Sandri MT, et al. Prevention of high-dose chemotherapy-induced cardiotoxicity in high-risk patients by angiotensin-converting enzyme inhibition. Circulation 2006;114:2474–81.

early detection and prompt prophylactic treatment initiation. Measurement of serum cardio-specific biomarkers has emerged in the last 15 years, resulting in a cost-effective diagnostic tool for early identification of patients more prone to developing cardiotoxicity, in whom a preventive pharmacological strategy and a closer cardiac monitoring are pivotal.

REFERENCES

[1] Bird BR, Swain SM. Cardiac toxicity in breast cancer survivors: review of potential cardiac problems. Clin Cancer Res 2008;14:14–24.

[2] Dolci A, Dominici R, Cardinale D, et al. Biochemical markers for prediction of chemotherapy-induced cardiotoxicity: systematic review of the literature and recommendations for use. Am J Clin Pathol 2008;130:688–95.

[3] Eschenhagen T, Force T, Ewer MS, et al. Cardiovascular side effects of cancer therapies: a position statement from the Heart Failure Association of the European Society of Cardiology. Eur J Heart Fail 2011;13(1):1–10.

[4] Yeh ET, Bickford CL. Cardiovascular complications of cancer therapy: incidence, pathogenesis, diagnosis, and management. J Am Coll Cardiol 2009;53(24):2231–47.

[5] Giantris A, Abdurrahman L, Hinkle A, Asselin B, Lipshultz SE. Anthracycline-induced cardiotoxicity in children and young adults. Crit Rev Oncol Hematol 1998;27:53–68.

[6] Grenier MA, Lipshultz SE. Epidemiology of anthracycline cardiotoxicity in children and adults. Semin Oncol 1998;25(4 suppl 10):72–85.

[7] Cardinale D, Colombo A, Bacchiani G, Tedeschi I, Meroni CA, Veglia F, Civelli M, Lamantia G, Colombo N, Curigliano G, Fiorentini C, Cipolla CM. Early detection of anthracycline cardiotoxicity and improvement with heart failure therapy. Circulation 2015;131(22):1981–8.

[8] Jones LW, Haykowsky MJ, Swartz JJ, et al. Early breast cancer therapy and cardiovascular injury. J Am Coll Cardiol 2007;50:1435–41.

[9] Shapiro CL, Haedenbergh PH, Gelman R, et al. Cardiac effects of adjuvant doxorubicin and radiation therapy in breast cancer patients. J Clin Oncol 1998;16:3493–501.

[10] Hershman DL, McBride RB, Eisenberger A, et al. Doxorubicin, cardiac risk factors, and cardiac toxicity in elderly patients with diffuse B-cell non-Hodgkin's lymphoma. J Clin Oncol 2008;26:3159–65.

[11] Tarantini L, Cioffi G, Gori S, et al. Trastuzumab adjuvant chemotherapy and cardiotoxicity in real-world women with breast cancer. J Card Fail 2012;18:113–9.

[12] Plana JC, Galderisi M, Barac A, Ewer MS, Ky B, Scherrer-Crosbie M, Ganame J, Sebag IA, Agler DA, Badano LP, Banchs J, Cardinale D, Carver J, Cerqueira M, DeCara JM, Edvardsen T, Flamm SD, Force T, Griffin BP, Jerusalem G, Liu JE, Magalhães A, Marwick T, Sanchez LY, Sicari R, Villarraga HR, Lancellotti P. Expert consensus for multimodality imaging evaluation of adult patients during and after cancer therapy: a report from the American Society of Echocardiography and the European Association of Cardiovascular Imaging. Eur Heart J Cardiovasc Imaging 2014 Oct;15(10):1063–93.

[13] Kalyanaraman B, Joseph J, Kalivendi S, et al. Doxorubicin-induced apoptosis: implications in cardiotoxicity. Mol Cell Biochem 2002;234–235:119–24.

[14] Barry E, Alvarez JA, Scully RE, et al. Anthracycline-induced cardiotoxicity: course, pathophysiology, prevention and management. Expert Opin Pharmacother 2007;8:1039–58.

[15] Kersting G, Tzvetkov MV, Huse K, Kulle B, Hafner V, Brockmöller J, Wojnowski L. Topoisomerase II beta expression level correlates with doxorubicin-induced apoptosis in peripheral blood cells. Naunyn Schmiedebergs Arch Pharmacol 2006;374:21–30.

[16] Ky B, Vejpongsa P, Yeh ET, Force T, Moslehi JJ. Emerging paradigms in cardiomyopathies associated with cancer therapies. Circ Res 2013;113(6):754–64.

[17] Vejpongsa P, Yeh ET. Topoisomerase 2β: a promising molecular target for primary prevention of anthracycline-induced cardiotoxicity. Clin Pharmacol Ther 2014;95(1):45–52.

[18] Hayes DF, Picard MH. Heart of darkness: the downside of trastuzumab. J Clin Oncol 2006;24:4056–8.

[19] Salmon DJ, Leyland-Jones B, Shak S, et al. Use of chemotherapy plus monoclonal antibody against HER2 for metastatic breast cancer that overexpresses HER2. N Engl J Med 2001;344:783–92.

[20] Seidman A, Hudis C, Pierri MK, et al. Cardiac dysfunction in the trastuzumab clinical trial experience. J Clin Oncol 2002;20:1215–21.

[21] Ewer MS, Lippman SM. Type II chemotherapy-related cardiac dysfunction: time to recognize a new entity. J Clin Oncol 2005;23:2900–2.

[22] Criscitello C, Metzger-Filho O, Saini KS, et al. Targeted therapies in breast cancer: are heart and vessels also being targeted? Breast Cancer Res 2012;14:209.

[23] Choueiri TK, Mayer EL, Je Y, et al. Congestive heart failure risk in patients with breast cancer treated with bevacizumab. J Clin Oncol 2011;29:632–68.

[24] Hunt SA, Abraham WT, Chin MH, et al. Focused update incorporated into the ACC/AHA 2005guidelines for the diagnosis and management of heart failure in adults. A report of the American College of Cardiology Foundation/American Heart Association Task Force on Practice Guidelines developed in collaboration with the International Society for Heart and Lung Transplantation. J Am Coll Cardiol 2009;53:e1–90.

[25] Altena R, Perik PJ, van Veldhuisen DJ, et al. Cardiovascular toxicity caused by cancer treatment: strategies for early detection. Lancet Oncol 2009;10:391–9.

[26] Thygesen K, Alpert JS, Jaffe AS, Simoons ML, Chaitman BR, White HD; Joint ESC/ACCF/AHA/WHF Task Force for Universal Definition of Myocardial Infarction; Authors/Task Force Members Chairpersons, Thygesen K, Alpert JS, White HD; Biomarker Subcommittee, Jaffe AS, Katus HA, Apple FS, Lindahl B, Morrow DA; ECG Subcommittee, Chaitman BR, Clemmensen PM, Johanson P, Hod H; Imaging Subcommittee, Underwood R, Bax JJ, Bonow JJ, Pinto F, Gibbons RJ; Classification Subcommittee, Fox KA, Atar D, Newby LK, Galvani M, Hamm CW; Intervention Subcommittee, Uretsky BF, Steg PG, Wijns W, Bassand JP, Menasche P, Ravkilde J; Trials & Registries Subcommittee, Ohman EM, Antman EM, Wallentin LC, Armstrong PW, Simoons ML; Trials & Registries Subcommittee, Januzzi JL, Nieminen MS, Gheorghiade M, Filippatos G; Trials & Registries Subcommittee, Luepker RV, Fortmann SP, Rosamond WD, Levy D, Wood D; Trials & Registries Subcommittee, Smith SC, Hu D, Lopez-Sendon JL, Robertson RM, Weaver D, Tendera M, Bove AA, Parkhomenko AN, Vasilieva EJ, Mendis S; ESC Committee for Practice Guidelines (CPG), Bax JJ, Baumgartner H, Ceconi C, Dean V, Deaton C, Fagard R,

Funck-Brentano C, Hasdai D, Hoes A, Kirchhof P, Knuuti J, Kolh P, McDonagh T, Moulin C, Popescu BA, Reiner Z, Sechtem U, Sirnes PA, Tendera M, Torbicki A, Vahanian A, Windecker S; Document Reviewers, Morais J, Aguiar C, Almahmeed W, Arnar DO, Barili F, Bloch KD, Bolger AF, Botker HE, Bozkurt B, Bugiardini R, Cannon C, de Lemos J, Eberli FR, Escobar E, Hlatky M, James S, Kern KB, Moliterno DJ, Mueller C, Neskovic AN, Pieske BM, Schulman SP, Storey RF, Taubert KA, Vranckx P, Wagner DR. Third universal definition of myocardial infarction. J Am Coll Cardiol. 2012;60(16):1581–98.

[27] O'Brien PJ. Cardiac troponin is the most effective translational safety biomarker for myocardial injury in cardiotoxicity. Toxicology 2008;245(3):206–18.

[28] Newby LK, Jesse RL, Babb JD, et al. ACCF 2012 expert consensus document on practical clinical consider- ations in the interpretation of troponin elevations: a report of the American College of Cardiology Foundation task force on Clinical Expert Consensus Documents. J Am Coll Cardiol 2012;60:2427–63.

[29] Herman EH, Zhang J, Lipshultz SE, et al. Correlation between serum levels of cardiac troponin-T and the severity of the chronic cardiomyopathy induced by doxorubicin. J Clin Onc 1999;17: 2237–43.

[30] Lipshultz SE, Rifai N, Sallan SE, et al. Predictive value of cardiac troponin T in pediatric patients at risk for myocardial injury. Circulation 1997;96:2641–8.

[31] Cardinale D, Sandri MT, Martinoni A, et al. Left ventricular dysfunction predicted by early troponin I release after high-dose chemotherapy. J Am Coll Cardiol 2000;36:517–22.

[32] Cardinale D, Sandri MT, Martinoni A, et al. Myocardial injury revealed by plasma troponina I in breast cancer treated with high-dose chemotherapy. Ann Oncol 2002;13:710–5.

[33] Auner HW, Tinchon C, Brezinschek RI, et al. Monitoring of cardiac function by serum cardiac troponin T levels, ventricular repolarisation indices, and echocardiography after conditioning with fractionated total body irradiation and high-dose cyclophosphamide. Eur J Haematol 2002;69:1–6.

[34] Sandri MT, Cardinale D, Zorzino L, Passerini R, Lentati P, Martinoni A, Martinelli G, Cipolla CM. Minor increases in plasma troponin I predict decreased left ventricular ejection fraction after high-dose chemotherapy. Clin Chem. 2003 Feb;49(2):248–52.

[35] Cardinale D, Sandri MT, Colombo A, et al. Prognostic value of troponin I in cardiac risk stratification of cancer patients undergoing high-dose chemotherapy. Circulation 2004;109:2749–54.

[36] Lipshultz SE, Rifai N, Dalton VM, et al. The effects of dexrazoxane on myocardial injury in doxorubicin-treated children with acute lymphoblastic leukemia. N Engl J Med 2004;351:1451–2.

[37] Specchia G, Buquicchio C, Pansini N, et al. Monitoring of cardiac function on the basis of serum troponin levels in patients with acute leukemia treated with anthracyclines. J Lab Clin Med 2005;145(4):212–20.

[38] Kilickap S, Barista I, Akgul E, et al. cTnT can be a useful marker for early detection of anthracycline cardiotoxicity. Ann Oncol 2005;16(5):798–804.

[39] Lee HS, Son CB, Shin SH, Kim YS. Clinical correlation between brain natriutetic peptide and anthracyclin-induced cardiac toxicity. Cancer Res Treat 2008;40(3):121–6.

[40] Schmidinger M, Zielinski CC, Vogl UM, et al. Cardiac toxicity of sunitinib and sorafenib in patients with metastatic renal cell carcinoma. J Clin Oncol 2008;26(32):5204–12.

[41] Cardinale D, Colombo A, Torrisi R, et al. Trastuzumab-induced cardiotoxicity: clinical and prognostic implications of troponin I evaluation. J Clin Oncol 2010;28:3910–6.

[42] Morris PG, Chen C, Steingart R, Troponin I, et al. and C-reactive protein are commonly detected in patients with breast cancer treated with dose-dense chemo-therapy incorporating trastuzumab and lapatinib. Clin Cancer Res 2011;17:3490–9.

[43] Sawaya H, Sebag IA, Plana JC, Januzzi JL, Ky B, Cohen V, Gosavi S, Carver JR, Wiegers SE, Martin RP, Picard MH, Gerszten RE, Halpern EF, Passeri J, Kuter I, Scherrer-Crosbie M. Early detection and prediction of cardiotoxicity in chemotherapy-treated patients. Am J Cardiol 2011;107(9):1375–80.

[44] Lipshultz SE, Scully RE, Lipsitz SR, et al. Assessment of dexrazoxane as a cardioprotectant in doxorubicintreated children with high-risk acute lymphoblastic leukaemia: long-term follow-up of a prospective, randomised, multicentre trial. Lancet Oncol 2010;11(10):950–61.

[45] Sawaya H, Sebag IA, Plana JC, et al. Assessment of echocardiography and biomarkers for the extended prediction of cardiotoxicity in patients treated with anthracyclines, taxanes, and trastuzumab. Circ Cardiovasc Imaging 2012;5(5):596–603.

[46] Geiger S, Stemmler HJ, Suhl P, Stieber P, Lange V, Baur D, Hausmann A, Tischer J, Horster S. Anthracycline-induced cardiotoxicity: cardiac monitoring by continuous wave-Doppler ultrasound cardiac output monitoring and correlation to echocardiography. Onkologie 2012;35(5):241–6.

[47] Mornoş C, Petrescu L. Early detection of anthracycline-mediated cardiotoxicity: the value of considering both global longitudinal left ventricular strain and twist. Can J Physiol Pharmacol 2013;91(8):601–7.

[48] Mavinkurve-Groothuis AM, Marcus KA, Pourier M, Loonen J, Feuth T, Hoogerbrugge PM, de Korte CL, Kapusta L. Myocardial 2D strain echocardiography and cardiac biomarkers in children during and shortly after anthracycline therapy for acute lymphoblastic leukaemia (ALL): a prospective study. Eur Heart J Cardiovasc Imaging 2013;14(6):562–9.

[49] Ky B, Putt M, Sawaya H, French B, Januzzi JL Jr, Sebag IA, Plana JC, Cohen V, Banchs J, Carver JR, Wiegers SE, Martin RP, Picard MH, Gerszten RE, Halpern EF, Passeri J, Kuter I, Scherrer-Crosbie M. Early increases in multiple biomarkers predict subsequent cardiotoxicity in patients with breast cancer treated with doxorubicin, taxanes, and trastuzumab. J Am Coll Cardiol 2014;63(8):809–16.

[50] Putt M, Hahn VS, Januzzi JL, Sawaya H, Sebag IA, Plana JC, Picard MH, Carver JR, Halpern EF, Kuter I, Passeri J, Cohen V, Banchs J, Martin RP, Gerszten RE, Scherrer-Crosbie M, Ky B. Longitudinal changes in multiple biomarkers are associated with cardiotoxicity in breast cancer patients treated with doxorubicin, taxanes, and trastuzumab. Clin Chem 2015;61(9):1164–72.

[51] Ewer MS, Ewer SM. Troponin I provides insight into cardiotoxicity and the anthracycline-trastuzumab interaction. J Clin Oncol 2010;28(25):3901–4394.

[52] Apple FS, Collinson PO. IFCC Task Force on Clinical Applications of Cardiac Biomarkers. Analytical characteristics of High-Sensitivity Cardiac Troponin Assays. Clin Chem 2012;58:54–61.

[53] Salvatici M, Cardinale D, Botteri E, Bagnardi V, Mauro C, Cassatella MC, Lentati P, Bottari F, Zorzino L, Passerini R, Cipolla CM, Sandri MT. TnI-Ultra assay measurements in cancer patients: comparison with the conventional assay and clinical implication. Scand J Clin Lab Invest 2014;74(5):385–91.

[54] Kismet E, Varan A, Ayabakan C, et al. Serum Troponin T levels and echocardiographic evaluation in children treated with doxorubicin. Pediatr Blood Cancer 2004;42:220–4.

[55] Soker M, Kervancioglu M. Plasma concentrations of NT-pro-BNP and cardiac troponin-I in relation to doxorubicin-induced cardiomyopathy and cardiac function in childhood malignancy. Saudi Med J. 2005;26:1197–202.

[56] Christenson ES, James T, Agrawal V, et al. Use of biomarkers for the assessment of chemotherapy-induced cardiac toxicity. Clin Biochem 2015;48:223–35.

[57] Chowdhury P, Kehl D, Choudhary R, Maisel A. The use of biomarkers in the patient with heart failure. Curr Cardiol Rep 2013;15(6):372.

[58] Xin W, Lin Z, Mi S. Does B-type natriuretic peptide-guided therapy improve outcomes in patients with chronic heart failure? A systematic review and meta-analysis of randomized controlled trials. Heart Fail Rev 2015;20(1):69–80.

[59] Suzuki T, Hayashi D, Yamazaki T, et al. Elevated Btype natriuretic peptide levels after anthracycline administration. Am Heart J 1998;136(2):362–3.

[60] Pichon MF, Cvitkovic F, Hacene K, et al. Drug-induced cardiotoxicity studied by longitudinal B-type natriuretic peptide assays and radionuclide ventriculography. In Vivo 2005;19(3):567–76.

[61] Ekstein S, Nir A, Rein AJ, et al. N-terminal-proB-type natriuretic peptide as a marker for acute anthracycline cardiotoxicity in children. J Pediatr Hematol Oncol 2007;29:440–4.

[62] Dodos F, Halbsguth T, Erdmann E, et al. Usefulness of myocardial performance index and biochemical markers for early detection of anthracycline-induced cardiotoxicity in adults. Clin Res Cardiol 2008;97:318–26.

[63] Roziakova L, Bojtarova E, Mistrik M, et al. Serial measurements of cardiac biomarkers in patients after allogeneic hematopoietic stem cell transplantation. J Exp Clin Cancer Res 2012;31:13.

[64] Sandri MT, Salvatici M, Cardinale D, et al. N-terminal pro-B-type natriuretic peptide after high-dose chemotherapy: a marker predictive of cardiac dysfunction? Clin Chem 2005;51:1405–10.

[65] Romano S, Fratini S, Ricevuto E, et al. Serial measurements of NT-proBNP are predictive of not-high-dose anthracycline cardiotoxicity in breast cancer patients. Br J Cancer 2011;105:1663–2168.

[66] Perik PJ, Lub-De Hooge MN, Gietema JA, et al. Indium-111-labeled trastuzumab scintigraphy in patients with human epidermal growth factor receptor 2-positive metastatic breast cancer. J Clin Oncol 2006;24:2276–82.

[67] Knobloch K, Tepe J, Lichtinghagen R, et al. Simultaneous hemodynamic and serological cardiotoxicity monitoring during immunotherapy with trastuzumab. Int J Cardiol 2008;125:113–5.

[68] Onitilo AA, Engel JM, Stankowski RV, et al. High-sensitivity C-reactive protein (hs-CRP) as a biomarker for trastuzumab-induced cardiotoxicity in HER2-positive early-stage breast cancer: a pilot study. Breast Cancer Res Treat 2012;134:291–8.

[69] Force T, Krause DS, Van Etten RA. Molecular mechanisms of cardiotoxicity of tyrosine kinase inhibition. Nat Rev Cancer 2007;7:332–44.

[70] Baldus S, Heeschen C, Meinertz T, Zeiher AM, Eiserich JP, Münzel T, Simoons ML, Hamm CW. CAPTURE Investigators. Myeloperoxidase serum levels predict risk in patients with acute coronary syndromes. Circulation 2003;108(12):1440–5.

[71] Tang WH, Tong W, Troughton RW, Martin MG, Shrestha K, Borowski A, Jasper S, Hazen SL, Klein AL. Prognostic value and echocardiographic determinants of plasma myeloperoxidase levels in chronic heart failure. J Am Coll Cardiol 2007;49(24):2364–70.

[72] O'Donoghue M, de Lemos JA, Morrow DA, et al. Prognostic utility of heart-type fatty acid binding protein in patients with acute coronary syndromes. Circulation 2006;114:550–7.

[73] Shortt CR, Worster A, Hill SA, Kavsak PA. Comparison of hs-cTnI, hscTnT, hFABP and GPBB for identifying early adverse cardiac events in patients presenting within six hours of chest pain-onset. Clin Chim Acta 2013;419:39–41.

[74] ElGhandour AH, ElSorady M, Azab S, ElRahman M. Human heart-type fatty acid-binding protein as an early diagnostic marker of doxorubicin cardiac toxicity. Hematol Rev 2009;1:29–32.

[75] Horacek JM, Tichy M, Jebavy L, Pudil R, Ulrychova M, Maly J. Use of multiple biomarkers for evaluation of anthracycline-induced cardiotoxicity in patients with acute myeloid leukemia. Exp Oncol 2008;30:157–9.

[76] Yancy CW, Jessup M, Bozkurt B, Butler J, Casey DE Jr, Drazner MH, Fonarow GC, Geraci SA, Horwich T, Januzzi JL, Johnson MR, Kasper EK, Levy WC, Masoudi FA, McBride PE, McMurray JJ, Mitchell JE, Peterson PN, Riegel B, Sam F, Stevenson LW, Tang WH, Tsai EJ, Wilkoff BL. American College of Cardiology Foundation; American Heart Association Task Force on Practice Guidelines. 2013 ACCF/AHA guideline for the management of heart failure: a report of the American College of Cardiology Foundation/American Heart Association Task Force on Practice Guidelines. J Am Coll Cardiol 2013 Oct 15;62(16):e147–239.

[77] van Dalen EC, Caron HN, Dickinson HO, et al. Cardioprotective interventions for cancer patients receiving anthracyclines. Cochrane Database Syst Rev 2011;(6):15–7.

[78] Huh WW, Jaffe N, Durand JB, et al. Comparison of doxorubicin cardiotoxicity in pediatric sarcoma patients when given with dexrazoxane versus as continuous infusion. Pediatr Hematol Oncol 2010;27(7):546–57.

[79] Hensley ML, Hagerty KL, Kewalramani T, Green DM, Meropol NJ, Wasserman TH, Cohen GI, Emami B, Gradishar WJ, Mitchell RB, Thigpen JT, Trotti A 3rd, von Hoff D, Schuchter LM. American Society of Clinical Oncology 2008 clinical practice guideline update: use of chemotherapy and radiation therapy protectants. J Clin Oncol 2009;27(1):127–45.

[80] Barry EV, Vrooman LM, Dahlberg SE, et al. Absence of secondary malignant neoplasms in children with high-risk acute lymphoblastic leukemia treated with dexrazoxane. J Clin Oncol 2008;26(7):1106–11.

[81] Kalay N, Basar E, Ozdogru I, et al. Protective effects of carvedilol against anthracycline-induced cardiomyopathy. J Am Coll Cardiol 2006;48(11):2258–62.

[82] Bosch X, Esteve J, Sitges M, et al. Prevention of chemotherapy-induced left ventricular dysfunction with enalapril and carvedilol: rationale and design of the OVERCOME trial. J Card Fail 2011;17:643–8.

[83] Heck SL, Gulati G, Ree AH, Schulz-Menger J, Gravdehaug B, Røsjø H, Steine K, Bratland A, Hoffmann P, Geisler J, Omland T. Rationale and design of the prevention of cardiac dysfunction during an Adjuvant Breast Cancer Therapy (PRADA) Trial. Cardiology 2012;123(4):240–7.

[84] Acar Z, Kale A, Turgut M, Demircan S, Durna K, Demir S, Meriç M, Ağaç MT. Efficiency of atorvastatin in the protection of anthracycline-induced cardiomyopathy. J Am Coll Cardiol 2011;58(9):988–9.

[85] Seicean S, Seicean A, Plana JC, Budd GT, Marwick TH. Effect of statin therapy on the risk for incident heart failure in patients with breast cancer receiving anthracycline chemotherapy: an observational clinical cohort study. J Am Coll Cardio 2012;60(23): 2384–90.

[86] Chotenimitkhun R, D'Agostino R Jr, Lawrence JA, Hamilton CA, Jordan JH, Vasu S, Lash TL, Yeboah J, Herrington DM, Hundley WG. Chronic statin administration may attenuate early anthracycline-associated declines in left ventricular ejection function. Can J Cardiol 2015;31(3):302–7.

[87] Kaya MG, Ozkan M, Gunebakmaz O, Akkaya H, Kaya EG, Akpek M, Kalay N, Dikilitas M, Yarlioglues M, Karaca H, Berk V, Ardic I, Ergin A, Lam YY. Protective effects of nebivolol against anthracycline-induced cardiomyopathy: a randomized control study. Int J Cardiol 2013;167(5):2306–10.

[88] Nakamae H, Tsumura K, Terada Y, et al. Notable effects of angiotensin II receptor blocker, valsartan, on acute cardiotoxic changes after standard chemotherapy with cyclophosphamide, doxorubicin, vincristine, and prednisolone. Cancer 2005;104(11):2492–8.

[89] Cadeddu C, Piras A, Mantovani G, et al. Protective effects of the angiotensin II receptor blocker telmisartan on epirubicin-induced inflammation, oxidative stress, and early ventricular impairment. Am Heart J 2010;160(3):487.e1–7.

[90] Akpek M, Ozdogru I, Sahin O, Inanc M, Dogan A, Yazici C, Berk V, Karaca H, Kalay N, Oguzhan A, Ergin A. Protective effects of spironolactone against anthracycline-induced cardiomyopathy. Eur J Heart Fail 2015;17(1):81–9.

[91] Cardinale D, Colombo A, Sandri MT, et al. Prevention of high-dose chemotherapy-induced cardiotoxicity in high-risk patients by angiotensin-converting enzyme inhibition. Circulation 2006;114: 2474–81.

[92] Spallarossa P, Garibaldi S, Altieri P, et al. Carvedilol prevents doxorubicin-induced free radical release and apoptosis in cardiomyocytes in vitro. J Mol Cell Cardiol 2004;37(4):837–46.

[93] Vaynblat M, Shah HR, Bhaskaran D, et al. Simultaneous angiotensin converting enzyme inhibition moderates ventricular dysfunction caused by doxorubicin. Eur J Heart Fail 2002;4:583–6.

[94] Sacco G, Bigioni M, Evangelista S, Goso C, Manzini S, Maggi CA. Cardioprotective effects of zofenopril, a new angiotensin-converting enzyme inhibitor, on doxorubicin-induced cardiotoxicity in the rat. Eur J Pharmacol 2001;414:71–8.

[95] al-Shabanah O, Mansour M, el-Kashef H, al-Bekairi A. Captopril ameliorates myocardial and hematological toxicities induced by adriamycin. Biochem Mol Biol Int 1998;45:419–27.

[96] Tokudome T, Mizushige K, Noma T, et al. Prevention of doxorubicin (adriamycin)-induced cardiomyopathy by simultaneous administration of angiotensin-converting enzyme inhibitor assessed by acoustic densitometry. J Cardiovasc Pharmacol 2000;36:361–8.

[97] Toko H, Oka T, Zou Y, et al. Angiotensin II type 1a receptor mediates doxorubicin-induced cardiomyopathy. Hypertens Res 2000;25: 597–603.

[98] Riad A, Bien S, Westermann D, Becher PM, Loya K, Landmesser U, Kroemer HK, Schultheiss HP, Tschöpe C. Pretreatment with statin attenuates the cardiotoxicity of Doxorubicin in mice. Cancer Res 2009;69(2):695–9.

[99] Dessì M, Madeddu C, Piras A, et al. Long-term, up to 18 months, protective effects of the angiotensin II receptor blocker telmisartan on Epirubin-induced inflammation and oxidative stress assessed by serial strain rate. Springerplus 2013;2(1):198.

[100] Ederhy S, Massard C, Dufaitre G, et al. Frequency and management of troponin I elevation in patients treated with molecular targeted therapies in Phase 1 trials. Investig New Drugs 2010;30(2):611–5.

Chapter 8

Myocardial Ischemia and Cancer Therapy

S. Chandra and J. Carver

Abramson Cancer Center of the University of Pennsylvania, Philadelphia, PA, United States

INTRODUCTION

Patients with cancer frequently present with chest pain that can be due to underlying coronary artery disease (CAD), related to their cancer (local extension of their tumor, pericardial, or pleural involvement and/or metastatic disease to bone), be an ischemic manifestation due to increased myocardial demand (anemia, sepsis, pain) or directly-induced by their treatment [chemotherapy or radiation therapy (XRT)] [1–3]. In this chapter, we will limit discussion to treatment-induced ischemia.

Myocardial ischemia is most typically manifested by chest pressure or pain with or without dynamic changes on the electrocardiogram (ECG). Other manifestations of ischemia include biomarker leaks, arrhythmias and conduction delay, transient left ventricular dysfunction, mitral regurgitation, and sudden death. Ischemic chest pain may present during or immediately following treatment (acute treatment-related) or as a late effect surfacing months to years after treatment completion (late treatment-related). For the purposes of this chapter, we will use chest pain as a descriptor for all ischemic manifestation.

RADIATION INDUCED ISCHEMIC HEART DISEASE

XRT has been an integral part of stand-alone or adjuvant therapy in the treatment of certain types of cancers including early stage breast cancers, certain types of lymphomas (primarily Hodgkin's disease), thoracic malignancies, and pediatric solid tumors. Forty percent of curative cancer treatments involve XRT [2]. However, the use of therapeutic radiation can lead to a spectrum of radiation-induced cardiovascular disease (RIHD) including CAD, congestive heart failure (CHF), valvular heart disease, pericardial disease, conduction abnormalities, and sudden cardiac death [3] (Fig. 8.1). It is agreed that the incidence of cardiotoxicity varies with the extent of radiation exposure to the heart, the estimated aggregate incidence of radiation-induced cardiac disease is 10–30% by 5–10 years posttreatment and increases almost linearly thereafter, although the incidence may be lower with modern techniques [4]. In specific populations, estimates of relative risk of fatal CV events after mediastinal irradiation for Hodgkin's disease ranges between 2 and 7 and after irradiation for left-sided breast cancer from 1.0 to 2.25. [5].

Pathology and Mechanism

The first reports of XRT induced cardiotoxicity were reported as early as 1929 in an autopsy series examining hearts from 10 patients who underwent wide-field radiation. A varied spectrum of myocardial injury was demonstrated from slight interstitial fibrosis to hyaline and fatty degeneration of the muscle fibers with pathologic necrosis [6]. With the advent of coronary angiography in the late 1970s, physicians began to evaluate the incidence, type, and extent of radiation-induced premature CAD in young patients who had wide-field mediastinal radiation [7]. Throughout the 1980s, several case reports and cohort studies [8–10] observed the development of radiation induced coronary artery disease distant from the completion of treatment.

The primary mechanism underlying both early and late effects of XRT induced cardiotoxicity has been that radiation exposure leads to endothelial cell damage and subsequent microvascular dysfunction due to fibrosis (Fig. 8.2). Fibrosis from tissue radiation is thought to be secondary to multiple converging pathways including inflammation, oxidative stress, and chronic changes in gene expression [11]. Correspondingly, the initiation of RIHD in the coronary arteries is similar to that of most other tissues with radiation leading to microvascular damage, inflammation, and subsequent fibrosis.

In general, the pathologic changes observed in RIHD are morphologically similar to atherosclerotic disease in large vessels (100–500 mm and >500 mm, respectively). These lesions consist of lipid deposits (atheromas) and fibrosis and are typically histologically indistinguishable from those that occur as a result of the generalized spontaneous process of atherosclerosis [11–13]. In small-sized arteries, there is often subendothelial fibrosis, accumulation

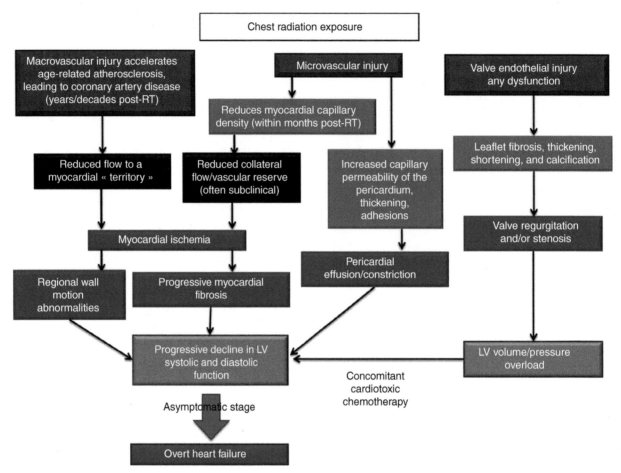

FIGURE 8.1 **Radiation induced ischemic heart disease.** *From Lancellotti P, et al. Expert consensus for multi-modality imaging evaluation of cardiovascular complications of radiotherapy in adults: a report from the European Association of Cardiovascular Imaging and the American Society of Echocardiography. J Am Soc Echocardiogr 2013;26(9):1013–32.*

of a cellular collagenous material in the media, and accumulation of lipid-laden macrophages (foam cells) in the intima. In medium-sized arteries, foam cells, fibroblasts, and collagen accumulate in the intima [14]. Moreover, in an autopsy study of 27 patients with CAD, 16 of whom had previous radiation, Veinot and Edwards demonstrated some morphologic differences in the coronary vessel between the irradiated patient and the general population including increased fibrosis in the adventitia [15].

The early histologic studies have given way to more mechanistic studies of radiation induced vascular disease. Recently Weintraub et al. proposed a mechanism of inflammation involving oxidative stress leading to the activation of the nuclear factor-kappa B (NF-κB) leading to the activation of inflammatory cytokines and adhesion molecules which ultimately leads to the development of inflammatory cells and foam cell formation (Fig. 8.2) [1,11].

In addition to the traditional model of atherosclerosis, mural, or occlusive thrombosis composed of platelets and fibrin in arterioles and larger arteries occurs at various stages after radiation, but its incidence is not known [12]. Also unknown is the contribution of platelets to the atheromatous

plaques associated with radiation. Morphologically, it is postulated that accumulation of lipid-containing macrophages along with intimal proliferation of myofibroblasts result in the formation of plaques that may eventually thrombose [12]. The complex mechanism of thrombosis in the vascular bed with preexisting atheromas remains to be elucidated.

While the XRT-induced coronary plaques are histologically virtually indistinguishable from traditional coronary atherosclerotic disease, the locations of XRT-induced plaques are focal and typically occur in the anterior arteries, that is, those closest to the typical radiation field. The left main coronary artery is most commonly affected in patients subjected to mediastinal radiation [14] and left anterior descending artery and right coronary arteries are typically also involved [16]. Furthermore, ostial and proximal lesions are common thus making subsequent management of RIHD more challenging (Fig. 8.3).

Several large survivorship studies in Hodgkin's lymphoma and breast cancer have sought to associate risk factors with RIHD. Risk factors for radiation-associated cardiac toxicity can be divided into radiation specific and patient

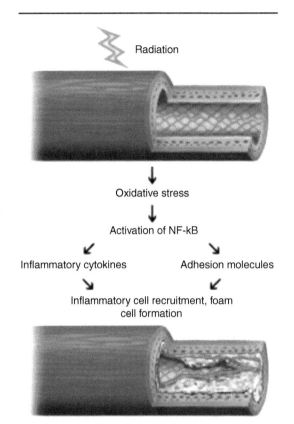

FIGURE 8.2 **Proposed mechanism of involvement of NF-kB in RIHD.** *From Weintraub et al. Understanding radiation-induced vascular disease. J Am Coll Cardiol 2010;55(12):1237–9.*

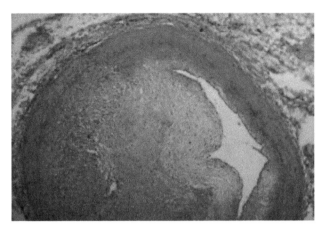

FIGURE 8.3 **Significant fibrosis of the left anterior descending (LAD) artery after XRT.** *From Lenihan and Cardinale. Late cardiac effects of cancer treatment. J Clin Oncol 2012;30(30):3657–64.*

specific factors (Table 8.1). Radiation factors include doses higher than 30 Gy, fractionated dose greater than 2 Gy/day, large volume of irradiated heart, younger age at exposure, longer time after the exposure, and concomitant adjuvant anthracycline-based chemotherapy [5,18]. Patient-specific factors include age >65 years, the presence of comorbidity, that is, diabetes, hypertension, and preexisting cardiac disease [5].

Beginning in the mid-1980s, newer techniques in delivering radiation came into practice with the increased awareness of RIHD especially as oncologic survivorship increased and late effects of XRT therapy were beginning to be seen [4].

These techniques focused on decreasing radiation doses to the heart, using image-guided therapy, breath holding during treatment and decreasing radiation fields (Table 8.2). Further development of three-dimensional treatment planning with dose volume histograms has been used to accurately quantitate dose volume and cardiac volume exposure. Linear accelerator photons and multiple-field conformal or intensity-modulated radiotherapy (IMRT) have enabled more precise localization of radiation dosing to limit cardiac exposure [6]. For example, it is recommended that for left breast/chest wall XRT, 6 MV, or occasionally higher energy photons (for large breasts) from a linear accelerator should be used [19]. The introduction of cardiac-sparing lead block during treatment has become the standard of care to shield the heart and reduce the amount of cardiac tissue exposed to XRT. The use of a four-field IMRT technique can offer better sparing than the partial shielding technique as the maximum heart depth is increased. It has been proposed that maximum heart distance (MHD), that is, the maximal distance between anterior cardiac contour and posterior tangential field edges as seen on beam's eye view is a reliable predictor of the mean heart dose in left-tangential breast or chest wall irradiation, and may be useful in centers where three-dimensional cardiac dose assessment is not routinely available [5,19]. *A strong*

TABLE 8.1 Risk Factors for Development of RIHD

Radiation Specific Risk Factors	Patient Specific Risk Factors
Anterior or left chest irradiation	Age > 65 years
Doses higher than 30–35 Gy	Cardiovascular risk factors
Fractionated dose greater than 2 Gy/day	Diabetes
Lack of shielding	Hypertension
Large volume of irradiated heart	Smoking
Younger age at exposure (<50)	Elevated BMI
Longer time after the exposure	Hypercholesterolemia
Concomitant adjuvant chemotherapy (the use of anthracyclines considerably increases the risk)	Preexisting cardiac disease

TABLE 8.2 Modern Radiation Therapy Techniques

Three-dimensional treatment planning
Intensity-modulated radiation therapy in selected cases
Positron emission tomography-computed tomography fusion planning in selected cases
Reducing total dose (being tested in randomized trials)
Reducing treatment field size
Daily fraction size 2 Gy

Source: Carver JR, et al. American society of clinical oncology clinical evidence review on the ongoing care of adult cancer survivors: cardiac and pulmonary late effects. J Clin Oncol 2007;25(25):3991–4008.

linear correlation was found between the MHD and the mean heart dose: for every 1-cm increase in MHD, the mean heart dose increased by 2.9% on average (95% CI 2.5–3.3). Electron beams can be used for the treatment of superficial structures such as in the internal mammary lymph nodes or the boost dose on the breast after surgery, in the treatment of breast cancer. For mediastinal XRT, high-energy photons from a linear accelerator should be used to treat patients with equal weighting of anterior and posterior portals (instead of anterior weighting), all fields should be treated on each XRT fraction, use of a subcarinal block after a dose of 30 Gy, and use of shrinking-field technique are the most important parameters to minimize heart exposure [5,20].

Clinical Considerations

Patients with RIHD can present with any manifestation of ischemia, chest pain being the most common. Symptoms are typically similar to those due to atherosclerotic CAD. There should be a high index of suspicion for any patient previously exposed to chest XRT that any "supply-demand" associated chest symptom may reflect underlying CAD and lead to appropriate CAD investigation according to the best test available at your institution or your practice pattern, see section "Monitoring and Treatment of Ischemic Cardiac Toxicity."

Numerous studies have demonstrated that XRT therapy leads to increased incidence of premature ischemic heart disease. There is a higher rate of silent ischemia in those who have had XRT therapy secondary to associated neuropathic changes and alterations in pain perception. While the focus of this section is on the coronary ischemic complications of XRT, it is important to realize that XRT-induced cardiotoxicity has a spectrum of cardiotoxicity where abnormalities rarely occur in isolation, that is, CAD tends to be present coincident with possible pericardial/myocardial/conduction system fibrosis, and valvular lesions. The incidence of RIHD has been steadily decreasing as XRT techniques have improved. Regardless, given the late presentation often up to decades after incident XRT exposure, it is imperative that those with XRT exposure be closely screened, diagnosed and aggressively treated.

CHEMOTHERAPY-INDUCED ISCHEMIC HEART DISEASE

Radiation as a cause of CAD has been well documented. Many chemotherapeutic agents have also been implicated in causing myocardial ischemia or exacerbating underlying coronary artery disease either through a direct effect on the coronary vasculature with or without coincident pro-thrombotic state (supply) or through indirect effects that increase demand. The latter include changes in blood pressure, fluid status, sepsis, anemia, chemotherapy-associated sinus tachycardia, and circulating cytokines. For reduction of coronary blood flow (the supply side), the mechanism of action is varied but mainly due to drug-induced coronary vasospasm, which can cause angina, acute coronary syndromes, or myocardial infarction [21]. The following section addresses the existing literature focused on chemotherapeutic agents that cause coronary artery spasm. As opposed to RIHD that is generally a late effect, these drugs are responsible for early or acute syndromes. A detailed list of chemotherapy drugs implicated in chest pain syndromes is presented in Table 8.3 [22].

TABLE 8.3 Chemotherapeutic Agents Implicated in Ischemic Heart Disease

Antimetabolites
Capecitabine (Xeloda)
Fluorouracil (Adrucil)
Microtubule targeting agents
Paclitaxel (Taxol) [23,24]
Docetaxel (Taxotere) (<*TAXOTERE (docetaxel) Drug label. pdf*>) [25]
Monoclonal antibody-based tyrosine kinase inhibitor
Bevacizumab (Avastin)
Ramucirumab
Small molecule tyrosine kinase inhibitors
Erlotinib (Tarceva)
Sorafenib (Nexavar)
Alkylating agents
Cisplatin
Antitumor antibiotics
Bleomycin
Topoisomerase inhibitors
Etoposide
Biologic Response Modifiers
Interferon
Interleukin-2

Antimetabolites

The most common [22] chemotherapy-induced chest pain syndromes are secondary to the antimetabolite chemotherapy agents 5-fluorouracil (5-FU, Adrucil) (*<5FU drug label. pdf>*), and the oral capecitabine, a prodrug that is converted to 5-FU (Xeloda) (*<XELODA (capecitabine) Drug Insert. pdf>*) [26]. Additionally, cisplatin (Platinol) (*<PLATINOL (cisplatin for injection, USP) Insert.pdf>*) and other platinum-based agents used have also demonstrated significant IHD toxicities. Symptoms with use of these agents have been reported to vary greatly from typical angina to transient vasospasm.

5-FU/Capecitabine

5-fluorouracil and capecitabine are a class of chemotherapeutic agents known as fluoropyrimidines and are used in the treatment of solid tumors including colorectal and breast cancers. 5-FU has been known to cause a spectrum of cardiovascular toxicities including most commonly chest pain, acute coronary syndrome, coronary vasospasm, arrhythmias, heart failure, hypertension, hypotension, cardiogenic shock, and sudden death [27]. The true incidence of ischemic heart disease and cardiotoxicity associated with 5-FU is varied. A large meta-analysis by Polk et al. looked at the frequency of fluorouracil-induced cardiotoxicity in 30 studies with different study designs, patient selection criteria, and treatment schedules. They found that the incidence ranged between 0% and 35% [27]. In larger studies with >400 patients, the estimated incidence of symptomatic cardiotoxicity has been estimated to be 1.2–4.3% and the frequency of treatment-related sudden death varied from 0% to 8% but clustered around 0–0.5% [27].

The most common cardiac symptom due to 5-FU is chest pain, which can be either nonspecific or typical angina [27,28]. The relative incidence of chest pain is variably reported in the literature and occurs with an incidence of 0–18.6% with concurrent ECG changes [27,29]. There is a wide variability in mode of administration of both 5-FU as bolus versus continuous infusion and in various combination regimens. In a large meta-analysis there was some evidence that continuous infusion had a higher incidence of chest pain [27]. Moreover, the temporal relation between symptom onset and medication exposure varied widely as well. Cardiac events may occur during initial bolus infusion but tend to occur within 2–5 days of starting prolonged (typically 72–96 h) infusional therapy, and may last up to 48 h after stopping the drug [30–32]. The pain typically occurs at rest, unlike classical angina, and is generally resolves after stopping the drug with or without nitrates or calcium blocker therapy [29].

Chest pain may or may not be accompanied by ECG changes that are typical of ischemia with ST segment

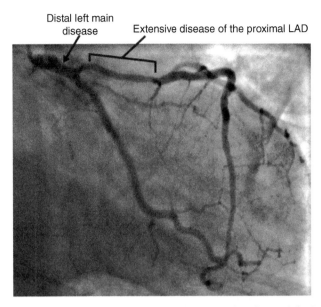

FIGURE 8.4 **Angiographic evidence of RIHD.** This patient had distal left main CAD and diffused LAD disease localized to areas subject to radiation. The more distal vessels were normal. The distal coronary arteries are larger than the more proximal areas [35].

elevation in the leads reflecting the distribution of the affected coronary artery. The accompanying ECG (Fig. 8.5) shows classical evidence of spasm in the distribution of the left anterior descending coronary artery. Typical anginal chest pain can also be present without any ST segment change in the ECG or there can be just be arrhythmias in patients with chest pain or there maybe evidence of silent myocardial ischemia and arrhythmias in otherwise asymptomatic patients [33,34] (Fig. 8.4).

Capecitabine is an oral agent that when metabolized in the liver becomes active 5-FU (*<XELODA (capecitabine) Drug Insert.pdf>*). All of the presentations and mechanisms described for 5-FU above are also relevant and consistent for capecitabine.

Although symptoms and electrocardiographic changes could mimic acute myocardial infarction with ST segment changes, myocardial necrosis is not usual. A systemic review by Polk et al. showed that most patients had CK-MB and troponin levels below the cut-off points for myocardial infarction [27]. However, Jensen et al. showed that there was an increase in NT-proBNP and lactic acid was significantly higher in patients with symptoms [28]. These biomarker changes were transient and did not differ between patients who had clinical signs of cardiotoxicity and those who did not [27,28]. There is little consensus on the role or utility of routine biomarker surveillance in patients receiving 5-FU or capecitabine. The take-home message is that vasospasm can potentially lead to myocardial damage.

Additionally, there is variability to what extent that a background of CAD and traditional risk factors have on predisposing patients with IHD from 5-FU and capecitabine

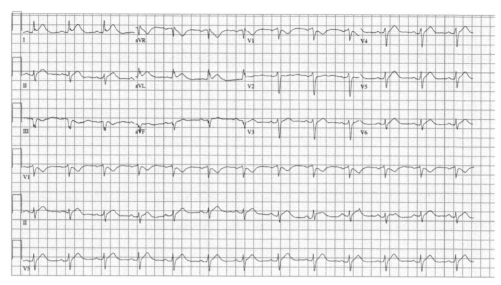

FIGURE 8.5   **EKG showing ST elevation in the anterolateral and inferior leads during infusion of 5-FU.**

exposure. However, Meyer et al. describe patient groups with an elevated risk of cardiotoxicity: those with preexisting cardiac disease (RR = 6.83, p = 0.0023); patients receiving calcium channel blockers (RR = 4.75, p = 0.014); those receiving nitrates (RR = 9.18, p = 0.007) for preexisting CAD; and patients receiving concomitant etoposide (RR = 10.32, p = 0.022) [30]. Thus, we recommend cautious use and close cardiac monitoring of 5-FU and capecitabine in those patients with known history of coronary artery disease.

Although we currently do not recommend pretreatment evaluation for CAD, anyone with suggestive symptoms after treatment evaluation is routinely evaluated either with coronary CT angiography or coronary angiography.

The treatment of chest pain and cardiac symptoms that develop with the use of 5-FU and capecitabine has short- and long-acting nitrates (sublingual nitroglycerine and isosorbide dinitrates) along with calcium channel blockers as the cornerstone. Typically, there is resolution of symptoms with 5-FU and capecitabine by stopping the drug. The diagnosis of an acute coronary syndrome is based upon the patient's clinical presentation, ECG changes, and elevations in cardiac enzymes; patients should be assessed and treated for underlying CAD per standard of care for all noncancer patients [22,36,37]. Rechallenge for those individuals who experienced cardiotoxicity related to these agents remains controversial. Some centers have been successful in pretreating patients with nitrates and calcium channel blockers in an effort to prevent coronary vasospasm [38]. There have been small series case reports of using calcium channel blockers in rechallenge with 5-FU continuing chemotherapy. In a single patient experience, Cerny et al. reported a 57-year-old male with node-positive colon cancer who was treated with 5-FU, leucovorin, and oxaliplatin (FOLFOX

regimen). The patient experienced significant chest pain related to infusion of 5-FU but was able to be monitored closely and treated with a calcium channel blocker to prevent coronary vasospasm [39]. A larger case series by Ambrosy et al. described five patients with primary colorectal adenocarcinoma or anal squamous cell carcinoma who experienced chest pain and/or dyspnea at rest or with exertion who were able to successfully continue retreatment with secondary prophylaxis with diltiazem [40]. Notably in all five patients there were acute electrocardiographic findings suggestive of ischemia at initial chest-pain presentation, and one patient had troponin elevation consistent with an acute ST-segment elevation myocardial infarction. All patients underwent subsequent ischemic evaluation with either stress echocardiograms (4/5 patients) or coronary angiography (1/5 patients) prior to rechallenge.

The mechanism of action has been proposed to be primarily due to coronary vasospasm but other postulated causative mechanisms involved in 5-FU cardiotoxicity include: an autoimmune response to damaged cells; an increased oxygen demand in patients receiving 5-FU; coronary spasm caused by protein kinase C-mediated vasoconstriction and dihydropyrimidine dehydrogenase deficiency [38,41,42]. Sudhoff et al. have documented coronary vasospasm during infusion of 5-fluorouracil in animal and human models [43]. Work remains to further elucidate the mechanism of action of 5-FU and capecitabine-induced IHD and to find a marker to predict toxicity prior to treatment.

Cisplatin

Acute cisplatin cardiotoxicity manifests in a variety of ways including arrhythmias (supraventricular tachycardias, bradycardias) ST-T wave changes, left bundle branch block, acute ischemic events, myocardial infarction, and ischemic cardiomyopathy [25,44–48]. The mechanism of chest pain may be large vessel spasm or related to thrombosis. Jafri and Protheroe reported a case of cisplatin-associated thrombosis which manifested as ACS in a young testicular cancer patient without other atherosclerotic risk factors [45]. They proposed that cisplatin has a direct effect on the endovascular milieu; with a possible mechanism of decreased protein C activity and elevated von Willebrand factor levels leading to acute thrombosis and ischemia. Moreover, Nuver et al. looked at 65 testicular cancer patients treated with cisplatin-based chemotherapy and found an increase in plasma von Willebrand factor levels and in the intima-media thickness of the carotid artery [49].

It is well known that platinum-based chemotherapy also leads to late cardiovascular effects through a continued direct effect of platinum on the vascular endothelium (that can be present for decades) and the association of increased risk of hypertension, hyperlipidemia, and the metabolic syndrome [50]. Thus, patients exposed to platinum-based chemotherapy are at increased risk for atherosclerosis and an in increased risk of late vascular events compared to age-matched cohorts [51].

Microtubule Targeting Agents (Taxanes and Vinca Alkaloids)

Paclitaxel

Paclitaxel (Taxol) (<*Paclitaxel (TAXOL) Drug Insert. pdf*>) is a chemotherapeutic agent typically used in the treatment of ovarian cancer, breast cancer, lung cancer, and pancreatic cancer among others. Studies of treatment courses of patients who participated in four clinical trials of paclitaxel at Johns Hopkins Oncology from 1983 to 1990 demonstrated a diverse spectrum of cardiac toxicity including ventricular arrhythmias, bradycardia, several degrees of atrioventricular conduction block, bundle branch block, and cardiac ischemia during paclitaxel administration (<*Paclitaxel (TAXOL) Drug Insert.pdf*>) [24]. The rate of cardiac ischemia was approximately 5%. A subsequent study by Arbuck et al. assessed the incidence of myocardial infarction and cardiac ischemia in a database of 3400 patients reported an incidence of 0.26% of significant adverse cardiac events [23]. The author went on to explain that the autopsy studies of these affected patients had significant coronary artery disease risk factors and atherosclerotic burden. Notably, there was a significant incidence of arrhythmias with the most common being asymptomatic sinus bradycardia with an incidence of up to 30% [23].

The mechanism of action of paclitaxel-induced coronary ischemia is not well known. Myocardial ischemia associated with paclitaxel is thought to be multifactorial in etiology, with other coadministered drugs and predrug underlying heart disease as possible contributing factors. In addition, the Cremophor EL vehicle in which paclitaxel is formulated may be responsible for its cardiac toxicity, and the mechanism is likely due to its induction of histamine release which may induce coronary artery vasospasm [23].

Docetaxel

According to the package insert for docetaxel (Taxotere) (<*TAXOTERE (docetaxel) Drug label.pdf*>) there are postmarket reports of myocardial infarction. Per Yeh et al. [22], the incidence of these events is approximately 1.7% based on a large Phase II clinical trial published by Vermorken et al. [22,25]. However, details regarding the mechanism and risk factors are unknown, and clinically this is a very unusual complication of using this drug.

Vinca Alkaloids

The vinca alkaloids, including vincristine, vinblastine, and venorelbine, have been used in the treatment of many hematologic and solid tumor malignancies. There are multiple case reports dating back to 1975 that describe acute myocardial infarction associated with the infusion of each of these agents, with a predominance of reports associated with vincristine infusion. Associated arterial hypertension has also been reported. The mechanism for coronary ischemia favors coronary vasospasm. Because all of the literature consists of isolated case reports, the absolute incidence and CV risk associated with these drugs is not known [52–54].

Monoclonal Antibodies (MABS)
Rituximab

Rituximab (Rituxan), a chimeric anti-CD20 monoclonal antibody, is a commonly used component of the treatment of various lymphoproliferative and rheumatologic disorders (<*Rituxan (rituximab) Drug Insert.pdf*>). The mechanism of action of rituximab is through complement-mediated cell lysis and antibody-dependent cellular cytotoxicity through activation of $Fc\gamma$ receptors. The product insert for rituximab (<*Rituxan (rituximab) Drug Insert.pdf*>) refers to myocardial infarction as a complication of the infusion of rituximab. Data are largely extrapolated from pooled, placebo-controlled studies of rituximab given to rheumatoid arthritis (RA) patients; the proportion of patients with serious cardiovascular reactions was 1.7% and 1.3% in the rituximab and placebo treatment groups, respectively. Three cardiovascular deaths occurred during the double-blind period of the RA studies including all rituximab regimens (3/769 = 0.4%) as compared to none in the placebo treatment group (0/389) (<*Rituxan (rituximab) Drug Insert.pdf*>).

Additionally, Armitage et al. reported three cases of acute coronary syndromes in a cohort of 818 patients during the first rituximab infusion [55]. One patient had known previous coronary artery disease and the other two patients had independent risk factors for CAD. All three patients demonstrated elevated cardiac enzymes consistent with myocardial ischemia but only one had accompanying ECG changes of acute myocardial ischemia. The patient with known previous coronary artery disease experienced a cardiac arrhythmia, developed asystole, and died. Both surviving patients had coronary angiography: subsequently one was treated medically and the other received a percutaneous intervention. Numerous case reports [56–62] have also reported typical chest pain and myocardial infarction following rituximab infusions. In a larger cohort study assessing the safety data of global rituximab RA clinical trial in 3194 patients with 11,962 patient-years of follow-up, MI was the most common serious cardiac event in the All Exposure population (49 events in 42 patients; 1.3%). The event rate was 0.41/100 patient-years (95% CI 0.31–0.54) versus 0.27/100 patient-years (95% CI 0.09–0.84) in the placebo + MTX population. Of the 42 patients, 17 had at least one conventional risk factor [63]. The authors concluded that the rate of myocardial infarction in RA patients given rituximab was the same as in the general rheumatoid arthritis population, which is at increased risk for coronary events [64].

The mechanism of cardiac toxicity of rituximab is suggested to be secondary to cytokine release leading to increased myocardial demand. Armitage et al. and others propose that the mechanism of these ischemic cardiac events associated with the initial infusion of rituximab may be secondary to alterations in blood pressure and heart rate (again, increased demand), leading to myocardial ischemia in those perhaps with preexisting plaque or via coronary artery vasospasm [55]. This is not a direct effect of rituximab on the coronary vasculature, that is, not a cause of coronary spasm, but a reflection of increased demand in patients with either underlying CAD or with predilection for CAD. This can be managed by aggressive pretreatment for all patients to avoid cytokine release, slowing or stopping the infusion with any hint of sensitivity, and aggressive pretreatment management of known CAD and cardiac risk factors.

Bevacizumab

Bevacizumab (Avastin) is a vascular endothelial growth factor-specific angiogenesis inhibitor indicated for the treatment of metastatic colorectal cancer, nonsquamous non-small cell lung cancer, metastatic breast cancers, glioblastomas, and other solid tumors (<*AVASTIN (bevacizumab) Package Insert.pdf*>). It has been widely reported that arterial thrombotic events (ATEs) tend to occur more frequently in patients treated with bevacizumab as compared with patients treated with chemotherapy alone [65,66]. Per the package insert, ATEs with bevacizumab including cerebral infarction, transient ischemic attacks, myocardial infarction, angina, and others occurred at an incidence of 2.6% in patients receiving bevacizumab compared to 0.8% those in the control arm (<*AVASTIN (bevacizumab)*

Package Insert.pdf>). The mechanism of bevacizumab-induced ATE is unclear but it is suspected to involve vascular endothelial growth factor (VEGF). VEGF stimulates endothelial cell proliferation, promotes endothelial cell survival, and helps maintain vascular integrity. VEGF inhibition is thought to lead to a prothromobotic state.

Scapatti et al. performed a pooled analysis of five randomized controlled trials with a total of 1,745 patients with metastatic colorectal, breast, or non-small cell lung carcinoma. Bevacizumab use was associated with increased risk for an arterial thromboembolic event (HR = 2.0, 95% confidence interval [CI] = 1.05 to 3.75; $p = 0.031$) but not for a venous thromboembolic event (HR = 0.89, 95% CI = 0.66–1.20; $p = .44$). The absolute rate of developing arterial thromboembolism was 5.5 events per 100 person-years for those receiving combination therapy and 3.1 events per 100 person-years for those receiving chemotherapy alone (ratio = 1.8, 95% CI = 0.94–3.33; $p = .076$) [65]. In a meta-analysis of 16 randomized trials by Ranpura et al. with a total of 10,217 patients with a variety of advanced solid tumors, bevacizumab was associated with an increased risk of fatal adverse events (FAEs) in patients receiving taxanes or platinum agents (RR, 3.49; 95% CI, 1.82-6.66; incidence, 3.3% vs. 1.0%) but not when used in conjunction with other agents (RR, 0.85; 95% CI, 0.25–2.88; incidence, 0.8% vs. 0.9%). The most common causes of FAEs were not cardiac: hemorrhage (23.5%), neutropenia (12.2%), and gastrointestinal tract perforation (7.1%) [67]. Finally, another meta-analysis by Shutz et al. in 2011 assessed 13,026 patients from 20 randomized trials and found no difference between low- and high-dose groups.

Among patients receiving bevacizumab in combination with chemotherapy, the risk of developing ATE during therapy was increased in patients with a history of arterial thromboembolism or age greater than 65 years (<*AVASTIN (bevacizumab) Package Insert.pdf*>) [65]. Bevacizumab-associated ATEs were reported to occur at any time during therapy; the median time to event was approximately 3 months. Events did not seem to be associated with dose or cumulative exposure [22,65]. The actual incidence of coronary artery thromboembolism is not known but there is a potential and the take-home message is that in patients being treated with bevacizumab who present with coronary syndromes, there should be a high level of suspicion that bevacizumab is the culprit and that bevacizumab therapy should be discontinued in these patients [22].

TYROSINE KINASE INHIBITORS (TKIS)

Sorafenib

Sorafenib is a multitargeted tyrosine kinase inhibitor (TKI) of tumor cell proliferation and angiogenesis used to treat patients with advanced clear cell renal cell carcinoma.

In the seminal trial validating the efficacy and safety of sorafenib, the authors reported that cardiac ischemia or infarction occurred in 12 patients in the sorafenib group (3%) and 2 patients in the placebo group (<1%) (p = 0.01) [68]. The authors did not report if these patients had predisposing cardiovascular risk factors or previous coronary artery disease. The mechanism of sorafenib-induced myocardial ischemia is unknown. There has been one case report in the literature by Aramia et al. [69] of a 65-year-old male who experienced a non-ST elevation myocardial infarction without angiographic significant coronary stenosis. With no definite evidence, the authors postulated that this was sorafenib-induced coronary vasospasm secondary to the downstream effects on Raf, VEGF, and platelet-derived growth factor receptor tyrosine kinase signaling pathways. This is the only MI case report to our knowledge and the events may not be causally related beyond ischemia secondary to the increased demand of hypertension associated with this drug.

Sunitinib, another TKI approved for treatment of renal cell carcinoma and gastrointestinal stromal tumor, has been reported to have a increased risk of congestive heart failure [70]. Hypertension leading to increased myocardial demand and possible ischemia is plausible but documentation of primary coronary ischemia has not been reported. However, the clinical trials for sunitinib have largely excluded patients with known preexisting hypertension and coronary artery disease which are risk factors for cardiac toxicity [71].

BCR-ABL 1 Targeted Therapy

The TKIs nilotinib and ponatinib are second-generation drugs that target BCR-ABL 1 in the treatment of CML. Both have been associated with vascular toxicity. Nilotinib has been associated with hyperglycemia and hyperlipidemia and both drugs have been associated with hypertension [72]; documented primary coronary ischemia has not been reported. Vascular toxicity can affect any arterial circulation including the coronary arteries with associated angina, ACS and acute myocardial infarction as well as peripheral arterial disease. The mechanism behind these vascular toxicities is unclear and toxicity appears to be dose dependent and is increased in patients with underlying vascular disease and cardiac risk factors and in older patients.

Topoisomerase Inhibitors—Etoposide

Etoposide has been used in the treatment of hematologic and solid tumors. It is a major component of the treatment of germ cell tumors along with bleomycin and cisplatin. There are multiple single case reports of infusion-related myocardial infarction ascribed to etoposide. However, in all of them coadministration of cisplatin obscures causality.

Cytokines

Interferon Alpha

Interferon has used in the treatment of advanced melanoma and renal cell carcinoma. With newer immunotherapy and TKIs, the use of this drug for cancer has decreased dramatically. The most common side effect of interferon alpha is a flu-like syndrome and there have been different manifestations of interferon-induced cardiotoxicity including supraventricular arrhythmias, interferon-induced congestive heart failure, and myocardial ischemia. In a review of 44 case reports of cardiotoxicity associated with interferons alpha, alpha 2, and beta, 10 patients suffered myocardial infarction with 6 deaths [73]. Notably 5 out of the 10 patients had underlying coronary artery disease. The postulated mechanism of action has been secondary to increased myocardial demand in the setting of vascular stress.

Interleukin-2

Interleukin-2 (IL-2) and its commercially available recombinant form aldesleukin (Proleukin) (<PROLEUKIN (aldesleukin) Package insert.pdf>) are biologic agents used in the treatment of renal cell carcinoma and melanomas. Like Interferon, newer effective treatments have virtually replaced these drugs for cancer therapy. In a small series of 10 patients who received recombinant IL-2, arterial, and pulmonary artery catheters were used to monitor the cardiopulmonary effects of IL-2 given i.v. at a dose of 100,000 U/kg every 8 h for 5 days. A severe capillary leak syndrome developed in all patients. Myocardial infarction occurred unexpectedly in 3 patients, as evidenced by a focal injury pattern on ECG and elevations of creatinine phosphokinase myocardial band fractions. All patients receiving rIL-2 exhibited major reductions in their left ventricular stroke work index (47 ± 11 to 29 ± g.m/m^2), an index of cardiac contractility [74]. In another larger series of 1241 metastatic cancer patients treated with intravenous bolus infusions of IL-2 (720,000 IU/kg every 8 h), patients were evaluated for the incidence of specific treatment-related toxicities and overall found to have an increased incidence of cardiac ischemia of 3% versus 0% in controls Moreover, Kammula et al. suggested that the improvement in safety seen in more recent trials compared with the initial experience most likely reflects the development of strategies to screen eligible patients, including prechemo cardiac and coronary screening for patients over the age of 50 years and those with other risk factors [75].

Treatment with IL-2 is associated with significant cardiorespiratory effects, as well as capillary leak syndrome (<PROLEUKIN (aldesleukin) Package insert.pdf>) [76], which is characterized by a loss of vascular tone and extravasation of plasma proteins and fluid into the extravascular space. Capillary leak syndrome results in hypotension and reduced organ perfusion, which may be severe and can result in death. Patients presenting with capillary leak syndrome have associated with cardiac arrhythmias (supraventricular and ventricular), angina, myocardial infarction, and other systemic manifestations. Because of the increase in myocardial demand and hemodynamic changes associated with the use of Interferons and Interleukins, screening for CAD is an essential part of pretreatment evaluation.

CANCER COHORT STUDIES—ISCHEMIC HEART DISEASE

Several cancer cohort studies of specific populations across have looked at risk of cardiovascular disease in survivor populations. Specifically those patients with Hodgkin's lymphoma, breast cancer, and testicular cancer have been widely studied in large survivorship studies.

Hodgkin's Lymphoma

Multiple large cohort studies have been conducted in various national databases [77–81]. In a seminal study by Swerdlow et al. of a cohort of 7,033 Hodgkin's disease patients treated in Britain from November 1, 1967, through September 30, 2000 (with a median follow up of 9.9 years), risk of myocardial infarction mortality was compared with that of the general population of England and Wales [81]. There were 166 deaths from myocardial infarction, and the increased risk of death from myocardial infarction remained high for at least 25 years after treatment. The overall standardized mortality ratio (SMR) was 2.5, and the absolute excess risk was approximately 0.13% per year (125.8 per 100,000 person-years). On a relative scale, the risk of death from myocardial infarction was highest among patients who were younger than 25 years at first treatment and within the first year of treatment. On an absolute scale, however, risk was highest among patients who were older than 45 years at first treatment because of the higher rates of heart disease that occur at older ages. They found that the risk of death from myocardial infarction was high in the year after first treatment, peaked 15–19 years after treatment was first received and remained statistically significantly increased 20–24 years after treatment, with some evidence suggesting that the increased risk may persist for even 25 years or longer after treatment. Risk at 20 or more years after first treatment was particularly high for patients who had received supradiaphragmatic radiotherapy and vincristine without anthracylines (SMR = 14.8, 95% CI = 4.8–34.5).

In another retrospective study conducted from 1962 to 1998 at a university-based referral center with a matched general population Hull et al. [80] used the Surveillance, Epidemiology, and End Results (SEER) and National Hospital Discharge Survey (NHDS) data. They looked for observed-to-expected ratios for cardiac valve surgery, coronary artery bypass graft surgery (CABG), and percutaneous coronary intervention (PCI). 42 patients (10.4%) developed coronary artery disease at a median of 9 years after treatment, 30 patients (7.4%) developed carotid and/or subclavian artery disease at a median of 17 years after treatment, and 25 patients (6.2%) developed clinically significant valvular dysfunction (predominantly aortic stenosis) at a median of 22 years. Observed-to Expected Ratio for valve surgery was 8.42 (95% CI, 3.20–13.65) and CABG or PCI was 1.63 (95% CI, 0.98–2.28). There was at least one cardiac risk factor present in all patients who developed coronary artery disease. They found that the only treatment-related factor associated with the development of coronary artery disease was utilization of a radiation technique that resulted in a higher total dose to a portion of the heart (RR, 7.8; 95% CI, 1.1–53.2; $p = 0.04$). In this study cohort, freedom from any cardiovascular morbidity was 88% at 15 years and 84% at 20 years.

In summary, these and other large studies have shown that myocardial infarction has been identified as a major contributor to higher long-term mortality in survivors of Hodgkin's disease. Death due to cardiac causes is estimated to be responsible for about one-quarter of the mortality for reasons other than Hodgkin's disease itself, which equals 2–5% of overall mortality in those with Hodgkin's disease.

The first actual demonstration of a linear dose-response relationship for mean heart dose and coronary heart disease was recently published [82]. They found that they overall risk of coronary heart disease increased by 7.4% per Gy resulting in a 2.5-fold increased risk at a mean dose of 20 Gy. These retrospective studies all emerge from an era of pre-modern radiation delivery techniques that may overestimate the cardiotoxicity risks in patients being treated today.

Breast Cancer

In the breast cancer cohort studies, cardiac doses from XRT have been lower and risks smaller and subsequently the phenomenon of RIHD is less obvious in breast cancer patients than in Hodgkin lymphoma patients [83]. However, a reliable indication of the effect of radiotherapy on heart disease can be obtained by comparing the experience of irradiated women with left-sided tumors with that of women with right-sided tumors. The Early Breast Cancer Trialists' Collaborative Group (EBCTCG) has performed the largest meta-analysis exploring the impact of XRT on breast cancer mortality and on mortality from other causes (*<darby 2005 lancet.pdf>*) [83–85]. The most recently updated EBCTCG data relate mortality from heart disease to estimated cardiac XRT doses in over 30,000 women followed for up to 20 years. In the last update of this group's meta-analysis on loco-regional XRT, with 178,000 woman-years of follow-up, the annual mortality rate from breast cancer was reduced by 13.2% [standard error (SE), 2.5%], but the

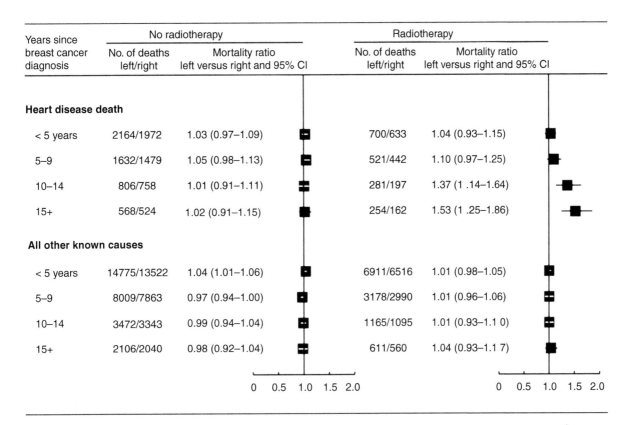

Years since breast cancer diagnosis	No radiotherapy		Radiotherapy	
	No. of deaths left/right	Mortality ratio left versus right and 95% CI	No. of deaths left/right	Mortality ratio left versus right and 95% CI
Heart disease death				
< 5 years	2164/1972	1.03 (0.97–1.09)	700/633	1.04 (0.93–1.15)
5–9	1632/1479	1.05 (0.98–1.13)	521/442	1.10 (0.97–1.25)
10–14	806/758	1.01 (0.91–1.11)	281/197	1.37 (1.14–1.64)
15+	568/524	1.02 (0.91–1.15)	254/162	1.53 (1.25–1.86)
All other known causes				
< 5 years	14775/13522	1.04 (1.01–1.06)	6911/6516	1.01 (0.98–1.05)
5–9	8009/7863	0.97 (0.94–1.00)	3178/2990	1.01 (0.96–1.06)
10–14	3472/3343	0.99 (0.94–1.04)	1165/1095	1.01 (0.93–1.10)
15+	2106/2040	0.98 (0.92–1.04)	611/560	1.04 (0.93–1.17)

FIGURE 8.6   **Cardiovascular mortality in breast cancer therapy with and without XRT in left-sided versus right-sided breast cancer.** Mortality ratios by radiotherapy status, cause, and years since diagnosis in 300,000 women with breast cancer and registered in the Surveillance Epidemiology and End Results (SEER) cancer registries, 1973 to 2001 [82,84].

annual mortality rate from other causes was increased by 21.2% (SE, 5.4%). In the absence of other causes of death, the 20-year survival would have been 53.4% among women treated with XRT versus 48.6% among controls. In the absence of any breast cancer deaths, the 20-year survival would have been 69.5% among those randomized to XRT versus 73.8% for controls. Moreover, comparison of CV mortality between patients treated with and without XRT has shown a statistically significant relative risk of 1.37 in 10–14 years after XRT. A similar latent time was estimated in an overview of trials started before 1975 [5]. In a Swedish study that included 55,000 patients with a history of breast cancer, there was an increased mortality ratio of 1.10 (95% CI, 1.03–1.18) for all CV diseases and 1.13 (95% CI 1.03–1.25) for deaths from ischemic disease for left versus right side radiation in a period of >10 years after treatment [5]. Moreover, the role of ischemic heart disease specifically was investigated by some of the authors from the EBCTCG with 2,168 women who underwent radiotherapy for breast cancer between 1958 and 2001 in Sweden and Denmark, and the study included 963 women with major coronary events and 1,205 controls [84]. They found that the rates of major coronary events increased linearly with the mean dose to the heart by 7.4% per Gy (95%, 2.9–14.5;

$p < 0.001$), with no apparent threshold. The increase was apparent within the first 5 years after radiotherapy and continued into the third decade after radiotherapy (<*darby 2005 lancet.pdf*>).

In summary, Darby et al. and other large national breast cancer registries have shown (Fig. 8.6), that in breast cancer patients who were not treated with radiotherapy, the subsequent risk of heart disease was independent of tumor laterality, while for irradiated patients, the heart disease mortality ratio, left-sided versus right-sided tumors, increased with increasing time since diagnosis (i.e., with increasing time since irradiation). The increase was specific to heart disease as, for mortality from all other known causes, the left-sided versus right-sided mortality ratio was close to unity in both irradiated and nonirradiated patients [83]. These data suggest that the increasing trend in the left-sided versus right-sided mortality ratio for heart disease shown in Fig. 8.6 is caused by radiotherapy, with the bulk of the risk occurring more than a decade after exposure.

Testicular Cancer

In young men with testicular cancer, early studies from the United Kingdom between 1982 and 1992 looking at 992 patients with a median follow-up of 10.2 years showed a twofold or greater risk of developing cardiovascular disease [85]. Additionally, a large study looking at the incidence of ischemic heart disease in 2,512 long-term survivors in the Netherlands was compared with that of the general population [86]. Van den Belt-Dusebout et al. reported that the standardized incidence ratio (SIR) for coronary heart disease was 1.17 (95% CI, 1.04–1.31), with 14 excess cases per 10,000 person-years. The SIR for MI was significantly increased in nonseminoma survivors with attained ages of less than 45 (SIR = 2.06) and 45–54 years (SIR = 1.86) but significantly decreased for survivors with attained ages of 55 years or older (SIR = 0.53). In Cox analysis, mediastinal irradiation was associated with a 3.7-fold (95% CI, 2.2–6.2-fold) increased MI risk compared with surgery alone, whereas infradiaphragmatic irradiation was not associated with an increased MI risk. Cisplatin, vinblastine, and bleomycin chemotherapy was associated with a 1.9-fold (95% CI, 1.7–2.0-fold) increased MI risk, and bleomycin, etoposide, and cisplatin (BEP) cardiotoxicity was associated with a 1.5-fold (95% CI, 1.0–2.2-fold) increased CVD risk and was not associated with increased MI risk (hazard ratio = 1.2; 95% CI, 0.7–2.1). The authors concluded that nonseminomatous testicular cancer survivors experience a moderately increased MI risk at young ages secondary to a combination of both chemotherapy and radiation exposures.

Similarly, Haugnes et al. reviewed the late cardiovascular risk of treatment with infradiaphragmatic XRT and/or cisplatin-based chemotherapy, particularly the BEP regimen. Treatment with BEP alone had a 5.7-fold higher risk (95% CI, 1.9–17.1 fold) for coronary artery disease compared with surgery only and a 3.1-fold higher risk (95% CI, 1.2–7.7 fold) for myocardial infarction compared with age-matched controls [87]. Additional studies from Germany [88] and the Netherlands [89] showed similar increased observed-to-expected ratio for coronary artery disease compared to national age-matched controls.

MONITORING AND TREATMENT OF ISCHEMIC CARDIAC TOXICITY

Prevention, monitoring, and treatment of RIHD mirrors that of patients with nonradiation-induced IHD. Given the increased incidence in patients exposed to chest XRT and especially those with associated risk factors, it is recommended to aggressively monitor and treat all risk factors to achieve secondary prevention targets. The time interval for IHD development in RIHD is approximately 5–10 years [3]. The controversial issue is related to detection of ischemia—should it be different than guideline recommendations for atherosclerotic CAD and what studies should be done and how frequently should patients be monitored?

Recently, several practice guidelines have recommended screening for cardiovascular diseases [3,4,18,20] (Table 8.4) and specifically for ischemic heart disease in those with XRT. In addition to annual history and physical examinations, specific recommendations have been made on screening and aggressively treating hypertension with a goal blood pressure <140/90 mmHg, as well as other well-known risk factors for the development of coronary artery disease (i.e., diabetes mellitus, hyperlipidemia, renal disease). Certainly risk factor modification including a healthy diet and exercise regimens are encouraged. Additionally the use of aspirin 81 mg is encouraged unless strongly contraindicated, cardiac medications, and lipid lowering agents are recommended per national guidelines.

Moreover, recommendations for routine ECGs every 2–3 years in those with previous XRT have been proposed as many patients have silent conduction abnormalities [18]. Specific focus on the screening of cancer survivors treated as children, adolescents, and young adults, especially those who had higher volumes of radiation to the heart and those with other concomitant chemotherapy has been emphasized. Additional simple laboratory tests including lipid profile and thyroid monitoring have been recommended.

TABLE 8.4 JCO Recommendations for Practical Screening Tools for CVD in Cancer Survivors

Test	Test Timing Interval
Fasting lipid profile	Yearly, if abnormal
TSH (especially with neck irradiation)	Every several years, unless symptoms occur
Self-measurement of blood pressure	Several times per week in high-risk patients
Careful history and physical examination	At least yearly
Echocardiography (especially with any mediastinal irradiation or previous cardiotoxic chemotherapy)	Every 1–2 years in high-risk patients
Carotid ultrasound (particularly with mantle or neck irradiation)	Every 2 years in high-risk patients
Cardiac biomarkers (troponin, BNP)	Every 1–2 years in high-risk patients, unless symptoms occur
ECG	At least once every 2–3 years

Source: Kupeli S, et al. Evaluation of coronary artery disease by computed tomography angiography in patients treated for childhood Hodgkin's lymphoma. J Clin Oncol 2010;28(6):1025–30.

There are less formal recommendations on the use of adjuvant use of imaging modalities such as echocardiography, myocardial oxygen consumption, and stress testing, and clinical practice is largely based on expert consensus [3]. Echocardiography is a readily available, noninvasive method for global cardiac assessment including the development of cardiomyopathy and regional wall motion abnormalities from RIHD. Maximal myocardial oxygen consumption during exercise has prognostic significance in patients with cardiomyopathy and provides additional information about myocardial health [18]. Myocardial oxygen consumption has been observed to be low in patients with prior mediastinal irradiation, including those who did not have symptoms of cardiac dysfunction [89], yet there are limited data on the long-term significance of this important but subclinical finding; the use of myocardial oxygen consumption studies is not routinely recommended.

Tests of inducible ischemia including physiologic (exercise) or pharmacologic (e.g., dobutamine, persantine) stress testing augments the diagnosis of ischemic heart disease and cardiac dysfunction. However, the prognostic value of stress echocardiography and stress myocardial perfusion scanning in this population has not been well studied [18]. Radionuclide myocardial perfusion (or SPECT) scanning during exercise has 90% sensitivity and specificity in the general population to detect ischemic heart disease, but it also appears to detect radiation-induced microvascular damage in the myocardium of those whose hearts were exposed to irradiation and is therefore a less reliable tool for screening CAD [90]. These limited studies indicate that the perfusion defects often seen with previous XRT may be due to the microvascular fibrosis rather than epicardial coronary atherosclerosis and therefore, the ability of perfusion scanning to distinguish microvascular abnormalities from coronary artery disease in this population is unclear. The detection of microvascular damage, however, may potentially identify those who are at highest risk for cardiomyopathy and death, although this requires further study.

The use of coronary computed tomography angiogram (CTA) has been used in the general population to assess for the presence of coronary lesions and attain a coronary calcium score. The role of CTA in the Cardio-Oncology population is less clearly defined but may be considered an adjunct tool in the risk stratification of coronary artery disease. Coronary CT angiography has been used for follow-up in small groups of patients after radiation therapy for Hodgkin's disease. These studies demonstrated advanced coronary calcification and advanced obstructive CAD in relatively young patients [35]. However, current imaging guidelines argue that there are currently insufficient data to recommend a systematic use of these new tools after chest irradiation [3].

In those patients who present with typical anginal symptoms, recommendations for the diagnosis and treatment of CAD are similar to the general population including targeted revascularization [91]. Radiation-related CAD is managed conventionally, with medical control of risk factors as per the national guidelines [92–95]. Surgery may be technically challenging due to the presence of mediastinal scarring, friability of the vessels, and a possible increased rate of underlying atherosclerosis and higher restenosis rates for irradiated internal mammary vessels when they are chosen for CABG [96].

CONCLUSIONS

Cancer treatment-induced cardiotoxicity has been well established and accompanies chest radiation and a variety of chemotherapeutic agents [97]. Most clinicians are knowledgeable about cardiomyopathy risk, but many forget the less common complication of treatment-induced early and late coronary ischemia that has substantial risk on early and late non-cancer-related morbidity and mortality in the cancer population [98]. We endorse not only awareness, but an aggressive approach to detection and management, including diligent risk factor management in this population.

REFERENCES

[1] Weintraub NL, Jones WK, Manka D. Understanding radiation-induced vascular disease. J Am Coll Cardiol 2010;55(12):1237–9.

[2] Martinou M, Gaya A. Cardiac complications after radical radiotherapy. Semin Oncol 2013;40(2):178–85.

[3] Lancellotti P, et al. Expert consensus for multi-modality imaging evaluation of cardiovascular complications of radiotherapy in adults: a report from the European Association of Cardiovascular Imaging and the American Society of Echocardiography. J Am Soc Echocardiogr 2013;26(9):1013–32.

[4] Carver JR, et al. American society of clinical oncology clinical evidence review on the ongoing care of adult cancer survivors: cardiac and pulmonary late effects. J Clin Oncol 2007;25(25):3991–4008.

[5] Bovelli D, et al. Cardiotoxicity of chemotherapeutic agents and radiotherapy-related heart disease: ESMO clinical practice guidelines. Ann Oncol 2010;21(Suppl. 5):v277–82.

[6] Thibaudeau AA, Mattick WL. Histological findings in hearts which have been exposed to radiation in the course of treatment of adjacent organs. J Cancer Res 1929;13(3):251–9.

[7] Tracy GP, et al. Radiation-induced coronary artery disease. JAMA 1974;228(13):1660–2.

[8] Dunsmore LD, LoPonte MA, Dunsmore RA. Radiation-induced coronary artery disease. J Am Coll Cardiol 1986;8(1):239–44.

[9] Simon EB, et al. Radiation-induced coronary artery disease. Am Heart J 1984;108(4 Pt. 1):1032–4.

[10] Audebert AA, et al. Radiation-induced coronary artery disease. One observation (author's transl). Ann Med Interne (Paris) 1982;133(4):269–71.

[11] Taunk NK, et al. Radiation-induced heart disease: pathologic abnormalities and putative mechanisms. Front Oncol 2015;5:39.

[12] Fajardo LF. Is the pathology of radiation injury different in small vs large blood vessels? Cardiovasc Radiat Med 1999;1(1):108–10.

[13] Virmani R, et al. Pathology of radiation-induced coronary artery disease in human and pig. Cardiovasc Radiat Med 1999;1(1):98–101.

[14] Glanzmann C, et al. Cardiac risk after mediastinal irradiation for Hodgkin's disease. Radiother Oncol 1998;46(1):51–62.

[15] Veinot JP, Edwards WD. Pathology of radiation-induced heart disease: a surgical and autopsy study of 27 cases. Hum Pathol 1996;27(8):766–73.

[16] van Rijswijk S, et al. Mini-review on cardiac complications after mediastinal irradiation for Hodgkin lymphoma. Neth J Med 2008;66(6):234–7.

[17] Lenihan DJ, Cardinale DM. Late cardiac effects of cancer treatment. J Clin Oncol 2012;30(30):3657–64.

[18] Adams MJ, et al. Radiation-associated cardiovascular disease: manifestations and management. Semin Radiat Oncol 2003;13(3): 346–56.

[19] Aebi S, et al. Primary breast cancer: ESMO clinical practice guidelines for diagnosis, treatment and follow-up. Ann Oncol 2010;21(Suppl. 5):v9–v14.

[20] Eichenauer DA, Engert A, Dreyling M. Hodgkin's lymphoma: ESMO clinical practice guidelines for diagnosis, treatment and follow-up. Ann Oncol 2011;22(Suppl. 6):vi55–8.

[21] Khakoo AY, Yeh ET. Therapy insight: management of cardiovascular disease in patients with cancer and cardiac complications of cancer therapy. Nat Clin Pract Oncol 2008;5(11):655–67.

[22] Yeh ET, Bickford CL. Cardiovascular complications of cancer therapy: incidence, pathogenesis, diagnosis, and management. J Am Coll Cardiol 2009;53(24):2231–47.

[23] Arbuck SG, et al. A reassessment of cardiac toxicity associated with Taxol. J Natl Cancer Inst Monogr 1993;(15):117–30.

[24] Rowinsky EK, et al. Cardiac disturbances during the administration of taxol. J Clin Oncol 1991;9(9):1704–12.

[25] Vermorken JB, et al. Cisplatin, fluorouracil, and docetaxel in unresectable head and neck cancer. N Engl J Med 2007;357(17): 1695–704.

[26] McKendrick J, Coutsouvelis J. Capecitabine: effective oral fluoropyrimidine chemotherapy. Expert Opin Pharmacother 2005;6(7): 1231–9.

[27] Polk A, et al. Cardiotoxicity in cancer patients treated with 5-fluorouracil or capecitabine: a systematic review of incidence, manifestations and predisposing factors. Cancer Treat Rev 2013;39(8):974–84.

[28] Jensen SA, et al. Fluorouracil induces myocardial ischemia with increases of plasma brain natriuretic peptide and lactic acid but without dysfunction of left ventricle. J Clin Oncol 2010;28(36):5280–6.

[29] Anand AJ. Fluorouracil cardiotoxicity. Ann Pharmacother 1994;28(3):374–8.

[30] Meyer CC, et al. Symptomatic cardiotoxicity associated with 5-fluorouracil. Pharmacotherapy 1997;17(4):729–36.

[31] Patel B, et al. 5-Fluorouracil cardiotoxicity: left ventricular dysfunction and effect of coronary vasodilators. Am J Med Sci 1987;294(4):238–43.

[32] Saif MW, et al. Capecitabine vs continuous infusion 5-FU in neoadjuvant treatment of rectal cancer. A retrospective review. Int J Colorectal Dis 2008;23(2):139–45.

[33] Rezkalla S, et al. Continuous ambulatory ECG monitoring during fluorouracil therapy: a prospective study. J Clin Oncol 1989;7(4): 509–14.

[34] Yilmaz U, et al. 5-fluorouracil increases the number and complexity of premature complexes in the heart: a prospective study using ambulatory ECG monitoring. Int J Clin Pract 2007;61(5):795–801.

[35] Kupeli S, et al. Evaluation of coronary artery disease by computed tomography angiography in patients treated for childhood Hodgkin's lymphoma. J Clin Oncol 2010;28(6):1025–30.

[36] Braunwald E, et al. ACC/AHA guidelines for the management of patients with unstable angina and non-ST-segment elevation myocardial infarction: executive summary and recommendations. A report of the American College of Cardiology/American Heart Association task force on practice guidelines (committee on the management of patients with unstable angina). Circulation 2000;102(10):1193–209.

[37] O'Gara PT, et al. 2013 ACCF/AHA guideline for the management of ST-elevation myocardial infarction: a report of the American College of Cardiology Foundation/American Heart Association Task Force on Practice Guidelines. Circulation 2013;127(4):e362–425.

[38] Cianci G, et al. Prophylactic options in patients with 5-fluorouracil-associated cardiotoxicity. Br J Cancer 2003;88(10):1507–9.

[39] Cerny J, et al. Coronary vasospasm with myocardial stunning in a patient with colon cancer receiving adjuvant chemotherapy with FOLFOX regimen. Clin Colorectal Cancer 2009;8(1):55–8.

[40] Ambrosy AP, et al. Capecitabine-induced chest pain relieved by diltiazem. Am J Cardiol 2012;110(11):1623–6.

[41] Milano G, et al. Dihydropyrimidine dehydrogenase deficiency and fluorouracil-related toxicity. Br J Cancer 1999;79(3–4):627–30.

[42] Polk A, et al. A systematic review of the pathophysiology of 5-fluorouracil-induced cardiotoxicity. BMC Pharmacol Toxicol 2014;15:47.

[43] Sudhoff T, et al. 5-Fluorouracil induces arterial vasocontractions. Ann Oncol 2004;15(4):661–4.

[44] Berliner S, et al. Acute coronary events following cisplatin-based chemotherapy. Cancer Invest 1990;8(6):583–6.

[45] Jafri M, Protheroe A. Cisplatin-associated thrombosis. Anticancer Drugs 2008;19(9):927–9.

[46] Karabay KO, Yildiz O, Aytekin V. Multiple coronary thrombi with cisplatin. J Invasive Cardiol 2014;26(2):E18–20.

[47] Tomirotti M, et al. Ischemic cardiopathy from cis-diamminedichloro-platinum (CDDP). Tumori 1984;70(3):235–6.

[48] Mortimer JE, et al. A phase II randomized study comparing sequential and combined intraarterial cisplatin and radiation therapy in primary brain tumors. A Southwest Oncology Group study. Cancer 1992;69(5):1220–3.

[49] Nuver J, et al. Acute chemotherapy-induced cardiovascular changes in patients with testicular cancer. J Clin Oncol 2005;23(36):9130–7.

[50] Strumberg D, et al. Evaluation of long-term toxity in patients after cisplatin-based chemotherapy for non-seminomatous testicular cancer. Ann Oncol 2002;13(2):229–36.

[51] Feldman DR, Schaffer WL, Steingart RM. Late cardiovascular toxicity following chemotherapy for germ cell tumors. J Natl Compr Canc Netw 2012;10(4):537–44.

[52] Cargill RI, Boyter AC, Lipworth BJ. Reversible myocardial ischaemia following vincristine containing chemotherapy. Respir Med 1994;88(9):709–10.

[53] Lejonc JL, et al. Myocardial infarction following vinblastine treatment. Lancet 1980;2(8196):692.

[54] Zabernigg A, Gattringer C. Myocardial infarction associated with vinorelbine (Navelbine). Eur J Cancer 1996;32A(9):1618–9.

[55] Armitage JD, et al. Acute coronary syndromes complicating the first infusion of rituximab. Clin Lymphoma Myeloma 2008;8(4):253–5.

[56] Roy A, Khanna N, Senguttuvan NB. Rituximab-vincristine chemotherapy-induced acute anterior wall myocardial infarction with cardiogenic shock. Tex Heart Inst J 2014;41(1):80–2.

[57] Renard D, Cornillet L, Castelnovo G. Myocardial infarction after rituximab infusion. Neuromuscul Disord 2013;23(7): 599–601.

[58] Mehrpooya M, et al. Delayed myocardial infarction associated with rituximab infusion: a case report and literature review. Am J Ther 2015;23(1):e283–7.

[59] Keswani AN, et al. Rituximab-induced acute ST elevation myocardial infarction. Ochsner J 2015;15(2):187–90.

[60] Gogia A, Khurana S, Paramanik R. Acute myocardial infarction after first dose of rituximab infusion. Turk J Haematol 2014;31(1): 95–6.

[61] Arunprasath P, et al. Rituximab induced myocardial infarction: a fatal drug reaction. J Cancer Res Ther 2011;7(3):346–8.

[62] van Sijl AM, van der Weele W, Nurmohamed MT. Myocardial infarction after rituximab treatment for rheumatoid arthritis: Is there a link? Curr Pharm Des 2014;20(4):496–9.

[63] van Vollenhoven RF, et al. Long-term safety of rituximab in rheumatoid arthritis: 9.5-year follow-up of the global clinical trial programme with a focus on adverse events of interest in RA patients. Ann Rheum Dis 2013;72(9):1496–502.

[64] Lindhardsen J, et al. The risk of myocardial infarction in rheumatoid arthritis and diabetes mellitus: a Danish nationwide cohort study. Ann Rheum Dis 2011;70(6):929–34.

[65] Scappaticci FA, et al. Arterial thromboembolic events in patients with metastatic carcinoma treated with chemotherapy and bevacizumab. J Natl Cancer Inst 2007;99(16):1232–9.

[66] Ranpura V, et al. Risk of cardiac ischemia and arterial thromboembolic events with the angiogenesis inhibitor bevacizumab in cancer patients: a meta-analysis of randomized controlled trials. Acta Oncol 2010;49(3):287–97.

[67] Ranpura V, Hapani S, Wu S. Treatment-related mortality with bevacizumab in cancer patients: a meta-analysis. JAMA 2011;305(5): 487–94.

[68] Escudier B, et al. Sorafenib in advanced clear-cell renal-cell carcinoma. N Engl J Med 2007;356(2):125–34.

[69] Arima Y, et al. Sorafenib-induced acute myocardial infarction due to coronary artery spasm. J Cardiol 2009;54(3):512–5.

[70] Richards CJ, et al. Incidence and risk of congestive heart failure in patients with renal and nonrenal cell carcinoma treated with sunitinib. J Clin Oncol 2011;29(25):3450–6.

[71] Chu TF, et al. Cardiotoxicity associated with tyrosine kinase inhibitor sunitinib. Lancet 2007;370(9604):2011–9.

[72] Moslehi JJ, Deininger M. Tyrosine kinase inhibitor-associated cardiovascular toxicity in chronic myeloid leukemia. J Clin Oncol 2015;33(35):4210–8.

[73] Sonnenblick M, Rosin A. Cardiotoxicity of interferon. a review of 44 cases. Chest 1991;99(3):557–61.

[74] Nora R, et al. Myocardial toxic effects during recombinant interleukin-2 therapy. J Natl Cancer Inst 1989;81(1):59–63.

[75] Kammula US, White DE, Rosenberg SA. Trends in the safety of high dose bolus interleukin-2 administration in patients with metastatic cancer. Cancer 1998;83(4):797–805.

[76] Lee RE, et al. Cardiorespiratory effects of immunotherapy with interleukin-2. J Clin Oncol 1989;7(1):7–20.

[77] Aleman BMP, et al. Late cardiotoxicity after treatment for Hodgkin lymphoma. Blood 2007;109(5):1878–86.

[78] Aleman BMP, et al. Long-term cause-specific mortality of patients treated for Hodgkin's disease. J Clin Oncol 2003;21(18):3431–9.

[79] Castellino SM, et al. Morbidity and mortality in long-term survivors of Hodgkin lymphoma: a report from the childhood cancer survivor study. Blood 2011;117(6):1806–16.

[80] Hull MC, et al. Valvular dysfunction and carotid, subclavian, and coronary artery disease in survivors of hodgkin lymphoma treated with radiation therapy. JAMA 2003;290(21):2831–7.

[81] Swerdlow AJ, et al. Myocardial infarction mortality risk after treatment for hodgkin disease: a collaborative British cohort study. J Natl Cancer Inst 2007;99(3):206–14.

[82] van Nimwegen FA, et al. Radiation dose-response relationship for risk pf coronary heart disease in survivors of hodgkin lymphoma. J Clin Oncol 2016;34(3):235–43.

[83] Darby SC, et al. Radiation-related heart disease: current knowledge and future prospects. Int J Radiat Oncol Biol Phys 2010;76(3): 656–65.

[84] Darby SC, et al. Risk of ischemic heart disease in women after radiotherapy for breast cancer. N Engl J Med 2013;368(11):987–98.

[85] Darby SC, et al. Long-term mortality from heart disease and lung cancer after radiotherapy for early breast cancer: prospective cohort study of about 300,000 women in US SEER cancer registries. Lancet Oncol 2005;6(8):557–65.

[86] van den Belt-Dusebout AW, et al. Long-term risk of cardiovascular disease in 5-year survivors of testicular cancer. J Clin Oncol 2006;24(3):467–75.

[87] Haugnes HS, et al. Cardiovascular risk factors and morbidity in long-term survivors of testicular cancer: a 20-year follow-up study. J Clin Oncol 2010;28(30):4649–57.

[88] Dieckmann KP, et al. Myocardial infarction and other major vascular events during chemotherapy for testicular cancer. Ann Oncol 2010;21(8):1607–11.

[89] Meinardi MT, et al. Cardiovascular morbidity in long-term survivors of metastatic testicular cancer. J Clin Oncol 2000;18(8):1725–32.

[90] Maunoury C, et al. Myocardial perfusion damage after mediastinal irradiation for Hodgkin's disease: a thallium-201 single photon emission tomography study. Eur J Nucl Med 1992;19(10):871–3.

[91] Schutz FA, et al. Bevacizumab increases the risk of arterial ischemia: a large study in cancer patients with a focus on different subgroup outcomes. Ann Oncol 2011;22(6):1404–12.

[92] White DA, et al. Acute chest pain syndrome during bleomycin infusions. Cancer 1987;59(9):1582–5.

[93] Vogelzang NJ, Frenning DH, Kennedy BJ. Coronary artery disease after treatment with bleomycin and vinblastine. Cancer Treat Rep 1980;64(10–11):1159–60.

[94] House KW, Simon SR, Pugh RP. Chemotherapy-induced myocardial infarction in a young man with Hodgkin's disease. Clin Cardiol 1992;15(2):122–5.

[95] Edwards GS, Lane M, Smith FE. Long-term treatment with cis-dichlorodiammineplatinum(II)-vinblastine-bleomycin: possible association with severe coronary artery disease. Cancer Treat Rep 1979;63(4):551–2.

[96] Huddart RA, et al. Cardiovascular disease as a long-term complication of treatment for testicular cancer. J Clin Oncol 2003;21(8): 1513–23.

[97] Pihkala J, et al. Cardiopulmonary evaluation of exercise tolerance after chest irradiation and anticancer chemotherapy in children and adolescents. Pediatrics 1995;95(5):722–6.

[98] Fajardo LF. Radiation-induced coronary artery disease. Chest 1977;71(5):563–4.

Chapter 9

Radiation Therapy and Cardiovascular Risk

M.P. Sittig* and S.L. Shiao*,**,†

*Department of Radiation Oncology, Cedars-Sinai Medical Center, Los Angeles, CA, United States; **Department of Biomedical Sciences, Cedars-Sinai Medical Center, Los Angeles, CA, United States; †Department of Medicine, University of California, Los Angeles, CA, United States

INTRODUCTION

In 1896, a German physics professor named Wilhelm Conrad Roentgen gave a lecture regarding the recent discovery of a new kind of ray [1]. He described the utility of the new physical phenomena, including its use in diagnosis as he produced the first two-dimensional radiograph. In that same year, the first radiation therapy (RT) treatment was delivered by a young physician named Emil Grubbe who convinced his superiors to allow him to treat a woman with recurrent breast carcinoma to good effect. The technology was crude at best in the early days and, in fact, early radiologists would often test the output of their machines by holding their arms under the beam and waiting for erythema to develop [2]. Thankfully since that time, the field of radiation oncology has changed remarkably with advances in technology allowing the sophisticated delivery of both curative and palliative doses of ionizing radiation.

The evolution of the field has been mirrored by a rise in the number of patients undergoing RT [3]. In general, approximately two-thirds of patients diagnosed with cancer in the United States undergo treatment with radiation [4]. With the dramatic successes of radiation treatments and systemic therapy, many patients are living as cancer survivors. Estimates by some agencies suggest that by 2020, there will be nearly 12 million cancer survivors, three times the number seen in the mid-2000s [5]. These cancer survivors have unique concerns resulting from late toxicities of chemotherapy and radiation treatment [6]. In particular, treatment-related cardiovascular complications have been increasingly recognized and, in fact, in survivors of certain cancers including breast and lung cancers, cardiovascular disease is the leading nonmalignant cause of death.

Cardiovascular complications from radiation largely arise from treatments in which radiation is delivered to the heart and/or major vessels. Radiation to these locations have well-documented increases in risk for cardiovascular disease (including stroke) from radiation-mediated accelerated atherosclerosis and loss of vascular integrity. As the number of cancer survivors grows, it is increasingly important that clinicians involved in the care of oncology patients have an appreciation of the radiation-related complications and how to best manage these issues as they arise.

MECHANISM OF CARDIOVASCULAR INJURY IN THE SETTING OF RADIATION THERAPY

The interaction between ionizing radiation and normal tissues rests upon an understanding of how radiation energy deposited in tissues (measured in Gray, abbreviated Gy) affects the biological function of that given tissue. The effect of radiation depends on a number of tissue-intrinsic variables, one of which is the type and number of vessels contained within the tissue. In the context of the vascular system, the arterial system represents the area of greatest interest in both the treatment and prevention of vascular-related complications from radiation including both stroke and heart disease. Other sites, including the venous system, heart valves, and lymphatic channels can also be affected by radiation therapy in a dose-dependent fashion [7–9].

Cellular Radiobiology

At a cellular level, high energy X-rays, such as those used in radiation treatment, mediate their effect by damaging the DNA of cells through the production of free radicals (hence the name "ionizing"). Interestingly, though cells damaged by radiation do undergo apoptotic and necrotic cell death, a significant number also enters a unique state of mitotic senescence [10]. For those cells which are either permanently mitotically arrested or undergo mitosis at a very low rate, many of these cells exhibit a loss of a cell-specific functioning. Cardiac myocytes, for example, require the production of energy in the form of ATP and the regulation of calcium for their ongoing function and although myocytes do not typically undergo routine division, they often exhibit dose-dependent impairment in these two functions following irradiation. In famous experiments performed by Bergonie and Tribondeau, cells which were dividing more rapidly, such as malignant tumor cells, were found to be more susceptible to the damaging effects of RT [11,12]. Slower-proliferating tissues or those that were better differentiated, such as vascular cells and cardiac myocytes underwent fewer adverse changes in response to therapeutic doses of radiation. The relative difference in cell death rates between malignant and normal cells underlies the current treatment paradigm of fractionated RT, in which a small portion or fraction of the total prescribed dose of radiation is delivered in multiple consecutive treatments. Though many of these doses were determined empirically to be safe, it has become apparent in cancer survivors, that doses once thought to be safe can still carry significant long-term consequences particularly on the cardiovascular system.

Dose–Response Relationship

As exposure to ionizing radiation increases, so does the risk of developing cellular dysfunction, which can lead to clinically meaningful toxicity, including cardiovascular disease [13]. The Childhood Cancer Survivor Study has tracked posttreatment complications in patients who had previously undergo chemotherapy and RT, and in a 2009 study, data regarding radiation doses and rates of heart disease were published. Over 14,000 patients were followed and compared to a group of siblings without an oncologic history [14]. The authors found that there was an increase rate in heart failure, myocardial infarction, and valvular dysfunction following radiotherapy to the chest. There did not appear to be a clinically meaningful risk for patients receiving less than 5 Gy, whereas those patients who received more than 15 Gy were at significantly higher risk.

In women treated with whole-breast RT as a part of breast conserving therapy, an increased risk of heart disease occurred proportional to the dose received by the heart. Examination of older trials comparing women with right-sided tumors in which the heart receives little dose versus left-sided tumors in which portions of heart may have received full dose showed that women with right-sided tumors have significantly less risk of cardiac morbidity and mortality compared with women with left-sided tumors [15–17]. As such, modern RT has focused tremendous effort to reduce dose delivered to normal structures, particularly the heart, with sophisticated computerized planning and advanced dose delivery. However, patients treated prior to 2000 would likely have received significant radiation dose to the heart.

Specific Mechanisms of Cardiovascular Damage

Atherosclerosis

The precise pathophysiologic mechanism mediating vascular damage following RT remains elusive. Two mechanisms have been proposed: accelerated atherosclerosis and endothelial damage, both of which may not be mutually exclusive [18]. On the basis of a traditional understanding of the development of atherosclerotic lesions, several groups have suggested that radiation causes atherosclerotic plaques to develop at an accelerated rate [19,20]. This is a multistep process that begins with inflammation, which leads to endothelial irritation and recruitment of immune cells, which subsequently consumes low-density lipoprotein (LDL) and forms atheromas. In this view, radiation exposure acts as the initiating inflammatory step, and causes a similar cascade of events as atherosclerotic lesions which develop in the absence of radiation exposure.

A competing theory by Fonkalsrud et al. theorizes that radiation initially disrupts endothelial cells and the vasa vasorum [21]. Examination of canine femoral arteries by electron microscopy after a dose that was similar to what a patient might receive during treatment (40 Gy) found early endothelial dysfunction, including breakdown of intracellular structures, early thrombosis formation, and adventitial damage. At 4 months following radiation, areas of the media had undergone fibrosis and necrosis. These studies suggest that the main initial target of vascular damage following radiation are the endothelial cells.

Regardless of the etiology, RT-induced atherosclerosis and native plaques have a number of important differences. In the setting of RT, the atherosclerotic lesion is seen "in-field," meaning only in the area in which radiation is delivered to the patient, which is consistent with the local nature of the treatment. Radiation-induced atherosclerotic lesions also tend to be longer than those which develop de novo, and the regions which have maximal stenosis are typically seen at the ends of the lesions [22]. Microscopically, the plaques are seen more commonly in medium and large arteries than in smaller arteries [23]. A useful and commonly cited marker of atherosclerosis is the intima-media thickness, which is seen in RT-naïve lesions as well as those related to therapy [24,25].

Biochemical changes that occur following radiation have also been demonstrated in vivo, including the acute upregulation of proinflammatory biomarkers and cytokines within the vascular endothelium and oxidative injury from free radicals produced by radiation. This process is accompanied by a more chronic process in which the upregulation of cellular adhesion molecules, changes in cytokine expression, smooth muscle proliferation, and the decreased expression of nitric oxide are all thought to contribute to the chronicity of RT-induced atherosclerosis [26]. Additional factors including DNA damage, endothelial and smooth muscle cell NF-kB activation, mitochondrial dysregulation, and vascular senescence may also play a role in endothelial dysfunction and subsequent atherosclerosis [27–29].

Once endothelial cell damage has occurred, the process of radiation-induced atherosclerosis mimics the nonradiation mediated atherosclerotic process with intimal thickening causing an intrinsic compression of the normal laminar blood flow. In addition to endothelial damage, radiation to vessels may also cause micro- and macroscopic changes to the tissues surrounding the vessel, including the adventitia. Vessel hardening can occur through the replacement of elastic tissue with fibrous tissue, mediated by fibroblast activation [30]. The net result of the process is reduced vascular elasticity leading to more extrinsic compression, increasing the likelihood of hemodynamic compromise in combination with inflammatory intimal thickening [31].

Valvular Disease and Dysfunction

In addition to atherosclerotic lesions, RT to the heart may also cause valvular dysfunction. In particular, valvular thickening, retraction, and calcification may occur in the leaflets of the valve and the regions surrounding each valve. Consequently, for cancer survivors stenosis occurs at a higher rate in those exposed to therapeutic radiation as compared to the general population. Valvular complications generally only become apparent more than a decade after completion of RT, and continue to present up to three decades after treatment. Other than the radiation dose received by the valve, women also have been reported to have a higher risk for the development of valvular dysfunction following RT [32].

Echocardiographic studies have demonstrated that patients who received RT to the mediastinum were at an increased likelihood of valvular stenosis, regurgitation, systolic dysfunction, and diastolic dysfunction. Following radiation, valvular insufficiency is most commonly seen in the aortic and mitral valves, and less commonly in the tricuspid valve [33]. The rate of valvular dysfunction increased with time; in one series, patients who had been assessed for cardiac function with EKG and echocardiogram were found to have categorically dysfunctional aortic valves even into the third decade after treatment [33].

In a series involving both surgical patients and autopsy specimens from patients who had previously undergone thoracic irradiation, valve leaflet thickening was noted to be present in 12 of 17 hearts, with those demonstrating thickening receiving an average radiation dose of 46 Gy to the heart [34]. The mean time from treatment to development of clinically significant symptoms was just over 8 years. Each of the seven dissected valves (three mitral and four aortic) and 18 postmortem specimens (six mitral, five tricuspid, four aortic, and three pulmonary) demonstrated

radiation-related fibrosis. Of note, despite the presence of tricuspid and pulmonary valve fibrosis, these changes were not deemed by the authors to be clinically significant. Further studies have also corroborated the relative infrequency of right-sided heart valve involvement in radiation-related toxicity, despite the relative proximity of these valves to the anterior mediastinum [35]. Despite the frequency of valvular abnormalities seen in this series and others, it is important to note that overt valvular dysfunction in patients undergoing thoracic radiation remains rare [36]. Cutter et al. performed a study of patients who were treated with thoracic radiation for Hodgkin's lymphoma and evaluated rates of valvular heart disease. The authors found that patients receiving between 20 and 30 Gy to the heart had 1.4% risk of developing clinically significant valvular dysfunction at 30 years [37].

For those patients who have severely dysfunctional valves, replacement may be indicated. This is typically indicated in patients who have poor cardiac function (NYHA Class III or IV). In a series from the Mayo Clinic, cardiac patients undergoing valve replacement who had received radiation treatment to the mediastinum (mean heart dose of 46 Gy, range 25–70 Gy) for a variety of malignancies (Hodgkin's lymphoma, non-Hodgkin's lymphoma, breast cancer, lung cancer, thymoma, and seminoma) were reviewed [38]. In this series, most patients requiring valvular surgery also required a simultaneous coronary artery bypass, a notable finding, given the relative likelihood that these disease processes would occur simultaneously as both the coronary arteries and valves would fall within a typical thoracic radiation treatment field. The most common type of operation was aortic valve replacement, followed by mitral valve replacement. In 12 of 60 patients, multiple valves required repair simultaneously. Despite successful surgeries in 82% of treated patients, the authors warn that surgical candidates must be selected carefully, as it is unlikely that valve replacement will fully eliminate the decline in cardiac function following RT which is a progressive and dynamic process.

Pericardial Disease

RT can also affect the pericardium, and unlike the changes seen in the coronary arteries and valves, radiation-induced pericardial disease may develop both acutely and chronically. Pericardial effusions postradiation exist on a spectrum of presentations, from minimal and asymptomatic to severe cardiac tamponade, leading to hemodynamic compromise. Animal experiments have demonstrated that with 20 Gy to the heart, significant changes occur to both the visceral and parietal layers of the pericardium [39]. In these experiments, mimicking what is seen in some patients, effusions were either serous or hemorrhagic, with the possibility of fibrous adhesions developing after many months to 1 year [40].

Radiation-induced pericarditis may present with symptoms which are similar to pericardial effusion, but the time course is initially faster [41]. Shortness of breath, fever, and chest pain are common. A Kussmaul sign (paradoxical rise in jugular venous pressure) and a friction rub may be observed on physical exam. EKG changes, including diffuse ST segment changes, may be present [42]. Ultrasonography often demonstrates a hypodense layer between the pericardium and the adjacent cardiac tissue, whereas chest radiography can demonstrate a "globular" heart if the effusion is of considerable size [41]. Pericardiocentesis can be both diagnostic (to distinguish between radiation-induced and malignant effusions) and therapeutic (if large enough to cause clinically relevant symptoms). Patients who have recurrent effusions may require drain placement or surgery for the creation of a pericardial window. Low-to-moderate severity effusions can be treated with nonsteroidal antiinflammatory drugs (NSAIDs). Although acute pericarditis can be easily linked causally to RT, often RT-induced pericarditis is delayed and may occur months to years after the treatment, and typically occurring with less severe symptoms, such as isolated dyspnea [43]. Historically, pericarditis occurred in up to 20% of patients receiving thoracic RT; however, modern RT methods (post-2000), which include CT planning for heart avoidance, have reduced the incidence to 2.5% [44,45].

For some patients, particularly those with either pericardial effusion or pericarditis following RT, constrictive pericarditis may develop in the years following therapy [46]. In this process, the fibrous, stiff pericardium is unable to accommodate volume changes and leads to a constrictive physiology, with impaired ventricular filling and diminished cardiac output [47]. Systolic function is typically preserved until late in the disease course. Clinically, patients present with recurrent dyspnea and volume overload, and with refractory heart failure which does not respond to the usual medications. There is no known treatment to halt this process, and ultimately, patients with this condition require a pericardiectomy.

Conduction System Abnormalities

Like other structures of the heart, the conduction system including both the nodes and conduction bundles may be adversely affected by RT [48]. First, second, and third atrioventricular blocks, as well as incomplete and complete bundle branch blocks have been reported following radiation. The etiology is multifactorial; decreased blood flow caused by atherosclerotic lesions and fibrosis caused by irradiation are likely causal factors for the development of conduction abnormalities. Effects on the conduction system like most of the other radiation-related cardiovascular problems typically begin to occur one to two decades after treatment [48]. The dose required to cause clinically significant

arrhythmias is reported to be approximately 40 Gy [49]. Rates of conduction abnormalities vary by studies series, from between 0% and 45% at 15 years of follow-up. For patients who develop bundle branch blocks, the right bundle is more commonly affected, likely due to the proximity of the right bundle to radiation fields entering the chest cavity anteriorly, which has traditionally been weighted more heavily in mediastinal RT for Hodgkin's lymphoma where most of the reported conduction abnormalities have been observed.

In a study of 48 long-term survivors of Hodgkin's disease who had previously undergone RT, Adams et al. examined a subset of patients with ECG ($n = 47$), ambulatory Holter monitor ($n = 42$), and exercise stress test ($n = 46$). With median follow-up time of 14.3 years (range: 5.9–27.5 years), 19% had sinus tachycardia, three patients had bradycardia, a monotonous or noncircadian heart rate in 57%, and abnormal exercise stress test in 21% of patients [50]. As with those with other cardiac abnormalities seen in patients who have undergone RT, the rates of these findings happen at an increased frequency in previously irradiated patients when compared with the general population [51].

Patients who develop clinically significant bradyarrhythmias from radiation require a pacemaker similar to those patients with nonradiation-related conduction abnormalities or arrhythmias [46]. For patients requiring pacing, a small series suggests the mean time between initial RT and development of clinically significant arrhythmia to be 12 years (range: 10–18). One other consideration for patients requiring pacemaker placement, is for the cardiologist to evaluate the patient for pericardiectomy as conduction abnormalities and constrictive pericarditis occurred together in as many as half the patients, and a small benefit to concurrent pacer placement and pericardiectomy was seen in this small cohort.

Heart Failure

Both diastolic and systolic heart failure have been associated with thoracic RT and more worrisome, patients with heart failure related to cancer treatment are at a 3.5-fold increased risk of death when compared to patients with idiopathic cardiomyopathy [52]. Retrospective and population-based studies have demonstrated that patients who have undergone thoracic irradiation for diseases including breast cancer and lymphoma have higher rates of heart failure [53,54]. In a systematic review by Nolan et al., systolic and diastolic dysfunction were explored. Patients with a prior history of thoracic irradiation for Hodgkin's lymphoma were found to have an increased likelihood of abnormal resting left ventricular ejection fraction (LVEF), ranging from 5% to 29%. Worse LVEF was associated with older treatment [55].

A number of studies have examined diastolic function using echocardiography and nuclear imaging, with

TABLE 9.1 Cardiovascular Risks Following Radiation Therapy

Tissue at Risk	Complication	Typical Time Course
Cerebral vasculature	Moyamoya (with increased risk of intracranial hemorrhage), small vessel ischemic disease	~3 years
Carotid arteries	Transient ischemic attack, stroke	6 months–20 years
Coronary arteries	Accelerated atherosclerosis, ischemic heart disease, stable/unstable angina, myocardial infarction, ischemic cardiomyopathy/heart failure	5–30 years
Myocardium	Radiation-related diastolic dysfunction, fibrosis, restrictive cardiomyopathy/heart failure	5–30 years
Pericardium	Pericarditis, small effusion to chronic large effusion/tamponade, pericardial fibrosis, and constriction	Acute: 2–12 months Chronic: 1–20 years
Cardiac valves	Valvular insufficiency (most commonly affecting aortic and mitral valves), aortic stenosis	8–30 years
Cardiac conduction system	1st degree, 2nd degree, or 3rd degree AV block, sick sinus/ bradycardia, RBBB, supraventricular and ventricular tachyarrhythmias, QT prolongation	10–18 years
Renal, iliac, and femoral arteries	Renal insufficiency/failure, intermittent claudication, extremity necrosis, peripheral arterial disease	2–16 years

inconsistent results. Heidenreich et al. examined patients treated for Hodgkin's lymphoma with at least 35 Gy of thoracic irradiation and found mild to moderate dysfunction in 14% of patients. Those with diastolic dysfunction were also more likely to have exercise-induced ischemia [56]. In contrast, Glanzmann et al. found that that Hodgkin's patients without any history of hypertension or coronary artery disease had no statistically significant increase in diastolic dysfunction following thoracic radiotherapy [57].

A number of chemotherapeutic regimens including alkylating agents, anthracyclines, and certain targeted antibodies are known to cause heart failure [58]. Worsening systolic heart function is seen in patients who undergo treatment with both modalities, when compared to radiotherapy alone [59]. Newer targeted therapies, including trastuzumab (Herceptin) used in the treatment of Her2-amplified breast cancers, is known to cause both reversible and irreversible changes in systolic function [60,61]. This effect is typically exacerbated by the addition of cytotoxic therapies and RT [62,63].

Time Course for Vascular Changes Following Radiation Therapy

A number of studies have examined the time course of normal tissue damage from RT and have found that the highest risk of developing cardiovascular complications within the first 10 years after treatment, but this risk continues out beyond 20 years from treatment [15]. Patients with pre-existing cardiovascular disease or risk factors have earlier onset and may require earlier intervention. Aside from the unique

scenarios involving tumor encroachment into vascular structures, acute vascular toxicity (those occurring within 3 months of treatment) is an exceedingly rare complication of RT with the exception of pericarditis for patients receiving high dose radiation to the heart directly [64]. However, cardiovascular toxicities vary by patient's age, disease site, amount of radiation delivered, and technique used to deliver radiation [65]. These toxicities are briefly summarized in Table 9.1, where specific risks by disease site are reviewed.

CARDIOVASCULAR RISK BY DISEASE SITE

Due to the wide number of body sites and disease indications in which RT can be used to treat cancer, each location has unique potential risks faced by patients as they undergo treatment, and there is a wide variation in radiation dose delivered to vascular structures. Thus, we review here the relevant studies by disease site and the vasculature and/or organs at risk. It should be noted that certain cancers associated with a more limited prognosis (e.g., locally advanced lung cancer) are less likely to have established long-term data regarding associated cardiovascular toxicities. Also, cancers affecting regions of the where there is relatively low risk of vascular complications (e.g., distal extremities) are also less likely to produce clinically evident cardiovascular toxicities.

Intracranial Lesions

RT is regularly used for primary brain tumors, both benign and malignant, as well as for metastatic intracranial lesions.

Many patients with metastatic disease or high-grade primary brain tumors have limited prognoses, and thus do not have a lifespan that would allow for chronic atherosclerotic changes or strokes to occur. A review of the current literature reveals a very limited number of cases in patients treated for primary glioma [66]. However, radiation treatment for benign intracranial diseases, such as pituitary adenomas have found some associations between radiation treatment and stroke risk though the implications for patients remain unclear.

Pituitary adenomas treated with radiotherapy have an established risk of stroke in the years following treatment. In 331 patients with pituitary adenomas treated with radiation in the United Kingdom from 1970 to 1980, 64 patients had a stroke with an actuarial incidence of 21% at 20 years following treatment. The authors of the study concluded that patients treated with radiotherapy had a relative risk for stroke of 4.1 when compared with the general UK population [67]. In contrast, a study from the University of Pittsburgh reported on 156 patients treated with radiation for pituitary adenoma from 1980 to 1989. Older age was the only factor that predicted stroke, and not at a higher rate than predicted in the general population [68]. Given the rapidity with which radiation treatment has changed in the last decade, these results should be interpreted with caution as much lower doses are currently delivered to the brain with modern techniques; the two studies highlight the effect of improved radiation techniques over two different eras reducing overall risk of stroke.

The incidence of vascular disease in patients treated definitively or with adjuvant radiotherapy for meningiomas which also typically have a very long survival postradiation treatment remains low. Review of the available literature finds only a small number of case reports which report transient ischemic attacks (TIA) following radiotherapy for meningioma [69].

Intracranial Vascular Malformations

In addition to stroke risk, brain irradiation has also been linked to a rare cerebrovascular malformation called "moyamoya" (meaning "puff of smoke" in Japanese), in which the terminal portion of the internal carotid artery progressively narrows [70]. The disease may occur sporadically, and is more common among people living in East Asian countries, particularly Korea and Japan and can lead to stroke. Although moyamoya is a rare complication of radiotherapy, it has been reported in childhood survivors of brain cancer who underwent treatment with radiotherapy, including both photons and protons [71,72]. Young patients (<9 years of age), those with a history of neurofibromatosis type 1 (NF1), and tumor location adjacent to the circle of Willis are all considered risk factors for the development of this condition [73]. The typical time course for the development of moyamoya in the reported cases is approximately 3 years and may be a precursor for intracranial hemorrhages later in life. Thus, for young patients who may need brain irradiation, the possibility of vascular disease should be discussed along with potential alternatives.

Cancers of the Head and Neck

Carotid Risk and RT

Carotid artery disease is well established as causative factor in ischemic stroke with almost 140,000 carotid endarterectomies performed each year in the United States [74]. Patients diagnosed with head and neck cancers have an increased risk of developing a carotid-related stroke due to both their primary disease causing procoagulation changes systemically and for radiation-induced accelerated atherosclerotic plaque development in the carotid arteries.

In a trial by Pereira Lima et al, patients undergoing treatment for head and neck cancer were identified and prospectively enrolled in a trial to follow levels of intimal-medial thickness via ultrasound, previously demonstrated as a surrogate marker of atherosclerotic change [75]. These patients underwent evaluation with sonography at the time of study enrollment prior to treatment, within 90 days of completing RT, and 6 months from completing therapy. Treatment consisted of 6 MV (megavolt) photons delivered in 2 Gy per daily fraction, delivered 5 days per week, to the primary disease and bilateral draining lymphatics, to a total dose of 44 Gy. A boost dose followed was administered to a smaller region with gross disease, for an additional 16–26 Gy. A significant change was noted in the intimal-medial thickness in the early posttreatment period (within 90 days), but further changes were not statistically significant in the latter follow-up period (beyond 6 months). The authors note that the changes seen on imaging suggest that intima-media thickening begins early following treatment, but does not change appreciably in the intermediate period.

Young patients face a particularly large treatment-related burden, as they have potentially more life years in which they can be affected by both their primary malignancy and treatment-related toxicity. In a 2002 study examining risk of ischemic stroke in head and neck cancer patients, Dorresteijn et al. examined 367 patients (including those with larynx carcinomas, pleomorphic adenomas, and parotid carcinomas) who underwent RT prior to the age of 60 [76]. The patient population was predominantly male (61%) with a median age of 49.3 years. RT doses were between 50 and 66 Gy, delivered at between 2 and 2.4 Gy per day (five fractions per week). Treated patients were compared with a population-based cohort matched for age and gender. Relative risks were calculated for the irradiation treatment group and compared with the expected number of strokes. Of 367 patients included in the trial, 14 patients developed an ischemic stroke after completing RT, giving an overall relative risk of developing ischemic stroke as compared with a matched nonirradiated population of 5.6 (95% confidence interval: 3.1–9.4). Of the included cancers analyzed, larynx carcinomas had the lowest relative risk (5.1), whereas parotid carcinomas had the highest (8.5). The authors note that age at the time of treatment may be an important factor when considering posttreatment vascular complications, suggesting that the relative young age of their head and neck cohort may face different toxicities when compared to older patients [54]. Other factors, including hypertension, smoking, and hyperlipidemia were also noted to likely play a role in addition to undergoing RT based on prior studies [77]. In summary, the authors conclude that physicians should pay particular attention to risk reduction including smoking cessation, adequate control of hypertension and/or hyperlipidemia. Carotid lesions may be evaluated using sonography, and will differ from typical atherosclerotic lesions in their location, typically with involvement of the distal carotid artery, and lack of confinement to the arterial bifurcation. They also suggest that indications for post-RT surgery be limited as much as possible, as surgical salvage of irradiated carotids arteries is potentially complicated. Medical management is preferred for carotid disease, including the use of antiplatelet therapies, angiotensin converting enzyme inhibitors, and statins though data is limited on the efficacy and safety of these agents in the post-RT setting.

Trends in Head and Neck Cancer

Historically, squamous cell carcinomas of the head and neck have been associated with the chronic use of alcohol and tobacco, and have typically affected older patients, with relatively poor survival despite combined modality therapy (chemotherapy, RT, and surgery) [78]. With decreased tobacco use seen in the United States, this group of patients has decreased over time. Simultaneously, there has been an emerging category of patients seen with tumors linked to infection with the human papillomavirus (HPV), specifically subtypes 16 and 18, involving the oral cavity [79]. These patients fit a different profile than traditional head and neck cancer patients: they are typically younger, nonsmokers, are more frequently Caucasian and present with early nodal metastases [80]. These patients also have a significantly better outcomes compared to non-HPV related head and neck cancers. As the proportion of these patients with HPV-induced head and neck malignancies increases, it will be especially important to consider their long-term toxicity as many of them will be long-term survivors. Given that many of these patients will otherwise have an additional 20–40 years, consideration should be given to try to eliminate or reduce treatment-related risk of vascular complications. In a Taiwanese study of young patients (age less than 55 years) with head and neck cancers, there was an elevated risk of stroke following combined chemoradiotherapy

compared to the general population (relative risk: 1.8) [81]. As HPV+ tumors of the head and neck appear much more radiosensitive, ongoing trials are examining whether this subpopulations of patients can safely undergo treatment with a reduced amount of radiation in an attempt to lower both short- and long-term toxicity [82].

Treatment Recommendations for Vascular Complications Following Irradiation of the Head and Neck

Given the elevated risks seen in patients who have been treated with RT for head and neck malignancies, patients who have undergone RT of the head and neck should be evaluated with ultrasonography of the carotid arteries at regular intervals starting 2–5 years after treatment in order to assess patients for risk and need for intervention. Furthermore, additional cardioprotective treatments should be implemented given the accelerated nature of radiation-induced atherosclerotic disease. This would include annual lipid monitoring and management, blood pressure control, smoking cessation, weight loss, and regular physical activity.

Cancers of the Thorax

Lymphoma

RT was first used in 1902 for the palliative treatment of bulky lymphadenopathy associated with lymphoma [83]. The patient responded rapidly, but the effect was short-lived and the limited reproducibility of the technology at the time prevented early pioneers from using ionizing radiation to cure their patients. Nearly a half century later, Peters described a technique in which larger radiation fields were utilized, which yielded excellent long-term survival [84]. It was not long before Dollinger et al. published a case of coronary artery fibrosis in a patient who was treated 18 years earlier for Hodgkin lymphoma; this case was considered the first report of late vascular toxicity following RT [85]. Subsequent studies of the Dutch experience found a similar time frame for the development of cardiac disease. In this review of 2617 Hodgkin's lymphoma patients treated between 1965 and 1995, van Nimwegen et al. found that the median time between therapeutic radiation and development of coronary heart disease (CHD) was 19 years [86].

Since that time, additional studies have demonstrated that treatment of mediastinal structures has a causal relationship with increased risk of cardiac complications, including increased risk of cardiac mortality due to the radiation dose to cardiac structures [87,88]. Many early long-term survivors of Hodgkin's disease present with ongoing cardiac problems resulting from early crude, but curative, administration of radiation. Recognition of this toxicity has led to the transformation of the treatment of the disease with chemotherapeutic regimens taking the forefront, and reduction in radiation dose and field size in selected patients, significantly reducing the rate of mediastinal radiation [89]. In fact, current trials suggest that certain patients with Hodgkin's lymphoma can forego radiation all together without sacrificing freedom from disease progression or overall survival, thus radiation-induced cardiac disease from Hodgkin's disease will likely become increasingly rare [90].

With advances in our understanding, radiation fields and doses to the mediastinum have continued to decrease. Many patients still receive radiation for lymphomas and as such, have cardiac radiation exposure, but these doses have diminished significantly. Patients diagnosed and treated prior to 1990, would have received total lymphoid irradiation which would have included the supradiaphragmatic lymph nodes of the mediastinum, bilateral axillae, infradiaphragmatic nodes, and spleen [91]. These patients are at the highest risk for cardiac complications; treatments after 1990 treated much smaller volumes by limiting treatment to the involved lymph node chain, and after 2000 even smaller volumes were used to specifically target the involved lymph nodes only. The decrease in field size has significantly reduced the amount of normal tissue exposed to ionizing radiation including the heart, though patients who have involvement of mediastinal nodes still cannot fully avoid irradiating of the cardiac structures [92]. In addition to field size changes, the amount of dose also decreased over time due in large part to the recognition of the long-term treatment-related toxicity faced by lymphoma patients including cardiac toxicity [93,94]. Through a series of trials conducted in the 1990s and early 2000s, the dose delivered has been reduced from 40 to 20 Gy without compromising disease control [89,95]. Although longer follow-up remains to be completed, most radiation oncologists believe that with the reductions in dose and field size, the cardiovascular risk is likely significantly less compared to prior treatment methods.

Breast Cancer

In the 1980s, treatment for early-stage breast cancer was undergoing a revolution with multiple randomized trials being conducted comparing mastectomy to lumpectomy followed by chest wall radiation (breast-conserving therapy). These trials encompassing thousands of women found no difference in overall survival between mastectomy and breast-conserving therapy, and thus lumpectomy followed by chest-wall radiation became an accepted standard of care and in the modern era more than half of all women diagnosed with stage-I and -II breast cancer undergo breast-conserving therapy in lieu of mastectomy [96,97].

Traditionally, adjuvant RT has been delivered via opposed tangential beams designed to cover the entire breast (Fig. 9.1). Typical doses are in the range of 50–54 Gy often with a boost dose of 10–14 Gy to the lumpectomy cavity. Patients with right-sided breast cancer infrequently receive significant dose to the heart, whereas patients with left-sided cancers often have the apex and anterior aspect of the heart at risk in the field, depending on patient's anatomy. Studies have taken advantage of this anatomical difference to analyze the effect of radiation on the heart. In a SEER analysis by Darby et al., women with breast cancer diagnosed between 1973 and 2001 were evaluated for cause of mortality [98]. Over 300,000 women were diagnosed with breast cancer in that time period with 37% receiving RT. The authors found the most common cause of death was due to cancer recurrence, but the second most common

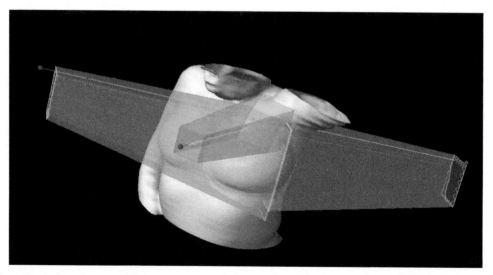

FIGURE 9.1   **Example of a three-dimensional body contour derived from CT simulation used in the radiotherapy treatment planning for treatment of a left-sided breast cancer and supraclavicular lymph nodes following lumpectomy.** Careful planning and individualized field design is needed to minimize radiation to the heart and vascular structures. The *yellow* regions represent the medial and lateral tangential fields, whereas the *blue* represents the supraclavicular field. (Eclipse™ Treatment Planning System, Varian Medical Systems, Palo Alto, California.)

cause of death was heart disease. Women treated in the years 1973–1982 faced the greatest risk of cardiac-related mortality as the technology used in treatment was less sophisticated and included larger volumes of the heart within the treatment field. The authors concluded that the risk of heart disease was significant even 20 years after treatment, and that although treatment planning had improved, there was still risk of heart disease following treatment.

Multiple observational studies supported the SEER analysis and showed an increased risk of cardiac morbidity and mortality in women treated for breast cancer, especially left-sided breast cancers. In a recent study from Oxford, the medical records and radiotherapy plans of women treated for breast cancer in Denmark and Sweden of these patients were reviewed, and compared with healthy controls to evaluate for differences in heart disease [15]. Using estimates of the heart dose, the authors reported that there was a linear association between radiation dose received by the heart and risk for major coronary events, including myocardial infarction, coronary revascularization, or death from ischemic heart disease. The risks of one of these events increased 7.4% per Gray delivered to the heart, with radiation-induced changes occurring within the first 5 years after treatment. The excess cardiac risk was seen beyond 20 years from treatment. Risks of radiation-related coronary events were higher in patients who had a prior history of heart disease.

To better understand the etiology of the excess cardiac mortality, Nilsson et al. reviewed a group of Swedish women with a history of breast cancer diagnosed between 1970 and 2003; these women were examined and linked with a registrar of coronary angiography [99]. This allowed the investigators to examine the association between left-breast radiotherapy and development of specific coronary artery lesions. The two identified areas at higher risk of developing stenosis: the mid and distal left anterior descending artery and the diagonal artery. These areas coincide anatomically with regions likely treated with traditional opposed tangential fields. Inclusion of the internal mammary chain within the treatment field, as is seen with patients who have high-risk or node-positive disease, increases the dose delivered to the right-sided vasculature.

There is little doubt that radiation to the heart increases the risk of heart disease; therefore, much of the research efforts in breast radiation oncology have been devoted to strategies reducing the dose of radiation to the heart. Techniques including 3D CT-based planning and respiratory gating discussed further subsequently have dramatically reduced the dose to the heart such that the cardiotoxic risk in appropriately treated patients can be largely mitigated.

Lung Cancer

Although the incidence of lung cancer has been decreasing since the 1990s, the disease still remains the largest contributor to cancer deaths, greater than the cumulative number of breast, prostate, and colon deaths annually [100]. Most patients become symptomatic only with advanced disease, which makes effective therapy more challenging. Despite recent improvements in therapeutic regimens for patients with both small-cell and non-small-cell lung cancers (SCLC and NSCLC), the 5-year survival remains below 20% [101]. Thus, given this dismal prognosis, it is not surprising that studies examining cardiovascular risk in lung cancer patients do not suggest a demonstrable increased risk of heart disease following treatment for advanced lung cancers.

In an effort to improve lung-cancer-specific survival, a large-scale clinical trial was developed to evaluate the utility of low-dose chest computed tomography (CT) compared to chest X-rays to identify asymptomatic lung cancers in at-risk populations [102]. Ultimately, the trial was a success; current smokers or former smokers with a significant smoking history saw a benefit in identifying early-stage lesions. For these early patients, surgery or radiation can be utilized for curative intent. As many of these patients cannot tolerate surgery, stereotactic ablative body radiotherapy (SABR), also called stereotactic body radiotherapy (SBRT), has become an increasingly common alternative to surgery. SABR/SBRT, unlike previous conventionally fractionated radiation courses, delivers much higher doses per fraction, typically 10 Gy or more per fraction over a much shorter period of time. With the rise in the number of early-stage diagnoses, use of SABR/SBRT for lung cancer has risen sharply highlighting the need to understand the risks more completely [103].

Delivering high dose per fraction treatments is likely to expose patients to similar risks of cardiotoxicity over the long term, including a dose-dependent accelerated development of atherosclerotic lesions as for conventionally fractionated courses, such as those used for breast cancer. In a recent dose-escalation trial (RTOG 0813) for NSCLC; toxicities occurring within 1 year of treatment included bradycardia, hypoxia, pneumonitis, and death have been reported, but the rates of these complications was found to be low (7.2% at a median dose of 12 Gy per fraction) [104]. The only unusual complication from these very high doses of RT has been with treatment of central lesions adjacent to the proximal bronchial tree and heart, as there had been reports of some patients developing marked toxicity including aorta–esophageal fistula leading to exsanguination [105,106]. As a result, the safe dose of radiation for the region surrounding the proximal bronchial tree and great vessels is currently being explored in several trials. Long-term data regarding the outcome for patients treated with SBRT for early-stage lung cancers is not yet available and it will likely be a decade or more before the data matures [107].

Treatment Considerations for Thoracic Radiation

RT for various thoracic malignancies including, lymphoma, lung, and breast remains an essential part of many treatment courses. As overall survival for many of these cancers has increased, the risks to vascular structures from radiation have become increasingly appreciated. Therefore, radiation oncologists have adopted increasingly sophisticated technology to reduce dose to the heart including advanced dosimetric calculation, three-dimensional planning, innovative treatment delivery utilizing highly conformal techniques to reduce the dose to the heart and other vascular structures at risk. One particular technique that has dramatically improved dose to the heart has been motion management. By monitoring the respiration and cardiac cycles in thoracic and breast malignancies, radiation oncologists can now account quantify and account for motion-related changes allowing for more precise delivery to tumors and reduced normal tissue dose [108,109]. Through monitoring of external movement of the chest or of tidal volume it is possible to reduce radiation treatment fields such that the dose to the cardiovascular structures can be significantly curtailed.

By treating patients only when they are in a certain phase of the respiratory cycle (aka respiratory gating), dose to the heart can be reduced by as much as half depending on specific patient anatomy [110–112]. For instance, in dosimetric studies comparing whole-breast RT delivered using opposed tangential fields, the use of deep inspiratory breath hold has been demonstrated to decreased mean heart dose by over 55% and left anterior descending artery dose by over 72% [113]. Those undergoing regional nodal irradiation including the internal mammary chain nodes typically have higher heart doses, but heart dose is reduced with the use of motion management. Thus, though not always widely available due to the complexity of the current technique, patients treated with modern radiation often have significantly reduced heart doses; the effect of these dramatically reduced radiation doses on cardiovascular morbidity remains to be elucidated.

Perfusion scans offer insight into the functional status of the cardiac tissue following radiotherapy. In a study by Marks et al., left-sided breast cancer patients were prospectively enrolled for cardiac perfusion studies using technetium 99m or tetrofosmin [114]. They were evaluated prior to RT and at 6, 12, 18, and 24 months after treatment. Cardiac perfusion defects were found in 27, 29, 38, and 42%, respectively. The authors found that patients with less than 5% of the left ventricle within the treatment field have a rate of new perfusion defects ranging from 10% to 20%, whereas those with more than 5% of the left ventricle faced a 50–60% rate. The clinical effect of lower dose remains to be seen as perfusion studies using respiratory gating showed no benefit in perfusion for the reduced dose. In a randomized, prospective phase-III trial of women testing respiratory gating to reduce heart does for left-sided breast cancer patients, Zellars et al. found that women with left-sided breast tumors developed perfusion defects regardless of the lower RT dose delivered to the heart with respiratory gating. This suggests that respiratory gating may not necessarily provide adequate cardiac protection and that even

very low doses of radiation can impact cardiac function [115]. Thus, given the uncertain cardiovascular effects of even low doses of RT, patients receiving thoracic radiation should be considered at elevated risk for cardiac disease.

Cancers of the Abdomen

RT plays an integral role in the treatment of a number of intraabdominal malignancies, including esophageal, gastric, pancreatic, and renal cancers; however, like primary lung cancers, the poor prognosis for many of these diseases historically meant that few patients survived long enough to realize the late effects of radiation. The exception to this has been survivors of lymphoma, particularly Hodgkin's disease, many of whom received radiation to the entire subdiaphragmatic lymph node chains in addition to their cervical and thoracic lymph node chains. In these survivors, both iliofemoral and aortic atherosclerosis have been observed in patients who received total lymphoid irradiation [116]. The most common arteries affected include the femoral, superficial femoral, and popliteal arteries. In these arteries, stenosis, thrombosis, and aneurysmal dilatation occur and have been attributed to a late effect of RT. Mesenteric insufficiency from celiac, superior mesenteric, or inferior mesenteric artery vascular damage, intermittent claudication and limb ischemia have also been described and, like other vascular beds, these changes can occur in the years and even decades following treatment [116–119]. Traditional risk factors, such as pre-existing vascular disease, smoking, and sedentary lifestyle are thought to accelerate this process; therefore, aggressive management of these factors postradiation is critical. Otherwise, treatment for these conditions mimics that for nonradiation-related vascular changes.

In addition to direct vascular damage, radiation-induced renal damage can occur following abdominal RT and manifests as secondary hypertension. A small case series suggests that ionizing radiation directly causes atherosclerotic damage to the renal artery, and that smaller vessels within the kidney can also be affected. In a report by Staab et al., two cases of renal artery stenosis following radiation presented with secondary hypertension with markedly elevated systolic blood pressures and elevated creatinine levels, suggestive of renal dysfunction. Both patients received greater than 30 Gy to the retroperitoneum and presented at 6 and 12 years postradiation with treatment-resistant hypertension. In both cases, endarterectomies with venous stenting were the preferred treatment modalities [120].

Cancers of the Pelvis

The treatment for gynecologic, prostate, and lower gastrointestinal tract malignancies often involves significant radiation to the pelvic vasculature in order to treat the tumor and involved lymph nodes. Although the vessels are typically considered highly resistant to both the acute and chronic effects of radiation, a number of cases demonstrate that irradiation of major arteries involving the pelvis can lead to limb ischemia, though this remains quite rare relative to the number of treated patients. In a case series published by Moutardier et al., four patients with treatment to the pelvis for gynecologic cancers subsequently required bypass (femoropopliteal and axillofemoral), angioplasty with stent, and medical management [121]. Ischemic symptoms were variable, and ranged from intermittent claudication to toe necrosis, with the time course of symptoms ranging from 2 to 7 years postradiation. Another case series by Pherwani et al. demonstrated similar symptoms in three patients treated for testicular tumors who underwent pelvic and periaortic radiation (which is rarely done now for treatment of testicular cancer). Symptoms developed between 5 and 16 years after treatment with one requiring iliofemoral bypass, whereas two required angioplasty, all with symptomatic relief [122]. Treatment doses in both case series ranged from 30 to 65 Gy. In both case series, patients responded well to treatment, without persistent symptoms following correction. Of note, both authors mentioned that fibrosis of surrounding tissue could complicate stenting, as the targeted vessel segment may be under external compression.

There have also been more severe cases of vascular compromise following pelvic radiation. Levenback et al. published a series of six cases of arterial occlusion following treatment for gynecologic malignancies, two of whom underwent adjuvant RT; one was treated with mixed energy neutrons and the other with photons and neutrons [123]. In both cases, the patients had late effects related to RT, at 16 and 18 years following treatment. Both of the patients experienced chronic worsening arterial disease in the femoral artery before ultimately requiring partial limb amputation for gangrenous changes. The severe fibrosis experienced by these patients might be attributed to their unusual radiation treatment modality with neutrons, which has been described to cause this toxicity [124]. It remains unknown how more modern techniques with better control of the dose distribution will affect long-term vascular changes in the pelvis. As it is unavoidable that that pelvic vasculature receives full treatment dose due to the distribution of the lymph nodes that drain the pelvis, it is likely that the low, but persistent risk of pelvic vascular compromise will remain unchanged and thus survivors of malignancies that required pelvic radiation should be aware of this risk and take appropriate measures to avoid other causes of vascular damage that may aggravate a strong existing risk from radiation.

TREATMENT RECOMMENDATIONS

The most important treatment for reducing cardiovascular risk in patients following radiation is to minimize radiation exposure whenever possible to vascular structures. To this end, radiation oncologists have developed a multitude of new technologies to reduce radiation dose including brachytherapy, computer-aided three-dimensional planning, and proton therapy. For breast, prostate, and gynecologic malignancies, brachytherapy, which uses radiation sources delivered internally, can limit dose to the tumor and significantly reduce dose to normal tissues though its use is limited to specific settings [125]. Photon-based external beam radiation is more widely used and, as outlined previously, advanced planning techniques have allowed for both better delineation of dose to cardiovascular structures and the ability to limit dose though individual anatomy of both the tumor and normal tissue structures remain the primary determinants of cardiovascular radiation dose [126]. Finally, use of proton radiotherapy has increased, and a number of studies have shown dosimetric advantages to using proton therapies for esophageal, lung, and breast cancers as a means of sparing additional dose to the heart [127–129]. However, there have not been studies in adults to demonstrate a clinically meaningful reduction in cardiac or other normal tissue toxicity, though benefit has been seen in children treated with radiation. Long-term follow-up from ongoing studies will be critical to determine if the reduced cardiac dose from protons will ultimately decrease long-term cardiovascular morbidity.

Although avoiding excess radiation dose provides the best means of reducing cardiovascular risk from radiation, irradiation of many of the cardiovascular structures remains inevitable due to the proximity of those structures to areas requiring treatment, thus the importance of identifying patients who have received prior radiation and their potential risk depending on their treatment fields. For those patients, who have received significant dose to the heart or significant vascular structures (i.e., carotids, aorta, femoral arteries), aggressive management of cardiac risk factors, such as blood pressure, diabetes, and lipid levels is critical. Further, assessing cardiovascular risk following treatment is likely beneficial.

Pediatric oncologic societies have published guidelines on the management of survivors of childhood cancers [130]. These include evaluation with physical exam yearly with consideration of Doppler for pediatric patients who have undergone radiotherapy to a dose more than 40 Gy anywhere involving the head, neck, or thorax, with a further recommendation to establish a baseline carotid evaluation with bilateral Doppler 10 years after completing RT. For pediatric patients undergoing chest radiotherapy, echocardiogram is recommended prior to treatment and then "periodically," depending on RT dose and use of anthracycline-based chemotherapy [131]. Hemoglobin A1c is also recommended to be checked every 2 years.

Unfortunately, there are no internationally recognized guidelines for the monitoring and management of cardiovascular complications seen in adult cancer survivors. On

TABLE 9.2 Treatment Recommendations for Cardiovascular Tissues at Risk

Tissue at Risk	Treatment Recommendations
All disease sites	• Smoking cessation • Adequate physical activity • Mediterranean-style diet • Blood glucose control (for diabetics)
Cerebral vasculature	• Careful selection of patients who require cerebral RT, especially children • Consider alternatives to RT for nonmalignant conditions
Carotid arteries	• Pretreatment assessment with ultrasound for patients with pre-existing cardiovascular risk factors • Aggressive blood-pressure management • Cholesterol management (may use ACC/AHA atherosclerotic cardiovascular heart disease risk calculator) • Weight management • Consider posttreatment surveillance 1 year after radiotherapy for patients with risk factors, then routinely as indicated
Cardiac structures include coronary arteries, pericardium, valves, and conduction system	• Careful selection of patients who require thoracic RT • Utilization of technology to radiotherapy dose to heart • Aggressive blood-pressure management • Cholesterol management • Weight management
Renal, iliac, and femoral arteries	• Careful selection of patients who require abdominal/pelvic RT • Aggressive blood-pressure management • Cholesterol management • Weight management

RT, radiation therapy

the basis of available data, we recommend that patients with any known pre-existing cardiovascular disease (prior myocardial infarction, stroke, TIA, angioplasty, or bypass) who are being considered for thoracic or head/neck irradiation undergo evaluation by a cardiologist, including baseline EKG, echocardiogram, metabolic panel, and hemoglobin A1c (Table 9.2). These patients should be followed and treatment should be informed by the severity of their disease and degree of vascular involvement in the radiotherapy field. In many cases, optimal management will include aggressive medical management including LDL-lowering mediation, blood pressure management, weight loss, exercise, smoking cessation, and routine monitoring with echocardiography and/or Doppler ultrasonography.

For patients who are undergoing chest or head/neck radiotherapy, it is reasonable to initially screen them and determine their cardiovascular risk based on the American College of Cardiology/American Heart Association guidelines (ref) [132,133]. Patients should be evaluated for hypertension, hyperlipidemia, diabetes, tobacco use, weight, physical activity, and family history (defined as heart disease in first degree relative, female <65 years old and male <55 years old). Framingham risk score may inform clinical decision-making to help determine optimal medical management. A patient with high risk of 10 year CHD event (as noted by a >20% Framingham score) suggests that stringent LDL and blood-pressure management should

be pursued, whereas the patient with a less than 10% risk may pursue less aggressive therapy. The Framingham risk score underestimates cardiovascular risk in women, and the Reynold's risk score has been proposed for risk stratification in women [134].

CONCLUSIONS

Radiation remains a critical component of treatment for many types of malignancies. Advances in radiation delivery have dramatically reduced radiation dose to cardiovascular structures, particularly in the treatment of breast cancer and lymphomas. These are only two malignancies in which remarkable improvements have been made with decreasing dose to vascular and cardiac structures; other disease sites remain. Additionally, advances in therapies and an aging population will likely yield an increasing number of cancer survivors and a higher burden of radiation-related cardiovascular disease. Thus, it is critical to identify those patients at increased risk in order to ensure that they receive earlier cardiovascular screening as well as more aggressive management of their other cardiovascular risk factors. Coordination with radiation, medical oncology, and preventive cardiologist may be useful to help identify appropriate patients and their potential sites of cardiovascular risk.

REFERENCES

[1] Scatliff JH, Morris PJ. From Roentgen to magnetic resonance imaging: the history of medical imaging. N C Med J 2014;75(2):111–3.

[2] Belisario JC. A discussion on the skin erythema dose with roentgen rays; some biological implications. Br J Radiol 1952;25(294):326–35.

[3] Smith BD, Smith GL, Hurria A, Hortobagyi GN, Buchholz TA. Future of cancer incidence in the United States: burdens upon an aging, changing nation. J Clin Oncol 2009;27(17):2758–65.

[4] Smith BD, Haffty BG, Wilson LD, Smith GL, Patel AN, Buchholz TA. The future of radiation oncology in the United States from 2010 to 2020: will supply keep pace with demand? J Clin Oncol 2010;28(35):5160–5.

[5] Parry C, Kent EE, Mariotto AB, Alfano CM, Rowland JH. Cancer survivors: a booming population. Cancer Epidemiol Biomarkers Prev 2011;20(10):1996–2005.

[6] Hewitt M, Greenfield S, Stovall E. From cancer patient to cancer survivor: lost in transition; 2006. Available from: https://www.nap.edu/catalog/11468/ from-cancer-patient-to-cancer-survivor-lost-in-transition

[7] Elerding SC, Fernandez RN, Grotta JC, Lindberg RD, Causay LC, McMurtrey MJ. Carotid artery disease following external cervical irradiation. Ann Surg 1981;194(5):609–15.

[8] Kim JH, Choi JH, Ki EY, et al. Incidence and risk factors of lower-extremity lymphedema after radical surgery with or without adjuvant radiotherapy in patients with FIGO stage I to stage IIA cervical cancer. Int J Gynecol Cancer 2012;22(4):686–91.

[9] Jaworski C, Mariani JA, Wheeler G, Kaye DM. Cardiac complications of thoracic irradiation. J Am Coll Cardiol 2013;61(23):2319–28.

[10] Held KD. Radiobiology for the Radiologist, 6th ed., by Eric J. Hall and Amato J Giaccia Radiat Res 2006;166(5):816–817.

[11] Jackson SP. Sensing and repairing DNA double-strand breaks. Carcinogenesis 2002;23(5):687–96.

[12] Haber AH, Rothstein BE. Radiosensitivity and rate of cell division: "Law of Bergonié and Tribondeau". Science 1969;163(3873):1338–9.

[13] Travis LB, Ng AK, Allan JM, et al. Second malignant neoplasms and cardiovascular disease following radiotherapy. JNCI J Natl Cancer Inst 2012;104(5):357–70.

[14] Mulrooney DA, Yeazel MW, Kawashima T, et al. Cardiac outcomes in a cohort of adult survivors of childhood and adolescent cancer: retrospective analysis of the Childhood Cancer Survivor Study cohort. BMJ 2009;339:b4606.

[15] Darby SC, Ewertz M, Hall P. Ischemic heart disease after breast cancer radiotherapy. N Engl J Med 2013;368(26):2527.

[16] Taylor CW, Nisbet A, McGale P, Darby SC. Cardiac exposures in breast cancer radiotherapy: 1950s–1990s. Int J Radiat Oncol Biol Phys 2007;69(5):1484–95.

[17] Taylor CW, Wang Z, Macaulay E, Jagsi R, Duane F, Darby SC. Exposure of the heart in breast cancer radiotherapy: a systematic review of heart doses published during 2003-2013. Int J Radiat Oncol 2015;93(4):845–53.

[18] Plummer C, Henderson RD, O'Sullivan JD, Read SJ. Ischemic stroke and transient ischemic attack after head and neck radiotherapy: a review. Stroke 2011;42(9):2410–8.

[19] King LJ, Hasnain SN, Webb JA, et al. Asymptomatic carotid arterial disease in young patients following neck radiation therapy for Hodgkin lymphoma. Radiology 1999;213(1):167–72.

[20] Loftus CM, Biller J, Hart MN, Cornell SH, Hiratzka LF. Management of radiation-induced accelerated carotid atherosclerosis. Arch Neurol 1987;44(7):711–4.

[21] Fonkalsrud EW, Sanchez M, Zerubavel R, Mahoney A. Serial changes in arterial structure following radiation therapy. Surg Gynecol Obstet 1977;145(3):395–400.

[22] Shichita T, Ogata T, Yasaka M, et al. Angiographic characteristics of radiation-induced carotid arterial stenosis. Angiology 2009;60(3):276–82.

[23] Weintraub NL, Jones WK, Manka D. Understanding radiation-induced vascular disease. J Am Coll Cardiol 2010;55(12):1237–9.

[24] Polak JF, Pencina MJ, Pencina KM, O'Donnell CJ, Wolf PA, D'Agostino RB. Carotid-wall intima-media thickness and cardiovascular events. N Engl J Med 2011;365(3):213–21.

[25] Gujral DM, Chahal N, Senior R, Harrington KJ, Nutting CM. Radiation-induced carotid artery atherosclerosis. Radiother Oncol 2014;110(1):31–8.

[26] Zhao W, Diz DI, Robbins ME. Oxidative damage pathways in relation to normal tissue injury. Br J Radiol 2007; 80 Spec No:S23–31.

[27] Martinet W, Knaapen MWM, De Meyer GRY, Herman AG, Kockx MM. Elevated levels of oxidative DNA damage and DNA repair enzymes in human atherosclerotic plaques. Circulation 2002;106(8):927–32.

[28] Andreassi MG. Coronary atherosclerosis and somatic mutations: an overview of the contributive factors for oxidative DNA damage. Mutat Res 2003;543(1):67–86.

[29] Mercer J, Mahmoudi M, Bennett M. DNA damage, p53, apoptosis and vascular disease. Mutat Res 2007;621(1-2):75–86.

[30] Taunk NK, Haffty BG, Kostis JB, Goyal S. Radiation-induced heart disease: pathologic abnormalities and putative mechanisms. Front Oncol 2015;5:39.

[31] Sidhu PS, Naoumova RP, Maher VM, et al. The extracranial carotid artery in familial hypercholesterolaemia: relationship of intimal-medial thickness and plaque morphology with plasma lipids and coronary heart disease. J Cardiovasc Risk 1996;3(1):61–7.

[32] Lund MB, Ihlen H, Voss BM, et al. Increased risk of heart valve regurgitation after mediastinal radiation for Hodgkin's disease: an echocardiographic study. Heart 1996;75(6):591–5.

[33] Ng AK. Review of the cardiac long-term effects of therapy for Hodgkin lymphoma. Br J Haematol 2011;154(1):23–31.

[34] Veinot JP, Edwards WD. Pathology of radiation-induced heart disease: a surgical and autopsy study of 27 cases. Hum Pathol 1996;27(8):766–73.

[35] Carlson RG, Mayfield WR, Normann S, Alexander JA. Radiation-associated valvular disease. Chest 1991;99(3):538–45.

[36] Carlson RG. Radiation-associated valvular disease. Chest J 1991;99(3):538.

[37] Cutter DJ, Schaapveld M, Darby SC, et al. Risk of valvular heart disease after treatment for Hodgkin lymphoma. J Natl Cancer Inst 2015;107(4). pii: djv008.

[38] Handa N, McGregor CG, Danielson GK, et al. Valvular heart operation in patients with previous mediastinal radiation therapy. Ann Thorac Surg 2001;71(6):1880–4.

[39] Fajardo LF, Stewart JR. Pathogenesis of radiation-induced myocardial fibrosis. Lab Invest 1973;29(2):244–57.

[40] Maisch B, Seferović PM, Ristić AD, et al. Guidelines on the diagnosis and management of pericardial diseases executive summary; The Task force on the diagnosis and management of pericardial diseases of the European society of cardiology. Eur Heart J 2004;25(7):587–610.

[41] Byhardt R, Brace K, Ruckdeschel J, Chang P, Martin R, Wiernik P. Dose and treatment factors in radiation-related pericardial effusion associated with the mantle technique for Hodgkin's disease. Cancer 1975;35(3):795–802.

[42] Yusuf SW, Sami S, Daher IN. Radiation-induced heart disease: a clinical update. Cardiol Res Pract 2011;2011:317659.

[43] Morton DL, Glancy DL, Joseph WL, Adkins PC. Management of patients with radiation-induced pericarditis with effusion: a note on the development of aortic regurgitation in two of them. Chest 1973;64(3):291–7.

[44] Carmel RJ, Kaplan HS. Mantle irradiation in Hodgkin's disease. An analysis of technique, tumor eradication, and complications. Cancer 1976;37(6):2813–25.

[45] Mauch PM, Weinstein H, Botnick L, Belli J, Cassady JR. An evaluation of long-term survival and treatment complications in children with Hodgkin's disease. Cancer 1983;51(5):925–32.

[46] Ling LH, Oh JK, Schaff HV, et al. Constrictive pericarditis in the modern era: evolving clinical spectrum and impact on outcome after pericardiectomy. Circulation 1999;100(13):1380–6.

[47] Bertog SC, Thambidorai SK, Parakh K, et al. Constrictive pericarditis: etiology and cause-specific survival after pericardiectomy. J Am Coll Cardiol 2004;43(8):1445–52.

[48] Benoff LJ, Schweitzer P. Radiation therapy-induced cardiac injury. Am Heart J 1995;129(6):1193–6.

[49] Slama MS, Le Guludec D, Sebag C, et al. Complete atrioventricular block following mediastinal irradiation: a report of six cases. Pacing Clin Electrophysiol 1991;14(7):1112–8.

[50] Adams MJ, Lipsitz SR, Colan SD, et al. Cardiovascular status in long-term survivors of Hodgkin's disease treated with chest radiotherapy. J Clin Oncol 2004;22(15):3139–48.

[51] Lee MS, Finch W, Mahmud E. Cardiovascular complications of radiotherapy. Am J Cardiol 2013;112(10):1688–96.

[52] Felker GM, Thompson RE, Hare JM, et al. Underlying causes and long-term survival in patients with initially unexplained cardiomyopathy. N Engl J Med 2000;342(15):1077–84.

[53] Boekel NB, Schaapveld M, Gietema JA, et al. Cardiovascular disease risk in a large, population-based cohort of breast cancer survivors. Int J Radiat Oncol 2015;94(5):1061–72.

[54] Hancock SL, Tucker MA, Hoppe RT. Factors affecting late mortality from heart disease after treatment of Hodgkin's disease. JAMA 1993;270(16):1949–55.

[55] Nolan MT, Russell DJ, Marwick TH. Long-term risk of heart failure and myocardial dysfunction after thoracic radiotherapy: a systematic review. Can J Cardiol 2015;32(7):908–20.

[56] Heidenreich PA, Hancock SL, Vagelos RH, Lee BK, Schnittger I. Diastolic dysfunction after mediastinal irradiation. Am Heart J 2005;150(5):977–82.

[57] Glanzmann C, Kaufmann P, Jenni R, Hess OM, Huguenin P. Cardiac risk after mediastinal irradiation for Hodgkin's disease. Radiother Oncol 1998;46(1):51–62.

[58] Shakir DK, Rasul KI. Chemotherapy induced cardiomyopathy: pathogenesis, monitoring and management. J Clin Med Res 2009;1(1):8–12.

[59] Tsai HR, Gjesdal O, Wethal T, et al. Left ventricular function assessed by two-dimensional speckle tracking echocardiography in long-term survivors of hodgkin's lymphoma treated by mediastinal radiotherapy with or without anthracycline therapy. Am J Cardiol 2011;107(3):472–7.

[60] Ewer MS, Vooletich MT, Durand JB, et al. Reversibility of trastuzumab-related cardiotoxicity: new insights based on clinical course and response to medical treatment. J Clin Oncol 2005;23(31):7820–6.

[61] Tham YL, Verani MS, Chang J. Reversible and irreversible cardiac dysfunction associated with trastuzumab in breast cancer. Breast Cancer Res Treat 2002;74(2):131–4.

[62] Belkacémi Y, Gligorov J, Ozsahin M, et al. Concurrent trastuzumab with adjuvant radiotherapy in HER2-positive breast cancer patients: acute toxicity analyses from the French multicentric study. Ann Oncol 2008;19(6):1110–6.

[63] Tan-Chiu E, Yothers G, Romond E, et al. Assessment of cardiac dysfunction in a randomized trial comparing doxorubicin and cyclophosphamide followed by paclitaxel, with or without trastuzumab as adjuvant therapy in node-positive, human epidermal growth factor receptor 2-overexpressing breast can. J Clin Oncol 2005;23:7811–9.

[64] Rockman CB, Riles TS, Fisher FS, Adelman MA, Lamparello PJ. The surgical management of carotid artery stenosis in patients with previous neck irradiation. Am J Surg 1996;172(2):191–5.

[65] McCready RA, Hyde GL, Bivins BA, Mattingly SS, Griffen WO. Radiation-induced arterial injuries. Surgery 1983;93(2):306–12.

[66] Fraum TJ, Kreisl TN, Sul J, Fine HA, Iwamoto FM. Ischemic stroke and intracranial hemorrhage in glioma patients on antiangiogenic therapy. J Neurooncol 2011;105(2):281–9.

[67] Brada M, Burchell L, Ashley S, Traish D. The incidence of cerebrovascular accidents in patients with pituitary adenoma. Int J Radiat Oncol Biol Phys 1999;45(3):693–8.

[68] Flickinger JC, Nelson PB, Taylor FH, Robinson A. Incidence of cerebral infarction after radiotherapy for pituitary adenoma. Cancer 1989;63(12):2404–8.

[69] Cameron EW. Transient ischaemic attacks due to meningioma—report of 4 cases. Clin Radiol 1994;49(6):416–8.

[70] Kim JS, Moyamoya Disease:. Epidemiology, clinical features, and diagnosis. J Stroke 2016;18(1):2–11.

[71] Zwagerman NT, Foster K, Jakacki R, Khan FH, Yock TI, Greene S. The development of Moyamoya syndrome after proton beam therapy. Pediatr Blood Cancer 2014;61(8):1490–2.

[72] Wang C, Roberts KB, Bindra RS, Chiang VL, Yu JB. Delayed cerebral vasculopathy following cranial radiation therapy for pediatric tumors. Pediatr Neurol 2014;50(6):549–56.

[73] Murphy ES, Xie H, Merchant TE, Yu JS, Chao ST, Suh JH. Review of cranial radiotherapy-induced vasculopathy. J Neurooncol 2015;122(3):421–9.

[74] Go AS, Mozaffarian D, Roger VL, et al. Heart disease and stroke statistics—2014 update: a report from the American Heart Association. Circulation 2014;129(3):e28–e292.

[75] Pereira Lima MN, Biolo A, Foppa M, da Rosa PR, Rohde LEP, Clausell N. A prospective, comparative study on the early effects of local and remote radiation therapy on carotid intima-media thickness and vascular cellular adhesion molecule-1 in patients with head and neck and prostate tumors. Radiother Oncol 2011;101(3):449–53.

[76] Dorresteijn LDA, Kappelle AC, Boogerd W, et al. Increased risk of ischemic stroke after radiotherapy on the neck in patients younger than 60 years. J Clin Oncol 2002;20(1):282–8.

[77] Silverberg GD, Britt RH, Goffinet DR. Radiation-induced carotid artery disease. Cancer 1978;41(1):130–7.

[78] Deschler DG, Richmon JD, Khariwala SS, Ferris RL, Wang MB. The "new" head and neck cancer patient–young, nonsmoker, nondrinker, and HPV positive: evaluation. Otolaryngol Head Neck Surg 2014;151(3):12–7.

[79] Marur S, D'Souza G, Westra WH, Forastiere AA. HPV-associated head and neck cancer: a virus-related cancer epidemic. Lancet Oncol 2010;11(8):781–9.

[80] Goon PKC, Stanley MA, Ebmeyer J, et al. HPV & head and neck cancer: a descriptive update. Head Neck Oncol 2009;1:36.

[81] Huang YS, Lee CC, Chang TS, et al. Increased risk of stroke in young head and neck cancer patients treated with radiotherapy or chemotherapy. Oral Oncol 2011;47(11):1092–7.

[82] Kimple RJ, Harari PM. Is radiation dose reduction the right answer for HPV-positive head and neck cancer? Oral Oncol 2014;50(6):560–4.

[83] Bonadonna G. Historical review of Hodgkin's disease. Br J Haematol 2000;110(3):504–11.

[84] Peters MV. Prophylactic treatment of adjacent areas in Hodgkin's disease. Cancer Res 1966;26(6):1232–43.

[85] Dollinger MR, Lavine DM, Foye LV. Myocardial infarction due to postirradiation fibrosis of the coronary arteries. Case of successfully treated Hodgkin's disease with lower esophageal involvement. JAMA 1966;195(4):316–9.

[86] van Nimwegen FA, Schaapveld M, Cutter DJ, et al. Radiation dose–response relationship for risk of coronary heart disease in survivors of Hodgkin lymphoma. J Clin Oncol 2016;34(3):235–43.

[87] Schellong G, Riepenhausen M, Bruch C, et al. Late valvular and other cardiac diseases after different doses of mediastinal radiotherapy for Hodgkin disease in children and adolescents: report from the longitudinal GPOH follow-up project of the German-Austrian DAL-HD studies. Pediatr Blood Cancer 2010;55(6):1145–52.

[88] Tukenova M, Guibout C, Oberlin O, et al. Role of cancer treatment in long-term overall and cardiovascular mortality after childhood cancer. J Clin Oncol 2010;28(8):1308–15.

[89] Engert A, Plütschow A, Eich HT, et al. Reduced treatment intensity in patients with early-stage Hodgkin's lymphoma. N Engl J Med 2010;363(7):640–52.

[90] Meyer RM, Gospodarowicz MK, Connors JM, et al. ABVD alone versus radiation-based therapy in limited-stage Hodgkin's lymphoma. N Engl J Med 2012;366(5):399–408.

[91] Glatstein E, Fuks Z, Goffinet DR, Kaplan HS. Non-Hodgkin's lymphomas of stage III extent. Is total lymphoid irradiation appropriate treatment? Cancer 1976;37(6):2806–12.

[92] Yahalom J, Mauch P. The involved field is back: issues in delineating the radiation field in Hodgkin's disease. Ann Oncol 2002;13(Suppl. 1):79–83.

[93] Swerdlow AJ, Higgins CD, Smith P, et al. Myocardial infarction mortality risk after treatment for Hodgkin disease: a collaborative British cohort study. J Natl Cancer Inst 2007;99(3):206–14.

[94] Ng AK, LaCasce A, Travis LB. Long-term complications of lymphoma and its treatment. J Clin Oncol 2011;29(14):1885–92.

[95] Dühmke E, Franklin J, Pfreundschuh M, et al. Low-dose radiation is sufficient for the noninvolved extended-field treatment in favorable early-stage Hodgkin's disease: long-term results of a randomized trial of radiotherapy alone. J Clin Oncol 2001;19(11):2905–14.

[96] Blichert-Toft M, Rose C, Andersen JA, et al. Danish randomized trial comparing breast conservation therapy with mastectomy: six years of life-table analysis. Danish Breast Cancer Cooperative Group. J Natl Cancer Inst Monogr 1992;(11):19–25.

[97] van Dongen JA, Voogd AC, Fentiman IS, et al. Long-term results of a randomized trial comparing breast-conserving therapy with mastectomy: European Organization for Research and Treatment of Cancer 10801 trial. J Natl Cancer Inst 2000;92(14):1143–50.

[98] Darby SC, McGale P, Taylor CW, Peto R. Long-term mortality from heart disease and lung cancer after radiotherapy for early breast cancer: prospective cohort study of about 300,000 women in US SEER cancer registries. Lancet Oncol 2005;6(8):557–65.

[99] Nilsson G, Holmberg L, Garmo H, et al. Distribution of coronary artery stenosis after radiation for breast cancer. J Clin Oncol 2012;30(4):380–6.

[100] Howlander N, Noone A, Krapcho M, et al. Cancer of the Lung and Bronchus - SEER Stat Fact Sheets. SEER Cancer Statistics Review, 1975–2012, National Cancer Institute. Available from: http://seer.cancer.gov/statfacts/html/lungb.html.

[101] Siegel R, Naishadham D, Jemal A. Cancer statistics. CA Cancer J Clin 2012;62(1):10–29.

[102] Aberle DR, Adams AM, Berg CD, et al. Reduced lung-cancer mortality with low-dose computed tomographic screening. N Engl J Med 2011;365(5):395–409.

[103] Lagerwaard FJ, Verstegen NE, Haasbeek CJA, et al. Outcomes of stereotactic ablative radiotherapy in patients with potentially operable stage I non-small cell lung cancer. Int J Radiat Oncol Biol Phys 2012;83(1):348–53.

[104] Bezjak A, Paulus R, Gaspar LE, et al. Primary study endpoint analysis for NRG oncology/RTOG 0813 trial of stereotactic body radiation therapy for centrally located non-small cell lung cancer (NSCLC). Int J Radiat Oncol Biol Phys 2016;94(1):5–6.

[105] Kilburn JM, Kuremsky JG, Blackstock AW, et al. Thoracic re-irradiation using stereotactic body radiotherapy (SBRT) techniques as first or second course of treatment. Radiother Oncol 2014;110(3):505–10.

[106] Timmerman R, McGarry R, Yiannoutsos C, et al. Excessive toxicity when treating central tumors in a phase II study of stereotactic body radiation therapy for medically inoperable early-stage lung cancer. J Clin Oncol 2006;24(30):4833–9.

[107] Benedict SH, Yenice KM, Followill D, et al. Stereotactic body radiation therapy: the report of AAPM Task Group 101. Med Phys 2010;37(8):4078–101.

[108] Giraud P, Yorke E, Ford EC, et al. Reduction of organ motion in lung tumors with respiratory gating. Lung Cancer 2006;51(1):41–51.

[109] Wang W, Li J, Bin, Hu HG, et al. Correlation between target motion and the dosimetric variance of breast and organ at risk during whole breast radiotherapy using 4DCT. Radiat Oncol 2013;8:111.

[110] Aznar MC, Maraldo MV, Schut DA, et al. Minimizing late effects for patients with mediastinal Hodgkin lymphoma: deep inspiration breath-hold, IMRT, or both? Int J Radiat Oncol Biol Phys 2015;92(1):169–74.

[111] Jagsi R, Moran JM, Kessler ML, Marsh RB, Balter JM, Pierce LJ. Respiratory motion of the heart and positional reproducibility under active breathing control. Int J Radiat Oncol Biol Phys 2007;68(1):253–8.

[112] Scotti V, Marrazzo L, Saieva C, et al. Impact of a breathing-control system on target margins and normal-tissue sparing in the treatment of lung cancer: experience at the radiotherapy unit of Florence University. Radiol Med 2014;119(1):13–9.

[113] Yeung R, Conroy L, Long K, et al. Cardiac dose reduction with deep inspiration breath hold for left-sided breast cancer radiotherapy patients with and without regional nodal irradiation. Radiat Oncol 2015;10:200.

[114] Marks LB, Yu X, Prosnitz RG, et al. The incidence and functional consequences of RT-associated cardiac perfusion defects. Int J Radiat Oncol Biol Phys 2005;63(1):214–23.

[115] Zellars R, Bravo PE, Tryggestad E, et al. SPECT analysis of cardiac perfusion changes after whole-breast/chest wall radiation therapy with or without active breathing coordinator: results of a randomized phase 3 trial. Int J Radiat Oncol Biol Phys 2014;88(4):778–85.

[116] Jurado JA, Bashir R, Burket MW. Radiation-induced peripheral artery disease. Catheter Cardiovasc Interv 2008;72(4):563–8.

[117] Chun CL, Joye J, Triadafilopoulos G. Holiday pains: a case of radiation-induced mesenteric ischemia. Dig Dis Sci 2013;58(2): 349–53.

[118] White CJ. Chronic mesenteric ischemia: diagnosis and management. Prog Cardiovasc Dis 2011;54(1):36–40.

[119] Beaulieu RJ, Arnaoutakis KD, Abularrage CJ, Efron DT, Schneider E, Black JH. Comparison of open and endovascular treatment of acute mesenteric ischemia. J Vasc Surg 2014;59(1):159–64.

[120] Staab GE, Tegtmeyer CJ, Constable WC. Radiation-induced renovascular hypertension. AJR Am J Roentgenol 1976;126(3):634–7.

[121] Moutardier V, Christophe M, Lelong B, Houvenaeghel G, Delpero JR. Iliac atherosclerotic occlusive disease complicating radiation therapy for cervix cancer: a case series. Gynecol Oncol 2002;84(3):456–9.

[122] Pherwani AD, Reid JA, Keane PF, Hannon RJ, Soong CV, Lee B. Synergism between radiotherapy and vascular risk factors in the accelerated development of atherosclerosis: a report of three cases. Ann Vasc Surg 2002;16(5):671–5.

[123] Levenback C, Burke TW, Rubin SC, Curtin JP, Wharton JT. Arterial occlusion complicating treatment of gynecologic cancer: a case series. Gynecol Oncol 1996;63(1):40–6.

[124] Douglas JG, Koh W, Austin-Seymour M, Laramore GE. Treatment of salivary gland neoplasms with fast neutron radiotherapy. Arch Otolaryngol Head Neck Surg 2003;129(9):944–8.

[125] Stewart AJ, O'Farrell DA, Cormack RA, et al. Dose volume histogram analysis of normal structures associated with accelerated partial breast irradiation delivered by high dose rate brachytherapy and comparison with whole breast external beam radiotherapy fields. Radiat Oncol 2008;3:39.

[126] Gunderson LL, Tepper JE, editors. Clinical radiation oncology. 3rd ed. Philadelphia: Elsevier Saunders; 2012.

[127] Takada A, Nakamura T, Takayama K, et al. Preliminary treatment results of proton beam therapy with chemoradiotherapy for stage I-III esophageal cancer. Cancer Med 2016;5(3):506–15.

[128] Chang JY, Li H, Zhu XR, et al. Clinical implementation of intensity modulated proton therapy for thoracic malignancies. Int J Radiat Oncol Biol Phys 2014;90(4):809–18.

[129] Bradley JA, Dagan R, Ho MW, et al. Initial report of a prospective dosimetric and clinical feasibility trial demonstrates the potential of protons to increase the therapeutic ratio in breast cancer compared with photons. Int J Radiat Oncol 2015;95(1):411–21.

[130] Nathan PC, Amir E, Abdel-Qadir H. Cardiac outcomes in survivors of pediatric and adult cancers. Can J Cardiol 2016;32.

[131] Children's Oncology Group. Long-term follow-up guidelines for survivors of childhood, adolescent and young adult cancers, Version 4.0. Monrovia, CA; 2013. Available from: http://www.survivorshipguidelines.org/

[132] Eckel RH, Jakicic JM, Ard JD, et al. 2013 AHA/ACC guideline on lifestyle management to reduce cardiovascular risk: a report of the American College of Cardiology/American Heart Association Task Force on practice guidelines. J Am Coll Cardiol 2013;63(25 Pt B):2960–84.

[133] Goff DC, Lloyd-Jones DM, Bennett G, et al. 2013 ACC/AHA guideline on the assessment of cardiovascular risk: a report of the American College of Cardiology/American Heart Association Task Force on practice guidelines. Circulation 2014;129(25 Suppl. 2): S49–73.

[134] Ridker PM, Buring JE, Rifai N, Cook NR. Development and validation of improved algorithms for the assessment of global cardiovascular risk in women. J Am Med Assoc 2007;297(6):611–9.

Chapter 10

Identification of At-Risk Patients and Comorbidities That Increase Risk

A. Silver*, A. Palomo* and T.M. Okwuosa**

*Rush University Medical Center, Chicago, IL, United States; **Division of Cardiology, Rush University Medical Center, Chicago, IL, United States

CANCER AND CARDIOVASCULAR DISEASE

The most recent vital statistics from the United States show cardiovascular disease (CVD) and cancer as the leading causes of death from 1935 through 2010 [1]. In 2013, heart disease and cancer accounted for almost half of all deaths in the United States [2]. According to the Surveillance Epidemiology and End Results (SEER) Program registry, the incidence of cancer diagnosis from 2006 to 2010 was 463.0 per 100,000 men and women per year, with a survival rate of 65.8% in 5 years—a significant improvement from prior years, attributed to chemo and radiotherapy [3]. On the basis of 2014 National Cancer Institute (NCI) data, there are about 14.5 million cancer survivors living in the United States currently (expected to rise to 19 million by year 2024) [http://www.cancer.gov/about-cancer/what-is-cancer/statistics]; and ~2 of 3 persons diagnosed with cancer are expected to live at least 5 years after diagnosis [3].

As cancer patients live longer, many of them are dying from CVD because of major complications of the intense oncologic treatments [4–6]. Decades after diagnosis, cancer survivors had 15-fold increased rates of congestive heart failure (CHF), 10-fold higher rates of CVD, and 9-fold higher rates of stroke as compared to controls [7]. In fact, the risk of cardiovascular morbidity has been shown to be higher than that of tumor recurrence in cancer survivors [8,9]. Cancer-related cardiovascular morbidity and mortality is attributed to cancer therapy with radiation and chemotherapy, and risks may persist up to 45 years after therapy [10]. In addition, long-term cancer survivors have higher incidence of hypertension, dyslipidemia, acute coronary syndromes, and strokes compared with the general population [11].

Chemotherapy is associated with significant cardiovascular morbidity and mortality, including heart failure, arrhythmias, hypertension, and cardiovascular death [12–14]. Comparatively, radiotherapy creates an inflammatory milieu which leads to a myriad of cardiac dysfunction, including pericardial disease, coronary artery disease (CAD), valvular heart disease, heart block/arrhythmia, and cardiomyopathy [15].

Given the higher prevalence of CVD in cancer survivors and cancer patients undergoing treatment, early identification of at-risk persons—prior to development of cardiovascular problems—and knowledge of comorbidities that increase risk become crucial to circumventing cardiovascular morbidity/mortality that may arise during cancer treatment, or in the long term of cancer survivorship. In this chapter, we discuss how patients at risk for cardiovascular side effects/complications resulting from cancer therapy can be identified. We will also discuss comorbidities that increase the risk of cardiovascular events secondary to oncologic treatment. *We employ the term cardiomyopathy to define the principal cardiotoxicity observed with cancer therapies; both terminologies are used interchangeably in this chapter.*

OVERLAPPING RISK FACTORS

For the reason that both cancer and heart disease have overlapping risk factors (such as smoking, obesity, unhealthy diet, physical inactivity, and aging), patients with heart disease have higher risk of cancer compared with the general population.

Obesity

Overweight and obesity are associated with the various risk factor components that make up the metabolic syndrome [16], which in turn leads to increased risk of CVD even in the absence of diabetes (CHD equivalent) [17,18]. Similarly, in a UK cohort study of 5.24 million adults, elevated or increasing body mass index (BMI) was associated with 11 of 22 studied cancers (including gastrointestinal, pelvic malignancies, kidney cancer, and leukemias), irrespective of smoking status [19]. Some proposed mechanisms are linked to changes in hormone metabolism, including insulin, insulin-like growth factors, sex hormones, and adipokines, even though the precise roles and interactions of these mechanisms are not fully understood.

Smoking

Each puff of cigarette contains a mixture of over 60 well-established carcinogens [20] so that while smoking is a known as major risk factor for lung cancer [21], it has also been implicated in a variety of GI malignancies [22,23]. Smoking, including light and intermittent smoking as well as second hand smoke exposure, is likewise associated with increased risk of myocardial infarction (MI) and CVD [24,25]. Smoking contributes to the development of atherosclerotic plaque, and induces a hypercoagulable state that leads to coronary thrombosis.

Physical Inactivity and Diet

Physical inactivity is a modifiable risk factor for CVD, cancer (particularly colorectal, breast, and endometrial), as well as CVD and cancer-related deaths and recurrence [26,27]. In a meta-analysis of 15 datasets from 14 articles, including 7873 incident cases, there were inverse associations between leisure time physical activity and colon cancer: RR: 0.80; 95% CI: 0.67–0.96 for men, and 0.86; 0.76–0.98 for women [28]; with similar findings in another meta-analysis of observational studies involving both colon and rectal cancers [29]. Likewise, a study of a cohort of over 34,000 participants showed significant associations between beef consumption and ischemic heart disease (IHD) as well as bladder cancer, with nonvegetarians more likely to develop colon and prostate cancers. Furthermore, nuts and legumes consumption were associated with lower risks of certain cancers, in addition to IHD [30]. Conversely, consumption of high fiber diet is associated with approximately 10% decrease in the risk of colon cancer [31].

Inflammation

Chronic low-grade inflammation, noted by circulating, is associated with CVD, and is a major contributor to cancer initiation and progression [32,33]. As such, inflammation appears to be central to the pathophysiologic mechanisms of both processes, and higher circulating levels of IL-1, IL-6, C-reactive protein (CRP), tumor necrosis factor (TNF), and serum amyloid A (SAA) are associated with tumor growth [34], and known to be poor prognostic indicators for a number of solid tumors [35,36]. The higher levels of inflammation associated with the common risk factors associated with both cancer and CVD could be markers, and to some extent, causative.

CHEMOTHERAPY AND HEART DISEASE RISK

Many chemotherapeutic agents are associated with two types of cardiotoxicity. More than 50% of all patients exposed to anthracycline chemotherapy—utilized in many cancers, including breast cancer, lymphomas, leukemias, endometrial and ovarian cancers, and sarcomas—will show some degree of cardiac dysfunction 10–20 years (or more) after chemotherapy, 5% will develop overt heart failure with up to 60% mortality, and 40% will experience arrhythmias [12,13]. The risk of anthracycline-associated cardiomyopathy varies on the basis of a variety of factors to be discussed later in the chapter.

Other commonly utilized chemotherapeutic drugs that have been implicated in cardiac toxicity and heart failure include tyrosine kinase inhibitors (TKIs), such as trastuzumab, bevacizumab, sunitinib, sorafenib, imatinib, dasatinib, and nilotinib. Trastuzumab is a monoclonal antibody which targets the human epidermal growth factor receptor 2 protein (HER-2) receptor, and leads to mostly reversible ErbB2 signaling-mediated type-II cardiac dysfunction without ultrastructural changes [14]. The incidence of trastuzumab-associated cardiac dysfunction is about 5–10% with 2–3% incidence of clinical heart failure. However, used in combination with doxorubicin, trastuzumab leads to great than sevenfold increased risk of heart failure [37].

Left ventricular ejection fraction (LVEF) assessment by cardiac imaging with 2D echocardiography, MUGA and more recently, cardiac magnetic resonance (CMR), is used to detect cardiotoxicity. Unfortunately, only 42% of patients are able to recover *some* cardiac function by the time these imaging modalities detect LV dysfunction [38], thus underscoring the need for early identification of those at risk for cardiac dysfunction with chemotherapy.

Early Identification of Risk

LVEF can identify patients with cardiotoxicity; however, a change in LVEF is sometimes a late manifestation of myocardial damage. As such, methods to detect myocardial toxicity before a decline are necessary. In addition, there is limited accuracy and lack of reproducibility of 2D echocardiography for LVEF assessment, as well as a lack of consensus in defining what constitutes a clinically significant reduction in cardiac function during and after chemotherapy. Furthermore, serial LVEF monitoring, although accepted, has never been validated for this purpose. Of note, 2D echocardiography exhibits low sensitivity for detection of small changes in LV function, and is affected by changes in loading conditions associated with chemotherapy which may then affect the LVEF value. Otterstad et al. showed that 2D echocardiography detected differences close to 10% in LVEF. Since this is the same magnitude of change that is used to adjudicate cancer therapy-induced cardiomyopathy by most groups, the sensitivity of 2D echocardiography in this setting has been questioned [39]. Accordingly, the development of strategies for early detection of cardiotoxicity has been the focus of more recent research efforts. These strategies fall largely into three main categories: myocardial strain imaging, cardiac biomarkers, or a combination of imaging and biomarkers. Early studies involving these strategies have focused on alterations in imaging or biomarkers during chemotherapy as a means of detecting subclinical myocardial dysfunction, whereas more recent studies have sought to establish the predictive power of early detection approaches.

Diastolic Function

Diastolic dysfunction may precede the onset of systolic dysfunction in some pathological processes. Tassan-Mangina et al. [40] assessed diastolic using tissue Doppler imaging (TDI) of the LV basal lateral and posterior walls in 20 patients at baseline (prior to receiving doxorubicin chemotherapy) 1–3 months after completion of chemotherapy

in 18 of 20 patients, and a mean of 3.5 ± 0.6 years after chemotherapy in 16 of 20 patients. There was no change in LVEF during treatment or in early follow-up but there was a 16% point decline in LVEF by 3.5 years of follow-up. Of note, despite the early changes in diastolic parameters followed by a subsequent change in LVEF, there were no CHF events in the patient population during the follow-up period.

Myocardial Strain Imaging by Speckle Tracking Echocardiography for Risk Identification

Speckle tracking echocardiography (STE) for detection of LV myocardial strain is a novel cardiac imaging technique assessed by echocardiography. It measures LV regional and global deformations in response to force as a marker of contractility and elasticity. Change in LV strain measures precedes change in LVEF [41], and strain has been shown to be a very specific predictor of cardiac dysfunction in cancer patients receiving chemotherapy [42] (Fig. 10.1A,B).

In a study by Stoodley et al. [43], an absolute global longitudinal strain (GLS) value of ≤ 17.2% obtained 6 months

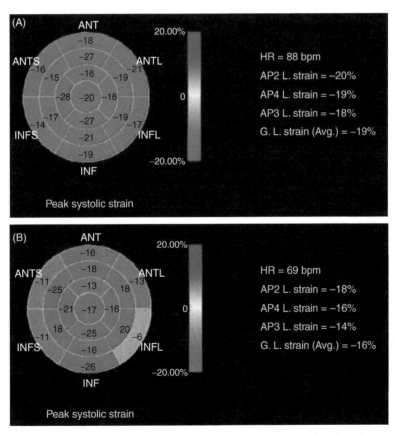

FIGURE 10.1   Myocardial global longitudinal strain images by STE (A) prechemotherapy and (B) during chemotherapy. A 41-year-old female requiring R-CHOP chemotherapy for a diagnosis of lymphoma. Change in GLS from baseline of −19% (A) to −16% within 6 weeks into doxorubicin-based chemotherapy (B). This patient's troponin-I also increased from a baseline level of less than 0.01–0.16 by 6 weeks of chemotherapy. Her LVEF was 60% at baseline and 56% at 6 weeks of chemotherapy; but dropped to 45% at reimaging 1 month later. In this case, her GLS and troponin-I predicted her subsequent reduction in LVEF.

after anthracycline (doxorubicin or epirubicin) therapy was predictive of abnormal longitudinal strain at 1-year follow-up, with a sensitivity of 100% and specificity of 80%. Strain alterations were associated with higher doses of anthracycline although within the dose range considered to have an acceptable toxicity profile.

Myocardial GLS has excellent inter- and intraobserver variability compared with other cardiac imaging modalities [44], and is highly correlated with the relatively expensive and much less available cardiac MRI—the gold standard for the assessment of LV dysfunction [45]. In addition, strain imaging as obtained with echocardiography is less expensive and less time-consuming compared with other cardiac imaging modalities for LVEF assessment, such as 3D echocardiography, cardiac MRI and MUGA scanning. Unlike the nuclear MUGA scan, cardiac angiography or cardiac catheterization, strain does not confer any radiation risk to the patient; and since myocardial strain imaging does not employ intravenous contrast, it extinguishes the concern for contrast-induced nephropathy and renal damage, such as seen with CMR imaging or cardiac CT angiography or cardiac catheterization.

Other strain imaging modalities including circumferential and radial strain have higher inter- and intraobserver variability and have consequently remained mostly in the research phase. GLS has stronger clinical data and has become a useful tool for risk profiling, particularly in chemotherapy patients.

Cardiac MRI

Studies have been inconsistent with regard to the presence of late gadolinium enhancement (LGE) as a marker of cardiotoxicity in patients receiving chemotherapy [46–50]. When present, several but not all reports suggest a propensity for the lateral wall for unclear reasons. Some have theorized that the lack of consistent LGE in anthracycline-related cardiomyopathy is because the fibrosis pattern is diffuse whereas LGE is a technique that identifies discrete areas of fibrosis relative to the normal surrounding areas of myocardium. One study [51] showed that myocardial fibrosis was present in patients treated with anthracyclines compared to controls correlated with echocardiographic measures of diastolic dysfunction because of expansion of the extracellular matrix as measured by extracellular volume using T1-weighted imaging. In another study using a T1-weighted technique, myocardial enhancement relative to skeletal muscle enhancement early after gadolinium was associated with a reduction in LVEF 28 days after anthracycline administration that was sustained at the 6-month follow-up in the majority of patients [52]. Further investigation using cardiac MRI techniques to discern early myocardial changes during or after chemotherapy is likely forthcoming. The additive value of MRI to biomarkers or strain is yet to be determined.

Biomarkers as Risk Markers of Cancer Therapy-Induced Cardiomyopathy

The role of biomarkers in this setting lies in the prediction of cardiomyopathy/detection of subclinical cardiomyopathy. Several studies have evaluated the role of cardiac biomarkers [particularly, brain natriuretic peptide (BNP), and troponin-I which accurately reflect myocardial injury] in the evaluation of cardiotoxicity associated with cancer therapy [53–58].

Troponin

The role of troponin rise in the detection of cardiac-marker-induced cardiomyopathy has been studied in recent times, and is being further defined in other studies. Troponin-I is a well-established, highly sensitive, and specific marker of myocardial injury with a wide diagnostic window, and a robust chemical assay [59]. In a study by Cardinale et al., a rise in troponin-I within approximately 3 days of doxorubicin chemotherapy predicted a reduction in LVEF [60]. The same study showed that troponin-I had a negative predictive value of 99% in ruling out future development of LV systolic dysfunction from baseline prior to chemotherapy. Findings were similar in the study by Sawaya et al. which showed a negative predictive value of 90% for ruling out the possibility of doxorubicin-induced systolic dysfunction using troponin-I biomarker [42]. Troponin-I has also been successful in differentiating reversible and irreversible LV dysfunction associated with trastuzumab chemotherapy [61], and in the identification of cardiovascular outcomes [defined as death resulting from a cardiac cause, acute pulmonary edema, overt heart failure, asymptomatic LVEF reduction ($\geq 25\%$ from baseline), or life-threatening arrhythmias] in patients receiving various types and combinations of high dose chemotherapy. In contrast, Morris et al. demonstrated that troponin-I increases were common in patients receiving both trastuzumab and lapatinib, but were not associated with subsequent LV dysfunction by MUGA scans [62].

Although not as specific as troponin-I, troponin-T has also been shown to be predictive of chemotherapy-induced cardiomyopathy in children and adults [53,63]. Conversely, troponin-T was not associated with reduction in LVEF in another study [64].

Natriuretic Peptides

Although somewhat controversial, the natriuretic peptides (BNP and NT-pro-BNP) appear to be mostly useful in the prediction and diagnosis of cancer-therapy-induced systolic dysfunction. The studies by Sawaya et al. showed that NT-pro-BNP did not predict cardiotoxicity [42,65]. Likewise, Daugaard et al. showed only modest correlations between NT-ANP/BNP and LV systolic dysfunction [66]; however, this was not the case in a similar study carried out in a pediatric population where ANP and BNP were both indeed significantly correlated with systolic and diastolic dysfunction [67]. More recently, other studies in both children and adults have also supported the role of pro-BNP in the identification of these patients [68–76]. Of note, in a group of patients where most had received chemotherapy, BNP showed an AUC of 0.86 in the detection of asymptomatic LV systolic dysfunction [77]. Pitfalls associated with the use of natriuretic peptides include biological variation, and variance with age, renal function, and BMI. This calls for caution in the interpretation of data obtained using these serum markers.

The combination of troponin-I and BNP (or pro-BNP) has been useful in the identification of patients at risk for LV dysfunction post high-dose anthracyclines. As such, it elevations in each or both biomarkers might be useful in the identification of patients at risk of developing cardiotoxicity, with future need for cardiological follow-up [58,78].

Combination and Novel Biomarkers in Risk Identification

The need to identify newer metrics beyond the long-recognized factors of age and cardiovascular comorbidities has inspired investigators to seek innovative mechanisms by which risk for cardiotoxicity could be predicted. This has led to the advent of serum biomarker testing to increase sensitivity, and pharmacogenomic risk profiling to increase specificity of predicting high-risk patients for chemotherapy-induced cardiotoxicity. Data are limited on associations between novel biomarkers and cancer-therapy-related cardiac dysfunction. Recent considered heart-failure biomarkers of interest include serum galectin-3, ST-2, glycogen phosphorylase BB (GPBB), heart-type fatty-acid-binding protein (H-FABP), and hs-CRP. In their studies, Horacek et al. suggested some promise in GPBB [79–81], whereas another study has shown H-FASB and hs-CRP as possible future markers for consideration [82]. Whether these markers will predict cancer-therapy-related cardiac dysfunction or cardiovascular events in future is unclear. In one study, cardiac and inflammatory markers including NT-pro-BNP, MR-pro-ANP, mid-regional pro-atrial natriuretic peptide (MR-pro-ADM), C-terminal pro-endothelin-1 (CT-proET-1), copeptin, hs-troponin-T, IL-6, CRP and cytokines SAA, haptoglobin, and fibronectin, were all associated with all-cause mortality in cancer patients [83]. Conversely, in a pediatric population, NT-pro-BNP but not troponin-I, were useful indicators of LV systolic dysfunction [74]; and in the study by Dodos et al., neither BNP nor troponin-T was useful in the identification of chemotherapy-related LV (systolic or diastolic) dysfunction [64]. Of note, the study by Armenia et al. showed that BNP, but not other biomarkers (including troponin-T, ST-2 and Galectin-3), was a marker of LV dysfunction [68]. Furthermore, among a panel of biomarkers [troponin-I, CRP, pro-BNP, growth differentiation factor-15 (GDF-15), myeloperoxidase (MPO), PlGF, soluble fms-like tyrosine kinase receptor (sFlt-1), and gal-3] in 78

breast-cancer patients undergoing doxorubicin and trastuzumab chemotherapy, Ky et al. [84] found that troponin-I and MPO—but not the other biomarkers—improved risk prediction of chemotherapy-induced cardiotoxicity. In a longitudinal study of the same patients followed for up to 15 months, only MPO remained as a predictor [85]. Conversely, another biomarker panel of NT-pro-BNP, TNF-α, galectin-3, IL-6, Troponin I, ST2 and sFlt-1 showed only NT-pro-BNP as a predictor to detect subclinical cardiotoxicity after treatment with anthracyclines [86].

To date, the jury is still out on what combinations of biomarkers best predict cardiotoxicities associated with cancer therapy.

Use of Imaging Combined With Biomarkers

As described previously, alterations in either myocardial mechanics or biomarkers have both been linked to chemotherapy-related myocardial damage. Because they both are utilized as endpoints of the same pathological process, there may be value to using these methods conjointly to detect cardiotoxicity. In the study by Sawaya et al. [65], a change in longitudinal strain and troponin-I at 3 months after doxorubicin chemotherapy predicted cardiotoxicity at the 6-month follow-up. Cardiotoxicity was also predicted by the number of segments that showed a change in longitudinal strain at 3 months. In another seminal paper by Sawaya et al. [42], they further demonstrated that a combination of 10% decrease in longitudinal strain with troponin-I predicted cardiotoxicity following doxorubicin therapy with a specificity of 97%; whereas either marker showed a sensitivity of 89% and a negative predictive value of 97% in detecting cardiotoxicity. Therefore, the data suggest more benefit to the use of combinations of risk markers (strain imaging modality plus biomarkers in this case) in the identification of persons at risk for cardiotoxicity following chemotherapy.

The Role of Genetics

Data examining the role of genetics in the prediction of chemotherapy-induced cardiomyopathy are limited. The NRG1/erbB pathway is critical for the cardioprotective repair and maintenance of the myocardial structure in adults, and impaired NRG1 signaling exacerbates anthracycline-mediated cardiotoxicity. There is evidence that NRG1-deficient hearts are prone to anthracycline toxicity, and resulted in a deregulation of the ubiquitine–proteasome system, with a net result of the vacuolization of cardiomyocytes, such as seen with anthracycline-induced cardiotoxicity [87]. Another study found that among 2100 genes associated with de novo CVD, a common single nucleotide polymorphism (SNP) in the hyaluronan synthase 3 (HAS3) gene was found to have a modifying effect on anthracycline dose-dependent cardiomyopathy risk [88]. The rs2232228 AA genotype conferred an 8.9-fold (95% CI, 2.1–37.5-fold;

$P = 0.003$) increased cardiomyopathy risk compared with the GG genotype. The hyaluronan produced by HAS3 plays an active role in tissue remodeling, and is known to reduce reactive oxygen species (ROS)-induced cardiac injury. Another study of 2977 SNPs in 220 key drug biotransformation genes in children identified multiple genetic variants in SLC28A3 and other transporter (ABCB1, ABCB4, and ABCC1) genes associated with anthracycline cardiotoxicity—positive and negative predictive values of 75 and 95%, respectively [89]. Additional studies are required to uncover other genetic variants contributing to anthracycline—and other cancer-therapy-induced cardiotoxicity.

An article by Jensen and McLeod [90] focused on the role of using a "candidate-gene" approach to more specifically identify which patients are at risk of developing chemotherapy-induced cardiotoxicity. The authors note importantly that there is no clear relationship between cumulative dose of trastuzumab and the likelihood of developing cardiotoxicity. Furthermore, a significant number of adverse effects occur in patients without cardiac risk factors, suggesting a possible genetic predisposition that warrants a sophisticated exploration. Two small studies suggest that an ErbB2 polymorphism (Ile655Val) confers both increased growth potential in tumor cells and increased propensity for cardiotoxicity in patients treated with trastuzumab [91,92].

The limitation of the candidate-gene approach to genotyping cardiotoxicity risk is unveiled by the various efforts that have been undertaken to isolate a selection of SNPs in animal models to guide the mechanism of myocardial injury associated with anthracycline in human models. Accordingly, the candidate-gene approach to specify polymorphisms that predispose to chemotherapeutic cardiotoxicity has not been as fruitful as had been hoped.

RISK FACTORS SPECIFIC TO REPRESENTATIVE CHEMOTHERAPIES

Anthracyclines

A well-studied side effect of anthracyclines is cardiotoxicity in the form of cardiomyopathy with reduced LV systolic function. Anthracycline-induced cardiomyopathy occurs through a number of processes, including inhibition of topoisomerase II, generation of free oxygen radicals which induce DNA damage and cell apoptosis, inhibition cellular pathways initiating apoptosis, and DNA intercalation [93]. Cardiac myocytes are particularly sensitive to oxidative stress due to the aerobic metabolic demands of the heart. The risk factors that predispose to anthracycline toxicity are summarized in Table 10.1.

TABLE 10.1 Risk Factors, Strength of Evidence, and Aspects of Note for Anthracycline-Induced Cardiotoxicity

Risk Factor	Special Notes	Noted Increase in Risk
Cumulative dose	Significantly increased risk at doses over 500 mg/m^2	7.5–26% at 550 mg/m^2 [84,85] versus 1.7% at 300 mg/m^2 [84], and 3.0–5.0% at 400 mg/m^2 [84,85]; 9% increased risk for every 50 mg/m^2 added [94]
Age	Bimodal age distribution: higher risk noted in age younger than 4 years or older than 65 years	32% for less than age 4 years [86] and 125% at age greater than 65 years [84]; 7% increased risk for each additional 5 years of age [94]
Duration of time postchemotherapy	Incidence increases progressively postchemotherapy	Median time for cardiotoxicity postchemotherapy is 3.5 months [94]
Comorbid cardiac risk factors	Particularly hypertension, but also diabetes, coronary disease, obesity, renal dysfunction, pulmonary disease, electrolyte abnormalities, infection, and pregnancy	45–58% for hypertension [89,90], 27–74% for diabetes [89,90], 58% for coronary artery disease [90]
Concomitant cardiotoxic chemotherapy	Trastuzumab, taxanes, cyclophosphamide; either potentiating risk or overlapping toxicity	Dose and drug dependent
Chest wall radiation	High-dose radiation for left-sided breast cancer, lung cancer, mediastinal lymphomas with concomitant, or prior anthracycline therapy	23% for high-dose radiation versus low-dose radiation [87]
Female sex	Particularly in the pediatric population	100% increased risk in females compared with males at a given dose in pediatric patients [88], 61% for all age females [94]
Echocardiographic evidence of toxicity	Drop in LVEF postchemotherapy from baseline prior to starting chemotherapy	37% increased risk of cardiotoxicity for each percent unit drop in LVEF at the end of chemotherapy [94]
Infusion rates	Continuous infusion is less cardiotoxic	9.5% with continuous infusion versus 46.6% with bolus IV injection [95]

Cumulative Dose

One major factor predisposing to anthracycline toxicity is the cumulative dose delivered. Swain et al. retrospectively looked at three clinical trials to estimate the rate of cardiotoxicity as a function of dose [96]. A total of 630 patients had received doxorubicin, an estimated 26% of these patients who received a dose of 550 mg/m^2 developed CHF, with over 50% of the patients having severely reduced LVEF less than 30%. A similar retrospective study by Von Hoff et al. had a total of 4018 patients who had received doxorubicin and found similar results [97]. At a dose of 400 mg/m^2, the overall incidence was 0.14% versus 7% at 550 mg/m^2. Thus, it is surmised that cardiomyopathy associated with doxorubicin is noticeable at doses above 400 mg/m^2, and is quite significant at doses over 500 mg/m^2.

Age

The risk of anthracycline-induced cardiomyopathy exhibits a bimodal age distribution, with lower doses of anthracyclines affecting older as well as younger patients. The study by Swain et al. separated patients greater and less than 65 years of age, and determined that even a smaller cumulative dose of 400 mg/m^2 was associated with an increased incidence of CHF [96]. The hazard ratio at 400 mg/m^2 of anthracycline greater than 65 years of age was 2.25 compared with less than 65 years, indicating that older age is associated with higher sensitivity to cumulative doses of anthracycline.

On the other end of the age distribution, Lipshultz et al. characterized anthracycline cardiotoxicity risk in children with childhood leukemias by measuring electrocardiogram, echocardiography, and exercise stress testing to evaluate cardiac function approximately 6 years posttreatment [95]. The study had many major findings, reaffirming that cumulative dose is the most significant risk factor for cardiotoxicity, it also determined that those who are less than 4 years of age were at increased risk for cardiotoxicity, with up to 32% of patients of this age presenting with left ventricular (LV) dysfunction after anthracycline administration. With echocardiography, the authors concluded cumulative dose was correlated with decreased contractility and decreased ventricular wall thickness. The authors concluded that through loss of cardiac myocytes, the infant heart cannot adjust to the child's growth, subsequently leading to a dilated cardiomyopathy.

Concomitant Radiation Therapy

Chest wall radiation is commonly used with anthracyclines in the adjuvant setting to treat cases of breast, lung cancer, and mediastinal lymphomas, putting the heart at increased risk for cardiotoxicity due to the combination of both treatment modalities. High-dose radiation alone has been shown to increase cardiotoxicity, and when used with high-dose anthracyclines, puts patients at increased risk. Shapiro et al. retrospectively analyzed 299 patients and their individual risk for cardiomyopathy based on radiation dose to the heart [94]. The incidence of cardiac events was 12% in the high dose doxorubicin compared with the low dose group. Within the high-dose group, patients who received a moderate or high dose of radiation to the heart were at increased risk for cardiac events, compared with the no- or low-dose radiation group.

Female Sex

Females appear to be at increased risk for developing cardiotoxicity as well. Another study by Lipshultz et al. looked at 120 children who were treated with doxorubicin doses ranging from 244 to 550 mg/m^2 for leukemia or sarcoma [98]. It compared this cohort to 296 normal control patients and measured cardiac function with echocardiography. It determined that female patients were nearly at twice the risk of developing cardiomyopathy compared with males at a given dose. This study confirmed that cumulative dose appears to be the most significant risk factor for anthracycline-induced heart failure, with a higher predisposition in females. The mechanism for higher risk of anthracycline-induced cardiomyopathy in females is unknown, but could perhaps be due to higher body-fat percentage leading to increased concentration of anthracyclines within the systemic circulation.

Preexisting Cardiovascular Risk Factors

Preexisting cardiac risk factors appear to increase the incidence of CHF in patients receiving doxorubicin. Most notably, hypertension has the largest coacting negative effect with doxorubicin with up to 58% increased risk of developing CHF, with a hazard ratio of 1.8 [99]. Diabetes was significant in the noncontrolled model with a 27% increased risk. Results from a large cohort study evaluated 43,338 women with breast-cancer diagnosis, and showed that hypertension increased the risk of doxorubicin-induced cardiotoxicity by 45%, diabetes by 74%, and CAD by 58% [100].

Concomitant Chemotherapies

Chemotherapies often administered with anthracyclines (including trastuzumab, taxanes, and cyclophosphamide) also increase the risk of cardiotoxicity with his agent [101]. The cardiotoxicity of taxanes when used with anthracyclines was recognized early. The pharmokinetics of taxanes reduce the metabolism of anthracyclines leading to increased concentration of the anthracyclines. Phase-II studies of taxanes plus doxorubicin showed that the incidence of heart failure was potentiated by higher doses of anthracyclines [102]. A dose of 420 mg/m^2 of anthracycline when combined with paclitaxel had an incidence of 50% for heart failure when compared to 5.4% at a dose of less than 360 m/m^2 of anthracycline. Thus it is not recommended to exceed a dose of 360 mg/m^2 of anthracycline in patients receiving adjuvant taxane therapy.

Trastuzumab is a monoclonal antibody in HER-2 positive breast cancers and has been used as adjuvant therapy with anthracyclines for metastatic disease. A large-scale cohort study by Chen et al. of 45,537 women with breast cancer showed a 3-year incidence of heart failure due to trastuzumab plus anthracycline of 23.8% versus 14.0% with trastuzumab alone [103]. The original randomized controlled trial aiming to characterize trastuzumab by Slamon et al. randomly assigned 138 women to receive cyclophosphamide plus an anthracycline as a control versus the control plus trastuzumab [104]. It found an incidence of severe heart failure of 27% in the trastuzumab, anthracycline, plus cyclophosphamide versus 8% in the anthracycline plus cyclophosphamide group. Thus, anthracyclines play a role in potentiating the toxicity of trastuzumab.

The risk of cardiotoxicity is increased modestly when anthracyclines are combined with cyclophosphamide, compared with taxanes or trastuzumab–anthracycline combinations. Perez et al. reported on LVEF in 1576 patients who had received a total cumulative dose of doxorubicin of 240 mg/m^2 plus cyclophosphamide at 2400 mg/m^2 [105]. LVEF was measured using echocardiography before and after doxorubicin and cyclophosphamide delivery, and 6.6% of these patients developed grade-2 LV dysfunction, with 2.5% developing LVEF decrease of over 15%.

Other Risk Factors for Anthracycline-Induced Cardiotoxicity

Other risk factors that have been studied include route and speed of administration, with continuous infusions over prolonged periods of time favored over bolus intravenous injections which increase the risk of cardiotoxicity. Type of anthracycline agent used is also a risk factor (i.e., doxorubicin carries a higher risk than epirubicin or liposomal doxorubicin) [106].

A recent study by Cardinale et al. prospectively evaluated 2625 patients receiving anthracycline and evaluated LVEF every 3 months during chemotherapy treatment for a year, and then biannually [107]. Cardiotoxicity was defined as a drop in LVEF by 10% to less than 50%, and at the end of chemotherapy, every percentage drop in LVEF increased the risk of clinical heart failure by 37%. The results of this study imply that there remains an asymptomatic group where LVEF decreases before patients are symptomatic from heart failure.

Trastuzumab

Trastuzumab is a monoclonal antibody developed in the 1980s that binds to the extracellular domain of HER-2 and mediates antibody-dependent cytotoxicity by inhibiting proliferation of cells that overexpress HER-2 protein [108]. It is an oncogenic transmembrane tyrosine kinase receptor protein that mediates signaling of cellular proliferation and prevention of apoptosis. Trastuzumab was first approved in 1998 for the treatment of HER-2 positive metastatic breast cancer, which constitutes approximately 25% of all breast cancers.

The cardiotoxic effects of trastuzumab have been well studied. Most notably, a 2012 Cochrane review of over 10,000 patients from studies that compared the incidence of cardiotoxicity in trastuzumab-treated patients relative to control arms demonstrated significantly increased risk of symptomatic CHF and reduced LVEF [109]. In addition, studies of the incidence of cardiotoxicity from trastuzumab in community settings that applied less stringent inclusion criteria strongly echo these findings, offering important generalizability of the clinical trials to more heterogenous population settings [108]. The pathophysiology of trastuzumab-mediated cardiotoxicity is not completely understood. However, the mechanism is thought to involve inhibition of the normal physiologic action of HER-2 on cardiomyocytes and resident cardiac stem cells. When the HER-2 signaling pathway is blocked, cardiac dysfunction results from cardiomyocyte death due to accumulation of reactive oxygen species and subsequent impaired differentiation of microvascular networks by cardiac stem cells [110,111].

A number of risk factors that are known to potentiate the cardiovascular toxicity of trastuzumab (Table 10.2) have been challenging to identify, and are framed by two important historical considerations. First, while one may reasonably presume that a history of heart disease almost certainly predisposes patients to developing trastuzumab-induced cardiotoxicity, the majority of clinical trials exclude such patients from studying its occurrence. Second, when trastuzumab was undergoing clinical trials, cardiac events were not anticipated as adverse outcomes, and so the monitoring of cardiac function was not included in most of the initial studies. As such, a considerable degree of the data supporting the clinical and statistical significance of cardiovascular risk factors are limited by retrospective study design, small sample size, or publication bias associated with metaanalyses. Nonetheless, currently available literature offer indispensable insight into which patients are most at risk for the cardiotoxic effects of trastuzumab.

Prior or Concomitant Doxorubicin Exposure

The best-supported risk factor for trastuzumab-induced cardiotoxicity appears to be the cumulative effect observed with concomitant anthracycline and trastuzumab administration [112]. In a retrospective review of the original phase-II and -III trastuzumab clinical trials, Seidman et al. [112] found that the incidence of cardiomyopathy was greatest in

TABLE 10.2 Risk Factors and Aspects of Note for Trastuzumab-Induced Cardiotoxicity

Risk Factors	Aspects
Baseline left ventricular dysfunction	• Asymptomatic decrease in LVEF to <50%, decreased LVEF to 20% below baseline, or signs and symptoms of CHF in patients with metastatic cancer with >1 year trastuzumab therapy • Usually temporary decline, reassess LVEF after 1 month of therapy
Coronary artery disease	• Increases risk of symptomatic heart failure with adjuvant trastuzumab in early breast cancer • CAD risk equivalents (e.g., diabetes mellitus) increase risk of cardiotoxicity in elderly patients. • Increases risk for cardiac events in patients with stage I–III breast cancer receiving trastuzumab
Hypertension	• Increases risk of symptomatic heart failure with adjuvant trastuzumab in early breast cancer
Older age	• Patients over 60 years old and treated with adjuvant trastuzumab have an increased cardiovascular risk profile and are at higher risk for trastuzumab cardiotoxicity • Highest risk at age >80 years
Smoking	• Increased risk for systolic dysfunction in smokers receiving adjuvant trastuzumab
Heavy alcohol consumption	• Ten drinks or more per week during the course of trastuzumab treatment leads to higher risk of cardiotoxicity
Renal dysfunction	• GFR <78 mL/min per 1.73 m^2 was the strongest predictor of trastuzumab cardiotoxicity independent of doxorubicin treatment and baseline LVEF • Higher risk at 12-month follow-up for early breast cancer patients receiving adjuvant trastuzumab
Genetic polymorphisms	• HER2 Ile/Val carrier state was associated with a higher risk of cardiac toxicity compared to Ile/Ile genetic polymorphisms

patients receiving concomitant trastuzumab and anthracycline plus cyclophosphamide (27%). The risk was substantially lower in patients receiving paclitaxel and trastuzumab (13%) or trastuzumab alone (3–7%); however, most of these patients had received prior anthracycline therapy. Most trastuzumab-treated patients developing cardiac dysfunction were symptomatic (75%), and most improved with standard treatment for CHF (79%). Subsequently, Farolfi et al. [113] assessed the incidence of trastuzumab-induced cardiotoxicity and heart failure in a retrospective study in 179 patients, and identified 78 patients (44%) in which trastuzumab-induced cardiotoxicity occurred. They showed that a previous cumulative dose greater than 240 mg/m^2 of doxorubicin or greater than 500 mg/m^2 of epirubicin increased the risk of trastuzumab-induced cardiotoxicity threefold compared with lower doses. Nonetheless, the data regarding risk of trastuzumab-induced cardiotoxicity in relationship to prior epirubicin exposure has been conflicting. Russo et al. [114] did not observe a significant association with epirubicin, but redemonstrated the threefold increased risk of trastuzumab-induced cardiotoxicity after doxorubicin exposure, as outlined by Farolfi's group. In contrast, Cochet et al. [115] stratified patients on the basis of epirubicin doses of 0, 300, and 600 mg/m^2. Trastuzumab-induced cardiotoxicity was apparent in 9% of patients without any epirubicin exposure, whereas 35% prevalence was observed in those patients exposed to 600 mg/m^2 of epirubicin.

Baseline LV Dysfunction

Impaired LV diastolic function before treatment is a well-documented independent predictor of trastuzumab-mediated cardiotoxicity. This was shown in a prospective study that included 118 women presenting with HER-2 positive early-stage invasive breast cancer [115]. Of the patients that developed cardiomyopathy, no significant difference was observed in baseline systolic function as measured by LVEF and peak ejection rate. In contrast, patients with baseline diastolic dysfunction defined as prolonged time to peak filling rate greater than 180 ms were significantly more likely to develop clinically significant progression of impaired ventricular relaxation.

CAD and Risk Factors

The strongest evidence for CAD as an independent predictor of trastuzumab-induced cardiotoxicity comes from a small retrospective study of 45 patients [116] that aimed to assess the cardiac safety profile of trastuzumab in elderly breast cancer patients. Patients with trastuzumab-related cardiotoxicity presented more often with cardiovascular risk factors, such as history of cardiac disease (33% vs. 9.1%, $P = 0.017$) and diabetes (33.3% vs. 6.1%, $P = 0.010$), compared with those without. Consequently, given that the 5-year CHF mortality in patients of more than 65 years of age is approximately 50%, the authors advise that elderly patients, particularly those with one or more cardiac risk factor, warrant exceptional awareness of their risk for developing symptomatic and asymptomatic cardiotoxicity with trastuzumab exposure. Risk that preexisting CAD poses for the development of trastuzumab-associated cardiomyopathy in younger patients may remain elusive, as those patients with known history of cardiac disease are excluded from studies. As such, studies that evaluate known CAD risk factors, such as uncontrolled hypertension, dyslipidemia, and age as independent risk factors for trastuzumab-induced cardiotoxicity should be considered surrogates for CAD risk equivalent conditions.

Older patients have underwhelming representation in clinical trials. Nonetheless, many studies support an association of age-related comorbidities with increased risk of trastuzumab cardiotoxicity, and few have gone so far as to show the independent attributable impact of age alone. A study of the Italian Cardio-Oncologic network of 499 women with HER-2 positive early breast cancer found that patients over age 60 were three times more likely to develop clinical heart failure, 10% more likely to experience a greater than 10% decline in ejection fraction, 2.5 times as likely to discontinue trastuzumab, and 14% less likely to resume trastuzumab. In their study, 32% of HER-2 positive early breast cancer patients treated with adjuvant trastuzumab whom were greater than 60 years of age had an increased cardiovascular risk profile and commonly developed trastuzumab cardiotoxicity [117]. Findings were similar in a review of the over 2000 patients who were more than 66 years old taken from the SEER-Registry which found that age greater than 80 years, CAD, hypertension, and weekly trastuzumab administration increased the risk of heart failure with trastuzumab therapy [118].

Other Risk Factors for Trastuzumab Cardiotoxicity

Heavy alcohol consumption appears to be a risk factor for cardiotoxicity in breast cancer patients treated with trastuzumab as noted in a retrospective cohort study by Lemieux et al. where they observed that drinking 10 or more alcoholic beverages per week during trastuzumab treatment was significantly associated with cardiotoxicity [92]. It is hypothesized that the relationship between alcohol consumption and trastuzumab-induced cardiotoxicity is related to hypertension [92,108]. The proposed pathophysiologic mechanism of risk in this case is that ethanol may increase underlying oxidative stress and promote ongoing cardiac damage in the context of anthracycline or trastuzumab exposure.

Renal dysfunction may increase myocardial sensibility to the insult of anthracyclines, taxanes, and trastuzumab when used in combination. To this end, glomerular filtration rate (GFR) < 78 was shown to be a strong independent predictor of cardiotoxicity 1 year after trastuzumab-based adjuvant chemotherapy for early HER-2 positive breast cancer [114].

To date, factors associated with TKI-induced cardiotoxicity have not been satisfactorily elucidated.

Risk Prediction Modeling for Chemotherapy-Induced Cardiotoxicity

Until recently, clinical strategies for managing the cardiovascular comorbidities of anthracycline and trastuzumab chemotherapies have largely focused on surveillance rather than prevention. As such, experts agree across the board that increased risk prediction efforts are warranted. To this extent, a statistical model was proposed by Romond et al. [119], and aims to estimate the risk of developing severe CHF in patients enrolled in the phase-III adjuvant trial of the National Surgical Adjuvant Breast and Bowel Project (NASBP), protocol B-31. In the regression analysis, only age and baseline LVEF remained statistically significant. Using these baseline risk factors, a prediction model was developed for the cumulative probability of cardiac events up to year 5 in patients who postanthracycline therapy. On the basis of parametric regression on cause-specific subdistribution hazard, a cardiac risk score (CRS) can be calculated as follows:

$$\frac{[7.0 + (0.04 \times \text{Age in years}) - (0.1 \times \text{Baseline percent LVEF})] \times 100}{4.76}$$

The authors conclude that although their model conforms closely to the data collected from the B-31 protocol, the formula should be validated by other studies that implement similar chemotherapy regimens. They further assert that their model may be utilized to guide chemotherapy on an individualized bases, noting that for patients who have a higher CRS, there may be overall greater potential benefit from a regimen that has proven efficacy but excludes anthracyclines. Alternatively, patients with low cardiac risk and more advanced clinical features of their cancers may derive excellent overall benefit from the treatment regimen in B-31.

VEGF Inhibitors

Vascular endothelial growth factor (VEGF) is a central pro-angiogenic protein that is expressed and secreted by over 60% of human cancers [120]. VEGF activates a biomolecular cascade that mediates endothelial cell proliferation and survival; and tumorigenesis may be further disrupted by the ancillary effect of VEGF inhibitor-mediated "normalization" of leaky tumor vasculature [121]. This suggests that VEGF inhibitors may enhance the efficacy of additional chemotherapies by improving vascular function thereby allowing more efficient drug delivery to tumor targets. Bevacizumab, probably the most well-known VEGF inhibitor, was approved in 2004 after it was shown in a phase-III trial to increase overall survival of metastatic colon cancer by an average of 4 months when added to standard chemotherapy [122].

As might be expected by a class of medications whose major target is vascular endothelium, VEGF inhibitors have become notorious for their deleterious cardiovascular side effects, the most prevalent of which is hypertension, occurring in 30–80% of patients [123,124]. Other known adverse effects include proteinuria (35% of patients), gastrointestinal perforations (5–7% of patients), and arterial emboli (0.5–1% of patients). VEGF inhibitor-associated hypertension is mechanistically understood to represent opposition of the nitric-oxide-dependent relaxation of vascular endothelial smooth muscle cells, and resembles the pathophysiology of preeclampsia that also manifests as a result of reduced VEGF signaling and is similarly accompanied by proteinuria. Nonetheless, the risk factors that predispose patients to this effect remain less clear, and include age greater than 65 years, smoking, hypercholesterolemia, and history of hypertension [123].

A study of 22 patients exposed to bevacizumab (for rectal or colon cancer) over a 5-month period showed that in all three patients in whom hypertension developed, the following risk factors were present: atherosclerosis (defined by either a history of smoking or hypercholesterolemia), an increased heart rate (>90 beats per minute), and eosinophilia (>500/mm^3) at the onset of hypertension [122]. Beyond the results of the aforementioned meta-analysis and RCT that support dose-dependent risk for hypertension, and the theoretical posture of a prospective observational study, there remains a palpable paucity of evidence that illuminates the risk factors that predispose to VEGF-inhibitor-associated hypertension. It would not be an understatement to say that the most important work in this subject is ripe for further investigation. Patients who develop hypertension as a consequence of VEGF inhibition may be at increased risk of cardiac events [125], yet hypertension in this setting is a strong marker of response to therapy and improved clinical outcome [126].

LV dysfunction has been shown in experimental models to be an independent complication of VEGF blockade. Indeed, in animal models, VEGF levels among other cytokines are elevated following myocardial injury and promote cardiac remodeling [127]. A number of clinical trials have demonstrated that bevacizumab and sunitinib may act synergistically with anthracyclines and lead to cardiac dysfunction. In their review on cardiotoxicity associated with sunitinib, Chu et al. [128] suggested that LV dysfunction might be partially due to direct cardiomyocyte toxicity, and is exacerbated by hypertension. They further identified patients with a history of CAD and prior heart failure as those being most at risk for the development of major adverse cardiac events caused by the multigated kinase inhibitor.

Various multigated kinase inhibitors have been reported to prolong the QT interval. Sunitinib in particular was shown to exhibit a dose-dependent increase on the risk of ventricular arrhythmia associated with prolonged QT interval [129]. As such, clinicians should obtain baseline ECGs in patients prior to initiating VEGF or multitarget kinase inhibitors with a cutoff of QTc > 450 s in men and > 470 s

in women to warrant close monitoring during therapy. Bagnes et al. [130] advise that an increase in QTc of more than 60 ms above baseline or to a time of more than 500 ms places patients at a significantly increased risk of arrhythmia with exposure to anti-VEGFs and multi targeted kinase inhibitors.

RISK FACTORS SPECIFIC TO RADIOTHERAPY

Radiotherapy significantly reduces rates of cancer recurrence and mortality due to cancer [131,132]. Nonetheless, with all of its benefits, radiotherapy is also associated with irradiation of surrounding organs, other than the area of tumor. Chest wall radiation as seen in patients with lung cancer, lymphoma, esophageal, and breast cancer is particularly associated with irradiation to the heart, especially when confined to the left chest wall as in left-sided breast cancer [133,134]. Radiotherapy creates an inflammatory milieu, and can lead to radiation-induced heart disease which occurs in up to 50% of patients, within the first 5 years after radiotherapy, up to the third decade post chest wall radiation [15,135]. This includes a myriad of cardiac abnormalities comprising valvular heart disease, pericardial disease (pericarditis, pericardial effusion, and constriction), conduction disturbances and arrhythmias, cardiomyopathy, which can occur up to 20–30 years after radiotherapy [15]. The magnitude of radiation-induced atherosclerosis is demonstrated in the evaluation of 294 young non-Hodgkin's lymphoma patients (mean age 42 years) a mean of 15 years after radiotherapy. Despite their youth, 40 of these patients (14%) had abnormal stress tests, out of which 55% had significant CAD and 16% had severe triple-vessel CAD or left main CAD that required coronary artery bypass grafting [136]. These cardiac complications of radiotherapy eventually lead to higher cardiac morbidity and mortality, and are essentially worsened in the setting of preexisting cardiac disease (heart failure or CAD); concomitant chemotherapy; and traditional cardiovascular risk factors, such as hypertension and diabetes, higher cumulative doses of radiotherapy, anterior or left-sided chest wall location (as in Hodgkin's lymphoma and left-sided breast cancer), and among younger and older age groups [15,135].

Radiation Dose

The study by Darby et al. [135] investigated the risk of major coronary events associated with radiotherapy in women treated for breast cancer, and found that risk of coronary events increased with higher doses of radiation. This risk began within the first 5 years after radiotherapy, and continued until the third decade postradiotherapy. Pericarditis used to be the most common side effect of traditional radiotherapy for Hodgkin's disease [137]. More recent dose restrictions to 30 Gy with lower daily fraction, different weighting of radiation fields, and blocking of the subcarinal region have reduced that incidence from 20% to 2.5% [138,139].

Age at Irradiation

Patients younger than 35 years have a 6.5 higher relative risk for radiation-induced cardiotoxicity, compared with the general population [140]. Similar observations have been made in the case of Hodgkin's lymphoma [141,142]. One study showed that age, combined with cardiovascular risk factors, in addition to dose of radiotherapy combined to significantly increase the risk of IHD. This study showed an exponential increase in risk with advancing age [135]. The risk of acute MI associated with radiotherapy appears to be highest at younger ages—irradiation before 20 years of age in one study, which decreased with increasing age at treatment [139].

Concomitant Chemotherapy

As previously discussed, radiation-induced cardiotoxicity (particularly cardiomyopathy) appears to be higher, predominantly with total cumulative doses of anthracyclines [94].

BIOMARKERS IN THE IDENTIFICATION OF RADIATION-INDUCED CARDIOTOXICITY

A few studies to date have evaluated biomarkers in patients undergoing radiotherapy with conflicting results (Table 10.3). One early study of 50 women with breast cancer did not find any change in serum troponin after a total dose of 45–46 Gy of radiation [143]. Similarly, another study of 30 patients receiving radiotherapy did not show any significant elevations in creatine kinase-myocardial band (CK-MB), troponin, or NT-pro BNP with radiotherapy [144]. Conversely, a more recent study found both troponin and BNP increased significantly with radiation, even though the absolute and mean values remained on a relatively low level [145]. Yet in another recent study of 58 patients receiving radiotherapy for left-sided breast cancer, hs-troponin-T increased during radiotherapy from baseline in 12 patients (21%). In this study, those with higher hs-troponin-T values had received significantly increased radiation doses for the whole heart and left ventricle (LV) than those with stable hs-troponin-T values [146]. Similarly, another study of 43 left-sided breast cancer patients showed that normalized BNP (current BNP at time t, divided by baseline BNP) correlated significantly with V20, V25, V30, V45, mean dose, and median heart dose. In the only subject who developed MI, V20, V25, V30, and V45 were the highest and BNP increased from 1 month after radiation, and was persistently high even at 12 months [147]. Hence, cardiac biomarkers might be useful for evaluation of radiation-induced cardiotoxicity but remain a research tool. Our current knowledge suggests that normalized values of these biomarkers could prove more useful for monitoring of subclinical CVD associated with radiotherapy, than absolute elevations in values.

CONCLUSIONS

This review highlights the lack of high-level evidence to guide clinical decision-making with respect to the detection and management of cardiotoxicity associated with cancer treatment. Consequently, there are no clear, consistent guidelines or recommendations for monitoring or identification of persons at risk for chemotherapy-induced cardiotoxicity. Likewise, there is paucity of data to guide clinical decision-making regarding the prevention, detection or management of radiation-induced cardiotoxicity. Part of the problem is that optimal timing of measurements has not been clearly established. In addition, data are limited on associations between novel biomarkers and cancer-therapy-related cardiotoxicity.

For now, the use of combinations of biomarkers (particularly troponin and BNP/pro-BNP), added to LV GLS assessment by STE—particularly when interpreted

TABLE 10.3 Markers Associated With Cardiotoxicity in Breast-Cancer Patients, and Strength of Evidence

Markers	Strength of Evidence on Radiotherapy[a]	Strength of Evidence on Chemotherapy[b]	Strength of Overall Evidence[c]
GLS[d]	+++++ (5)	+++++ (6)	+++++
Troponin-I[e]	+++ (5)	+++ (20)	+++
Troponin-T[e]	++ (3)	+++ (18)	+++
BNP[e]	+++++ (5)	++++ (8)	+++++
NT-pro-BNP[e]	++++ (3)	++++ (25)	++++

The numbers in parenthesis represent the number of articles providing each strength of evidence.
[a]Studies involved radiotherapy alone, or radiation plus anthracycline-based chemotherapy.
[b]Anthracycline-based (mostly doxorubicin) chemotherapy.
[c]Both chemotherapy and radiotherapy.
[d]Reduction in strain (not LV parameters) with chemotherapy or radiation therapy.
[e]Strength of evidence calculated based on fraction of studies showing significant associations between markers and parameters of LV dysfunction studied.

in the context of prior CVD/risk factors—hold reasonable promise in the early recognition of persons at risk for cardiotoxicity during therapy, and possibly into early survivorship years. However, the identification of these persons prior to cancer therapy, and well into the survivorship years remains to be fully determined. To this end, the role of genetics for the determination of persons at risk for cardiotoxicity because of cancer therapy is yet in its early phases, and deserves further investigation. With deeper understanding of the pathophysiology and genetic pathways, screening for genetic substrates could be integrated with established clinical and demographic factors to mitigate risk of developing cardiotoxicity associated with cancer therapy.

REFERENCES

[1] Hoyert DL. 75 years of mortality in the United States. NCHS Data Brief 1935–2010;2012:1–8.

[2] Kochanek KD, Murphy SL, Xu J, Arias E. Mortality in the United States. NCHS Data Brief 2013;2014:1–8.

[3] Howlader N NA, Krapcho M, Garshell J, Neyman N, Altekruse SF, Kosary CL, Yu M, Ruhl J, Tatalovich Z, Cho H, Mariotto A, Lewis DR, Chen HS, Feuer EJ, Cronin KA. SEER Cancer Statistics Review, 1975–2010. Bethesda, MD: National Cancer Institute; 2015. Based on November 2012 SEER data submission.

[4] Mertens AC, Liu Q, Neglia JP, Wasilewski K, Leisenring W, Armstrong GT, Robison LL, Yasui Y. Cause-specific late mortality among 5-year survivors of childhood cancer: the Childhood Cancer Survivor Study. J Natl Cancer Inst 2008;100:1368–79.

[5] Patnaik JL, Byers T, DiGuiseppi C, Dabelea D, Denberg TD. Cardiovascular disease competes with breast cancer as the leading cause of death for older females diagnosed with breast cancer: a retrospective cohort study. Breast Cancer Res 2011;13:R64.

[6] Armstrong GT, Liu Q, Yasui Y, Neglia JP, Leisenring W, Robison LL, Mertens AC. Late mortality among 5-year survivors of childhood cancer: a summary from the Childhood Cancer Survivor Study. J Clin Oncol 2009;27:2328–38.

[7] Menna P, Salvatorelli E, Minotti G. Cardiotoxicity of antitumor drugs. Chem Res Toxicol 2008;21:978–89.

[8] Schultz PN, Beck ML, Stava C, Vassilopoulou-Sellin R. Health profiles in 5836 long-term cancer survivors. Int J Cancer 2003;104: 488–95.

[9] Oeffinger KC, Mertens AC, Sklar CA, Kawashima T, Hudson MM, Meadows AT, Friedman DL, Marina N, Hobbie W, Kadan-Lottick NS, Schwartz CL, Leisenring W, Robison LL, Childhood Cancer Survivor S. Chronic health conditions in adult survivors of childhood cancer. New Engl J Med 2006;355:1572–82.

[10] Reulen RC, Winter DL, Frobisher C, Lancashire ER, Stiller CA, Jenney ME, Skinner R, Stevens MC, Hawkins MM. British Childhood Cancer Survivor Study Steering G. Long-term cause-specific mortality among survivors of childhood cancer. JAMA 2010;304:172–9.

[11] Cardinale D, Bacchiani G, Beggiato M, Colombo A, Cipolla CM. Strategies to prevent and treat cardiovascular risk in cancer patients. Semin Oncol 2013;40:186–98.

[12] Steinherz LJ, Steinherz PG, Tan CT, Heller G, Murphy ML. Cardiac toxicity 4 to 20 years after completing anthracycline therapy. JAMA 1991;266:1672–7.

[13] Kilickap S, Akgul E, Aksoy S, Aytemir K, Barista I. Doxorubicin-induced second degree and complete atrioventricular block. Europace 2005;7:227–30.

[14] Ewer MS, Lippman SM. Type II chemotherapy-related cardiac dysfunction: time to recognize a new entity. J Clin Oncol 2005;23: 2900–2.

[15] Lancellotti P, Nkomo VT, Badano LP, Bergler J, Bogaert J, Davin L, Cosyns B, Coucke P, Dulgheru R, Edvardsen T, Gaemperli O, Galderisi M, Griffin B, Heidenreich PA, Nieman K, Plana JC, Port SC, Scherrer-Crosbie M, Schwartz RG, Sebag IA, Voigt JU, Wann S, Yang PC. European Society of Cardiology Working Groups on Nuclear C., Cardiac Computed T., Cardiovascular Magnetic R., American Society of Nuclear Cardiology SfCMR and Society of Cardiovascular Computed Tomography. Expert consensus for multimodality imaging evaluation of cardiovascular complications of radiotherapy in adults: a report from the European Association of Cardiovascular Imaging and the American Society of Echocardiography. J Am Soc Echocardiogr 2013;26:1013–32.

[16] Lloyd-Jones DM, Liu K, Colangelo LA, Yan LL, Klein L, Loria CM, Lewis CE, Savage P. Consistently stable or decreased body mass index in young adulthood and longitudinal changes in metabolic syndrome components: the Coronary Artery Risk Development in Young Adults Study. Circulation 2007;115:1004–11.

[17] Malik S, Wong ND, Franklin SS, Kamath TV, L'Italien GJ, Pio JR, Williams GR. Impact of the metabolic syndrome on mortality from coronary heart disease, cardiovascular disease, and all causes in United States adults. Circulation 2004;110:1245–50.

[18] Hunt KJ, Resendez RG, Williams K, Haffner SM, Stern MP, San Antonio Heart S. National Cholesterol Education Program versus World Health Organization metabolic syndrome in relation to all-cause and cardiovascular mortality in the San Antonio Heart Study. Circulation 2004;110:1251–7.

[19] Bhaskaran K, Douglas I, Forbes H, dos-Santos-Silva I, Leon DA, Smeeth L. Body-mass index and risk of 22 specific cancers: a population-based cohort study of 5.24 million UK adults. Lancet 2014;384:755–65.

[20] How tobacco smoke causes disease: the biology and behavioral basis for smoking-attributable disease. Atlanta, GA: Centers for Disease Control and Prevention; 2010. A Report of the Surgeon General.

[21] Bjartveit K, Tverdal A. Health consequences of smoking 1–4 cigarettes per day. Tob Control 2005;14:315–20.

[22] De Stefani E, Boffetta P, Carzoglio J, Mendilaharsu S, Deneo-Pellegrini H. Tobacco smoking and alcohol drinking as risk factors for stomach cancer: a case-control study in Uruguay. Cancer Causes Control 1998;9:321–9.

[23] Coughlin SS, Calle EE, Patel AV, Thun MJ. Predictors of pancreatic cancer mortality among a large cohort of United States adults. Cancer Causes Control 2000;11:915–23.

[24] Barnoya J, Glantz SA. Cardiovascular effects of secondhand smoke: nearly as large as smoking. Circulation 2005;111:2684–98.

[25] Schane RE, Ling PM, Glantz SA. Health effects of light and intermittent smoking: a review. Circulation 2010;121:1518–22.

[26] Warburton DE, Nicol CW, Bredin SS. Health benefits of physical activity: the evidence. CMAJ 2006;174:801–9.

[27] Friedenreich CM, Neilson HK, Lynch BM. State of the epidemiological evidence on physical activity and cancer prevention. Eur J Cancer 2010;46:2593–604.

[28] Harriss DJ, Atkinson G, George K, Cable NT, Reilly T, Haboubi N, Zwahlen M, Egger M, Renehan AG. and group CC. Lifestyle factors

and colorectal cancer risk (1): systematic review and meta-analysis of associations with body mass index. Colorectal Dis 2009;11:547–63.

[29] Cong YJ, Gan Y, Sun HL, Deng J, Cao SY, Xu X, Lu ZX. Association of sedentary behaviour with colon and rectal cancer: a meta-analysis of observational studies. Brit J Cancer 2014;110:817–26.

[30] Fraser GE. Associations between diet and cancer, ischemic heart disease, and all-cause mortality in non-Hispanic white California Seventh-day Adventists. Am J Clin Nutr 1999;70:532S–8S.

[31] Aune D, Chan DS, Lau R, Vieira R, Greenwood DC, Kampman E, Norat T. Dietary fibre, whole grains, and risk of colorectal cancer: systematic review and dose-response meta-analysis of prospective studies. BMJ 2011;343:d6617.

[32] Heikkila K, Harris R, Lowe G, Rumley A, Yarnell J, Gallacher J, Ben-Shlomo Y, Ebrahim S, Lawlor DA. Associations of circulating C-reactive protein and interleukin-6 with cancer risk: findings from two prospective cohorts and a meta-analysis. Cancer Causes Control 2009;20:15–26.

[33] Pradhan AD, Manson JE, Rossouw JE, Siscovick DS, Mouton CP, Rifai N, Wallace RB, Jackson RD, Pettinger MB, Ridker PM. Inflammatory biomarkers, hormone replacement therapy, and incident coronary heart disease: prospective analysis from the Women's Health Initiative observational study. JAMA 2002;288:980–7.

[34] Bruzzo J, Chiarella P, Fernandez G, Bustuoabad OD, Ruggiero RA. Systemic inflammation and experimental cancer in a murine model. Medicina (B Aires) 2007;67:469–74.

[35] Tarhini AA, Lin Y, Yeku O, LaFramboise WA, Ashraf M, Sander C, Lee S, Kirkwood JM. A four-marker signature of TNF-RII, TGF-alpha. TIMP-1 and CRP is prognostic of worse survival in high-risk surgically resected melanoma. J Transl Med 2014;12:19.

[36] Malle E, Sodin-Semrl S, Kovacevic A. Serum amyloid A: an acute-phase protein involved in tumour pathogenesis. Cell Mol Life Sci 2009;66:9–26.

[37] Bowles EJ, Wellman R, Feigelson HS, Onitilo AA, Freedman AN, Delate T, Allen LA, Nekhlyudov L, Goddard KA, Davis RL, Habel LA, Yood MU, McCarty C, Magid DJ, Wagner EH, Pharmacovigilance Study T. Risk of heart failure in breast cancer patients after anthracycline and trastuzumab treatment: a retrospective cohort study. J Natl Cancer Inst 2012;104:1293–305.

[38] Cardinale D, Colombo A, Lamantia G, Colombo N, Civelli M, De Giacomi G, Rubino M, Veglia F, Fiorentini C, Cipolla CM. Anthracycline-induced cardiomyopathy: clinical relevance and response to pharmacologic therapy. J Am Coll Cardiol 2010;55:213–20.

[39] Otterstad JE, Froeland G, St John Sutton M, Holme I. Accuracy and reproducibility of biplane two-dimensional echocardiographic measurements of left ventricular dimensions and function. Eur Heart J 1997;18:507–13.

[40] Tassan-Mangina S, Codorean D, Metivier M, Costa B, Himberlin C, Jouannaud C, Blaise AM, Elaerts J, Nazeyrollas P. Tissue Doppler imaging and conventional echocardiography after anthracycline treatment in adults: early and late alterations of left ventricular function during a prospective study. Eur J Echocardiogr 2006;7:141–6.

[41] Neilan TG, Jassal DS, Perez-Sanz TM, Raher MJ, Pradhan AD, Buys ES, Ichinose F, Bayne DB, Halpern EF, Weyman AE, Derumeaux G, Bloch KD, Picard MH, Scherrer-Crosbie M. Tissue Doppler imaging predicts left ventricular dysfunction and mortality in a murine model of cardiac injury. Eur Heart J 2006;27:1868–75.

[42] Sawaya H, Sebag IA, Plana JC, Januzzi JL, Ky B, Tan TC, Cohen V, Banchs J, Carver JR, Wiegers SE, Martin RP, Picard MH, Gersten RE, Halpern EF, Passeri J, Kuter I, Scherrer-Crosbie M. Assessment of echocardiography and biomarkers for the extended prediction of cardiotoxicity in patients treated with anthracyclines, taxanes, and trastuzumab. Circ Cardiovasc Imaging 2012;5:596–603.

[43] Stoodley PW, Richards DA, Boyd A, Hui R, Harnett PR, Meikle SR, Byth K, Stuart K, Clarke JL, Thomas L. Left ventricular systolic function in HER2/neu negative breast cancer patients treated with anthracycline chemotherapy: a comparative analysis of left ventricular ejection fraction and myocardial strain imaging over 12 months. Eur J Cancer 2013;49:3396–403.

[44] Hare JL, Brown JK, Leano R, Jenkins C, Woodward N, Marwick TH. Use of myocardial deformation imaging to detect preclinical myocardial dysfunction before conventional measures in patients undergoing breast cancer treatment with trastuzumab. Am Heart J 2009;158:294–301.

[45] Brown J, Jenkins C, Marwick TH. Use of myocardial strain to assess global left ventricular function: a comparison with cardiac magnetic resonance and 3-dimensional echocardiography. Am Heart J 2009;157. 102 e1–e5.

[46] Fallah-Rad N, Walker JR, Wassef A, Lytwyn M, Bohonis S, Fang T, Tian G, Kirkpatrick ID, Singal PK, Krahn M, Grenier D, Jassal DS. The utility of cardiac biomarkers, tissue velocity and strain imaging, and cardiac magnetic resonance imaging in predicting early left ventricular dysfunction in patients with human epidermal growth factor receptor II-positive breast cancer treated with adjuvant trastuzumab therapy. J Am Coll Cardiol 2011;57:2263–70.

[47] Drafts BC, Twomley KM, D'Agostino R Jr, Lawrence J, Avis N, Ellis LR, Thohan V, Jordan J, Melin SA, Torti FM, Little WC, Hamilton CA, Hundley WG. Low to moderate dose anthracycline-based chemotherapy is associated with early noninvasive imaging evidence of subclinical cardiovascular disease. JACC Cardiovasc Imaging 2013;6:877–85.

[48] Neilan TG, Coelho-Filho OR, Pena-Herrera D, Shah RV, Jerosch-Herold M, Francis SA, Moslehi J, Kwong RY. Left ventricular mass in patients with a cardiomyopathy after treatment with anthracyclines. Am J Cardiol 2012;110:1679–86.

[49] Lawley C, Wainwright C, Segelov E, Lynch J, Beith J, McCrohon J. Pilot study evaluating the role of cardiac magnetic resonance imaging in monitoring adjuvant trastuzumab therapy for breast cancer. Asia Pac J Clin Oncol 2012;8:95–100.

[50] Wadhwa D, Fallah-Rad N, Grenier D, Krahn M, Fang T, Ahmadie R, Walker JR, Lister D, Arora RC, Barac I, Morris A, Jassal DS. Trastuzumab mediated cardiotoxicity in the setting of adjuvant chemotherapy for breast cancer: a retrospective study. Breast Cancer Res Treat 2009;117:357–64.

[51] Neilan TG, Coelho-Filho OR, Shah RV, Feng JH, Pena-Herrera D, Mandry D, Pierre-Mongeon F, Heydari B, Francis SA, Moslehi J, Kwong RY, Jerosch-Herold M. Myocardial extracellular volume by cardiac magnetic resonance imaging in patients treated with anthracycline-based chemotherapy. Am J Cardiol 2013;111:717–22.

[52] Wassmuth R, Lentzsch S, Erdbruegger U, Schulz-Menger J, Doerken B, Dietz R, Friedrich MG. Subclinical cardiotoxic effects of anthracyclines as assessed by magnetic resonance imaging-a pilot study. Am Heart J 2001;141:1007–13.

[53] Lipshultz SE, Miller TL, Scully RE, Lipsitz SR, Rifai N, Silverman LB, Colan SD, Neuberg DS, Dahlberg SE, Henkel JM, Asselin BL, Athale UH, Clavell LA, Laverdiere C, Michon B, Schorin MA, Sallan SE. Changes in cardiac biomarkers during doxorubicin treatment of pediatric patients with high-risk acute lymphoblastic leukemia: associations with long-term echocardiographic outcomes. J Clin Oncol 2012;30:1042–9.

[54] Mavinkurve-Groothuis AM, Marcus KA, Pourier M, Loonen J, Feuth T, Hoogerbrugge PM, de Korte CL, Kapusta L. Myocardial 2D strain echocardiography and cardiac biomarkers in children during and shortly after anthracycline therapy for acute lymphoblastic leukaemia (ALL): a prospective study. Eur Heart J Cardiovasc Imaging 2013;14:562–9.

[55] Goel S, Simes RJ, Beith JM. Exploratory analysis of cardiac biomarkers in women with normal cardiac function receiving trastuzumab for breast cancer. Asia Pac J Clin Oncol 2011;7:276–80.

[56] Pongprot Y, Sittiwangkul R, Charoenkwan P, Silvilairat S. Use of cardiac markers for monitoring of doxorubixin-induced cardiotoxicity in children with cancer. J Pediatr Hematol Oncol 2012;34:589–95.

[57] D'Errico MP, Grimaldi L, Petruzzelli MF, Gianicolo EA, Tramacere F, Monetti A, Placella R, Pili G, Andreassi MG, Sicari R, Picano E, Portaluri M. N-terminal pro-B-type natriuretic peptide plasma levels as a potential biomarker for cardiac damage after radiotherapy in patients with left-sided breast cancer. Int J Radiat Oncol Biol Phys 2012;82:e239–46.

[58] Roziakova L, Bojtarova E, Mistrik M, Dubrava J, Gergel J, Lenkova N, Mladosievicova B. Serial measurements of cardiac biomarkers in patients after allogeneic hematopoietic stem cell transplantation. J Exp Clin Cancer Res 2012;31:13.

[59] O'Brien PJ. Cardiac troponin is the most effective translational safety biomarker for myocardial injury in cardiotoxicity. Toxicology 2008;245:206–18.

[60] Cardinale D, Sandri MT, Martinoni A, Tricca A, Civelli M, Lamantia G, Cinieri S, Martinelli G, Cipolla CM, Fiorentini C. Left ventricular dysfunction predicted by early troponin I release after high-dose chemotherapy. J Am Coll Cardiol 2000;36:517–22.

[61] Cardinale D, Colombo A, Torrisi R, Sandri MT, Civelli M, Salvatici M, Lamantia G, Colombo N, Cortinovis S, Dessanai MA, Nole F, Veglia F, Cipolla CM. Trastuzumab-induced cardiotoxicity: clinical and prognostic implications of troponin I evaluation. J Clin Oncol 2010;28:3910–6.

[62] Morris PG, Chen C, Steingart R, Fleisher M, Lin N, Moy B, Come S, Sugarman S, Abbruzzi A, Lehman R, Patil S, Dickler M, McArthur HL, Winer E, Norton L, Hudis CA, Dang CT. Troponin I and C-reactive protein are commonly detected in patients with breast cancer treated with dose-dense chemotherapy incorporating trastuzumab and lapatinib. Clin Cancer Res 2011;17:3490–9.

[63] Schmidinger M, Zielinski CC, Vogl UM, Bojic A, Bojic M, Schukro C, Ruhsam M, Hejna M, Schmidinger H. Cardiac toxicity of sunitinib and sorafenib in patients with metastatic renal cell carcinoma. J Clin Oncol 2008;26:5204–12.

[64] Dodos F, Halbsguth T, Erdmann E, Hoppe UC. Usefulness of myocardial performance index and biochemical markers for early detection of anthracycline-induced cardiotoxicity in adults. Clin Res Cardiol 2008;97:318–26.

[65] Sawaya H, Sebag IA, Plana JC, Januzzi JL, Ky B, Cohen V, Gosavi S, Carver JR, Wiegers SE, Martin RP, Picard MH, Gerszten RE, Halpern EF, Passeri J, Kuter I, Scherrer-Crosbie M. Early detection and prediction of cardiotoxicity in chemotherapy-treated patients. Am J Cardiol 2011;107:1375–80.

[66] Daugaard G, Lassen U, Bie P, Pedersen EB, Jensen KT, Abildgaard U, Hesse B, Kjaer A. Natriuretic peptides in the monitoring of anthracycline induced reduction in left ventricular ejection fraction. Eur J Heart Failure 2005;7:87–93.

[67] Hayakawa H, Komada Y, Hirayama M, Hori H, Ito M, Sakurai M. Plasma levels of natriuretic peptides in relation to doxorubicin-induced cardiotoxicity and cardiac function in children with cancer. Med Pediatr Oncol 2001;37:4–9.

[68] Armenian SH, Gelehrter SK, Vase T, Venkatramani R, Landier W, Wilson KD, Herrera C, Reichman L, Menteer JD, Mascarenhas L, Freyer DR, Venkataraman K, Bhatia S. Screening for cardiac dysfunction in anthracycline-exposed childhood cancer survivors. Clin Cancer Res 2014;20(24):6314–23.

[69] Elbl L, Vasova I, Navratil M, Vorlicek J, Malaskova L, Spinar J. Comparison of plasmatic levels of B-natriuretic peptide with echocardiographic indicators of left ventricle function after doxorubicin therapy. Vnitr Lek 2006;52:563–70.

[70] Feola M, Garrone O, Occelli M, Francini A, Biggi A, Visconti G, Albrile F, Bobbio M, Merlano M. Cardiotoxicity after anthracycline chemotherapy in breast carcinoma: effects on left ventricular ejection fraction, troponin I and brain natriuretic peptide. Int J Cardiol 2011;148:194–8.

[71] Okumura H, Iuchi K, Yoshida T, Nakamura S, Takeshima M, Takamatsu H, Ikeno A, Usuda K, Ishikawa T, Ohtake S, Matsuda T. Brain natriuretic peptide is a predictor of anthracycline-induced cardiotoxicity. Acta Haematol 2000;104:158–63.

[72] Pichon MF, Cvitkovic F, Hacene K, Delaunay J, Lokiec F, Collignon MA, Pecking AP. Drug-induced cardiotoxicity studied by longitudinal B-type natriuretic peptide assays and radionuclide ventriculography. In Vivo 2005;19:567–76.

[73] Skovgaard D, Hasbak P, Kjaer A. BNP predicts chemotherapy-related cardiotoxicity and death: comparison with gated equilibrium radionuclide ventriculography. PloS One 2014;9:e96736.

[74] Soker M, Kervancioglu M. Plasma concentrations of NT-pro-BNP and cardiac troponin-I in relation to doxorubicin-induced cardiomyopathy and cardiac function in childhood malignancy. Saudi Med J 2005;26:1197–202.

[75] Tragiannidis A, Dokos C, Tsotoulidou V, Giannopoulos A, Pana ZD, Papageorgiou T, Karamouzis M, Athanassiadou F. Brain natriuretic peptide as a cardiotoxicity biomarker in children with hematological malignancies. Minerva Pediatr 2012;64:307–12.

[76] Gimeno E, Gomez M, Gonzalez JR, Comin J, Alvarez-Larran A, Sanchez-Gonzalez B, Molina L, Domingo-Domenech E, Garcia-Pallarols F, Pedro C, Abella E, Vilaplana C, de Sanjose S, Besses C, Salar A. NT-proBNP: a cardiac biomarker to assess prognosis in non-Hodgkin lymphoma. Leuk Res 2011;35:715–20.

[77] Tarantini L, Cioffi G, Di Lenarda A, Valle R, Pulignano G, Del Sindaco D, Frigo G, Soravia G, Tessier R, Catania G. Screening for asymptomatic left ventricular systolic dysfunction in high-risk patients. Preliminary experience with a program based on the use of ECG and natriuretic peptide. G Ital Cardiol (Rome) 2008;9:835–43.

[78] Roziakova L, Bojtarova E, Mistrik M, Krajcovicova I, Mladosievicova B. Abnormal cardiomarkers in leukemia patients treated with allogeneic hematopoietic stem cell transplantation. Bratisl Lek Listy 2012;113:159–62.

[79] Horacek JM, Tichy M, Jebavy L, Pudil R, Ulrychova M, Maly J. Use of multiple biomarkers for evaluation of anthracycline-induced cardiotoxicity in patients with acute myeloid leukemia. Exp Oncol 2008;30:157–9.

[80] Horacek JM, Tichy M, Pudil R, Jebavy L. Glycogen phosphorylase BB could be a new circulating biomarker for detection of anthracycline cardiotoxicity. Ann Oncol 2008;19:1656–7.

[81] Horacek JM, Vasatova M, Pudil R, Tichy M, Zak P, Jakl M, Jebavy L, Maly J. Biomarkers for the early detection of anthracycline-induced

cardiotoxicity: current status. Olomouc, Czechoslovakia: Biomedical papers of the Medical Faculty of the University Palacky; 2014.

[82] Ozturk G, Tavil B, Ozguner M, Ginis Z, Erden G, Tunc B, Azik MF, Uckan D, Delibas N. Evaluation of cardiac markers in children undergoing hematopoietic stem cell transplantation. J Clin Lab Anal 2014;29(4):259–62.

[83] Pavo N, Raderer M, Hulsmann M, Neuhold S, Adlbrecht C, Strunk G, Goliasch G, Gisslinger H, Steger GG, Hejna M, Kostler W, Zochbauer-Muller S, Marosi C, Kornek G, Auerbach L, Schneider S, Parschalk B, Scheithauer W, Pirker R, Drach J, Zielinski C, Pacher R. Cardiovascular biomarkers in patients with cancer and their association with all-cause mortality. Heart 2015;101:1874–80.

[84] Ky B, Putt M, Sawaya H, French B, Januzzi JL Jr, Sebag IA, Plana JC, Cohen V, Banchs J, Carver JR, Wiegers SE, Martin RP, Picard MH, Gerszten RE, Halpern EF, Passeri J, Kuter I, Scherrer-Crosbie M. Early increases in multiple biomarkers predict subsequent cardiotoxicity in patients with breast cancer treated with doxorubicin, taxanes, and trastuzumab. J Am Coll Cardiol 2014;63:809–16.

[85] Putt M, Hahn VS, Januzzi JL, Sawaya H, Sebag IA, Plana JC, Picard MH, Carver JR, Halpern EF, Kuter I, Passeri J, Cohen V, Banchs J, Martin RP, Gerszten RE, Scherrer-Crosbie M, Ky B. Longitudinal changes in multiple biomarkers are associated with cardiotoxicity in breast cancer patients treated with doxorubicin, taxanes, and trastuzumab. Clin Chem 2015;61:1164–72.

[86] van Boxtel W, Bulten BF, Mavinkurve-Groothuis AM, Bellersen L, Mandigers CM, Joosten LA, Kapusta L, de Geus-Oei LF, van Laarhoven HW. New biomarkers for early detection of cardiotoxicity after treatment with docetaxel, doxorubicin and cyclophosphamide. Biomarkers 2015;20:143–8.

[87] Vasti C, Hertig CM. Neuregulin-1/erbB activities with focus on the susceptibility of the heart to anthracyclines. World J Cardiol 2014;6:653–62.

[88] Wang X, Liu W, Sun CL, Armenian SH, Hakonarson H, Hageman L, Ding Y, Landier W, Blanco JG, Chen L, Quinones A, Ferguson D, Winick N, Ginsberg JP, Keller F, Neglia JP, Desai S, Sklar CA, Castellino SM, Cherrick I, Dreyer ZE, Hudson MM, Robison LL, Yasui Y, Relling MV, Bhatia S. Hyaluronan synthase 3 variant and anthracycline-related cardiomyopathy: a report from the children's oncology group. J Clin Oncol 2014;32:647–53.

[89] Visscher H, Ross CJ, Rassekh SR, Barhdadi A, Dube MP, Al-Saloos H, Sandor GS, Caron HN, van Dalen EC, Kremer LC, van der Pal HJ, Brown AM, Rogers PC, Phillips MS, Rieder MJ, Carleton BC, Hayden MR. Canadian Pharmacogenomics Network for Drug Safety Consortium. Pharmacogenomic prediction of anthracycline-induced cardiotoxicity in children. J Clin Oncol 2012;30:1422–8.

[90] Jensen BC, McLeod HL. Pharmacogenomics as a risk mitigation strategy for chemotherapeutic cardiotoxicity. Pharmacogenomics 2013;14:205–13.

[91] Beauclair S, Formento P, Fischel JL, Lescaut W, Largillier R, Chamorey E, Hofman P, Ferrero JM, Pages G, Milano G. Role of the HER2 [Ile655Val] genetic polymorphism in tumorogenesis and in the risk of trastuzumab-related cardiotoxicity. Ann Oncol 2007;18:1335–41.

[92] Lemieux J, Diorio C, Cote MA, Provencher L, Barabe F, Jacob S, St-Pierre C, Demers E, Tremblay-Lemay R, Nadeau-Larochelle C, Michaud A, Laflamme C. Alcohol and HER2 polymorphisms as risk factor for cardiotoxicity in breast cancer treated with trastuzumab. Anticancer Res 2013;33:2569–76.

[93] Volkova M, Russell R 3rd. Anthracycline cardiotoxicity: prevalence, pathogenesis and treatment. Curr Cardiol Rev 2011;7:214–20.

[94] Shapiro CL, Hardenbergh PH, Gelman R, Blanks D, Hauptman P, Recht A, Hayes DF, Harris J, Henderson IC. Cardiac effects of adjuvant doxorubicin and radiation therapy in breast cancer patients. J Clin Oncol 1998;16:3493–501.

[95] Lipshultz SE, Colan SD, Gelber RD, Perez-Atayde AR, Sallan SE, Sanders SP. Late cardiac effects of doxorubicin therapy for acute lymphoblastic leukemia in childhood. New Engl J Med 1991;324:808–15.

[96] Swain SM, Whaley FS, Ewer MS. Congestive heart failure in patients treated with doxorubicin: a retrospective analysis of three trials. Cancer 2003;97:2869–79.

[97] Von Hoff DD, Layard MW, Basa P, Davis HL Jr, Von Hoff AL, Rozencweig M, Muggia FM. Risk factors for doxorubicin-induced congestive heart failure. Ann Intern Med 1979;91:710–7.

[98] Lipshultz SE, Lipsitz SR, Mone SM, Goorin AM, Sallan SE, Sanders SP, Orav EJ, Gelber RD, Colan SD. Female sex and drug dose as risk factors for late cardiotoxic effects of doxorubicin therapy for childhood cancer. New Engl J Med 1995;332:1738–43.

[99] Hershman DL, McBride RB, Eisenberger A, Tsai WY, Grann VR, Jacobson JS. Doxorubicin, cardiac risk factors, and cardiac toxicity in elderly patients with diffuse B-cell non-Hodgkin's lymphoma. J Clin Oncol 2008;26:3159–65.

[100] Pinder MC, Duan Z, Goodwin JS, Hortobagyi GN, Giordano SH. Congestive heart failure in older women treated with adjuvant anthracycline chemotherapy for breast cancer. J Clin Oncol 2007;25:3808–15.

[101] Harake D, Franco VI, Henkel JM, Miller TL, Lipshultz SE. Cardiotoxicity in childhood cancer survivors: strategies for prevention and management. Future Cardiol 2012;8:647–70.

[102] Giordano SH, Booser DJ, Murray JL, Ibrahim NK, Rahman ZU, Valero V, Theriault RL, Rosales MF, Rivera E, Frye D, Ewer M, Ordonez NG, Buzdar AU, Hortobagyi GN. A detailed evaluation of cardiac toxicity: a phase II study of doxorubicin and one- or three-hour-infusion paclitaxel in patients with metastatic breast cancer. Clin Cancer Res 2002;8:3360–8.

[103] Chen J, Long JB, Hurria A, Owusu C, Steingart RM, Gross CP. Incidence of heart failure or cardiomyopathy after adjuvant trastuzumab therapy for breast cancer. J Am Coll Cardiol 2012;60:2504–12.

[104] Slamon DJ, Leyland-Jones B, Shak S, Fuchs H, Paton V, Bajamonde A, Fleming T, Eiermann W, Wolter J, Pegram M, Baselga J, Norton L. Use of chemotherapy plus a monoclonal antibody against HER2 for metastatic breast cancer that overexpresses HER2. New Engl J Med 2001;344:783–92.

[105] Perez EA, Suman VJ, Davidson NE, Kaufman PA, Martino S, Dakhil SR, Ingle JN, Rodeheffer RJ, Gersh BJ, Jaffe AS. Effect of doxorubicin plus cyclophosphamide on left ventricular ejection fraction in patients with breast cancer in the North Central Cancer Treatment Group N9831 Intergroup Adjuvant Trial. J Clin Oncol 2004;22:3700–4.

[106] Legha SS, Benjamin RS, Mackay B, Ewer M, Wallace S, Valdivieso M, Rasmussen SL, Blumenschein GR, Freireich EJ. Reduction of doxorubicin cardiotoxicity by prolonged continuous intravenous infusion. Ann Int Med 1982;96:133–9.

[107] Cardinale D, Colombo A, Bacchiani G, Tedeschi I, Meroni CA, Veglia F, Civelli M, Lamantia G, Colombo N, Curigliano G, Fiorentini C, Cipolla CM. Early detection of anthracycline cardiotoxicity and improvement with heart failure therapy. Circulation 2015;131:1981–8.

[108] Onitilo AA, Engel JM, Stankowski RV. Cardiovascular toxicity associated with adjuvant trastuzumab therapy: prevalence, patient characteristics, and risk factors. Ther Adv Drug Saf 2014;5: 154–66.

[109] Moja L, Tagliabue L, Balduzzi S, Parmelli E, Pistotti V, Guarneri V, D'Amico R. Trastuzumab containing regimens for early breast cancer. Cochrane Database Syst Rev 2012;4:CD006243.

[110] Zeglinski M, Ludke A, Jassal DS, Singal PK. Trastuzumab-induced cardiac dysfunction: a 'dual-hit'. Exp Clin Cardiol 2011;16:70–4.

[111] Barth AS, Zhang Y, Li T, Smith RR, Chimenti I, Terrovitis I, Davis DR, Kizana E, Ho AS, O'Rourke B, Wolff AC, Gerstenblith G, Marban E. Functional impairment of human resident cardiac stem cells by the cardiotoxic antineoplastic agent trastuzumab. Stem Cells Transl Med 2012;1:289–97.

[112] Seidman A, Hudis C, Pierri MK, Shak S, Paton V, Ashby M, Murphy M, Stewart SJ, Keefe D. Cardiac dysfunction in the trastuzumab clinical trials experience. J Clin Oncol 2002;20:1215–21.

[113] Farolfi A, Melegari E, Aquilina M, Scarpi E, Ibrahim T, Maltoni R, Sarti S, Cecconetto L, Pietri E, Ferrario C, Fedeli A, Faedi M, Nanni O, Frassineti GL, Amadori D, Rocca A. Trastuzumab-induced cardiotoxicity in early breast cancer patients: a retrospective study of possible risk and protective factors. Heart 2013;99:634–9.

[114] Russo G, Cioffi G, Di Lenarda A, Tuccia F, Bovelli D, Di Tano G, Alunni G, Gori S, Faggiano P, Tarantini L. Role of renal function on the development of cardiotoxicity associated with trastuzumab-based adjuvant chemotherapy for early breast cancer. Intern Emerg Med 2012;7:439–46.

[115] Cochet A, Quilichini G, Dygai-Cochet I, Touzery C, Toubeau M, Berriolo-Riedinger A, Coudert B, Cottin Y, Fumoleau P, Brunotte F. Baseline diastolic dysfunction as a predictive factor of trastuzumab-mediated cardiotoxicity after adjuvant anthracycline therapy in breast cancer. Breast Cancer Res Treat 2011;130:845–54.

[116] Serrano C, Cortes J, De Mattos-Arruda L, Bellet M, Gomez P, Saura C, Perez J, Vidal M, Munoz-Couselo E, Carreras MJ, Sanchez-Olle G, Tabernero J, Baselga J, Di Cosimo S. Trastuzumab-related cardiotoxicity in the elderly: a role for cardiovascular risk factors. Ann Oncol 2012;23:897–902.

[117] Tarantini L, Gori S, Faggiano P, Pulignano G, Simoncini E, Tuccia F, Ceccherini R, Bovelli D, Lestuzzi C, Cioffi G, Network I. Adjuvant trastuzumab cardiotoxicity in patients over 60 years of age with early breast cancer: a multicenter cohort analysis. Ann Oncol 2012;23:3058–63.

[118] Chavez-MacGregor M, Zhang N, Buchholz TA, Zhang Y, Niu J, Elting L, Smith BD, Hortobagyi GN, Giordano SH. Trastuzumab-related cardiotoxicity among older patients with breast cancer. J Clin Oncol 2013;31:4222–8.

[119] Romond EH, Jeong JH, Rastogi P, Swain SM, Geyer CE Jr, Ewer MS, Rathi V, Fehrenbacher L, Brufsky A, Azar CA, Flynn PJ, Zapas JL, Polikoff J, Gross HM, Biggs DD, Atkins JN, Tan-Chiu E, Zheng P, Yothers G, Mamounas EP, Wolmark N. Seven-year follow-up assessment of cardiac function in NSABP B-31, a randomized trial comparing doxorubicin and cyclophosphamide followed by paclitaxel (ACP) with ACP plus trastuzumab as adjuvant therapy for patients with node-positive, human epidermal growth factor receptor 2-positive breast cancer. J Clin Oncol 2012;30:3792–9.

[120] Folkman J. Tumor angiogenesis: therapeutic implications. New Engl J Med 1971;285:1182–6.

[121] Brown LF, Berse B, Jackman RW, Tognazzi K, Manseau EJ, Dvorak HF, Senger DR. Increased expression of vascular permeability factor (vascular endothelial growth factor) and its receptors in kidney and bladder carcinomas. Am J Pathol 1993;143:1255–62.

[122] Mir O, Mouthon L, Alexandre J, Mallion JM, Deray G, Guillevin L, Goldwasser F. Bevacizumab-induced cardiovascular events: a consequence of cholesterol emboli syndrome? J Natl Cancer Inst 2007;99:85–6.

[123] Robinson ES, Khankin EV, Karumanchi SA, Humphreys BD. Hypertension induced by vascular endothelial growth factor signaling pathway inhibition: mechanisms and potential use as a biomarker. Semin Nephrol 2010;30:591–601.

[124] Ranpura V, Hapani S, Wu S. Treatment-related mortality with bevacizumab in cancer patients: a meta-analysis. JAMA 2011;305:487–94.

[125] Yeh ET, Bickford CL. Cardiovascular complications of cancer therapy: incidence, pathogenesis, diagnosis, and management. J Am Coll Cardiol 2009;53:2231–47.

[126] Rini BI, Cohen DP, Lu DR, Chen I, Hariharan S, Gore ME, Figlin RA, Baum MS, Motzer RJ. Hypertension as a biomarker of efficacy in patients with metastatic renal cell carcinoma treated with sunitinib. J Natl Cancer Inst 2011;103:763–73.

[127] Heba G, Krzeminski T, Porc M, Grzyb J, Ratajska A, Dembinska-Kiec A. The time course of tumor necrosis factor-alpha, inducible nitric oxide synthase and vascular endothelial growth factor expression in an experimental model of chronic myocardial infarction in rats. J Vasc Res 2001;38:288–300.

[128] Chu TF, Rupnick MA, Kerkela R, Dallabrida SM, Zurakowski D, Nguyen L, Woulfe K, Pravda E, Cassiola F, Desai J, George S, Morgan JA, Harris DM, Ismail NS, Chen JH, Schoen FJ, Van den Abbeele AD, Demetri GD, Force T, Chen MH. Cardiotoxicity associated with tyrosine kinase inhibitor sunitinib. Lancet 2007;370:2011–9.

[129] Bello CL, Mulay M, Huang X, Patyna S, Dinolfo M, Levine S, Van Vugt A, Toh M, Baum C, Rosen L. Electrocardiographic characterization of the QTc interval in patients with advanced solid tumors: pharmacokinetic- pharmacodynamic evaluation of sunitinib. Clin Cancer Res 2009;15:7045–52.

[130] Bagnes C, Panchuk PN, Recondo G. Antineoplastic chemotherapy induced QTc prolongation. Curr Drug Saf 2010;5:93–6.

[131] Clarke M, Collins R, Darby S, Davies C, Elphinstone P, Evans E, Godwin J, Gray R, Hicks C, James S, MacKinnon E, McGale P, McHugh T, Peto R, Taylor C, Wang Y. Early Breast Cancer Trialists' Collaborative Group (EBCTCG). Effects of radiotherapy and of differences in the extent of surgery for early breast cancer on local recurrence and 15-year survival: an overview of the randomised trials. Lancet 2005;366:2087–106.

[132] Darby S, McGale P, Correa C, Taylor C, Arriagada R, Clarke M, Cutter D, Davies C, Ewertz M, Godwin J, Gray R, Pierce L, Whelan T, Wang Y, Peto R. Early Breast Cancer Trialists' Collaborative Group (EBCTCG). Effect of radiotherapy after breast-conserving surgery on 10-year recurrence and 15-year breast cancer death: meta-analysis of individual patient data for 10,801 women in 17 randomised trials. Lancet 2011;378:1707–16.

[133] Darby SC, McGale P, Taylor CW, Peto R. Long-term mortality from heart disease and lung cancer after radiotherapy for early breast cancer: prospective cohort study of about 300,000 women in US SEER cancer registries. Lancet Oncol 2005;6:557–65.

[134] Roychoudhuri R, Robinson D, Putcha V, Cuzick J, Darby S, Moller H. Increased cardiovascular mortality more than fifteen years after radiotherapy for breast cancer: a population-based study. BMC Cancer 2007;7:9.

[135] Darby SC, Ewertz M, Hall P. Ischemic heart disease after breast cancer radiotherapy. New Engl J Med 2013;368:2527.

[136] Heidenreich PA, Schnittger I, Strauss HW, Vagelos RH, Lee BK, Mariscal CS, Tate DJ, Horning SJ, Hoppe RT, Hancock SL. Screening for coronary artery disease after mediastinal irradiation for Hodgkin's disease. J Clin Oncol 2007;25:43–9.

[137] Carver JR, Shapiro CL, Ng A, Jacobs L, Schwartz C, Virgo KS, Hagerty KL, Somerfield MR, Vaughn DJ. Panel ACSE. American Society of Clinical Oncology clinical evidence review on the ongoing care of adult cancer survivors: cardiac and pulmonary late effects. J Clin Oncol 2007;25:3991–4008.

[138] Darby SC, Cutter DJ, Boerma M, Constine LS, Fajardo LF, Kodama K, Mabuchi K, Marks LB, Mettler FA, Pierce LJ, Trott KR, Yeh ET, Shore RE. Radiation-related heart disease: current knowledge and future prospects. Int J Radiat Oncol Biol Phys 2010;76:656–65.

[139] Hancock SL, Tucker MA, Hoppe RT. Factors affecting late mortality from heart disease after treatment of Hodgkin's disease. JAMA 1993;270:1949–55.

[140] Lee CK, Aeppli D, Nierengarten ME. The need for long-term surveillance for patients treated with curative radiotherapy for Hodgkin's disease: University of Minnesota experience. Int J Radiat Oncol Biol Phys 2000;48:169–79.

[141] Swerdlow AJ, Higgins CD, Smith P, Cunningham D, Hancock BW, Horwich A, Hoskin PJ, Lister A, Radford JA, Rohatiner AZ, Linch DC. Myocardial infarction mortality risk after treatment for Hodgkin disease: a collaborative British cohort study. J Natl Cancer Inst 2007;99:206–14.

[142] Hoppe RT. Hodgkin's disease: complications of therapy and excess mortality. Ann Oncol 1997;8(Suppl. 1):115–8.

[143] Hughes-Davies L, Sacks D, Rescigno J, Howard S, Harris J. Serum cardiac troponin T levels during treatment of early-stage breast cancer. J Clin Oncol 1995;13:2582–4.

[144] Kozak KR, Hong TS, Sluss PM, Lewandrowski EL, Aleryani SL, Macdonald SM, Choi NC, Yock TI. Cardiac blood biomarkers in patients receiving thoracic (chemo)radiation. Lung Cancer 2008;62:351–5.

[145] Nellessen U, Zingel M, Hecker H, Bahnsen J, Borschke D. Effects of radiation therapy on myocardial cell integrity and pump function: which role for cardiac biomarkers? Chemotherapy 2010;56:147–52.

[146] Skytta T, Tuohinen S, Boman E, Virtanen V, Raatikainen P, Kellokumpu-Lehtinen PL. Troponin T-release associates with cardiac radiation doses during adjuvant left-sided breast cancer radiotherapy. Radiat Oncol 2015;10:141.

[147] Palumbo I, Palumbo B, Fravolini ML, Marcantonini M, Perrucci E, Latini ME, Falcinelli L, Sabalich I, Tranfaglia C, Schillaci G, Mannarino E, Aristei C. Brain natriuretic peptide as a cardiac marker of transient radiotherapy-related damage in left-sided breast cancer patients: a prospective study. Breast 2015;25:45–50.

Chapter 11

Late Cardiac Effects in Childhood Cancer Survivors

S.E. Lipshultz*,**, N. Patel†, V.I. Franco* and S. Fisher†

*Department of Pediatrics, Wayne State University School of Medicine, Children's Hospital of Michigan, Detroit, MI, United States; **Karmanos Comprehensive Cancer Center, Detroit, MI, United States; †University of Maryland School of Medicine, Baltimore, MD, United States

INTRODUCTION

In the United States, the survival rate for children with cancer has increased to 83%, from 58% in the mid-1970s [1]. This success is the result, in part, to advances in treatment. However, treatments given at such a young age put survivors at a particularly vulnerable state for late adverse effects. Within the first 30 years after diagnosis, survivors of childhood cancers have an estimated 75% cumulative incidence of treatment-related chronic health problems [2]. In the United States, where 1 in 680 people between 20 and 50 years old are survivors of childhood cancer [3], the impact of long-term health consequences is concerning, particularly because this population is growing.

Some of the most common cancer drugs, such as the anthracyclines, are well known to be cardiotoxic. This cardiotoxicity is progressive and persistent if left untreated. It can lead to cardiomyopathy, clinical heart failure, the need for heart transplant, or death [4]. At 30 years after diagnosis, the number of cardiac-related deaths in survivors exceeds those caused by cancer recurrence [5]. Survivors also have a higher prevalence of cardiovascular events than that of healthy controls 5 years after diagnosis (Fig. 11.1). Furthermore, compared to controls, survivors are 15 times as likely to have heart failure [2], 10 times as likely to have coronary artery disease [2], 9 times as likely to have a cerebrovascular event [2], and 8 times as likely to die from cardiovascular-related disease [6].

This chapter summarizes what is known about the cardiotoxic effects of specific cancer treatments, their mechanisms or pathophysiology, risk factors and screening, and prevention and treatment.

ANTHRACYCLINE AND ANTHRACYCLINE-LIKE AGENTS

Among cancer therapies associated with adverse cardiac effects, the most well-known are the anthracyclines. Anthracycline cardiotoxicity can be acute or chronic. Acute cardiac effects occur within 1 week after beginning therapy and are less common. They include arrhythmias, ventricular dysfunction, pericarditis, and myocarditis, and are typically self-resolving [7]. Chronic progressive cardiac effects are more common and are divided into early-onset and late-onset. Early-onset effects occur less than 1 year after completing treatment, and late-onset effects occur more than 1 year later. Early-onset effects includes heart failure and, less commonly, pericardial effusion. Late-onset effects not only lead to long-term cardiac disease, they impair myocardial growth in children (Table 11.1) [8]. The most important cardiotoxic effects are associated with myocardial necrosis leading to long-term cardiomyopathy and heart failure.

Although the association between anthracyclines and cardiotoxicity is strong, its mechanisms remain unclear. A leading mechanism of cardiac insult from anthracyclines is likely related to oxidative stress and damage to cardiomyocytes [9]. Endomyocardial biopsy specimens show loss of myofibrils, distension of the sarcoplasmic reticulum, and vacuolization of the cytoplasm [7]. Doxorubicin itself can impair myocardial growth [10]. Interaction with topoisomerase 2-beta in cardiomyocytes, as opposed to topoisomerase 2-alpha, which is expressed in proliferating tumor cells and is a part of the therapeutic mechanism of anthracycline, is also a likely mechanism of its cardiac effects [11]. Radiation therapy and resulting endothelial damage potentiates the effects of anthracyclines. These patients are more likely

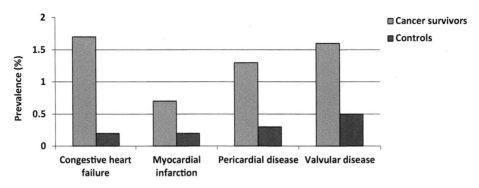

FIGURE 11.1 **Prevalence of cardiac conditions among 14,358, 5-year survivors of cancer diagnosed before the age of 21 years and a control group of 3,899 healthy siblings.** *From Lipshultz SE, et al. Dexrazoxane for reducing anthracycline-related cardiotoxicity in children with cancer: an update of the evidence. Prog Pediatr Cardiol 2014;36:39–49.*

TABLE 11.1 Characteristics of the Different Types of Anthracycline Cardiotoxicity

Characteristic	Acute Cardiotoxicity	Early-Onset Progressive Cardiotoxicity	Late-Onset Progressive Cardiotoxicity
Onset	Within the first week of anthracycline treatment	<1 year after completing anthracycline treatment	≥1 year after completing anthracycline treatment
Risk-factor dependence	Unknown	Yes[a]	Yes[a]
Clinical features in adults	Transient depression of myocardial contractility	Dilated cardiomyopathy	Dilated cardiomyopathy
Clinical features in children	Transient depression of myocardial contractility	Restrictive cardiomyopathy and/or dilated cardiomyopathy	Restrictive cardiomyopathy and/or dilated cardiomyopathy
Course	Usually reversible when anthracycline is discontinued	Can be progressive	Can be progressive

[a]Data from Giantris A, Abdurrahman L, Hinkle A, et al. Anthracycline induced cardiotoxicity in children and young adults. Crit Rev Oncol Hematol 1998;27:53–68. and Grenier MA, Lipshultz SE. Epidemiology of anthracycline cardiotoxicity in children and adults. Semin Oncol 1998;25:72–85.
Source: Adapted from Adams MJ, Lipshultz SE. Pathophysiology of anthracycline- and radiation-associated cardiomyopathies: implications for screening and prevention. Pediatr Blood Cancer 2005;44:600–6.

to experience heart failure and to present with peripheral or pulmonary edema, dyspnea, and exercise intolerance.

Anthracycline-related cardiac dysfunction progresses from asymptomatic systolic or diastolic dysfunction to severe clinical heart failure, indicating the importance of follow-up and screening. Adults typically develop dilated cardiomyopathy. Children may have nonischemic dilated or restricted cardiomyopathy and typically progress from one to the other [12]. Children experience heart failure more because of increased left ventricular (LV) afterload than because of reduced contractility [10]. Anthracyclines also have synergistic effects with nonanthracycline agents.

Monoclonal Antibodies

Monoclonal antibodies, namely HER2-targeted agents such as trastuzumab, are also well known for their cardiotoxic effects, which are even more severe when trastuzumab is combined with anthracyclines. Whether one potentiates the effects of the other or whether they each work independently

is unclear [13]. Evidence favors trastuzumab having its own mechanism of action because patients receiving it without anthracyclines also experience cardiac dysfunction.

Radiation therapy also leads to more severe cardiac toxicity. Unlike anthracyclines, however, the damage is not dose dependent and in fact may be reversible by discontinuing therapy and with medical management [14,15]. Trastuzumab-related cardiotoxicity alone is less severe because it causes an asymptomatic decrease in LV function as opposed to clinical heart failure. Its cardiotoxicity is thought to be directly related to its action on the HER2 receptor because studies in animal models have found that this gene is involved in embryogenesis of cardiac tissue [16]. Right ventricular dysfunction is less common but has been reported [17].

Tyrosine Kinase Inhibitors

Tyrosine kinase inhibitors, such as imatinib, are associated with heart failure. In animal models, heart failure is a consequence of inflammation and fibrosis involving myocyte vacuolization and interstitial lymphocytic infiltration [18]. Tyrosine kinase inhibitors are associated with hypertension and cardiomyopathy, and they inhibit vascular endothelial growth-factor receptors. Their toxicity is often acute, occurring within 2 weeks of starting therapy. The hypertension usually responds to antihypertensive medications, and the cardiomyopathy can often be reversed after therapy is stopped [19].

Other Anticancer Agents

Antimetabolites, such as fluorouracil and its precursor capecitabine, are associated with angina, myocardial infarction, and arrhythmia secondary to vasospasm, as well as to endothelial injury and occasionally to stress-induced cardiomyopathy [20]. Microtubule targeting agents, such as the vinca alkaloids, may cause hypertension and myocardial ischemia, as well as infarction, although the drug vinblastine is the most responsible agent. Taxanes, such as paclitaxel, may cause arrhythmias, such as asymptomatic bradycardia and heart block, but in conjunction with doxorubicin, they can lead to cardiomyopathy.

Alkylating agents, such as cyclophosphamide, may cause acute cardiomyopathy at high doses and fatal hemorrhagic myopericarditis as a consequence of endothelial capillary damage [21]. Several other drugs, through unclear mechanisms, have cardiotoxic effects, such as interleukin-2 myocarditis, etoposide-related vasospastic angina, and tamoxifen-related QT prolongation. With the prolonged survival of cancer patients, evaluating the risks and benefits of the possible cardiac consequences of these drugs that may occur later becomes essential.

THORACIC RADIATION

Radiation treatment of thoracic cancers can affect all structures and features of the heart. The primary mechanism is thought to be microvascular damage that leads to ischemia and fibrosis. Fibrosis can cause both acute and delayed cardiac changes, and it is potentiated by inflammation, oxidative stress, and changes in gene expression. Radiation-related heart disease has been studied in patients who have undergone mantle radiotherapy for Hodgkin lymphoma and breast cancer and in survivors of the atomic bombings in Japan [22,23]. The clinical and histologic features of radiation-induced tissue injury may lag behind the actual time or period of exposure. The type of injury is classified as acute, consequential, or late [24]. Acute radiation damage is most common in rapidly proliferating cells that are disrupted by the radiation, thus when functional cells are lost as part of normal tissue turnover they are not replaced. Consequential radiation effects are the result of acute damage that has not healed properly and persist to become chronic lesions. Late effects develop months or years later, are often progressive with follow-up as late as 20 to 34 years later, and more com-

monly occur in tissues with slow turnover [24]. The risk of late manifestations of cardiac dysfunction from radiation therapy is attributed to persistently elevated concentrations of inflammatory and proliferative markers in vascular endothelial cells beyond the period of exposure [25].

The spectrum of radiation-induced cardiac disease includes pericarditis, myocardial damage, coronary artery disease, valvular disease, and arrhythmia [26,27].

Damage to the Pericardium

Among the most common historic adverse effects of thoracic radiation on the heart is pericarditis. With modern radiotherapy techniques the incidence of clinically significant radiation-associated pericarditis has decreased. Acute pericarditis typically occurs during radiation therapy, whereas delayed pericarditis occurs at least 4 months after treatment. The most common symptoms are dyspnea, cough, fever, or pleuritic chest pain, but pericarditis can also be asymptomatic. The incidence after radiation therapy is dose related [28]. Pericarditis secondary to radiation is caused by protein-rich fluid accumulating in the pericardial sac, fibrosis, and the adipose layer being replaced by collagen. Further thickening of the fibrous pericardium may lead to constriction [22], which can be complicated by pericardial effusion or tamponade requiring pericardiocentesis or pericardiectomy. The risk of tamponade depends on the rate of fluid accumulation [29]. Most pericardial effusions resolve spontaneously over time, but effusion increases the risk of chronic pericarditis [30].

Damage to the Myocardium

Myocardial injury is marked by focal interstitial fibrosis caused by an increase in collagen. Activation of Rho and connective-tissue growth factor lead to fibrosis, but activated exchange nucleotide protein directly activated by cAMP (EPAC-1) leads to hypertrophy and amyloidosis, but not fibrosis [31]. Early injury to the myocardium is related to upregulated proinflammatory molecules, such as E-selectin, ICAM-1, and PECAM-1. These adhesion molecules are involved in changes in the microvasculature of the myocardium. Upregulation of cytokines, such as IL-6 and IL-8, enhances endothelial cell proliferation [32]. Endothelial cell proliferation in the microvasculature leads to localized cell death and consequently to cardiomyopathy and heart failure. Local insult to the myocardium is also potentiated by the prothrombotic nature of radiation that increases von Willebrand factor activity [33].

Myocardial damage begins with acute inflammation of the microvasculature and marked infiltration of neutrophils. Capillary damage from luminal narrowing and thrombus formation, as mentioned previously, causes ischemia, which leads to progressive fibrosis [34]. Myocardial fibrosis is a consequence of microvascular ischemia that results from endothelial cell proliferation. The foci of myocardial ischemia and necrosis are centered at areas of capillary loss, and these areas are preceded by endothelial proliferation [35]. Myocardial damage is also related to injury to the endothelial cells of the capillaries, as well as to the effects of fibrinous exudate, which both damages surrounding vasculature and disrupts fibrinolysis [29].

Arrhythmias

The cause of arrhythmias associated with radiation is unclear, but it is likely a consequence of the microvascular damage that affects conducting cardiac cells and ischemia in the electrical pathways. Radiation can cause nodal bradycardia or any type of heart block, including bundle branch blocks, by injuring any point in the conduction system. Among bundle branch blocks, right bundle branch block is most common, indicating that the most anterior portions of the heart are at highest risk for fibrosis [36]. Patients in whom complete AV node block develops require pacemaker implantation.

Coronary Artery Disease

The pathophysiology of coronary artery disease in patients who have undergone radiation treatment is similar to that of the general population, but the disease can develop at younger ages. However, ostial lesions are more common, as is fibrosis of the smooth muscle in the vascular walls. As with radiation-related pericardial and myocardial disease, the injury begins with damage to the adjacent microvasculature and leads to intimal hyperplasia and consequently to lipid deposition and potential thrombus formation. The oxidative stress from free radical formation may also contribute to the vascular wall damage [37].

Valvular Disease

Although less common than pericardial and myocardial disease, diseases of the mitral, aortic, tricuspid, and pulmonic valves can also be caused by radiation [38]. The mechanism is likely related to microvascular ischemia because these diseases are avascular but still related to fibrosis. The spectrum of valvular disease ranges from asymptomatic thickening to severe fibrosis. The changes are progressive and may become severe enough to require surgery [39]. With radiation-related cardiac disease, increases in cardiac mortality may be related to older radiation therapy equipment and techniques involved with dosing, frequency, and localization [40].

RISK FACTORS OF CARDIOTOXICITY

The degree and progression of cancer treatment-related cardiotoxicity differ among children. For example, some children may experience severe LV dysfunction, whereas others have no effects, despite receiving the same cumulative dose. Thus, in addition to presenting with different modifiable and nonmodifiable risk factors, a genetic predisposition might also be present [4].

Treatment-Related Risk Factors of Cardiotoxicity

Cumulative doses of anthracycline, chest-directed radiotherapy, and cranial irradiation all increase the risks for adverse cardiac effects. However, cumulative dose of anthracyclines has the biggest impact in late cardiac effects. The risk is 11 times as high with cumulative doses greater than 300 mg/m^2 than with lower doses [41,42].

In a sample of long-term survivors of childhood acute lymphoblastic leukemia (ALL), at higher cumulative anthracycline doses, there was LV dilation and LV fractional shortening (LVFS) declined [10]. Furthermore, in anthracycline-treated survivors of childhood cancer, after a median follow-up of 8 years, the LV was dilated at a cumulative anthracycline dose greater than 320 mg/m^2, and LVFS was significantly reduced at cumulative doses of 280 mg/m^2 or greater [41]. However, cardiac damage has been found even in patients who received doses less than 240 mg/m^2, suggesting that there is no true "safe" dose of anthracycline, especially with longer follow-up [4].

The association between chest-directed radiotherapy and long-term cardiac morbidity is well established. The average radiation dose was linearly related to the risk of cardiac mortality (60% estimated relative risk at 1 Gy) in a multicenter study of 4122 French and British childhood cancer survivors [43,44]. Other studies have shown an additive increased risk of cardiac mortality when high cumulative anthracycline doses were combined with radiotherapy [45,46].

Cranial irradiation is a standard of treatment for childhood leukemia or brain cancers and to prevent brain metastases. Compared to similar patients unexposed to cranial irradiation, those exposed had lower LV mass and LV dimensions over a 10-year follow-up [45]. These changes in LV structure were associated with a decrease in insulin-like growth factor-1 concentrations, which were possibly related to growth hormone deficiency, suggesting that cranial irradiation could be an additional risk factor for cardiotoxicity.

Modifiable and Nonmodifiable Risk Factors for Cardiotoxicity

Additional risk factors for cardiotoxicity include female sex, younger age at treatment, longer follow-up after treatment, trisomy 21, genetic mutations, pre-existing cardiovascular disease, and comorbidities (Table 11.2) [46].

Female survivors have a higher risk of cardiotoxicity than male survivors. Among 120 children receiving anthracyclines for ALL or sarcoma, girls had a higher cardiac

TABLE 11.2 Risk Factors for Cardiotoxicity in Childhood Cancer Survivors

Risk Factors	Comment
Cumulative anthracycline dose	Cumulative doses >300 mg/m^2 are associated with significantly elevated long-term risk [10,47,96,97]
Time after therapy	The incidence of clinically important cardiotoxicity increases progressively over decades [10,43,47,96]
Rate of anthracycline administration	Continuous infusion not cardioprotective in children [43,98]
Individual anthracycline dose	Higher individual doses are associated with increased late cardiotoxicity, even when cumulative doses are limited; no dose is risk-free [43,47,96]
Type of anthracycline	Liposomal encapsulated preparations may reduce cardiotoxicity. Data on anthracycline analogs and differences in cardiotoxicity are conflicting [99–101]
Radiation therapy	Cumulative cardiac radiation dose >30 Gy before or concomitant with anthracycline treatment increases risk; as little as 5 Gy increased the risk [8,43,102]
Concomitant therapy	Trastuzumab, cyclophosphamide, bleomycin, vincristine, amsacrine, and mitoxantrone, among others, may increase susceptibility or toxicity [101,102]
Pre-existing cardiac risk factors	Hypertension; ischemic, myocardial, and valvular heart disease; prior cardiotoxic treatment [101]
Personal health habits	Smoking; consumption of alcohol, energy drinks, stimulants, prescription, and illicit drugs [43]
Comorbidities	Diabetes, obesity, renal dysfunction, pulmonary disease, endocrinopathies, electrolyte and metabolic abnormalities, sepsis, infection, pregnancy, viruses, elite athletic participation, low vitamin D concentrations [43,51,101,103,104]
Age	Young (<1 year) and advanced age at treatment are associated with elevated risk [10,43,47]
Sex	Females are at greater risk than males [43,47]
Complementary therapies	More information needs to be collected to assess risk [43]
Additional factors	Trisomy 21 and African-American ancestry increase risk [97]

Source: Raj S, et al. Anthracycline-induced cardiotoxicity: a review of pathophysiology, diagnosis, and treatment. Curr Treat Options Cardiovasc Med 2014;16(6):315.

sensitivity to anthracyclines than did boys. Furthermore, this difference increased at higher cumulative doses [47].

Excess mortality is also significantly higher in long-term female survivors of childhood cancer than in their male counterparts [48]. Doxorubicin is poorly absorbed by fat, and girls tend to have a higher percentage of body fat than boys have. Therefore, because dosage is often calculated on the basis of body surface area [49], doxorubicin concentrations in intracellular cardiomyocytes may be higher in girls, perhaps increasing their susceptibility to anthracycline-induced cardiotoxicity [47].

As in the general population, long-term childhood cancer survivors can also have one or more of the traditional risk factors for atherosclerosis, such as obesity, diabetes, and tobacco use, which further increase the risk of cardiovascular complications beyond that directly related to cancer therapies.

The overall prevalence of obesity in survivors is similar to that in the general population [50], although survivors treated with cranial radiation have a greater risk of the condition [45]. Obesity is a serious health issue for survivors whose cardiovascular system might not be able to compensate for associated events, such as ischemia or atherosclerotic disease. The pathological determinants of atherosclerosis in youth is a validated, composite cardiovascular disease risk score. In survivors of different types of childhood cancer, these scores indicated that more than half the survivors had at least twice the odds of currently having an advanced coronary artery lesion than those of an individual of similar age and sex without cardiovascular disease risk factors. Risk was not strongly associated with a specific cancer type, cancer treatment, or marker of endocrine function, but it was marginally associated with physical inactivity and possibly cranial irradiation [51].

Physical inactivity is one of the leading modifiable risk factors of cardiovascular disease and other risks for atherosclerosis, such as metabolic syndrome. Childhood cancer survivors more often report having an inactive lifestyle and are less likely to meet physical activity guidelines than are their sibling or age- and sex-matched controls [52]. Older age at diagnosis, a higher percentage of body fat, a history of methotrexate exposure, and unusually high or low LV mass were all associated with lower maximum oxygen consumption in childhood cancer survivors [53]. Survivors with family histories of premature cardiovascular disease and genetic susceptibilities to cardiovascular diseases might also be at increased risk of treatment-related cardiotoxicity.

Individual variation in the risk of anthracycline-related cardiotoxicity at a given dose suggests a genetic predisposition [54]. In fact, the evidence of potential genetic risk factors is growing [54–58]. Hereditary hemochromatosis is a genetic disorder that can lead to iron overload. Among 184 high-risk ALL survivors screened for the frequency of HFE gene mutations, 10% had a mutation in the HFE C282Y allele. Among survivors in this 10%, the risk of doxorubicin-related myocardial injury was nine times higher than that of noncarriers [55]. Preliminary studies have also found that patients exposed to low-to-moderate doses of anthracyclines, who express homozygosity for the G allele of the CBR3 gene, which encodes carbonyl reductase 3, have an increased risk for cardiomyopathy [56,57].

Another study identified two genes, glucuronosyltransferase 1A6 (UGT1A6) and sodium-coupled nucleoside transporter SLC28A3, that may affect the risk of anthracycline-related cardiomyopathy [54]. Associations between cardiotoxicity and two other polymorphisms, the ABCC5 A-1629 T variant and the NOS3 G894T variant, have also been reported in children with high-risk ALL [97]. The ABCC5 gene is involved in the doxorubicin functional pathway and encodes for efflux transporters. Children with a polymorphism in the ABCC5 gene (the TT genotype of ABCC5 A-1629 T) have decreased left ventricular ejection fraction (LVEF) and LVFS. Furthermore, they were also more likely to have lower LVEF and LVFS values at the time of cancer diagnosis, which places them at higher risk of decreased LVEF and LVFS during and after cancer treatment.

The NOS3 gene modulates reactive oxygen or nitrogen species in the metabolic pathway of doxorubicin. In contrast to the ABCC5 variant, polymorphism in the homozygous T allele of NOS3 G894T was cardioprotective in high-risk patients who received a higher dose of doxorubicin without dexrazoxane: LVEF was 64% in those with the TT allele and 57% in those with the AA or AT alleles, indicating a clinically important difference in cardiac function. Furthermore, dexrazoxane prevented this effect in patients with any of the three alleles: 64.4% for TT and 66.5% for the others, further supporting the use of dexrazoxane in this high-risk group. Identifying these potential genetic risk factors may assist in screening, guiding treatment, and postchemotherapy monitoring [58].

An improved understanding of the lifetime cardiovascular risk associated with these factors in long-term childhood cancer survivors may help guide treatment and predict any potential additional cardiovascular risk of specific cancer therapies, such as anthracyclines [59].

RISK ASSESSMENT AND SCREENING FOR CARDIOTOXICITY

Echocardiography is likely to continue to be the mainstay of monitoring, given that it is portable, widely available, can usually be performed without sedation, and provides real-time data. Echocardiography provides a comprehensive assessment of cardiac structure and function. Its main limitation is the need for acoustic windows, which may be limited by lung disease, chest deformity, or obesity and that may be present to varying degrees in cancer survivors. Measurements of strain may improve early detection but are not validated predictors of outcomes.

Several studies have evaluated echocardiographic measures that may be more sensitive to early impairments in cardiac performance in children with cancer [60,61]. These measures include load-independent measures of systolic function (end-systolic wall stress and velocity of circumferential fiber shortening), diastolic function, tissue Doppler imaging, global function (myocardial performance index), and measures of cardiac mechanics (2-dimensional strain and strain rate). Acute cardiac measurements vary depending on loading conditions, which in turn may be sensitive to variations in chemotherapy. Long-term screening after chemotherapy has some justification [62]. Iarussi et al. [62] showed that increased end-systolic wall stress was associated with the effects of diastolic dysfunction in children after anthracycline treatment. Yildirim et al. reported that tissue Doppler imaging at rest and dobutamine stress echocardiography had a higher sensitivity than traditional measures of LV function for detecting early anthracycline-related toxicity in children [63]. Park et al. found abnormalities of regional wall motion using two-dimensional strain echocardiography and velocity vector imaging (which is angle independent) in children of 3–15 years of age after low-dose anthracycline therapy who had preserved global function [64].

Decreased longitudinal strain and increased high-sensitivity cardiac troponin I concentrations detected 3 months into therapy independently predicted cardiotoxicity, as defined previously, in a woman with breast cancer 6 months into therapy [65]. LVEF, measures of diastolic function, and N-terminal pro-B-type natriuretic peptide (NT-proBNP) concentrations did not predict cardiotoxicity.

Hare et al. showed that myocardial deformation, as identified by tissue Doppler echocardiography and two-dimensional strain imaging, detected myocardial cardiac deformation in women with normal ejection fractions (EF) receiving trastuzumab for breast cancer [66]. Sawaya et al. found that systolic longitudinal myocardial strain less than 19% and ultrasensitive troponin I concentrations measured during therapy predicted subsequent cardiotoxicity over 15 months in breast-cancer patients treated with anthracyclines, taxanes, and trastuzumab [65].

Although studies in adults have found useful positive predictive values for strain and cardiac biomarkers, these findings do not validate these screening methodologies. The positive predictive value is the probability that a positive screening test will correctly identify a condition of interest and depends partly on the prevalence of the condition. Further study is required to determine the validity of these measures, particularly with regard to their ability to predict patient outcomes and their cost-effectiveness [67].

Cardiac magnetic resonance imaging (C-MRI) is also increasingly used in pediatric cardiology to identify late cardiotoxicity characterized by abnormal longitudinal LV strain and regional strain, despite a normal LVEF, and with findings consistent with diffuse fibrosis. However, the prognostic value for late outcomes is unknown. Cardiac MRI offers great potential and several advantages over echocardiography and radionuclide angiography, including the lack of ionizing radiation. Measures of function and ventricular mass are highly reproducible and are not subject to variable image quality or affected by lung disease, chest shape, obesity, or assumptions of cardiac geometry. Accurate sequential monitoring of LV function, morphology, or changes in myocardial tissue detected with C-MRI can be used in clinical trials of prophylactic cardioprotective medications in patients receiving cancer therapy or in monitoring the response to cardiac therapy in patients with established cardiomyopathy. In a randomized controlled trial of β-blockers and angiotensin converting enzyme inhibitors in 90 patients with hematologic malignancies receiving anthracyclines, C-MRI documented a 3.4% decrease in LVEF in the control group and no change in the treatment group at 6 months [68].

C-MRI may detect myocardial inflammation and edema as the earliest changes of cardiotoxicity from cancer therapy and has the potential to predict subsequent ventricular dysfunction [69]. Although the prevalence of late gadolinium enhancement well after anthracycline therapy seems to be low, diffuse fibrosis detected using T1 mapping and extracellular volume may help detect late subclinical cardiotoxicity. The prognostic importance and cardiac treatment implications of these findings are unknown, but they may identify patients who may benefit from close cardiac follow-up.

European studies have recommended that patients treated with both anthracyclines and radiation for lymphomas be screened with coronary artery calcium measurements or computed tomographic (CT) angiography beginning 10 years after radiotherapy [70]. These studies also recommend an electrocardiogram at each cardiovascular screening visit to detect arrhythmias or conduction abnormalities. These screening tests can be repeated every 5 years or at the onset of cardiovascular signs or symptoms. Options for screening should include a cardiac-specific history for traditional risk factors, including a family history of heart disease, cholesterol concentrations, and a personal history of smoking or second-hand smoke exposure, hypertension, and diabetes or glucose intolerance [71].

Biomarkers of Cardiotoxicity

Serum cardiac troponin concentrations are a sensitive and specific marker of myocyte necrosis and are often used in diagnosing and managing ischemic heart disease in adults. This marker can be used during chemotherapy to identify myocyte necrosis. The Dana-Farber Cancer Institute Childhood Acute Lymphoblastic Leukemia Consortium Protocol 95-001 found that elevated serum cardiac troponin T (cTnT) concentrations during the first 90 days of anthracycline therapy were significantly associated with reduced echocardiographic measurements of LV mass and LV end-diastolic posterior wall thickness 4 years later [72].

Chronic elevations in proBNP concentrations indicate increased ventricular wall stress, in association with pressure or volume overload and elevated diastolic pressure [73]. In the aforementioned Dana-Farber Cancer Institute protocol 95-001, elevated concentrations of NT-proBNP during the first 90 days of therapy were associated with an abnormal LV thickness-to-dimension ratio 4 years later, suggesting pathologic ventricular remodeling. Additionally, a higher percentage of children had elevated concentrations of NT-proBNP than had elevated concentrations of cTnT before, during, and after treatment. This difference suggests that NT-proBNP may detect cardiac stress before any irreversible cell damage and death occurs, which may help identify children early in therapy who are at increased risk of eventual anthracycline-related cardiac abnormalities [72].

A nonspecific inflammatory marker, high-sensitivity C-reactive protein (hsCRP), is widely used to assess patient health. Systemic inflammation is associated with increased rates of cardiovascular disease in adults and may also be involved with the mechanisms of anthracycline-related cardiotoxicity and pediatric cardiomyopathy [73]. As such, elevated hsCRP concentrations may be a strong indicator of cardiac stress. Despite a small sample size, one study of 19 children with heart failure divided into three groups on the basis of symptom severity found that serum hsCRP concentrations were associated with decreased LV function and discriminated between the different groups of symptom severity [73]. However, as part of that same DFCI 95-01 study, elevated concentrations of hsCRP were not associated with echocardiographic changes [72]. These findings have encouraged further research on the use of serum hsCRP concentrations collected during therapy as potential predictors of late cardiac effects. Serum hsCRP concentrations may be a valuable screening tool for identifying long-term survivors at increased risk of subsequent cardiac disease. Currently, only serum concentrations of cTnT and NT-proBNP measured during active chemotherapy have been validated as surrogate endpoints for late cardiotoxicity in long-term survivors [4].

Nanoparticle-Capture Mass Spectrometry

The ability to identify heart-derived tissue proteins associated with myocardial injury that can be detected before marked elevations in cTnT concentrations could have profound implications on earlier detection and clinical monitoring for doxorubicin cardiotoxicity. One pilot study using nanoparticle-mass spectrometry identified several candidate protein biomarkers previously implicated in cardiac dysfunction, remodeling, fibrosis, and hypertrophy [74]. If validated, these candidate biomarkers might increase the predictive value of more routinely used markers, such as cTnT, to detect cardiac damage earlier, before it is irreparable and before cardiomyocytes are lost. However, larger studies evaluating the efficacy of nanoparticle-mass spectrometry are needed to verify and advance this novel diagnostic approach.

PREVENTING AND TREATING CARDIOTOXICITY

The goal of early treatment is to prevent pathological LV remodeling using drugs that target LV preload (diuretics) and LV afterload (angiotensin converting enzyme inhibitors or angiotensin-receptor blockers). Because anthracycline-related structural changes progress from dilated cardiomyopathy to a restrictive-like cardiomyopathy, it is critically important to understand the type of cardiomyopathy causing heart failure in these patients. Many treatments appropriate for heart failure caused by dilated cardiomyopathy are inappropriate for heart failure caused by restrictive cardiomyopathy [4].

Symptomatic patients may benefit from tailored precision therapy on the basis of hemodynamic monitoring or from heart transplantation. Cardiotoxicity may manifest as cardiomyopathy, pericarditis, heart failure, valvular heart disease, or premature coronary artery disease. Long-term cardiovascular monitoring of cancer survivors diagnosed in childhood, adolescence, and young adulthood should be aimed at early, preclinical detection, when interventions can be expected to have the greatest benefit.

Dexrazoxane

The most promising strategy for preventing anthracycline-related cardiotoxicity is the coadministration of dexrazoxane. Doxorubicin forms a complex with iron that is thought to facilitate the formation of toxic free radicals in tissues. Dexrazoxane is a chelating agent that reduces the formation of anthracycline–iron complexes, thus interfering with iron-mediated free radical generation [75–77]. It also reduces doxorubicin-induced DNA damage by inhibiting topoisomerase 2-beta [78]. Dexrazoxane is currently approved by the FDA only for use in adults with metastatic breast cancer who have received a cumulative dose of 300 mg/m^2 of doxorubicin and who may benefit from continued treatment with an anthracycline. However, in Aug. 2014, dexrazoxane was designated by the FDA as an orphan drug in children [79]. Dexrazoxane has reduced intermediate or surrogate endpoints of cardiotoxicity in several randomized trials of children [80].

Early debates about dexrazoxane increasing the risk of secondary malignancies [81,82] or reducing oncologic efficacy raised questions on the use of dexrazoxane in children, but since then, multiple studies have concluded just the opposite: that dexrazoxane can be safely administered without increasing the risk of second malignancies or decreasing treatment efficacy [83–88]. Among 206 children with high-risk, ALL randomly assigned to receive dexrazoxane before each dose of doxorubicin or doxorubicin alone, cTnT concentrations were elevated in 50% of those who received doxorubicin but in only 21% of those who were pretreated with dexrazoxane after a median follow-up of 2.7 years. This finding suggests that dexrazoxane prevents or reduces cardiac injury, as reflected by fewer episodes of elevated cTnT concentrations, without compromising the antileukemic efficacy of anthracyclines [76]. At 5 years after completing doxorubicin treatment, 134 of the original 206 children had echocardiographic evidence that dexrazoxane was cardioprotective (Fig. 11.1) [85]. Those who received doxorubicin alone had significantly abnormal mean z-scores for LVFS and LV end-systolic dimension, whereas those for the dexrazoxane group remained normal [85]. Other studies have found similar cardioprotective effects of dexrazoxane without compromised efficacy of cancer treatment or increased risk of second malignancies [87–90].

Similar to the study by Lipshultz et al. [85], Asselin et al. found in survivors of T-cell ALL and lymphoma that LV wall thickness and thickness-to-dimension ratio were worse than normal in those who received doxorubicin alone, but were normal in those who received dexrazoxane with doxorubicin 3–5 years after ALL diagnosis [84]. In another study in children with osteosarcoma, Schwartz et al. [88] examined the effect of dexrazoxane as a cardioprotectant to support doxorubicin dose escalation, its effects on tumor response, and increased risk of second malignancies. As hypothesized, dexrazoxane safely allowed escalating the cumulative doxorubicin dose of 450–600 mg/m^2, did not interfere with tumor response, and did not increase the risk of second malignancies [88].

The safety and feasibility of trastuzumab was tested in children with metastatic osteosarcoma and HER2 overexpression [89]. Dexrazoxane was added to the treatment protocol to protect patients from the cardiotoxic effects of doxorubicin combined with trastuzumab that are seen in adults. Although oncologic outcomes were poor in children who received trastuzumab, there was no measurable acute myocardial injury, indicating that dexrazoxane was cardioprotective and could be safely delivered in an anthracycline-based regimen in combination with trastuzumab [89].

Chow et al. [87] examined long-term overall and cause-specific mortality and relapse rates from the three Children's Oncology Group randomized clinical trials described previously [84,88], which were conducted between 1996 and 2001 [87]. In 1008 patients, of which 507 received dexrazoxane, overall mortality did not vary by dexrazoxane status (12.8% with dexrazoxane at 10 years versus 12.2% without; hazard ratio [HR], 1.03; 95% CI, 0.73–1.45 after a median follow-up of 12.6 years [87]. Thus, dexrazoxane did not appear to compromise long-term survival in survivors of childhood leukemia or lymphoma. Meanwhile, Vrooman et al. [86] pooled data from three large multicenter randomized trials from the DFCI ALL consortium to examine the incidence of secondary malignant neoplasms among patients with high-risk ALL treated with dexrazoxane and doxorubicin. After a median (range) follow-up of 3.8 years (0.2–13.6 years), only one secondary malignancy was observed among 553 patients [86].

In fact, the evidence in favor of dexrazoxane is so promising that the Dana–Farber Cancer Institute Childhood Acute Lymphoblastic Leukemia Consortium, applying the results from clinical trials, including its own studies, now incorporates dexrazoxane into current and future clinical trial protocols involving anthracycline therapy. Similarly, the Children's Oncology Group includes dexrazoxane in all its research protocols that require treatment with

doxorubicin doses of 150 mg/m^2 or more or that require an anthracycline at any dose with planned radiation treatment portals that may affect the heart. Because the cardiotoxic effects of anthracyclines can be immediate, and the damage to the cardiomyocytes can be irreversible and cumulative, dexrazoxane should be administered before the first anthracycline dose and before each therapy cycle [80].

It also appears that dexrazoxane has greater long-term cardioprotective effects in girls than in boys in one study, particularly with respect to changes in the LV end-diastolic thickness-to-dimension ratio, a marker of pathologic LV remodeling [85]. Mean LV thickness-to-dimension ratio and mean FS were significantly more impaired in girls not receiving dexrazoxane. However, there were no differences between boys treated with or without dexrazoxane (Fig. 11.2) [85]. In another study, both boys and girls

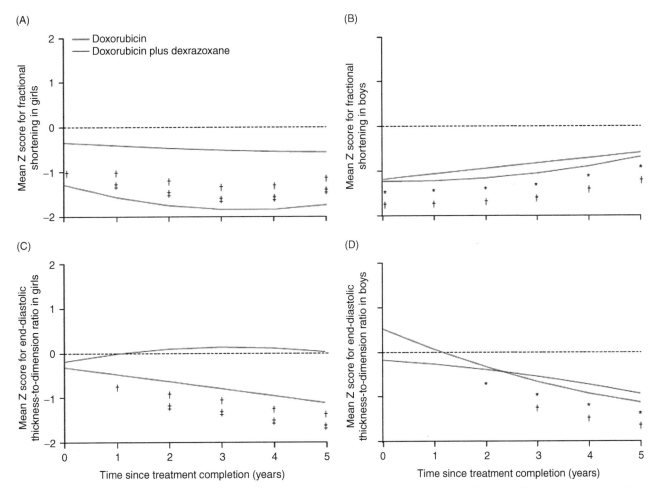

FIGURE 11.2 Mean left-ventricular echocardiographic Z scores in 134 boys and girls. Plots are adjusted for age. (A) is the mean Z score for fractional shortening in girls as a function of time since treatment completion in girls for both doxorubicin and doxorubicin plus dexrazoxane. (B) is the mean Z score for fractional shortening in boys as a function of time since treatment completion in years for both doxorubicin and doxorubicin plus dexrazoxane. (C) is the mean Z score for end-diastolic thickness-to-dimension ratio in girls as a function of time since treatment completion in years for both doxorubicin and doxorubicin plus dexrazoxane. (D) is the mean Z score for end-diastolic thickness-to-dimension ratio in boys as a function of time since treatment completion in years for both doxorubicin and doxorubicin plus dexrazoxane. *$P \leq 0.05$ for comparison of the mean Z score of the doxorubicin plus dexrazoxane group with zero. †$P \leq 0.05$ for comparison of the mean Z score for the doxorubicin group with zero. ‡$P \leq 0.05$ for comparisons of mean Z scores between the doxorubicin and doxorubicin plus dexrazoxane groups. *From Asselin BL, et al. Cardioprotection and safety of dexrazoxane in patients treated for newly diagnosed T-cell acute lymphoblastic leukemia or advanced-stage lymphoblastic Non-Hodgkin lymphoma: A report of the Children's Oncology Group Randomized Trial Pediatric Oncology Group 9404. J Clin Oncol 2016;34(8):854–62.*

showed cardioprotection when dexrazoxane was administered before doxorubicin doses [84].

Angiotensin-Converting Enzyme Inhibitors

Afterload reduction therapy with enalapril in 18 long-term survivors of childhood cancer treated with anthracyclines was associated with early improvements in LV dimension, afterload, mass, and FS. However, these improvements were lost after 6–10 years [90], by which time the six children with heart failure had either died or undergone cardiac transplantation. Thus, treatment with angiotensin-converting enzyme inhibitors improved structure and function in the short term in these children, but it did not prevent LV wall thinning, and it exacerbated the long-term consequences of inadequate cardiac hypertrophy (Fig. 11.3) [90].

Growth Hormone Therapy

Growth hormone therapy has been explored as a means to treat anthracycline-induced cardiotoxicity. One case-

control study compared 34 anthracycline-treated childhood cancer survivors treated with growth hormone to 86 childhood survivors of a similar cancer without growth hormone therapy [91]. Survivors who received growth-hormone therapy had improved LV wall thickness while on treatment, but these improvements were lost 4 years after therapy had been discontinued. Growth hormone replacement therapy did not reduce progressive LV dysfunction [91].

In survivors of childhood cancer, heart failure can progress rapidly to functional impairment that is refractory to drug therapy. In this situation, mechanical support may be considered. For patients who do not respond well to all other cardiac treatments, heart transplantation may be an option for end-stage anthracycline-induced cardiomyopathy [92].

Injury to the heart from radiation is complicated by infectious and inflammatory responses. Metabolic and genetic factors predispose to injury but are not well understood. Radiation injury can lead to restrictive cardiomyopathy, pericarditis, conduction and valvular disease, and

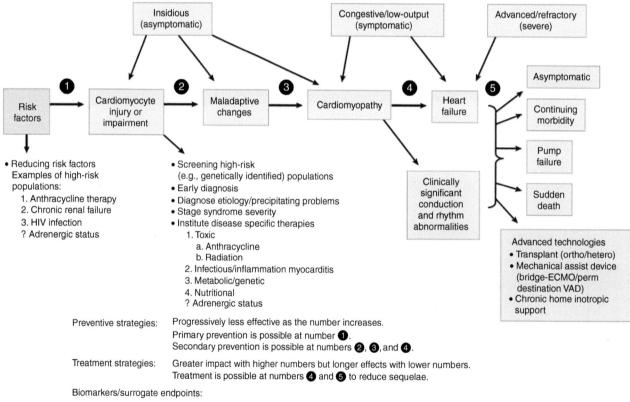

FIGURE 11.3 **Stages in the course of pediatric ventricular dysfunction.** These stages can be monitored by echocardiographic measurements of LV structure and function in combination with concentrations of validated cardiac biomarkers. Risk factors and high-risk populations for ventricular dysfunction are highlighted where preventive or early therapeutic strategies may be effective. Determining the cause of dysfunction may suggest cause-specific therapies. The circled numbers 1–5 indicate points of preventive or therapeutic interventions and where biomarker measurements may be helpful. ECMO, Extracorporeal membrane oxygenation; VAD, ventricular assist device. *From Lipshultz SE, Wilkinson JD. Beta-adrenergic adaptation in idiopathic dilated cardiomyopathy: differences between children and adults. Eur Heart J 2014;35:10–12.*

heart failure. Progressive findings may become apparent clinically 10 or more years after radiotherapy. Findings may be unsuspected but clinically important. Serial comprehensive cardiac testing is advised. Unlike the loss of cardiomyocytes related to anthracycline use, radiotherapy to the heart appears to be related to progressive fibrosis (scar tissue formation) years after therapy. Radiation therapy can also be associated with a higher risk of valvular heart disease and endocarditis and ostial coronary disease, in which stress testing, stress echocardiography, and myocardial perfusion imaging can be useful.

Intracardiac conduction defects caused by progressive scarring can be seen on electrocardiograms or cardiac event recording and are a risk for sudden death. Conduction defects have been reported in 75% of childhood survivors of cancer given thoracic radiation, where 60% had a conduction delay, 4% right bundle branch block, and 9% had a prolonged corrected QT interval on screening. This high prevalence supports electrocardiographic screening in this population [36].

New diagnostic tools, such as computed tomography angiography, magnetic resonance angiography, and coronary artery calcium scores, have been investigated in this population. Echocardiography is noninvasive and provides information on LV structure and function, the pericardium, and the cardiac valves. Measurements of diastolic function and the LV thickness-to-dimension ratio may be particularly valuable in patients at risk for a restrictive-like cardiomyopathy in which LV systolic dysfunction and dilation may not occur until later in the disease. Monitoring frequency has not been established. Assessment once every 1–5 years may help identify abnormalities early, depending on the patient's age at exposure, anthracycline dose, time since treatment, and the presence of other risk factors [8].

The development of coronary artery disease in survivors exposed to cardiac radiation should be assessed regularly after cancer treatment. This assessment should include traditional cardiovascular disease risk factors, such as dyslipidemia and hypertension, and cardiac stress testing with exercise electrocardiography, which can identify cardiac ischemia in asymptomatic patients. However, the results of the test should be interpreted with caution, because exercise electrocardiography may have false-positive and false-negative findings [93]. For patients with evidence of conduction abnormalities or an abnormal baseline electrocardiogram at rest, stress echocardiography or myocardial perfusion imaging is preferred. For patients unable to exercise, pharmacological stress induction should be considered. Because coronary events are rare in younger patients, even in those at increased risk, stress testing may be best used as survivors reach adulthood. These recommendations are also consistent with those of the Children's Oncology Group [94].

CONCLUSIONS

Adverse effects of chemotherapy can be either direct, by compromising myocardial structure and function, or indirect, by impairing vascular hemodynamics or other organ systems. Although many risk factors have been recognized, such as cumulative doxorubicin dose, younger age at diagnosis, and concomitant radiation therapy, childhood cancer survivors vary by who may or may not experience cardiotoxicity. Although dexrazoxane is a promising cardioprotectant when administered early during treatment before every dose of doxorubicin, it does not provide complete protection across different cancer types.

Clinicians must also review the evidence cautiously. The number of studies on cardiovascular toxicity and cancer in adults is large; however, the number in children is much smaller. Many pediatric treatment protocols are extrapolated from those for adults, which is not always appropriate, given the differences in body composition and developmental changes in children. Thus, more research is needed to find a balance between oncologic efficacy and reducing cardiac late effects [95].

REFERENCES

[1] Siegel RL, Miller KD, Jemal A. Cancer statistics, 2015. CA Cancer J Clin 2015;65:5–29.

[2] Oeffinger KC, Mertens AC, Sklar CA, et al. Chronic health conditions in adult survivors of childhood cancer. New Engl J Med 2006;355:1572–82.

[3] Mariotto AB, Rowland JH, Yabroff KR, et al. Long-term survivors of childhood cancers in the United States. Cancer Epidemiol Biomarkers Prev 2009;18:1033–40.

[4] Lipshultz SE, Franco VI, Miller TL, Colan SD, Sallan SE. Cardiovascular disease in adult survivors of childhood cancer. Annu Rev Med 2015;66:161–76.

[5] Mertens AC, Liu Q, Neglia JP, et al. Cause-specific late mortality among 5-year survivors of childhood cancer: the Childhood Cancer Survivor Study. JNCI 2008;100:1368–79.

[6] Mulrooney DA, Yeazel MW, Kawashima T, et al. Cardiac outcomes in a cohort of adult survivors of childhood and adolescent cancer: retrospective analysis of the Childhood Cancer Survivor Study cohort. BMJ 2009;339. b4606.

[7] Singal PK, Iliskovic N. Doxorubicin-induced cardiomyopathy. New Engl J Med 1998;339:900–5.

[8] Adams MJ, Lipshultz SE. Pathophysiology of anthracycline- and radiation-associated cardiomyopathies: implications for screening and prevention. Pediatr Blood Cancer 2005;44:600–6.

[9] Franco VI, Henkel JM, Miller TL, Lipshultz SE. Cardiovascular effects in childhood cancer survivors treated with anthracyclines. Cardiol Res Pract 2011;2011:134679.

[10] Lipshultz SE, Colan SD, Gelber RD, Perez-Atayde AR, Sallan SE, Sanders SP. Late cardiac effects of doxorubicin therapy for acute lymphoblastic leukemia in childhood. New Engl J Med 1991;324:808–8015.

[11] Martin E, Thougaard AV, Grauslund M, et al. Evaluation of the topoisomerase II-inactive bisdioxopiperazine ICRF-161 as a

protectant against doxorubicin-induced cardiomyopathy. Toxicology 2009;255:72–9.

[12] Raj S, Franco VI, Lipshultz SE. Anthracycline-induced cardiotoxicity: a review of pathophysiology, diagnosis, and treatment. Curr Treat Options Cardiovasc Med 2014;16(6):315.

[13] Seidman A, Hudis C, Pierri MK, et al. Cardiac dysfunction in the trastuzumab clinical trials experience. J Clin Oncol 2002;20:1215–21.

[14] Keefe DL. Trastuzumab-associated cardiotoxicity. Cancer 2002;95:1592–600.

[15] Pivot X, Suter T, Nabholtz JM, et al. Cardiac toxicity events in the PHARE trial, an adjuvant trastuzumab randomised phase III study. Eur J Cancer 2015;51:1660–6.

[16] Erickson SL, O'Shea KS, Ghaboosi N, et al. ErbB3 is required for normal cerebellar and cardiac development: a comparison with ErbB2-and heregulin-deficient mice. Development 1997;124:4999–5011.

[17] Bayar N, Kucukseymen S, Goktas S, Arslan S. Right ventricle failure associated with trastuzumab. Ther Adv Drug Saf 2015;6:98–102.

[18] Herman EH, Knapton A, Rosen E, et al. A multifaceted evaluation of imatinib-induced cardiotoxicity in the rat. Toxicol Pathol 2011;39:1091–106.

[19] Bair SM, Choueiri TK, Moslehi J. Cardiovascular complications associated with novel angiogenesis inhibitors: emerging evidence and evolving perspectives. Trends Cardiovasc Med 2013;23:104–13.

[20] Dalzell JR, Samuel LM. The spectrum of 5-fluorouracil cardiotoxicity. Anticancer Drugs 2009;20:79–80.

[21] Gottdiener JS, Appelbaum FR, Ferrans VJ, Deisseroth A, Ziegler J. Cardiotoxicity associated with high-dose cyclophosphamide therapy. Arch Intern Med 1981;141:758–63.

[22] Darby SC, Cutter DJ, Boerma M, et al. Radiation-related heart disease: current knowledge and future prospects. Int J Radiat Oncol Biol Phys 2010;76:656–65.

[23] Takahashi I, Ohishi W, Mettler FA Jr, et al. A report from the 2013 international workshop: radiation and cardiovascular disease, Hiroshima, Japan. J Radiol Prot 2013;33:869–80.

[24] Stone HB, Coleman CN, Anscher MS, McBride WH. Effects of radiation on normal tissue: consequences and mechanisms. Lancet Oncol 2003;4:529–36.

[25] Sievert W, Trott KR, Azimzadeh O, Tapio S, Zitzelsberger H, Multhoff G. Late proliferating and inflammatory effects on murine microvascular heart and lung endothelial cells after irradiation. Radiother Oncol 2015;117:376–81.

[26] Adams MJ, Hardenbergh PH, Constine LS, Lipshultz SE. Radiation-associated cardiovascular disease. Crit Rev Oncol Hematol 2003;45:55–75.

[27] Lipshultz SE, Scully RE, Stevenson KE, et al. Hearts too small for body size after doxorubicin for childhood leukemia: Grinch Syndrome. J Clin Oncol 2014;32:10021. (abstr.).

[28] Carmel RJ, Kaplan HS. Mantle irradiation in Hodgkin's disease. An analysis of technique, tumor eradication, and complications. Cancer 1976;37:2813–25.

[29] Stewart JR, Fajardo LF, Gillette SM, Constine LS. Radiation injury to the heart. Int J Radiat Oncol Biol Phys 1995;31:1205–11.

[30] Arsenian MA. Cardiovascular sequelae of therapeutic thoracic radiation. Prog Cardiovasc Dis 1991;33:299–311.

[31] Monceau V, Llach A, Azria D, et al. Epac contributes to cardiac hypertrophy and amyloidosis induced by radiotherapy but not fibrosis. Radiother Oncol 2014;111:63–71.

[32] Hendry JH, Akahoshi M, Wang LS, Lipshultz SE, Stewart FA, Trott KR. Radiation-induced cardiovascular injury. Radiat Environ Biophys 2008;47:189–93.

[33] Schultz-Hector S, Trott KR. Radiation-induced cardiovascular diseases: is the epidemiologic evidence compatible with the radiobiologic data? Int J Radiat Oncol Biol Phys 2007;67:10–8.

[34] Adams MJ, Lipshultz SE, Schwartz C, Fajardo LF, Coen V, Constine LS. Radiation-associated cardiovascular disease: manifestations and management. Semin Radiat Oncol 2003;13:346–56.

[35] Andratschke N, Maurer J, Molls M, Trott KR. Late radiation-induced heart disease after radiotherapy. Clinical importance, radiobiological mechanisms and strategies of prevention. Radiother Oncol 2011;100:160–6.

[36] Adams MJ, Lipsitz SR, Colan SD, et al. Cardiovascular status in long-term survivors of Hodgkin's disease treated with chest radiotherapy. J Clin Oncol 2004;22:3139–48.

[37] Senkus-Konefka E, Jassem J. Cardiovascular effects of breast cancer radiotherapy. Cancer Treat Rev 2007;33:578–93.

[38] Veinot JP, Edwards WD. Pathology of radiation-induced heart disease: a surgical and autopsy study of 27 cases. Human Pathol 1996;27:766–73.

[39] Carlson RG, Mayfield WR, Normann S, Alexander JA. Radiation-associated valvular disease. Chest 1991;99:538–45.

[40] Constine LS, Schwartz RG, Savage DE, King V, Muhs A. Cardiac function, perfusion, and morbidity in irradiated long-term survivors of Hodgkin's disease. Int J Radiat Oncol Biol Phys 1997;39:897–906.

[41] Nysom K, Holm K, Lipsitz SR, et al. Relationship between cumulative anthracycline dose and late cardiotoxicity in childhood acute lymphoblastic leukemia. J Clin Oncol 1998;16:545–50.

[42] Kremer LC, van Dalen EC, Offringa M, Ottenkamp J, Voute PA. Anthracycline-induced clinical heart failure in a cohort of 607 children: long-term follow-up study. J Clin Oncol 2001;19:191–6.

[43] Lipshultz SE, Adams MJ. Cardiotoxicity after childhood cancer: beginning with the end in mind. J Clin Oncol 2010;28:1276–81.

[44] Tukenova M, Guibout C, Oberlin O, et al. Role of cancer treatment in long-term overall and cardiovascular mortality after childhood cancer. J Clin Oncol 2010;28:1308–15.

[45] Landy DC, Miller TL, Lipsitz SR, et al. Cranial irradiation as an additional risk factor for anthracycline cardiotoxicity in childhood cancer survivors: an analysis from the cardiac risk factors in childhood cancer survivors study. Pediatric Cardiol 2013;34:826–34.

[46] Lipshultz SE, Adams MJ, Colan SD, et al. Long-term cardiovascular toxicity in children, adolescents, and young adults who receive cancer therapy: pathophysiology, course, monitoring, management, prevention, and research directions: a scientific statement from the American Heart Association. Circulation 2013;128:1927–95.

[47] Lipshultz SE, Lipsitz SR, Mone SM, et al. Female sex and drug dose as risk factors for late cardiotoxic effects of doxorubicin therapy for childhood cancer. New Engl J Med 1995;332:1738–43.

[48] Mertens AC, Yasui Y, Neglia JP, et al. Late mortality experience in five-year survivors of childhood and adolescent cancer: the Childhood Cancer Survivor Study. J Clin Oncol 2001;19:3163–72.

[49] Rodvold KA, Rushing DA, Tewksbury DA. Doxorubicin clearance in the obese. J Clin Oncol 1988;6:1321–7.

[50] Messiah SE, Lipshultz SE, Natale RA, Miller TL. The imperative to prevent and treat childhood obesity: why the world cannot afford to wait. Clin Obes 2013;3:163–71.

[51] Landy DC, Miller TL, Lopez-Mitnik G, et al. Aggregating traditional cardiovascular disease risk factors to assess the cardiometabolic health of childhood cancer survivors: an analysis from the Cardiac Risk Factors in Childhood Cancer Survivors Study. Am Heart J 2012;163:295–301. e2.

[52] Ness KK, Leisenring WM, Huang S, et al. Predictors of inactive lifestyle among adult survivors of childhood cancer: a report from the Childhood Cancer Survivor Study. Cancer 2009;115:1984–94.

[53] Miller AM, Lopez-Mitnik G, Somarriba G, et al. Exercise capacity in long-term survivors of pediatric cancer: an analysis from the Cardiac Risk Factors in Childhood Cancer Survivors Study. Pediatr Blood Cancer 2013;60:663–8.

[54] Visscher H, Ross CJ, Rassekh SR, et al. Validation of variants in SLC28A3 and UGT1A6 as genetic markers predictive of anthracycline-induced cardiotoxicity in children. Pediatr Blood Cancer 2013;60:1375–81.

[55] Lipshultz SE, Lipsitz SR, Kutok JL, et al. Impact of hemochromatosis gene mutations on cardiac status in doxorubicin-treated survivors of childhood high-risk leukemia. Cancer 2013;119:3555–62.

[56] Blanco JG, Leisenring WM, Gonzalez-Covarrubias VM, et al. Genetic polymorphisms in the carbonyl reductase 3 gene CBR3 and the NAD(P)H:quinone oxidoreductase 1 gene NQO1 in patients who developed anthracycline-related congestive heart failure after childhood cancer. Cancer 2008;112:2789–95.

[57] Blanco JG, Sun CL, Landier W, et al. Anthracycline-related cardiomyopathy after childhood cancer: role of polymorphisms in carbonyl reductase genes--a report from the Children's Oncology Group. J Clin Oncol 2012;30:1415–21.

[58] Krajinovic M, Elbared J, Drouin S, et al. Polymorphisms of ABCC5 and NOS3 genes influence doxorubicin cardiotoxicity in survivors of childhood acute lymphoblastic leukemia. Pharmacogenomics J 2015;doi: 10.1038/tpj.2015.63. (Epub ahead of print).

[59] LeClerc JM, Billett AL, Gelber RD, et al. Treatment of childhood acute lymphoblastic leukemia: results of Dana-Farber ALL Consortium Protocol 87-01. J Clin Oncol 2002;20:237–46.

[60] Kremer LC, van der Pal HJ, Offringa M, van Dalen EC, Voute PA. Frequency and risk factors of subclinical cardiotoxicity after anthracycline therapy in children: a systematic review. Ann Oncol 2002;13:819–29.

[61] Trachtenberg BH, Landy DC, Franco VI, et al. Anthracycline-associated cardiotoxicity in survivors of childhood cancer. Pediatric Cardiol 2011;32:342–53.

[62] Iarussi D, Galderisi M, Ratti G, et al. Left ventricular systolic and diastolic function after anthracycline chemotherapy in childhood. Clinical Cardiol 2001;24:663–9.

[63] Yildirim A, Sedef Tunaoglu F, Pinarli FG, et al. Early diagnosis of anthracycline toxicity in asymptomatic long-term survivors: dobutamine stress echocardiography and tissue Doppler velocities in normal and abnormal myocardial wall motion. Eur J Echocardiogr 2010;11:814–22.

[64] Park JH, Kim YH, Hyun MC, Kim HS. Cardiac functional evaluation using vector velocity imaging after chemotherapy including anthracyclines in children with cancer. Korean Circ J 2009;39:352–8.

[65] Sawaya H, Sebag IA, Plana JC, et al. Early detection and prediction of cardiotoxicity in chemotherapy-treated patients. Am J Cardiol 2011;107:1375–80.

[66] Hare JL, Brown JK, Leano R, Jenkins C, Woodward N, Marwick TH. Use of myocardial deformation imaging to detect preclinical myocardial dysfunction before conventional measures in patients undergoing breast cancer treatment with trastuzumab. Am Heart J 2009;158:294–301.

[67] Lipshultz SE, Cochran TR, Wilkinson JD. Screening for long-term cardiac status during cancer treatment. Circ Cardiovasc Imaging 2012;5:555–8.

[68] Bosch J. Carvedilol: the beta-blocker of choice for portal hypertension? Gut 2013;62:1529–30.

[69] Thavendiranathan P, Wintersperger BJ, Flamm SD, Marwick TH. Cardiac MRI in the assessment of cardiac injury and toxicity from cancer chemotherapy: a systematic review. Circ Cardiovasc Imaging 2013;6:1080–91.

[70] Tzonevska A, Chakarova A, Tzvetkov K. GSPECT-CT myocardial scintigraphy plus calcium scores as screening tool for prevention of cardiac side effects in leftsided breast cancer radiotherapy. Journal of BUON : official journal of the Balkan Union of Oncology 2014;19:667–72.

[71] van Leeuwen-Segarceanu EM, Bos W-JW, Dorresteijn LDA, et al. Screening Hodgkin lymphoma survivors for radiotherapy induced cardiovascular disease. Cancer Treat Rev 2011;37:391–403.

[72] Lipshultz SE, Miller TL, Scully RE, et al. Changes in cardiac biomarkers during doxorubicin treatment of pediatric patients with high-risk acute lymphoblastic leukemia: associations with long-term echocardiographic outcomes. J Clin Oncol 2012;30:1042–9.

[73] Ratnasamy C, Kinnamon DD, Lipshultz SE, Rusconi P. Associations between neurohormonal and inflammatory activation and heart failure in children. Am Heart J 2008;155:527–33.

[74] Petricoin EF, Ross MM, Zhou W, et al. Development and pilot evaluation of a new nanoparticle-capture workflow for doxorubicin-induced toxicity biomarker identification. Prog Pediatr Cardiol 2015;39:85–91.

[75] Hochster HS. Clinical pharmacology of dexrazoxane. Semin Oncol 1998;25:37–42.

[76] Lipshultz SE, Rifai N, Dalton VM, et al. The effect of dexrazoxane on myocardial injury in doxorubicin-treated children with acute lymphoblastic leukemia. New Engl J Med 2004;351:145–53.

[77] Lipshultz SE. Dexrazoxane for protection against cardiotoxic effects of anthracyclines in children. J Clin Oncol 1996;14:328–31.

[78] Lyu YL, Kerrigan JE, Lin CP, et al. Topoisomerase IIbeta mediated DNA double-strand breaks: implications in doxorubicin cardiotoxicity and prevention by dexrazoxane. Cancer Res 2007;67:8839–46.

[79] Prevention of cardiomyopathy for chilren and adolescents 0 through 16 years of age treated with anthracyclines. Federal Drug Administration, 2014. Available from: http://www.accessdata.fda.gov/scripts/opdlisting/oopd/listResult.cfm.

[80] Lipshultz SE, Franco VI, Sallan SE, et al. Dexrazoxane for reducing anthracycline-related cardiotoxicity in children with cancer: an update of the evidence. Prog Pediatr Cardiol 2014;36:39–49.

[81] Tebbi CK, London WB, Friedman D, et al. Dexrazoxane-associated risk for acute myeloid leukemia/myelodysplastic syndrome and other secondary malignancies in pediatric Hodgkin's disease. J Clin Oncol 2007;25:493–500.

[82] Lipshultz SE, Lipsitz SR, Orav EJ. Dexrazoxane-associated risk for secondary malignancies in pediatric Hodgkin's disease: a claim without compelling evidence. J Clin Oncol 2007;25:3179. author reply 80.

[83] Barry EV, Vrooman LM, Dahlberg SE, et al. Absence of secondary malignant neoplasms in children with high-risk acute lymphoblastic leukemia treated with dexrazoxane. J Clin Oncol 2008;26:1106–11.

[84] Asselin BL, Devidas M, Chen L, et al. Cardioprotection and safety of dexrazoxane in patients treated for newly diagnosed T-cell acute lymphoblastic leukemia or advanced-stage lymphoblastic Non-Hodgkin lymphoma: A report of the Children's Oncology Group Randomized Trial Pediatric Oncology Group 9404. J Clin Oncol 2016;34(8):854–62.

[85] Lipshultz SE, Scully RE, Lipsitz SR, et al. Assessment of dexrazoxane as a cardioprotectant in doxorubicin-treated children with high-risk acute lymphoblastic leukaemia: long-term follow-up of a prospective, randomised, multicentre trial. Lancet Oncol 2010;11:950–61.

[86] Vrooman LM, Neuberg DS, Stevenson KE, et al. The low incidence of secondary acute myelogenous leukaemia in children and adolescents treated with dexrazoxane for acute lymphoblastic leukaemia: a report from the Dana-Farber Cancer Institute ALL Consortium. Euro J Cancer (Oxford, England : 1990) 2011;47:1373–9.

[87] Chow EJ, Asselin BL, Schwartz CL, et al. Late mortality after dexrazoxane treatment: a report from the children's oncology group. J Clin Oncol 2015;33:2639–45.

[88] Schwartz CL, Wexler LH, Krailo MD, et al. Intensified chemotherapy with dexrazoxane cardioprotection in newly diagnosed nonmetastatic osteosarcoma: a report from the children's oncology group. Pediatr Blood Cancer 2016;63:54–61.

[89] Ebb D, Meyers P, Grier H, et al. Phase II trial of trastuzumab in combination with cytotoxic chemotherapy for treatment of metastatic osteosarcoma with human epidermal growth factor receptor 2 overexpression: a report from the children's oncology group. J Clin Oncol 2012;30:2545–51.

[90] Lipshultz SE, Lipsitz SR, Sallan SE, et al. Long-term enalapril therapy for left ventricular dysfunction in doxorubicin-treated survivors of childhood cancer. J Clin Oncol 2002;20:4517–22.

[91] Lipshultz SE, Vlach SA, Lipsitz SR, Sallan SE, Schwartz ML, Colan SD. Cardiac changes associated with growth hormone therapy among children treated with anthracyclines. Pediatrics 2005;115:1613–22.

[92] Lipshultz SE, Diamond MB, Franco VI, et al. Managing chemotherapy-related cardiotoxicity in survivors of childhood cancers. Paediatr Drugs 2014;16:373–89.

[93] Heidenreich PA, Schnittger I, Strauss HW, et al. Screening for coronary artery disease after mediastinal irradiation for Hodgkin's disease. J Clin Oncol 2007;25:43–9.

[94] Landier W, Bhatia S, Eshelman DA, et al. Development of risk-based guidelines for pediatric cancer survivors: the children's oncology group long-term follow-up guidelines from the Children's Oncology Group Late Effects Committee and Nursing Discipline. J Clin Oncol 2004;22:4979–90.

[95] Simbre VC, Duffy SA, Dadlani GH, Miller TL, Lipshultz SE. Cardiotoxicity of cancer chemotherapy: implications for children. Paediatr Drugs 2005;7:187–202.

[96] Lipshultz SE, Lipsitz SR, Sallan SE, et al. Chronic progressive cardiac dysfunction years after doxorubicin therapy for childhood acute lymphoblastic leukemia. J Clin Oncol 2005;23:2629–36.

[97] Krischer JP, Epstein S, Cuthbertson DD, Goorin AM, Epstein ML, Lipshultz SE. Clinical cardiotoxicity following anthracycline treatment for childhood cancer: the Pediatric Oncology Group experience. J Clin Oncol 1997;15:1544–52.

[98] Lipshultz SE, Miller TL, Lipsitz SR, et al. Continuous versus bolus infusion of doxorubicin in children with all: long-term cardiac outcomes. Pediatrics 2012;130:1003–11.

[99] Wouters KA, Kremer LC, Miller TL, Herman EH, Lipshultz SE. Protecting against anthracycline-induced myocardial damage: a review of the most promising strategies. Br J Haematol 2005;131:561–78.

[100] van Dalen EC, van der Pal HJ, van den Bos C, Caron HN, Kremer LC. Treatment for asymptomatic anthracycline-induced cardiac dysfunction in childhood cancer survivors: the need for evidence. J Clin Oncol 2003;21:3377. author reply -8.

[101] Barry E, Alvarez JA, Scully RE, Miller TL, Lipshultz SE. Anthracycline-induced cardiotoxicity: course, pathophysiology, prevention and management. Expert Opin Pharmacother 2007;8:1039–58.

[102] Giantris A, Abdurrahman L, Hinkle A, Asselin B, Lipshultz SE. Anthracycline-induced cardiotoxicity in children and young adults. Crit Rev Oncol Hematol 1998;27:53–68.

[103] Lipshultz SE, Landy DC, Lopez-Mitnik G, et al. Cardiovascular status of childhood cancer survivors exposed and unexposed to cardiotoxic therapy. J Clin Oncol 2012;30:1050–7.

[104] Miller TL, Lipsitz SR, Lopez-Mitnik G, et al. Characteristics and determinants of adiposity in pediatric cancer survivors. Cancer Epidemiol Biomarkers Prev 2010;19:2013–22.

[105] Lipshultz SE, Wilkinson JD. Beta-adrenergic adaptation in idiopathic dilated cardiomyopathy: differences between children and adults. Eur Heart J 2014;35:10–2.

Chapter 12

Chemotherapy-Induced Amenorrhea and Menopause: Cardiovascular Implications

C.L. Shufelt, D. Wall, R. Sarbaziha and E.T. Wang

Barbra Streisand Women's Heart Center, Cedars-Sinai Heart Institute, and Department of Obstetrics and Gynecology, Division of Reproductive Endocrinology and Infertility, Cedars-Sinai Medical Center, Los Angeles, CA, United States

MENOPAUSE

Menopause is the final menstrual period and results from the loss of ovarian follicular activity causing a permanent decline in gonadal hormone levels. Women are born with a fixed number of ovarian follicles, referred to as the ovarian reserve, that decline exponentially through atresia and ovulation until the onset of menopause. Menopause is confirmed by a serum follicle stimulating hormone (FSH) more than 30 mIU/mL and 12 consecutive months of amenorrhea [1]. The average age of menopause in the United States is 52 years; however, menopause may occur earlier in some women [1]. Different genetic disorders, illnesses, and ovotoxic treatments, such as certain chemotherapies are linked to ovarian dysfunction resulting in estrogen deficiency before the age of natural menopause. Premature menopause is defined as menopause before the age of 40 years, whereas early menopause occurs between the ages of 40 and 45 years [2].

Menopausal symptoms commonly include vasomotor symptoms (VMS), such as hot flashes and night sweats, urogenital atrophy, sleep disturbances, low libido, dyspareunia, and mood disturbance [3–6]. Hot flashes and night sweats are the most common symptoms; estimated to affect 14–51% in premenopause, 35–50% in perimenopause, and 30–80% in postmenopause [7]. Symptoms are also variable and based on a number of factors including culture, age, weight, smoking status, as well as physical and mental health [3,5,6,8]. Approximately one-third of women entering menopause at the age of 50 experience moderate-to-severe hot flashes; however, the rate of symptoms increases by 2–4% for each chronic physical disease (i.e., diabetes, hypertension) or mental disorder (i.e., depression, anxiety) [3]. Furthermore, women who smoke or are obese report more intense and frequent menopausal symptoms [3,8].

CHEMOTHERAPY-INDUCED MENOPAUSE

The average incidence of chemotherapy-induced menopause in premenopausal women treated for breast cancer with adjuvant chemotherapy is reportedly 68% with a wide range of 20–100% [9]. Chemotherapy-induced amenorrhea may lead to primary ovarian insufficiency (POI) if there is permanent damage to ovarian follicles defined as follicle depletion or dysfunction with cessation of menses before the age of 40 [10]. However, POI is a state of impaired ovarian function that may return with approximately 5–10% of women able to conceive [11]. The resumption of ovarian function may be short-lived with permanent loss of follicular activity eventually resulting in premature menopause. If amenorrhea lasts over a year, the vast majority of women will not regain ovarian function and are considered to have premature menopause [12].

An estimated 1% of reproductive-aged women will experience POI [13], however, the prevalence is higher in patients undergoing or who have received cancer treatment [12,14]. According to the Childhood Cancer Survivor Study of 2819 female childhood cancer survivors, approximately 6% developed acute ovarian failure shortly after cancer therapy, and another 8% developed premature menopause [15]. In another study, 30% of patients treated with a combination of alkylating agents and abdominopelvic radiation experienced premature menopause [16]. For many female-specific cancer therapies, POI is a common side effect even years after treatment, and women who do not experience acute ovarian failure still remain at an increased risk of developing premature menopause later in life [12].

Menopausal symptoms in cancer patients are common. Women receiving adjuvant chemotherapy may begin to experience VMS as early as 6–12 weeks posttreatment and symptoms may extend for years after treatment [17].

Menopausal symptoms may manifest differently in cancer patients compared to women who experience natural menopause. One study found that hot flashes were more prevalent, severe, and bothersome in cancer survivors compared to women seeking treatment for menopausal symptoms [18]. Additionally, research has shown that menopausal symptoms experienced by women with POI do not diminish over time, as with natural menopause [18,19]. Younger breast cancer patients also experience menopausal symptoms. Women who are premenopausal prior to the diagnosis of breast cancer report significantly higher vasomotor and dystrophic symptoms after the induction of ovarian failure, compared to women who are postmenopausal at the time of diagnosis [20].

Chemotherapy-induced amenorrhea has significant reproductive implications, such as loss of fertility and women who experience chemotherapy-induced menopause experience the psychological effects of understanding the potential loss of fertility. In 2012, 790,000 new cases of cancer were diagnosed in women in the United States, and 10% of these cases were in reproductive-age women under 45 years of age [21]. Fertility is an important issue in cancer survivorship, with 30–40% of reproductive-age survivors endorsing loss of control over reproductive future and inability to talk openly about fertility [22]. To this end, the American Society of Clinical Oncology has recommended that "As part of education and informed consent before cancer therapy, oncologists should address the possibility of infertility with patients treated during their reproductive years and be prepared to discuss possible fertility preservation options or refer patients to reproductive specialists" [23]. Fertility preservation options primarily focus on assisted reproductive technology, including cryopreservation of embryos or oocytes [24,25]. Studies have also demonstrated that the incidence of chemotherapy-induced amenorrhea underestimates infertility and reproductive impairment in cancer survivors who have resumption of menses [26]. Experimental methods of in vitro maturation, the process of maturing oocytes in the laboratory, or ovarian tissue cryopreservation are being explored as methods of fertility preservation in prepubertal girls facing gonadotoxic therapy [27,28].

CHEMOTHERAPY AND THE OVARIES

Certain chemotherapy agents can be gonadotoxic, or destructive to the finite number of primordial oocytes in the human ovary. Ovarian reserve, defined as the quantity and quality of oocytes, gradually decreases with age as primordial follicles undergo apoptotic loss over a woman's reproductive lifespan [29]. At the time of menopause, the ovarian reserve has been depleted. Thus, gonadotoxicity is dependent on age, the type of chemotherapy agent, and the dosage. Studies have demonstrated that among premenopausal women with early stage breast cancer, women who experience chemotherapy-induced amenorrhea have lower levels of serum anti-Mullerian hormone, an established ovarian reserve marker, than women who resume menses [30].

The most common histologic abnormalities in the ovaries of women who have received chemotherapy are fibrosis and destruction of the follicles. Chemotherapy can also result in inhibition or cessation of follicular maturation and decreased or apoptosis of primordial follicles [31,32]. Furthermore, ovarian aging is accelerated due to damage of the granulosa and theca cells which are responsible for sex steroid production. This leads to hormonal changes, such as an elevated FSH and LH and decrease in the levels of estradiol [31].

Chemotherapy agents are classified into three groups in terms of gonadotoxicity: high-risk (of inducing amenorrhea or menopause), intermediate-risk, and low-risk agents [33]. The high-risk agents include notably alkylating agents, such as cyclophosphamide and ifosfamide. Alkylating agents are not cell-cycle specific and do not require cell proliferation for cytotoxic action, which targets resting oocytes [34]. The effects of cyclophosphamide on the ovaries occur as early as 24 h after the administration of the drug, and after the first week of treatment 85% of the primordial follicles may be destroyed [35]. Rates of amenorrhea with cyclophosphamide range from 61–97%, whereas rates in younger women range from 18–61% [36]. In addition, older women require a shorter time to the induction of amenorrhea and the amenorrhea is more likely to be irreversible. Intermediate-risk agents include cisplatin, adriamycin, and doxorubicin. In an analysis of three prospective trials, the rate of amenorrhea was 80% in premenopausal women treated with doxorubicin. The studies also found that menses resumes in approximately 50% of women, however, this did not correlate with fertility in women below the age of 40 [36]. Low-risk agents include bleomycin, actinomycin D, vincristine, methotrexate, and 5-Fluorouracil. Because these agents target specific phases of the cell cycle, the ovarian follicles and granulosa cells are not as impacted and amenorrhea may not occur.

To protect ovarian function during chemotherapy, the concurrent administration of gonadotropin releasing hormone (GnRH) agonists has been evaluated extensively primarily in premenopausal breast cancer patients. Although it has been hypothesized that GnRH agonists suppress ovaries to a quiescent or prepubertal state, this has not been substantiated [37]. Other possible mechanisms include a decrease in ovarian perfusion and exposure of the ovaries to chemotherapy, pathways independent of gonadotropins as primordial oocytes are not yet responsive, or upregulation of intraovarian antiapoptotic molecules. The PROMISE-GIM6 Study, a randomized controlled trial of premenopausal women with stage-I to -III hormone receptor-positive or hormone receptor-negative breast cancer demonstrated that GnRH agonists during chemotherapy increases the incidence of menstrual resumption over 5 years (age-adjusted HR 1.48, 95% CI, 1.12–1.95) [38]. Another randomized trial of hormone-receptor-negative breast cancer concluded that the ovarian failure rate was 8% in the chemotherapy and GnRH agonists group compared to 22% in the chemotherapy alone group ($P = 0.04$) [39]. Systematic reviews have supported these conclusions with a higher rate of menstrual resumption after 6 months (OR 2.41, 95% CI 1.40–4.15) in the premenopausal breast cancer population [40,41]. However, the protective benefit of GnRH agonists on ovarian function has not been clearly established for other malignancies, such as Hodgkin or non-Hodgkin lymphoma [42], or for the purposes of fertility preservation [43].

THE CARDIOVASCULAR CONSEQUENCES OF MENOPAUSE

Heart disease is the leading cause of death in women and accounts for almost a quarter of female deaths in the United States annually [44]. CVD risk is lower in premenopausal women yet the incidence CVD mortality increases remarkably in the 5th decade of a woman's life, after the onset of menopause [45,46]. For every year menopause is delayed, CVD risk is reduced by 3% [47]. Furthermore, young women that enter menopause early experience a two- to sixfold higher incidence of CVD compared to age-matched premenopausal women [48]. CVD risk also occurs 10 years later in women compared to men; however, the dramatic increase in CVD at menopause closes the mortality gap between men and women [49]. The delayed CVD onset compared to men has largely been attributed to the protective effects of endogenous estrogen on the vasculature. However, a strong relationship remains between chronological age and CVD risk, making it difficult to determine the relative contribution of menopause to the increased CVD risk.

To date there is limited research evaluating the risk of CVD associated with chemotherapy-induced amenorrhea and menopause. There is some evidence that women who experience amenorrhea during and after chemotherapy treatment may have higher CVD risk due to a negative shift in serum lipids even if menstruation resumes [50,51]. Still, the current understanding is that regardless of the cause, women who experience menopause early have increased CVD morbidity and mortality [52,53].

Estrogen and the Vascular System

Estrogen has both positive and negative effects on the vascular system. Positive effects include the antiinflammatory response on injured blood vessels [54], and improving endothelial function which facilitates arterial vasodilation and

relaxation [55]. The presence of estrogen also enhances systemic fibrinolysis [56], has antioxidant effects within a healthy endothelium [57], and increases vascular reactivity [58]. Evidence suggests that the loss of ovarian estrogens activates both circulating and tissue renin–angiotensin–aldosterone system (RAAS) leading to hypertension [59], endothelial dysfunction and arterial stiffness [60], and is linked to the pathogenesis of diastolic dysfunction [61]. On the other hand, estrogen has a known procoagulant effect by inducing thrombin receptor expression [62]. Estrogen also increases the production of triglycerides and inflammatory markers, such as C-reactive protein [63].

In order to understand the effects of estrogen on the endothelium, one must consider the vascular age of the blood vessel. Estrogen activity on healthy endothelium is particularly different compared to its effect on diseased vessels where atherosclerotic plaque is present (Fig. 12.1). Estrogen readily binds to the estrogen receptors in a healthy endothelium producing nitric oxide, a powerful vasodilator [64]. In this setting, estrogen also reduces the progression of atherosclerosis, by decreasing cell adhesion and smooth muscle proliferation [64]. As aging occurs, atherosclerotic plaque forms over the endothelium obstructing vascular estrogen receptors. Estrogen cannot activate or bind to the receptors resulting in decreased nitric oxide production, decreased vasodilation, and endothelium dysfunction [65]. Furthermore, estrogen may contribute to plaque instability and increased neovascularization causing the fibrous cap of the atherosclerotic lesion to degrade and rupture.

Estrogen's effect on a healthy and diseased endothelium has come to be termed the "timing hypothesis." According to the timing hypothesis the beneficial effects of estrogen occur in younger blood vessels before advanced atherosclerosis develops, such as at the time of menopause. In older or diseased vessels no beneficial effects are seen and estrogen in this setting of an altered endothelium may be harmful [66]. Further support of the timing hypothesis was evident in the Women's Health Initiative, a double-blinded randomized clinical trial evaluating hormone-replacement therapy (HT) on the primary prevention of chronic disease, such as coronary heart disease (CHD). Results of this trial found an increased risk of CHD on hormone therapy compared to placebo (37 vs. 30 per 10,000 women per year), stroke (29 vs. 21 per 10,000 women per year), and venous thromboembolic events (34 vs. 16 per 10,000 women per year) [67]. Importantly and by design, women in this trial were on average 12 years postmenopausal and without menopausal symptoms. When data was further analyzed by age at study entry, it was found that women ages 50–59 years had a lower risk of CHD (RR 0.63 95% CI, 0.36–1.09) compared to older women in the 60–69 and 70–79 years cohorts (RR 0.94, 95% CI 0.71–1.24 and RR 1.13, 95% CI 0.82–1.54, respectively) [68]. This increased risk, however, was significantly reduced when HT

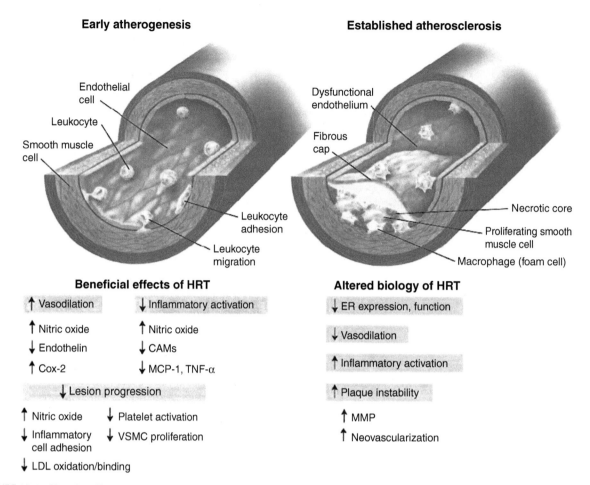

Early atherogenesis

Endothelial cell
Leukocyte
Smooth muscle cell

Leukocyte adhesion
Leukocyte migration

Established atherosclerosis

Dysfunctional endothelium
Fibrous cap

Necrotic core
Proliferating smooth muscle cell
Macrophage (foam cell)

Beneficial effects of HRT

↑ Vasodilation   ↓ Inflammatory activation

↑ Nitric oxide   ↑ Nitric oxide
↓ Endothelin   ↓ CAMs
↑ Cox-2   ↓ MCP-1, TNF-α

↓ Lesion progression

↑ Nitric oxide   ↓ Platelet activation
↓ Inflammatory   ↓ VSMC proliferation
  cell adhesion
↓ LDL oxidation/binding

Altered biology of HRT

↓ ER expression, function

↓ Vasodilation

↑ Inflammatory activation

↑ Plaque instability

↑ MMP

↑ Neovascularization

FIGURE 12.1   Vascular effects of estrogen in early versus established atherosclerosis. CAM, cell adhesion molecule; Cox-2, cycloxygenase 2; ER, estrogen receptor; HRT, hormone replacement therapy; LDL, low-density lipoprotein; MCP, monocyte chemoattractant protein; MMP, matrix metalloproteinase; TNF, tumor necrosis factor; VSMC, vascular smooth muscle cell. *From Ouyang P, Michos ED, Karas RH. Hormone replacement therapy and the cardiovascular system: lessons learned and unanswered questions. J Am Coll Cardiol 2006;47(9):1741–53.*

begins closer to the onset of menopause and in younger women, suggesting the blood vessels were less likely to be diseased [68,69].

Estrogen Deficiency and Lipids

Lipoproteins play a major role in atheroma formation. Estrogens have been found to clear low-density lipoprotein (LDL) particles from the vasculature and regulate LDL receptors in the liver. Therefore, it is unsurprising that women who experience premature menopause and POI also experience adverse changes in lipids at a younger age. A recent study comparing women with POI to age-matched controls found higher levels of total cholesterol and LDL, but no differences in HDL between groups [70]. In addition, the researchers also found a negative correlation between estrogen concentration and total cholesterol suggesting that as estrogen decreased, total cholesterol increased [70]. These results are consistent with other research measuring lipids in women with POI [71].

In an attempt to unveil the relative contributions of aging and menopause on CVD one study evaluated several known risk factors, such as blood pressure (BP) and cholesterol annually for 10 years and compared them to linear (reflective of chronological aging) and piecewise linear (reflective of ovarian aging) models [72]. Results found most risk factors including glucose, insulin, BP, fibrinogen, and C-reactive protein changed linearly consistent with the chronological aging model. However, total cholesterol, LDL, and apolipoprotein-B were associated with the loss of estrogen during menopause transition [72]. Another study comparing similar risk factors in pre- and postmenopausal women of the same age also found measureable differences only in total cholesterol, LDL, and apolipoprotein B [73]. These data suggest that cholesterol is the CVD risk factor that is most effected by menopause.

Similar changes to lipids have also been observed in women who experience chemotherapy-induced menopause. The destruction of germ cells by chemotherapy is well known, and the administration of especially alkylating agents, results in a reduction of estrogen and an unfavorable lipid profile shift. Premenopausal women who develop chemotherapy-induced ovarian dysfunction are found to have an increase in total cholesterol, LDL, HDL, and apolipoprotein B [51]. Changes to lipids also correlate significantly to whether or not menses is maintained during the treatment of adjuvant chemotherapy with a negative shift in serum lipids observed in patients with permanent amenorrhea [50,51]. Even women with irregular menstrual periods following adjuvant chemotherapy experience elevated serum total cholesterol and LDL [50]. An unhealthy lipid profile is a risk factor for CVD; therefore, the shift observed in women with chemotherapy-induced ovarian dysfunction possibly increases the risk of adverse cardiovascular outcomes, such as atherosclerosis, CHD, or ischemic heart disease (IHD), and stroke.

Estrogen Deficiency and Blood Pressure

BP increases after menopause. After the age of 60 years the prevalence of hypertension is approximately 65%, and 30% higher in women compared to men ($\geq 140/90$ mmHg) [74]. Women younger than 45 years have lower BP compared to men; however, after the age of 45 both systolic BP and pulse pressure is higher in women [75]. In contrast, diastolic BP is lower in women at all ages [75]. Furthermore, for each decade after the onset of menopause, there is a reported 5 mmHg increase in systolic BP likely due to the reduction of arterial compliance [76]. The loss of estrogen may be responsible for the increase in BP as estrogen is thought to regulate the RAAS by increasing angiotensinogen and suppressing renin, which activates the conversion of angiotensinogen to angiotensin I [59]. Additionally estrogen HT is found to reduce systolic BP, pulse pressure, and arterial stiffness indices when given to postmenopausal women [77].

The relationship between menopause and increased BP is difficult to determine because hypertension often clusters with several other factors associated with menopause, such as weight gain, hyperlipidemia, and chronological aging. Although studies have found a relationship between estrogen deficiency and increased BP [76,78], a large amount of evidence also indicates no connection between menopause and BP after the adjustment of age [46,72,73]. Interestingly, women with an early reduction of estrogen have measurable changes in BP after the onset of menopause. The Study on Hypertension Prevalence in Menopause in the Italian population (SIMONA) epidemiological study, one of the largest studies to investigate the relationship between menopause and BP, found a slight yet significant association between menopause and both systolic and diastolic BP in postmenopausal women between the ages of 46–49 years [78]. The youngest group of postmenopausal women in the study, those between the ages of 46–47 years, had the greatest

increase in BP compared to premenopausal women (SBP/DBP 3.4/3.1 mmHg higher) [78]. This study suggests that menopause is associated with changes to BP, however, because the changes are small, the effects of chronological age on BP may conceal the relationship.

Estrogen Deficiency and Weight Gain

Although weight gain alone is not a direct CVD risk factor, weight gain contributes to risk with respect to risk factors, such as hypertension and diabetes. Weight gain commonly occurs in breast-cancer patients undergoing chemotherapy and progresses over time with survivorship [79]. Women receiving adjuvant chemotherapy for early-stage breast cancer gain 2.5–6.0 kg in 50–96% of cases [80]. There is evidence that suggests that even a modest weight gain can affect future cardiovascular health. One study found that weight gain of 4–10 kg during adulthood is associated with a 27% increase in CHD risk compared to women with a stable weight [81]. There are several variables that may be responsible for the observed increase in weight including younger age, advanced cancer stage, cancer-related treatments, decreased physical activity, increased caloric intake, and menopausal status [82]. The use of adjuvant chemotherapy is connected to both increased weight gain and the onset of menopause. The onset of menopause during the first year after breast cancer diagnosis is shown to be a strong predictor of weight gain in patients treated with adjuvant chemotherapy [83].

Evidence also suggests that the onset of menopause is not connected with the weight gain observed in breast cancer. One study found women treated with adjuvant chemotherapy gained total body fat, truncal fat, and leg fat regardless of whether ovarian function was retained [84]. Though these results may indicate weight gain is more likely attributable to the use of adjuvant chemotherapies, it is also possible that differences in weight gain between women with and without induced ovarian failure could not be identified due to small sample size. However, studies with much larger populations also have not found a direct relationship between weight gain and menopausal status [85].

The association between weight gain and the onset of menopause or amenorrhea remains controversial in breast-cancer survivors likely due to the inaccuracy in defining treatment-related amenorrhea and induced menopause [85]. It is also likely that the differences in years since diagnosis, the different types of cancer treatment, and inaccuracy in reporting weight gain may also contribute to the observed inconsistencies. Regardless of the underlying cause, weight gain is a common occurrence in breast cancer, especially with the use of adjuvant chemotherapy. Furthermore, weight gain in breast cancer survivors may be connected to increase risk of CVD and all-cause mortality [86], as well as reoccurrence of the disease [87].

CONSIDERATIONS OF CARDIOVASCULAR DISEASE AND COMPLICATIONS DUE TO CHEMOTHERAPY-INDUCED MENOPAUSE

Women who experience chemotherapy-induced POI and premature menopause become estrogen deficient many years prior to the natural age of menopause. Female cancer survivors may therefore have higher risk of CVD outcomes independent of that caused by direct cardiotoxicity from chemotherapy and radiation. In a meta-analysis of 18 studies, the relationship between menopause status and CVD was significantly higher in women with early-onset menopause and bilateral oophorectomy after controlling for confounding variables, such as age and smoking [52]. Women who experience premature menopause also have an increased risk of long-term CVD. Women who enter menopause between the ages of 40–44 years have a 5.7% increased risk of CVD mortality by age 70 years and for every year delay in menopause a 1% decrease in risk of cardiovascular death is observed [53].

To date there is no research specifically evaluating the relationship between chemotherapy-induced menopause and CVD. Instead, the current understanding of risk is concluded from studies of women with bilateral oophorectomy [88], early-onset or premature menopause [89–91]. The findings may be applicable to cancer survivors with chemotherapy-induced ovarian failure as both result in decreased circulating estrogen; however, because chemotherapy-induced menopause is still not well characterized, unique cardiovascular consequences may exist that have not been identified.

Endothelial Dysfunction

Endothelial dysfunction is a marker of preclinical atherosclerosis characterized by both impaired endothelium-dependent vasodilation as well as a procoagulant and proinflammatory state that favors the development of atherosclerosis. Menopause marks an increase in endothelial dysfunction. Compared to men, age-related endothelial dysfunction is attenuated in both normotensive and hypertensive premenopausal women [92]. However, after menopause there is a sharp decline in endothelium-dependent vasodilation and by the age of 60 there are no observable sex-differences, indicating an association between endothelial dysfunction and reduced endogenous estrogen production [92].

Endothelial function is also impaired in women with POI. Women with POI experience impaired flow-mediated dilation, and reduced circulating endothelial progenitor cells compared to healthy age-matched controls [93]. Flow-mediated dilatation is significantly correlated to estradiol levels suggesting a relationship between endothelial dysfunction and estrogen deficiency [93]. Endothelial dysfunction in women with POI has been reversed with HT within 6 months of treatment further indicating the absence of ovarian hormones may result in impaired endothelial function and increased CVD risk [94].

Atherosclerosis and Coronary Heart Disease

Atherosclerosis is the most common long-term complication in both male and female cancer survivors. Though the relationship between atherosclerosis and cancer is still largely unknown, common etiological factors, such as smoking, and direct toxicity from anticancer therapy may explain the comorbidity of the two disorders [95]. There is limited research on atherosclerosis progression in female survivors of cancer. Still, breast cancer patients are found to have an increase in both atherosclerosis risk factors and progression determined by carotid intima-media thickness, after chemotherapy compared to controls [96]. It is unknown if the observed increase is connected to the induction of menopause.

Research consistently shows an inverse relationship between age of menopause and CHD or IHD mortality when looking at women between the ages of 35–55 [90,91,97]. A 3% increase in CHD has been observed for every 1-year decrease in age of menopause [90]. Later age of menopause may reduce the risk of CHD, with a 2% decrease for every year that age of menopause increases [98]. The relationship between CHD and early menopause remains after controlling for smoking, a habit that both reduces the age of menopause and is linked to heart disease [90,98]. A meta-analysis of 10 prospective studies found that women with the earliest age of natural menopause had an 11% greater risk of CHD mortality and an 18% greater risk of all-cause mortality compared to women who experience menopause at a normal age [89]. Interestingly, both cardiovascular and stroke mortality were not significantly related to early age of menopause, indicating early onset influences mortality mainly due to CHD [89].

Women who undergo bilateral oophorectomy during premenopausal years show an increased risk of CHD compared to women who experience natural premature menopause. Results from the Danish Nurse Cohort study showed that though both natural and surgically induced early menopause increased the risk for IHD, women who underwent bilateral oophorectomy before the age of 40 and did not use HT had the highest risk [97]. Another study looked at fatal and nonfatal cardiovascular health outcomes in women who underwent hysterectomy with and without bilateral oophorectomy for a follow-up period of 24 years [99]. All women had a statistically significant increase in CHD risk (HR 1.17; 95% CI: 1.02–1.35), however the risk was elevated in women oophorectomized before the age of 45 (HR 1.26; 95% CI: 1.04–1.54) [99]. These findings suggest the abrupt and permanent loss of ovarian hormones that occurs in surgical menopause is more detrimental to cardiovascular health than the more gradual decline observed in natural menopause.

Stroke

Evidence suggests that total cholesterol, LDL, and total to HDL cholesterol ratio are positively and significantly associated with increased risk of stroke in women, especially ischemic stroke [100]. Therefore, the adverse lipid profiles commonly observed in women with a premature reduction of estrogen may increase the risk of stroke. It is important to note that results from multiple studies suggest that HT actually increases the risk of stroke in postmenopausal women, especially in women over the age of 50 years [68,101,102].

Research suggests a relationship exists between younger age of menopause and increased risk of stroke. The Framingham study found that women who experience natural menopause before the age of 42 have double the stroke risk compared to women with menopause at a later age, even after adjusting for confounding variables (HR 2.03; 95% CI: 1.16–3.56) [103]. The incidence of cerebral infraction is 2.5 times higher in women who experienced menopause before the age of 40, compared to women with menopause between 50 and 54 years even after the adjustment of CVD risk factors, such as hypertension, BMI, and smoking (HR 2.57; 95% CI: 1.20–5.49) [104]. Women with surgically induced menopause have higher rates of stroke compared to nonsurgical premature menopause suggesting that the abrupt reduction of estrogen may have a stronger effect on stroke risk [104].

The relationship between stroke and premature menopause is not consistent, with a number of studies showing no connection between the two [47,89,105]. The Nurse's Health Study, a longitudinal analysis of over 35,000 women, found no association between age of menopause and total, ischemic, or hemorrhagic stroke [47]. Similarly, a large 37-year follow-up cohort study of close to 20,000 women found no definite relationship between age of natural menopause and mortality from stroke either ischemic or hemorrhagic [105]. However, most of the data that has shown no relationship between early-onset menopause and stroke with groups of women who experience premature or early menopause naturally, not induced by chemotherapy. Research using women with bilateral oophorectomy or "induced" premature or early menopause usually unveil a connection between estrogen deficiency and stroke [88,99]. For example, one study found a significant increase stroke risk by 149% in women who underwent bilateral oophorectomy before the age of 50 and did not receive HT [99]. Furthermore, the sudden loss of estrogen resulting from surgery and perhaps chemotherapy may be an important risk factor for stroke that is independent of the direct chemotoxic effect on the brain.

MENOPAUSE TREATMENT OPTIONS

There are several nonhormonal treatment options to help control menopausal symptoms in women with chemotherapy-induced menopause as treatment with estrogen after breast or other estrogen sensitive cancers remains controversial. Furthermore, the North American Menopause Society (NAMS) and American College of Cardiology/American Heart Association CVD treatment guidelines do not recommend the use of estrogen for primary or secondary prevention of CVD [106]. Paroxetine salt (trade name Brisdelle) is the only nonhormonal medication approved by the US Food and Drug Administration for the treatment of VMS. Research has shown that after 4 weeks hot flashes significantly decrease compared to placebo, and by week 12 women experience 5.6 less moderate-to-severe hot flashes per day with Brisdelle compared to a reduction of 3.9 per day with placebo [107]. Other selective serotonin reuptake/norepinephrine reuptake inhibitors may also be used in low dose for treatment although are considered an off-label indication. Other off-label treatment options include low-dose gabapentin and clonidine [108]. NAMS recommends cognitive behavioral therapy and hypnosis, and suggests weight loss, mindfulness-based meditation may be useful for the reduction of VMS [108]. Stellate ganglion blockade, a common anesthetic used for pain management, is emerging treatment option for VMS; however, further trials are needed to determine efficacy [108]. Due to negative or insufficient data, nonhormonal treatments that are not recommended by NAMS include cooling techniques, avoidance of triggers, exercise, yoga, over-the-counter supplements, and acupuncture [108]. It is important that practitioners carefully evaluate clinical history including previous chemotherapies, risk of deep vein thrombosis, risk of coronary artery disease, and risk for stroke before determining the best treatment option.

CONCLUSIONS

Prior to initiating chemotherapy, young women should be counseled about the possibilities of chemotherapy-induced amenorrhea, POI, and menopause. Clinicians should be aware of the changes to CVD risk factors, such as BP, lipids, weight gain as a result of chemotherapy-induced menopause and should monitor women that have been treated with higher risk chemotherapy agents closely both during and after treatment. The American Heart Association and American College of Cardiology treatment guidelines should be applied to all women with cardiovascular risk factors with special attention to monitoring women after chemotherapy. Future direction should focus on awareness and prevention by adapting chemotherapy-induced amenorrhea and menopause into guidelines for the prevention of CVD in women.

REFERENCES

[1] Shifren JL, Gass ML. The North American Menopause Society recommendations for clinical care of midlife women. Menopause 2014;21(10):1038–62.

[2] Rebar RW, Connolly HV. Clinical features of young women with hypergonadotropic amenorrhea. Fertil Steril 1990;53(5):804–10.

[3] Dennerstein L, Lehert P, Koochaki PE, Graziottin A, Leiblum S, Alexander JL. A symptomatic approach to understanding women's health experiences: a cross-cultural comparison of women aged 20 to 70 years. Menopause 2007;14(4):688–96.

[4] Dennerstein L, Dudley EC, Hopper JL, Guthrie JR, Burger HG. A prospective population-based study of menopausal symptoms. Obstet Gynecol 2000;96(3):351–8.

[5] Obermeyer CM, Sievert LL. Cross-cultural comparisons: midlife, aging, and menopause. Menopause 2007;14(4):663–7.

[6] Harlow SD, Gass M, Hall JE, et al. Executive summary of the Stages of Reproductive Aging Workshop + 10: addressing the unfinished agenda of staging reproductive aging. J Clin Endocrinol Metab 2012;97(4):1159–68.

[7] National Institutes of Health State-of-the-Science Conference statement. Management of menopause-related symptoms. Ann Int Med 2005;142(12 Pt 1):1003–13.

[8] Gold EB, Sternfeld B, Kelsey JL, et al. Relation of demographic and lifestyle factors to symptoms in a multi-racial/ethnic population of women 40-55 years of age. Am J Epidemiol 2000;152(5):463–73.

[9] Bines J, Oleske DM, Cobleigh MA. Ovarian function in premenopausal women treated with adjuvant chemotherapy for breast cancer. J Clin Oncol 1996;14(5):1718–29.

[10] Committee opinion, no., 605. primary ovarian insufficiency in adolescents and young women. Obstet Gynecol 2014;124(1):193–7.

[11] van Kasteren YM, Schoemaker J. Premature ovarian failure: a systematic review on therapeutic interventions to restore ovarian function and achieve pregnancy. Hum Reprod Update 1999;5(5):483–92.

[12] Partridge A, Gelber S, Gelber RD, Castiglione-Gertsch M, Goldhirsch A, Winer E. Age of menopause among women who remain premenopausal following treatment for early breast cancer: long-term results from International Breast Cancer Study Group Trials V and VI. Eur J Cancer 2007;43(11):1646–53.

[13] Luborsky JL, Meyer P, Sowers MF, Gold EB, Santoro N. Premature menopause in a multi-ethnic population study of the menopause transition. Human Reprod 2003;18(1):199–206.

[14] Sklar C. Maintenance of ovarian function and risk of premature menopause related to cancer treatment. J Natl Cancer Inst Monogr 2005;(34):25–7.

[15] Green DM, Sklar CA, Boice JD Jr, et al. Ovarian failure and reproductive outcomes after childhood cancer treatment: results from the Childhood Cancer Survivor Study. J Clin Oncol 2009;27(14):2374–81.

[16] Sklar CA, Mertens AC, Mitby P, et al. Premature menopause in survivors of childhood cancer: a report from the childhood cancer survivor study. J J Natl Cancer Inst 2006;98(13):890–6.

[17] Dnistrian AM, Schwartz MK, Fracchia AA, Kaufman RJ, Hakes TB, Currie VE. Endocrine consequences of CMF adjuvant therapy in premenopausal and postmenopausal breast cancer patients. Cancer 1983;51(5):803–7.

[18] Marino JL, Saunders CM, Emery LI, Green H, Doherty DA, Hickey M. Nature and severity of menopausal symptoms and their impact on quality of life and sexual function in cancer survivors compared with women without a cancer history. Menopause 2014;21(3):267–74.

[19] Allshouse AA, Semple AL, Santoro NF. Evidence for prolonged and unique amenorrhea-related symptoms in women with premature ovarian failure/primary ovarian insufficiency. Menopause 2015;22(2):166–74.

[20] Biglia N, Cozzarella M, Cacciari F, et al. Menopause after breast cancer: a survey on breast cancer survivors. Maturitas 2003;45(1):29–38.

[21] Siegel R, DeSantis C, Virgo K, et al. Cancer treatment and survivorship statistics, 2012. CA Cancer J Clin 2012;62(4):220–41.

[22] Wenzel L, Dogan-Ates A, Habbal R, et al. Defining and measuring reproductive concerns of female cancer survivors. J Natl Cancer Inst Monogr 2005;(34):94–8.

[23] Loren AW, Mangu PB, Beck LN, et al. Fertility preservation for patients with cancer: American Society of Clinical Oncology clinical practice guideline update. J Clin Oncol 2013;31(19):2500–10.

[24] Practice Committees of American Society for Reproductive, M., Society for Assisted Reproductive T. Mature oocyte cryopreservation: a guideline. Fertil Steril 2013;99(1):37–43.

[25] Ethics Committee of American Society for Reproductive M. Fertility preservation and reproduction in patients facing gonadotoxic therapies: a committee opinion. Fertil Steril 2013;100(5):1224–31.

[26] Letourneau JM, Ebbel EE, Katz PP, et al. Acute ovarian failure underestimates age-specific reproductive impairment for young women undergoing chemotherapy for cancer. Cancer 2012;118(7):1933–9.

[27] Practice Committees of the American Society for Reproductive, M., the Society for Assisted Reproductive T. In vitro maturation: a committee opinion. Fertil Steril 2013;99(3):663–6.

[28] Donnez J, Dolmans MM, Pellicer A, et al. Restoration of ovarian activity and pregnancy after transplantation of cryopreserved ovarian tissue: a review of 60 cases of reimplantation. Fertil Steril 2013;99(6):1503–13.

[29] Practice Committee of the American Society for Reproductive M. Testing and interpreting measures of ovarian reserve: a committee opinion. Fertil Steril 2012;98(6):1407–15.

[30] Anderson RA, Rosendahl M, Kelsey TW, Cameron DA. Pretreatment anti-Mullerian hormone predicts for loss of ovarian function after chemotherapy for early breast cancer. Eur J Cancer 2013;.

[31] Averette HE, Boike GM, Jarrell MA. Effects of cancer chemotherapy on gonadal function and reproductive capacity. CA Cancer J Clin 1990;40(4):199–209.

[32] Torino F, Barnabei A, De Vecchis L, Appetecchia M, Strigari L, Corsello SM. Recognizing menopause in women with amenorrhea induced by cytotoxic chemotherapy for endocrine-responsive early breast cancer. Endocr Relat Cancer 2012;19(2):R21–33.

[33] Rodriguez-Wallberg KA, Oktay K. Fertility preservation during cancer treatment: clinical guidelines. Cancer Manag Res 2014;6:105–17.

[34] Warne GL, Fairley KF, Hobbs JB, Martin FI. Cyclophosphamide-induced ovarian failure. New Engl J Med 1973;289(22):1159–62.

[35] Kalich-Philosoph L, Roness H, Carmely A, et al. Cyclophosphamide triggers follicle activation and "burnout"; AS101 prevents follicle loss and preserves fertility. Sci Transl Med 2013;5(185). 185ra162.

[36] Walshe JM, Denduluri N, Swain SM. Amenorrhea in premenopausal women after adjuvant chemotherapy for breast cancer. J Clin Oncol 2006;24(36):5769–79.

[37] Ben-Aharon I, Gafter-Gvili A, Leibovici L, Stemmer SM. Pharmacological interventions for fertility preservation during chemotherapy: a systematic review and meta-analysis. Breast Cancer Res Treat 2010;122(3):803–11.

[38] Lambertini M, Boni L, Michelotti A, et al. Ovarian suppression with triptorelin during adjuvant breast cancer chemotherapy and long-term ovarian function, pregnancies, and disease-free survival: a randomized clinical trial. JAMA 2015;314(24):2632–40.

[39] Moore HC, Unger JM, Albain KS. Ovarian protection during adjuvant chemotherapy. N Engl J Med 2015;372(23):2269–70.

[40] Munhoz RR, Pereira AA, Sasse AD, et al. Gonadotropin-releasing hormone agonists for ovarian function preservation in premenopausal women undergoing chemotherapy for early-stage breast cancer: a systematic review and meta-analysis. JAMA Oncol 2016;2(1):65–73.

[41] Shen YW, Zhang XM, Lv M, et al. Utility of gonadotropin-releasing hormone agonists for prevention of chemotherapy-induced ovarian damage in premenopausal women with breast cancer: a systematic review and meta-analysis. Onco Targets Ther 2015;8:3349–59.

[42] Demeestere I, Brice P, Peccatori FA, et al. Gonadotropin-releasing hormone agonist for the prevention of chemotherapy-induced ovarian failure in patients with lymphoma: 1-year follow-up of a prospective randomized trial. J Clin Oncol 2013;31(7):903–9.

[43] Behringer K, Wildt L, Mueller H, et al. No protection of the ovarian follicle pool with the use of GnRH-analogues or oral contraceptives in young women treated with escalated BEACOPP for advanced-stage Hodgkin lymphoma. Final results of a phase II trial from the German Hodgkin Study Group. Ann Oncol 2010;21(10): 2052–60.

[44] Kochanek KD, Xu J, Murphy SL, Minino AM, Kung HC. Deaths: final data for 2009. National vital statistics reports: from the Centers for Disease Control and Prevention, National Center for Health Statistics, National Vital Statistics System 2011;60(3):1–116.

[45] Mikkola TS, Gissler M, Merikukka M, Tuomikoski P, Ylikorkala O. Sex differences in age-related cardiovascular mortality. PloS One 2013;8(5):e63347.

[46] Kannel WB, Hjortland MC, McNAMARA PM, Gordon T. Menopause and risk of cardiovascular disease: the Framingham study. Ann Int Med 1976;85(4):447–52.

[47] Hu FB, Grodstein F, Hennekens CH, et al. Age at natural menopause and risk of cardiovascular disease. Arch Intern Med 1999;159(10):1061–6.

[48] Kannel WB, Wilson PF. RIsk factors that attenuate the female coronary disease advantage. Arch Int Med 1995;155(1):57–61.

[49] Anand SS, Islam S, Rosengren A, et al. Risk factors for myocardial infarction in women and men: insights from the INTERHEART study. Eur Heart J 2008;29(7):932–40.

[50] Vehmanen L, Saarto T, Blomqvist C, Taskinen M-R, Elomaa I. Tamoxifen treatment reverses the adverse effects of chemotherapy-induced ovarian failure on serum lipids. Brit J Cancer 2004;91(3):476–81.

[51] Saarto T, Blomqvist C, Ehnholm C, Taskinen MR, Elomaa I. Effects of chemotherapy-induced castration on serum lipids and apoproteins in premenopausal women with node-positive breast cancer. J Clin Endocrinol Metab 1996;81(12):4453–7.

[52] Atsma F, Bartelink M-LEL, Grobbee DE, van der Schouw YT. Postmenopausal status and early menopause as independent risk factors for cardiovascular disease: a meta-analysis. Menopause 2006;13(2):265–79.

[53] van der Schouw YT, van der Graaf Y, Steyerberg EW, Eijkemans JC, Banga JD. Age at menopause as a risk factor for cardiovascular mortality. Lancet 1996;347(9003):714–8.

[54] Miller AP, Feng W, Xing D, et al. Estrogen modulates inflammatory mediator expression and neutrophil chemotaxis in injured arteries. Circulation 2004;110(12):1664–9.

[55] Lieberman EH, Gerhard MD, Uehata A, et al. Estrogen improves endothelium-dependent, flow-mediated vasodilation in postmenopausal women. Ann Int Med 1994;121(12):936–41.

[56] Koh KK. Effects of hormone replacement therapy on coagulation and fibrinolysis in postmenopausal women. Int J Hematol 2002;76(Suppl 2):44–6.

[57] Sugishita K, Li F, Su Z, Barry W. Anti-oxidant effects of estrogen reduce $[Ca^{2+}]$ i during metabolic inhibition. J Mol Cell Cardiol 2003;35(3):331–6.

[58] Perregaux D, Chaudhuri A, Mohanty P, et al. Effect of gender differences and estrogen replacement therapy on vascular reactivity. Metabolism 1999;48(2):227–32.

[59] Schunkert H, Danser AJ, Hense H-W, Derkx FH, Ku S. Effects of estrogen replacement therapy on the renin-angiotensin system in postmenopausal women. Circulation 1997;95(1):39–45.

[60] Aroor AR, Demarco VG, Jia G, et al. The role of tissue renin–angiotensin–aldosterone system in the development of endothelial dysfunction and arterial stiffness. Front Endocrinol 2013;4:161.

[61] Zhao Z, Wang H, Jessup JA, Lindsey SH, Chappell MC, Groban L. Role of estrogen in diastolic dysfunction. Am J Physiol Heart Circ Physiol 2014;306(5):H628–640.

[62] Herkert O, Kuhl H, Sandow J, Busse R, Schini-Kerth VB. Sex steroids used in hormonal treatment increase vascular procoagulant activity by inducing thrombin receptor (PAR-1) expression role of the glucocorticoid receptor. Circulation 2001;104(23):2826–31.

[63] Hu P, Greendale GA, Palla SL, et al. The effects of hormone therapy on the markers of inflammation and endothelial function and plasma matrix metalloproteinase-9 level in postmenopausal women: the postmenopausal estrogen progestin intervention (PEPI) trial. Atherosclerosis 2006;185(2):347–52.

[64] Mendelsohn ME, Karas RH. The protective effects of estrogen on the cardiovascular system. New Engl J Med 1999;340(23):1801–11.

[65] Losordo DW, Kearney M, Kim EA, Jekanowski J, Isner JM. Variable expression of the estrogen receptor in normal and atherosclerotic coronary arteries of premenopausal women. Circulation 1994;89(4):1501–10.

[66] Clarkson TB, Melendez GC, Appt SE. Timing hypothesis for postmenopausal hormone therapy: its origin, current status, and future. Menopause 2013;20(3):342–53.

[67] Rossouw JE, Anderson GL, Prentice RL, et al. Risks and benefits of estrogen plus progestin in healthy postmenopausal women: principal results From the Women's Health Initiative randomized controlled trial. JAMA 2002;288(3):321–33.

[68] Rossouw JE, Prentice RL, Manson JE, et al. Postmenopausal hormone therapy and risk of cardiovascular disease by age and years since menopause. JAMA 2007;297(13):1465–77.

[69] Grodstein F, Manson JE, Stampfer MJ. Hormone therapy and coronary heart disease: the role of time since menopause and age at hormone initiation. J Womens Health 2006;15(1):35–44.

[70] Gulhan I, Bozkaya G, Uyar I, Oztekin D, Pamuk BO, Dogan E. Serum lipid levels in women with premature ovarian failure. Menopause 2012;19(11):1231–4.

[71] Knauff EA, Westerveld HE, Goverde AJ, et al. Lipid profile of women with premature ovarian failure. Menopause 2008;15(5):919–23.

[72] Matthews KA, Crawford SL, Chae CU, et al. Are changes in cardiovascular disease risk factors in midlife women due to chronological aging or to the menopausal transition? J Am Coll Cardiol 2009;54(25):2366–73.

[73] Peters HW, Westendorp IC, Hak AE, et al. Menopausal status and risk factors for cardiovascular disease. J Int Med 1999;246(6):521–8.

[74] Hajjar I, Kotchen TA. Trends in prevalence, awareness, treatment, and control of hypertension in the United States, 1988-2000. JAMA 2003;290(2):199–206.

[75] Martins D, Nelson K, Pan D, Tareen N, Norris K. The effect of gender on age-related blood pressure changes and the prevalence of isolated systolic hypertension among older adults: data from NHANES III. JGSM 2000;4(3):10–3. 20.

[76] Staessen JA, Ginocchio G, Thijs L, Fagard R. Conventional and ambulatory blood pressure and menopause in a prospective population study. J Hum Hypertens 1997;11(8):507–14.

[77] Scuteri A, Lakatta E, Bos A, Fleg J. Effect of estrogen and progestin replacement on arterial stiffness indices in postmenopausal women. Aging Clin Exp Res 2001;13(2):122–30.

[78] Zanchetti A, Facchetti R, Cesana GC, Modena MG, Pirrelli A, Sega R. Menopause-related blood pressure increase and its relationship to age and body mass index: the SIMONA epidemiological study. J Hypertens 2005;23(12):2269–76.

[79] Irwin ML, McTiernan A, Baumgartner RN, et al. Changes in body fat and weight after a breast cancer diagnosis: influence of demographic, prognostic, and lifestyle factors. J Clin Oncol 2005;23(4):774–82.

[80] Rimer BK, Winer EP. Weight gain in women diagnosed with breast cancer. J Am Diet Assoc 1997;97(5):519–29.

[81] Li TY, Rana JS, Manson JE, et al. Obesity as compared with physical activity in predicting risk of coronary heart disease in women. Circulation 2006;113(4):499–506.

[82] Rock CL, Flatt SW, Newman V, et al. Factors associated with weight gain in women after diagnosis of breast cancer. Women's Healthy Eating and Living Study Group. J Am Diet Assoc 1999;99(10):1212–21.

[83] Goodwin PJ, Ennis M, Pritchard KI, et al. Adjuvant treatment and onset of menopause predict weight gain after breast cancer diagnosis. J Clin Oncol 1999;17(1):120–9.

[84] Gordon AM, Hurwitz S, Shapiro CL, LeBoff MS. Premature ovarian failure and body composition changes with adjuvant chemotherapy for breast cancer. Menopause 2011;18(11):1244–8.

[85] Makari-Judson G, Judson CH, Mertens WC. Longitudinal patterns of weight gain after breast cancer diagnosis: observations beyond the first year. Breast J 2007;13(3):258–65.

[86] Nichols HB, Trentham-Dietz A, Egan KM, et al. Body mass index before and after breast cancer diagnosis: associations with all-cause, breast cancer, and cardiovascular disease mortality. Cancer Epidemiol Biomarkers Prev 2009;18(5):1403–9.

[87] Azrad M, Demark-Wahnefried W. The association between adiposity and breast cancer recurrence and survival: a review of the recent literature. Curr Nutr Rep 2014;3(1):9–15.

[88] Rivera CM, Grossardt BR, Rhodes DJ, et al. Increased cardiovascular mortality after early bilateral oophorectomy. Menopause 2009;16(1):15–23.

[89] Gong D, Sun J, Zhou Y, Zou C, Fan Y. Early age at natural menopause and risk of cardiovascular and all-cause mortality: a meta-analysis of prospective observational studies. Int J Cardiol 2016;203:115–9.

[90] Jacobsen BK, Knutsen SF, Fraser GE. Age at natural menopause and total mortality and mortality from ischemic heart disease: the Adventist Health Study. J Clin Epidemiol 1999;52(4):303–7.

[91] Jacobsen BK, Nilssen S, Heuch I, Kvale G. Does age at natural menopause affect mortality from ischemic heart disease? J Clin Epidemiol 1997;50(4):475–9.

[92] Taddei S, Virdis A, Ghiadoni L, et al. Menopause is associated with endothelial dysfunction in women. Hypertension 1996;28(4):576–82.

[93] Yorgun H, Tokgozoglu L, Canpolat U, et al. The cardiovascular effects of premature ovarian failure. Int J Cardiol 2013;168(1):506–10.

[94] Kalantaridou SN, Naka KK, Papanikolaou E, et al. Impaired endothelial function in young women with premature ovarian failure: normalization with hormone therapy. J Clin Endocrinol Metab 2004;89(8):3907–13.

[95] Nuver J, Smit AJ, Sleijfer DT, et al. Microalbuminuria, decreased fibrinolysis, and inflammation as early signs of atherosclerosis in long-term survivors of disseminated testicular cancer. Eur J Cancer 2004;40(5):701–6.

[96] Kalabova H, Melichar B, Ungermann L, et al. Intima-media thickness, myocardial perfusion and laboratory risk factors of atherosclerosis in patients with breast cancer treated with anthracycline-based chemotherapy. Med Oncol 2011;28(4):1281–7.

[97] Lokkegaard E, Jovanovic Z, Heitmann BL, Keiding N, Ottesen B, Pedersen AT. The association between early menopause and risk of ischaemic heart disease: influence of hormone therapy. Maturitas 2006;53(2):226–33.

[98] Ossewaarde ME, Bots ML, Verbeek AL, et al. Age at menopause, cause-specific mortality and total life expectancy. Epidemiology 2005;16(4):556–62.

[99] Parker WH, Broder MS, Chang E, et al. Ovarian conservation at the time of hysterectomy and long-term health outcomes in the nurses' health study. Obstet Gynecol 2009;113(5):1027–37.

[100] Kurth T, Everett BM, Buring JE, Kase CS, Ridker PM, Gaziano JM. Lipid levels and the risk of ischemic stroke in women. Neurology 2007;68(8):556–62.

[101] Magliano DJ, Rogers SL, Abramson MJ, Tonkin AM. Systematic review: hormone therapy and cardiovascular disease: a systematic review and meta-analysis. BJOG 2006;113(1):5–14.

[102] Wassertheil-Smoller S, Hendrix S, Limacher M, et al. Effect of estrogen plus progestin on stroke in postmenopausal women: the Women's Health Initiative: a randomized trial. JAMA 2003;289(20):2673–84.

[103] Lisabeth LD, Beiser AS, Brown DL, Murabito JM, Kelly-Hayes M, Wolf PA. Age at natural menopause and risk of ischemic stroke The Framingham Heart Study. Stroke 2009;40(4):1044–9.

[104] Baba Y, Ishikawa S, Amagi Y, Kayaba K, Gotoh T, Kajii E. Premature menopause is associated with increased risk of cerebral infarction in Japanese women. Menopause 2010;17(3):506–10.

[105] Jacobsen BK, Heuch I, Kvale G. Age at natural menopause and stroke mortality: cohort study with 3561 stroke deaths during 37-year follow-up. Stroke 2004;35(7):1548–51.

[106] Utian WH, Archer DF, Bachmann GA, et al. Estrogen and progestogen use in postmenopausal women: July 2008 position statement of The North American Menopause Society. Menopause 2007;15(4 Pt 1):584–602.

[107] Orleans RJ, Li L, Kim M-J, et al. FDA approval of paroxetine for menopausal hot flushes. New Engl J Med 2014;370(19):1777–9.

[108] Carpenter JS, Gass ML, Maki PM, et al. Nonhormonal management of menopause-associated vasomotor symptoms. Menopause 2015;22(11):1155–74.

[109] Ouyang P, Michos ED, Karas RH. Hormone replacement therapy and the cardiovascular system: lessons learned and unanswered questions. J Am Coll Cardiol 2006;47(9):1741–53.

Chapter 13

Cancer and Physical Activity

A. AlBadri*, R.H. Tank**, M.M. Johl**, D. Gupta†, S. Asier† and P.K. Mehta†

*Barbra Streisand Women's Heart Center, Cedars-Sinai Heart Institute, Los Angeles, CA, United States; **Internal Medicine Department, Cedars-Sinai Medical Center, Los Angeles, CA, United States; †Division of Cardiology, Emory University School of Medicine, Atlanta, GA, United States

INTRODUCTION

Progress in cancer screening, diagnosis, and treatment has resulted in a growing population of survivors, with an estimated 13.7 million cancer survivors in United States in 2012 [1]. Cancer survivors are at increased risk of cardiovascular disease (CVD), and many risk factors are common between cancer and CVD. Physical inactivity is an important CVD risk factor, which is highly prevalent in cancer patients and survivors. Several recent reviews are published on the beneficial impact of exercise on cardiovascular morbidity and mortality, on hospital admissions, and improved quality of life [2–4]. Emerging data indicate that exercise also decreases cancer specific mortality and risk of recurrence rates [5–8]. While undergoing treatment for cancer and during recovery, it is common for cancer patients to experience fatigue, loss of energy, and reduced physical functioning, which prevent adequate physical activity [5]. However, even after cancer treatment is completed, a majority of cancer survivors remain physically inactive which contributes to poor functional capacity [9].

Evidence of left ventricular (LV) dysfunction from cancer related treatment can be obvious, such as when there is a decline in LV ejection fraction on a postchemotherapy echocardiogram, but LV dysfunction can also be present with no obvious decrease in ejection fraction. Patients can develop a decline in physical functioning over a period of years postchemotherapy, when compensatory cardiopulmonary mechanisms start to fail, and overt clinical symptoms of coronary heart disease and congestive heart failure occur. While cardiotoxic effects from cancer treatment is a major contributor to impaired functional capacity, there are other factors, such as anemia, nutrition, loss of muscle mass, and psychosocial factors [10–12] that contribute to a decline in exercise performance. In this chapter we review the impact of chemotherapy on cardiopulmonary reserve and discuss physical activity in cancer patients.

PHYSICAL ACTIVITY

Physical activity is one of American Heart Association (AHA)'s seven components for ideal cardiovascular health, and current recommendations for all adults >20 years old for physical activity are to exercise ≥150 min per week (moderate intensity) or ≥75 min per week (vigorous intensity) [13]. To lower blood pressure and lipid levels, AHA recommends average of 40 min of moderate to vigorous intensity aerobic exercise 3 or 4 times per week. In 2014, according to the National Health Interview Survey in United States, only 47% of women and 53% of men reported meeting these guidelines. These numbers are likely an overestimate because people also tend to overestimate their physical activity levels when compared to objective data collected by pedometers or accelerometers [14]. Physical inactivity is associated with a low cardiopulmonary fitness, a low functional capacity, and a poor quality of life [15,16].

Given unique considerations for patients with cancer, there are exercise and physical activity guidelines for cancer survivors put forth by the American Cancer Society (ACS) [17,18]. Similar to physical activity guidelines for the general population, the ACS 2012 [18] guidelines also recommend exercising 150 min per week for cancer patients when they are able. Strength training is also recommended twice a week. Studies have shown that majority of cancer survivors do not participate in physical activity [10,19]. Furthermore, sedentary behavior may be an independent risk factor for CVD [20,21]. A person can engage in regular physical activity and still be considered sedentary if a majority of time is spent doing sedentary activities, such as sitting in front of the computer or watching television. In the Women's Health Initiative Observational Study (WHI-OS), in postmenopausal women, physical activity was associated with a lower incidence and mortality from lung cancer [8]. In a cross-sectional study in patients diagnosed with colorectal cancer, greater sedentary time was associated with lower quality of life and functioning [22]. Given the importance of physical activity and the prognostic value of functional capacity, it is important for clinicians who care for cancer survivors to address physical activity as a key component for cardiovascular risk reduction. In general, exercise is an underprescribed, cost-effective intervention to improve cardiopulmonary functioning, and to reduce cardiovascular morbidity and mortality [23]. Physicians who treat cancer patients should be aware of these guidelines and note that patients are more likely to exercise when recommended by a physician. Structural exercise training is used as a primary and secondary prevention in various clinical settings, but it not typically prescribed as a standard of care for cancer patients [24]. While some institutions provide unique cancer rehabilitation programs where patients can exercise in a supervised, group setting, most cancer patients do not have access to rehabilitation facilities that target exercise.

PHYSICAL ACTIVITY DURING CANCER TREATMENT

Exercise during treatment of cancer is safe and has beneficial effects on physical functioning, fatigue, and quality of life. Exercise during chemotherapy does not reduce effectiveness of chemotherapy. ACS guidelines recommend that cancer patients resume normal daily activity and be physically active following the diagnosis of cancer [17]. The duration and intensity of exercise while undergoing cancer treatment may be less, but it is recommended to maintain physical activity as much as possible. Keeping in mind that a majority of cancer patients experience reduced level of functioning during cancer treatment, clinicians should encourage physical activity whenever possible, and modified forms of low impact exercise can be considered. The amount and duration of exercise should be tailored to individual patient's condition and preferences. For patients who are sedentary prior to their cancer diagnosis, low intensity exercises, such as stretching and short, slow walks can be encouraged. Special consideration is required for patients who have peripheral neuropathy, gait instability, bone pain, arthritis, and osteoporosis to avoid the risk of injury or falls. For patients who require bed rest, guidelines recommend maintaining range of motion and strength exercises [18,25]. For older adults, supervised group-based therapy by a physical therapist can also be an effective strategy for fall prevention [26].

COMPLEMENTARY STRATEGIES

Complementary and integrative strategies, such as Tai Chi and Yoga can be considered in patients who have impaired mobility and are frail, which may prevent them from aerobic exercise. Based on traditional Chinese medicine, Tai Chi is a practice that combines gentle body movements, with breathing and meditation. While there are some studies that have reported on benefits of Tai Chi in patients with cancer, well conducted, randomized controlled clinical trials, and comparative-effectiveness trials of addition of Tai Chi to traditional cancer exercise rehabilitation programs are needed [27,28]. Yoga is another form of exercise that can be considered in cancer patients and survivors. Based on the ancient Ayurvedic medicine, Yoga combines various body movements and postures (called *asanas*) with breathing techniques and meditation to improve physical functioning and well-being. A majority of studies on yoga have been conducted in those with breast cancer, indicating some benefit for fatigue, but rigorous trials are needed to demonstrate impact on improvements in cardiopulmonary reserve and physical functioning, and whether there is benefit of yoga above and beyond regular aerobic activity in cancer patients [29,30].

EVALUATION OF PHYSICAL CAPACITY

Exercise Treadmill Testing

Exercise treadmill testing (ETT) is generally utilized to evaluate symptoms, myocardial ischemia, stress-induced arrhythmias, and functional capacity (i.e., exercise tolerance). ETT provides prognostic information for both men and women, and is relatively inexpensive and widely available. However, it is not routinely performed to evaluate functional capacity in asymptomatic patients for preventive CVD risk assessment. Furthermore, it requires that patients be able to walk/run on a treadmill via a ramp protocol that increases speed and incline of the treadmill every 3 min (Bruce protocol) [31]. During ETT, exercise intensity and oxygen consumption is measured in metabolic equivalent of task (MET) [32]; one MET is equal to 3.5 mL O_2 consumption per body weight (kg) per minute in an average adult. Two METs is equal to 2 times the basal oxygen consumption, and three METs is 3 times the basal oxygen consumption, and so on. MET is estimated during ETT based on the speed and incline of the treadmill. Bruce protocol exercise treadmill stress testing is the most widely used exercise testing protocol to determine patient's MET level [31], and while routine ETT is not done in asymptomatic cancer survivors, a patient's MET level can be estimated based on the activities that they report. For example, sitting and typing at desk is 1.5 METs, being able to do light housework is equated to 3–4 METs, and brisk walking is 5 METs. As MET levels increase on exercise testing, cardiovascular prognosis improves, and this holds true for both men and women [33]. In the St. James Women Take Heart study by Gulati et al., in 5721 asymptomatic women (mean age 52 ± 11), decrease exercise capacity measured by MET was an independent predictor of death [34], with each decline in MET level predicting a 17% increase in cardiovascular mortality. In addition to MET level, patients heart rate recovery postexercise is also a measure of fitness [33,35,36].

Cardiopulmonary Exercise Testing (CPET)

Cardiopulmonary exercise testing (CPET) provides a more integrative method of assessing cardiopulmonary fitness because it provides information related to oxygen consumption and anaerobic threshold during exercise. It can be useful in evaluating patients with dyspnea, and is routinely used clinically in evaluation of patients with heart failure. It provides simultaneous evaluation of cardiovascular, pulmonary, and musculoskeletal system. Patients are exercised on either a treadmill or stationary cycle while wearing a face mask attached to a metabolic cart. Information regarding oxygen used and carbon dioxide production before, during, and after exercise is relayed to the metabolic cart while electrocardiogram, pulse oximetry, and frequent blood pressure assessments continuously monitor the patient. Information related to peak oxygen consumption (VO_2 max) and aerobic capacity, anaerobic ventilator threshold, and respiratory gas exchange ratio (ratio of carbon dioxide output and oxygen uptake) is obtained [37]. Clinicians can differentiate if symptoms of dyspnea are related strictly to cardiac etiologies (chronotropic incompetence, poor cardiac output, hypotensive response to exercise), pulmonary issues (hypoxia with exercise), or deconditioning (inability to reach anaerobic threshold).

In patients with known cardiomyopathy and congestive heart failure, CPET provides the clinician with an assessment of severity of cardiomyopathy and its contribution to clinical decline, as well as determination of appropriate timing for evaluation for advanced therapies (heart transplant or LV assist device implantation). This test should be performed for patients who do not have a physical limitation to perform an exercise test (i.e., severe arthritis, wheelchair bound) and are showing signs and symptoms suggestive of worsening cardiomyopathy or when clinical symptoms are worse than physical findings on examination. This test is incorporated into current heart failure and transplantation guidelines [38]. Patients who are on waiting list for transplantation should be evaluated every 3–6 months using CPET and heart failure survival prognostic scores to assess their eligibility for transplant. Few patients might show improvement in exercise capacity with the maximal pharmacological and device therapy, these patients may be considered for delisting [38]. In patients with known cardiomyopathy, CPET can be helpful to guide treatment plan and for prognosis. In cardiomyopathy patients with a VO_2 max greater than 14 mL/kg/min after reaching anaerobic threshold (respiratory gas exchange ratio >1.05) were reported to have had 1- and 2-year survival of 94% and 84%, respectively. Those with a VO_2 max <14 mL/kg/min had

significantly worse survival and may be a group who would benefit from advanced therapies, such as LV assist device or heart transplantation [39]. Survival improved with the increased knowledge of medical management, decreasing the threshold predictive of need for advanced therapies to <12 mL/kg/min for patients on an optimal beta blocker regimen [40]. The minute ventilation-carbon dioxide production relationship (VE/VCO_2 slope) improves risk stratification for heart failure patients by providing an index of ventilatory response to exercise. Those with a VE/VCO_2 slope ≥35 had a 75% 1-year mortality, while those with a slope <35 had a 25% 1-year mortality [41]. With optimal medical therapy and exercise training, or cardiac rehabilitation, heart failure patients can improve their functional capacity. CPET can be performed to quantify the extent of this improvement. A drawback of CPET testing is that it is not widely available, and requires trained clinical technicians. It is not recommended for routine assessments of functional capacity in general cardiology population, where ETT and 6-min walk tests are usually used to assess functional capacity.

Risk of CPET Testing in Cancer Patients

In cancer survivors CPET is not routinely performed to assess physical functioning, however, a systematic review of 118 studies with 5529 patients conducted by Lee W. Jones [42] has reported on the safety of maximal and submaximal exercise testing. In this review, 88 adverse events were related to exercise testing and 13 adverse events were related to exercise training. One exercise-related death was reported [42]. In another study of 85 patients with inoperable non-small cell lung cancer or metastatic breast cancer, who were treated with chemotherapy, safety of CPET was evaluated. Out of the 85 patients, 26% of patients with non-small lung cell cancer and 43.6% of breast cancer patients developed asymptomatic ST segment changes during exercise. Two patients experienced a nonlife-threatening event during testing [43]. Thus, individualized CPET protocol was reported to be safe and feasible to assess physical functioning and exercise response [43]. A joint statement by The American Thoracic Society/American College of Chest Physicians on CPET reported that the risk of death during exercise testing is 2–5 per 100,000 exercise tests [44]. However, more evidence regarding which specific cancer patients would have a CVD mortality benefit and the optimal timing of when exercise training should be considered is needed.

CARDIOPULMONARY RESERVE IN CANCER

Neither ETT nor CPET is routinely used to assess functional capacity in cancer patients. Cancer patients have been demonstrated to have markedly reduced cardiopulmonary reserve and low physical fitness levels [45,46]. The process of delivering oxygen to active skeletal muscles requires intact functioning of pulmonary, cardiovascular, and autonomic systems [47]. Due to the difference in partial pressure between the atmosphere and lung alveoli, oxygen diffuses during inspiration to the alveoli, and binds to hemoglobin in red blood cells. Through pulmonary veins, oxygenated blood is carried to the left heart, which pumps blood to skeletal muscles. When hemoglobin reaches active skeletal muscles, oxygen diffuses to the intracellular space where it binds to myoglobin and is delivered to the mitochondria. In the mitochondria, oxygen is used to synthesize adenosine triphosphate (ATP), the energy storage molecule, which is essential for muscle function. During exercise, active skeletal muscles require more ATP synthesis. As a response, the pulmonary oxygen diffusion capacity and cardiac output increase significantly [16]. During chemotherapy, one or more of these components may be affected.

Impairments in various components of the oxygen cascade (pulmonary diffusing capacity, skeletal muscle function, vascular function) combined with comorbid conditions and cardiac risk factors can lead to reduced exercise tolerance in cancer patients who have undergone chemotherapy or radiation therapy [16]. Oxygen consumption determined by VO$_2$ max declines every decade starting at age 20 by 5–15%, and this age-related decline in cardiopulmonary reserve is further accelerated after anthracycline-based chemotherapy [48]. As reviewed in this textbook, anthracycline-induced cardiac toxicity can have subtle, subclinical effects on systolic function and diastolic filling, and with aging and other cardiac risk factor development, the cardiotoxicity can clinically manifest years later with dyspnea and decline in exercise tolerance [49]. Alterations in myocardial tissue result in impaired left ventricular ejection fraction (LVEF) and cardiac output, which in turn reduce oxygen delivery [16]. In a study evaluating exercise capacity in 84 asymptomatic young childhood cancer survivors (age <21) compared to 79 healthy controls, there were no differences detected in exercise responses between the two groups. Childhood cancer survivors had received either anthracycline and/or chest radiation, and testing occurred at a mean of 7.7 ± 3.4 years after diagnosis. It was noted that boys younger than age 13 years had a significantly lower VO$_2$ max compared to controls [50], and authors concluded that this finding was due to lower physical fitness in the cancer survivors. In lung cancer patients who undergo pneumonectomy, VO$_2$ max decreases by approximately 20% at 6 months, but is unchanged with lobectomy [51].

AUTONOMIC DYSFUNCTION

The autonomic nervous system modulates physiologic responses to stimuli and allows for appropriate heart rate and blood pressure response to exercise, stress, noise, temperature, and sleep. An altered sympathovagal balance is associated with adverse cardiovascular outcomes; for example, an elevated resting heart is associated with poor prognosis, as well as impaired heart rate recovery post exercise. A low heart rate variability in postmyocardial infarction patients is associated with sudden death and adverse outcomes [52–55]. Scott et al. recently reported that patients with breast cancer exhibit autonomic dysfunction with elevated resting tachycardia, low heart rate variability, and reduced baroreflex sensitivity [56]. Exercise training can improve autonomic function, and large, randomized controlled trials that evaluate the impact of exercise-related improved autonomic function on CVD outcomes are needed.

FUNCTIONAL CAPACITY IN CANCER

Exercise requires coordinated function of autonomic, cardiovascular, pulmonary, and musculoskeletal systems, and all these systems can be affected by chemotherapy or malignancy itself. A study by Jones et al. in 248 women (mean age 55 ± 8 years) with breast cancer showed marked impairments in cardiopulmonary function despite normal cardiac function (i.e., LVEF > 50%) [57]. On average, VO$_2$ max was 27% ± 17% less compared to that of age-matched sedentary, but otherwise, healthy women without a history of breast cancer. The impairments in VO$_2$ max were particularly during primary adjuvant chemotherapy and in those patients with metastatic disease, with VO$_2$ max 31% and 33% less than that of healthy sedentary women, respectively [46,49,57]. Cancer therapy can cause acute and late-occurring cardiovascular and autonomic toxicity manifested by impaired LV function and biochemical alternations that reduce O$_2$ delivery, impair oxygen utilization, and diminished exercise tolerance [57–62]. Furthermore, patients who are receiving certain regimen of chemotherapy may have subclinical cardiac dysfunction which can be undetectable at bedside evaluation.

DIASTOLIC FUNCTION

Resting echocardiograms that are typically obtained to assess cardiotoxicity in cancer patients, and have normal LV function do not provide information regarding a patient's functional capacity. Ejection fraction does not predict functional capacity. A person with moderately low ejection fraction with normal left atrial pressures and normal pulmonary pressures may have well-controlled symptoms compared to a person with preserved ejection fraction who has high left atrial and pulmonary pressures. There is an inverse relationship between diastolic dysfunction and exercise capacity, which has been described in patients with ischemic heart disease, and congestive heart failure [63,64]. The most common method of assessing diastolic function is by tissue Doppler echocardiography; myocardial speckle tracking, and strain imaging are new emerging techniques that may be particularly useful in assessing chemotherapy induced changes in LV function [65,66]. Accordingly, diastolic dysfunction is an important contributor for the decreased physical performance in cancer patients.

Chemotherapy related toxicity manifests as LV systolic and diastolic dysfunction, or combination of both. Anthracycline-based chemotherapy and/or radiation therapy are well known to cause impairment in diastolic function [67–69], which decrease exercise performance due to decreased stroke volume and cardiac index, which, for some time, is compensated by an increased heart rate [70,71]. In an observational study evaluating 100 patients with breast cancer treated with anthracycline-based chemotherapy alone or combined with trastuzumab, of the 85 patients who received anthracyclines, 49 (58%) developed diastolic dysfunction during the median follow-up period of 12 months. Of those, 36 (73%) had diastolic dysfunction that persisted through the final follow-up visit. In 13 patients, diastolic dysfunction reversed by the end of the study. In this study, patients older than 50 years were 4 times more likely than younger patients to develop diastolic dysfunction after anthracycline-based chemotherapy. In addition, diastolic dysfunction was 3 times more likely in overweight patients compared to normal weight patients, and it was more than 7 times more likely in obese patients [45].

ANEMIA

Anemia is highly prevalent and is a significant problem in cancer patients, impacting prognosis [72]; reduced hemoglobin levels contribute to fatigue, dyspnea, and a reduction in functional capacity. Anemia can be secondary to iron deficiency (from poor dietary intake or impaired gastrointestinal absorption), low bone marrow red blood cell production (due to chemotherapy related myelosupression or impaired erythropoiesis due to malignancy), or blood loss from surgery, gastrointestinal, or gynecologic bleeding [73]. Several studies have examined the use of intravenous iron in combination with erythropoiesis-stimulating agents (ESAs, such as epoetin alfa and darbepoetin alfa) [74–76], which are associated with venous thrombosis, stroke, and increased mortality. Addition of intravenous iron, which is more effective than oral iron supplementation, to ESAs is used to increase hemoglobin levels in those with chronic kidney disease and chemotherapy-related anemia and appears to be effective [77], but larger comparative trials that guide optimal therapy of anemia, and impact of these agents on functional capacity and quality of life are needed.

BENEFITS OF EXERCISE

Physical activity should be encouraged in cancer survivors during their healthcare visits. The American College of Cardiology (ACC)/AHA Lifestyle guidelines on managing cardiovascular risk published in 2013 report that with a typical exercise intervention of the recommended activity for at least 12 weeks (3–4 sessions per week), there is an average of 2–5 mm Hg systolic and 1–4 mm Hg diastolic blood pressure reduction. For cholesterol lowering, data with moderate strength of evidence indicate that aerobic exercise leads to an average low density lipoprotein cholesterol reduction of 3–6 mg/dL, with variable effects on high density lipoprotein and triglyceride levels [78]. Exercise also has many effects on cell-signaling pathways with known positive benefits including improved nitric oxide bioavailability and endothelial function, improvements in glucose metabolism, insulin sensitivity, inflammation, and visceral fat [79–81]. In addition, exercise improves mood, anxiety, depression, sleep, and quality of life [82]. Exercise may also play an important role in modulating cardiotoxicity caused by targeted therapies by its ability to inhibit TGF-B1 signaling, increase GATA4 signaling, and upregulate cardioprotective pathways [19].

Exercise training in rehabilitation programs has been shown to improve both quality of life and overall survival in various chronic diseases [83–87]. VO_2 max improves after exercise training in cancer patients, and improved VO_2 max has been shown to be associated with improved survival in certain cancer patients [24,88,89]. Exercise training is associated with improvement of 10–15% in various markers of cardiopulmonary reserve including VO_2 max [9,90]. In a meta-analysis conducted by Jones et al. in 571 adult cancer patients stratified to exercise and nonexercise groups, exercise was associated with a significant improvement in VO_2 max (+2.90 mL/kg/min) while nonexercise was associated with a significant decline in VO_2 max (−1.02mL/kg/min) [91]. Another meta-analysis performed by McNeely et al showed an even greater improvement of VO_2 max (+3.39 mL/kg/min) in breast cancer patients undergoing structured exercise training program [92]. Other studies report improvements in VO_2 max ranging from 10% to 12% in patients who underwent exercise training while receiving chemotherapy [24,93]. In a meta-analysis that included 14 studies on exercise and effects of breast cancer concluded that many studies on breast cancer patients have shown that exercise is safe and improves physical and psychological well-being [94]. Similarly, Segal et al. showed maintenance of VO_2 max in male prostate cancer patients receiving chemoradiation therapy who underwent a structured exercise program [95]. While the benefit of improving cardiopulmonary fitness from baseline varies, several studies suggest that exercise training helps maintain fitness in patients with cancer [91]. Courneya et al. studied effects of exercise in breast cancer patients who were undergoing adjuvant chemotherapy and showed that while aerobic or resistance training did not necessarily improve VO_2 max, it was associated with maintenance of VO_2 max. Conversely, the control group saw a significant decline in VO$_2$ max, suggesting that exercise may be responsible for mitigating the traditional cardiopulmonary decline seen in individuals who do not participate in regular exercise training [96].

In patients with non-small cell lung cancer, VO$_2$ max was shown to increase with aerobic training only when patients did not receive platinum-based chemotherapeutic regimens, suggesting that this particular therapy may play a role in interfering with the physiologic adaptations of training [16]. Cancer-specific studies that test-specific exercise prescriptive regimens regarding frequency, duration, and intensity are needed to help inform rehabilitation guidelines in this population [92]. In addition to improving cardiopulmonary reserve and physical functioning, exercise can also improve cancer-related fatigue and quality of life. In a recent meta-analysis of 42 trials (3816 adult patients diagnosed with various cancers), moderate intensity aerobic exercise was shown to be safe and an effective intervention to help reduce fatigue and increase stamina [100].

BARRIERS TO EXERCISE

Research on barriers to exercise among cancer patients has focused primarily on patients with breast and colon cancers [87–89]. Despite the evidence supporting exercise as an effective management strategy, there are numerous barriers which prevent exercise, both during and following cancer treatment [83]. The main barriers that cancer patients report could be linked to the side effects of treatment [101] or health factors, such as nausea, dyspnea, joint stiffness, pain, neuropathy, weakness, fatigue, and feelings of social isolation due to their medical condition. Chemotherapy decreases immune function, which can lead to recurrent infections and hospitalizations, which further contributes to physical deconditioning. Prolonged rest due to fatigue after chemotherapy can contribute to cardiopulmonary and muscular deconditioning causing increase sensation of fatigue [45]. Furthermore, cancer patients usually feel self-conscious of their self-image and experience lack of confidence, interest, and motivation after surgery. For example, breast cancer survivors who are wearing prostheses feel limited to their choice of exercise (swimming, aerobics, and gym).

The timing of starting an exercise program in cancer patients is also challenging. At the time of cancer diagnosis, scheduled chemotherapy sessions, doctors' appointments, and side effects of the treatment limit starting an exercise program. This influences patients' decisions on when is the most appropriate time to begin an exercise program following a diagnosis. Environmental factors, lack of motivation, and safety issues affect physical activity as well. Environmental factors include the cost to join exercise program and the lack of specialized exercise facilities for cancer patients are also important barriers [101,102]. Insurance reimbursement for cancer rehabilitation is inadequate due to the lack

of research supporting their use [103]. Although fatigue during treatment is reported to be one of the main barriers to exercise [104–106], most of the studies do not report the degree of fatigue and whether they were experiencing fatigue at the time the research was conducted. Even some years after completion of their treatment for cancer patients may experience fatigue.

CONCLUSIONS

Physical inactivity is highly prevalent in cancer patients and survivors. Patients who undergo treatment for cancer experience a decline in cardiopulmonary reserve, which impacts their physical activity, functional status, and quality of life. Resting LV ejection fraction on echocardiography does not provide information related to functional status. Submaximal stress testing and a peak VO$_2$ max is helpful to measure physical functioning, can help with prognosis, and is safe in this patient population. Exercise training can help improve cardiopulmonary function and quality of life; however, it is not routinely prescribed. Cancer-specific exercise interventions to inform cancer rehabilitation guidelines are needed.

REFERENCES

[1] de Moor JS, Mariotto AB, Parry C, Alfano CM, Padgett L, Kent EE, et al. Cancer survivors in the United States: prevalence across the survivorship trajectory and implications for care. Cancer Epidemiol Biomarkers Prev 2013;22(4):561–70.

[2] Bruning RS, Sturek M. Benefits of exercise training on coronary blood flow in coronary artery disease patients. Prog Cardiovasc Dis 2015;57(5):443–53.

[3] Merghani A, Malhotra A, Sharma S. The U-shaped relationship between exercise and cardiac morbidity. Trends Cardiovasc Med 2016;26(3):232–40.

[4] Anderson L, Oldridge N, Thompson DR, Zwisler AD, Rees K, Martin N, et al. Exercise-based cardiac rehabilitation for coronary heart disease: cochrane systematic review and meta-analysis. J Am Coll Cardiol 2016;67(1):1–12.

[5] Li T, Wei S, Shi Y, Pang S, Qin Q, Yin J, et al. The dose-response effect of physical activity on cancer mortality: findings from 71 prospective cohort studies. Br J Sports Med 2016;50(6):339–45.

[6] Barbaric M, Brooks E, Moore L, Cheifetz O. Effects of physical activity on cancer survival: a systematic review. Physiother Can 2010;62(1):25–34.

[7] Meyerhardt JA, Giovannucci EL, Holmes MD, Chan AT, Chan JA, Colditz GA, et al. Physical activity and survival after colorectal cancer diagnosis. J Clin Oncol 2006;24(22):3527–34.

[8] Wang A, Qin F, Hedlin H, Desai M, Chlebowski R, Gomez S, et al. Physical activity and sedentary behavior in relation to lung cancer incidence and mortality in older women: the women's health initiative. Int J Cancer 2016;139(10):2178–92.

[9] Schmitz KH, Courneya KS, Matthews C, Demark-Wahnefried W, Galvão DA, Pinto BM, et al. American College of Sports Medicine roundtable on exercise guidelines for cancer survivors. Med Sci Sports Exerc 2010;42(7):1409–26.

[10] Ahlberg K, Ekman T, Gaston-Johansson F, Mock V. Assessment and management of cancer-related fatigue in adults. Lancet (London, England) 2003;362(9384):640–50.

[11] Lawrence DP, Kupelnick B, Miller K, Devine D, Lau J. Evidence report on the occurrence, assessment, and treatment of fatigue in cancer patients. J Natl Cancer Inst Monogr 2004;32:40–50.

[12] Elbl L, Vasova I, Tomaskova I, Jedlicka F, Kral Z, Navratil M, et al. Cardiopulmonary exercise testing in the evaluation of functional capacity after treatment of lymphomas in adults. Leukemia & lymphoma. 2006;47(5):843–51.

[13] Lloyd-Jones DM, Hong Y, Labarthe D, Mozaffarian D, Appel LJ, Van Horn L, et al. Defining and setting national goals for cardiovascular health promotion and disease reduction: the American Heart Association's strategic Impact Goal through 2020 and beyond. Circulation 2010;121(4):586–613.

[14] Mozaffarian D, Benjamin EJ, Go AS, Arnett DK, Blaha MJ, Cushman M, et al. Heart disease and stroke statistics—2015 update: a report from the American Heart Association. Circulation 2015;131(4):e29–e322.

[15] Blanchard CM, Courneya KS, Stein K. American Cancer Society's SCS, II. Cancer survivors' adherence to lifestyle behavior recommendations and associations with health-related quality of life: results from the American Cancer Society's SCS-II. J Clin Oncol 2008;26(13):2198–204.

[16] Jones LW, Eves ND, Haykowsky M, Freedland SJ, Mackey JR. Exercise intolerance in cancer and the role of exercise therapy to reverse dysfunction. Lancet Oncol 2009;10(6):598–605.

[17] Kushi LH, Doyle C, McCullough M, Rock CL, Demark-Wahnefried W, Bandera EV, et al. American Cancer Society Guidelines on nutrition and physical activity for cancer prevention: reducing the risk of cancer with healthy food choices and physical activity. CA Cancer J Clin 2012;62(1):30–67.

[18] Rock CL, Doyle C, Demark-Wahnefried W, Meyerhardt J, Courneya KS, Schwartz AL, et al. Nutrition and physical activity guidelines for cancer survivors. CA Cancer J Clin 2012;62(4):243–74.

[19] Scott JM, Lakoski S, Mackey JR, Douglas PS, Haykowsky MJ, Jones LW. The potential role of aerobic exercise to modulate cardiotoxicity of molecularly targeted cancer therapeutics. Oncologist 2013;18(2):221–31.

[20] Tremblay MS, Leblanc AG, Carson V, Choquette L, Connor Gorber S, Dillman C, et al. Canadian physical activity guidelines for the early years (aged 0–4 years). Appl Physiol Nutr Metab 2012;37(2):345–69.

[21] Lee IM, Rexrode KM, Cook NR, Manson JE, Buring JE. Physical activity and coronary heart disease in women: is "no pain, no gain" passe? JAMA 2001;285(11):1447–54.

[22] van Roekel EH, Winkler EA, Bours MJ, Lynch BM, Willems PJ, Meijer K, et al. Associations of sedentary time and patterns of sedentary time accumulation with health-related quality of life in colorectal cancer survivors. Prev Med Rep 2016;4:262–9.

[23] Blaney JM, Lowe-Strong A, Rankin-Watt J, Campbell A, Gracey JH. Cancer survivors' exercise barriers, facilitators and preferences in the context of fatigue, quality of life and physical activity participation: a questionnaire-survey. Psychooncology 2013;22(1):186–94.

[24] Lakoski SG, Eves ND, Douglas PS, Jones LW. Exercise rehabilitation in patients with cancer. Nat Rev Clin Oncol 2012;9(5):288–96.

[25] Wolin KY, Schwartz AL, Matthews CE, Courneya KS, Schmitz KH. Implementing the exercise guidelines for cancer survivors. J Support Oncol 2012;10(5):171–7.

[26] Martin JT, Wolf A, Moore JL, Rolenz E, DiNinno A, Reneker JC. The effectiveness of physical therapist-administered group-based exercise on fall prevention: a systematic review of randomized controlled trials. J Geriatr Phys Ther 2013;36(4):182–93.

[27] Lee MS, Pittler MH, Ernst E. Is Tai Chi an effective adjunct in cancer care? A systematic review of controlled clinical trials. Support Care Cancer 2007;15(6):597–601.

[28] Zeng Y, Luo T, Xie H, Huang M, Cheng AS. Health benefits of qigong or tai chi for cancer patients: a systematic review and meta-analyses. Complement Ther Med 2014;22(1):173–86.

[29] Sadja J, Mills PJ. Effects of yoga interventions on fatigue in cancer patients and survivors: a systematic review of randomized controlled trials. Explore (NY) 2013;9(4):232–43.

[30] Samuel SR, Veluswamy SK, Maiya AG, Fernandes DJ, McNeely ML. Exercise-based interventions for cancer survivors in India: a systematic review. Springerplus 2015;4:655.

[31] Kaminsky LA, Whaley MH. Evaluation of a new standardized ramp protocol: the BSU/Bruce Ramp protocol. J Cardiopulm Rehabil 1998;18(6):438–44.

[32] Bruce RA, Kusumi F, Hosmer D. Maximal oxygen intake and nomographic assessment of functional aerobic impairment in cardiovascular disease. Am Heart J 1973;85(4):546–62.

[33] Mora S, Redberg RF, Cui Y, Whiteman MK, Flaws JA, Sharrett AR, et al. Ability of exercise testing to predict cardiovascular and all-cause death in asymptomatic women: a 20-year follow-up of the lipid research clinics prevalence study. JAMA 2003;290(12):1600–7.

[34] Gulati M, Pandey DK, Arnsdorf MF, Lauderdale DS, Thisted RA, Wicklund RH, et al. Exercise capacity and the risk of death in women: the St James Women Take Heart Project. Circulation 2003;108(13):1554–9.

[35] Gulati M, Shaw LJ, Thisted RA, Black HR, Bairey Merz CN, Arnsdorf MF. Heart rate response to exercise stress testing in asymptomatic women: the St. James women take heart project. Circulation 2010;122(2):130–7.

[36] Kohli P, Gulati M. Exercise stress testing in women: going back to the basics. Circulation 2010;122(24):2570–80.

[37] Balady GJ, Arena R, Sietsema K, Myers J, Coke L, Fletcher GF, et al. Clinician's guide to cardiopulmonary exercise testing in adults: a scientific statement from the American Heart Association. Circulation 2010;122(2):191–225.

[38] Mehra MR, Canter CE, Hannan MM, Semigran MJ, Uber PA, Baran DA, et al. The 2016 International Society for Heart Lung Transplantation listing criteria for heart transplantation: a 10-year update. J Heart Lung Transpl 2016;35(1):1–23.

[39] Mancini DM, Eisen H, Kussmaul W, Mull R, Edmunds LH Jr, Wilson JR. Value of peak exercise oxygen consumption for optimal timing of cardiac transplantation in ambulatory patients with heart failure. Circulation 1991;83(3):778–86.

[40] Peterson LR, Schechtman KB, Ewald GA, Geltman EM, de las Fuentes L, Meyer T, et al. Timing of cardiac transplantation in patients with heart failure receiving beta-adrenergic blockers. J Heart Lung Transpl 2003;22(10):1141–8.

[41] Sarullo FM, Fazio G, Brusca I, Fasullo S, Paterna S, Licata P, et al. Cardiopulmonary exercise testing in patients with chronic heart failure: prognostic comparison from peak VO_2 and VE/VCO_2 slope. Open Cardiovasc Med J 2010;4:127–34.

[42] Jones LW. Evidence-based risk assessment and recommendations for physical activity clearance: cancer. Appl Physiol Nutr Metab 2011;36(Suppl. 1):S101–12.

[43] Jones LW, Eves ND, Mackey JR, Peddle CJ, Haykowsky M, Joy AA, et al. Safety and feasibility of cardiopulmonary exercise testing in patients with advanced cancer. Lung Cancer 2007;55(2):225–32.

[44] American Thoracic S, American College of Chest P. ATS/ACCP statement on cardiopulmonary exercise testing. Am J Resp Crit Care Med 2003;167(2):211–77.

[45] Jones LW, Eves ND, Haykowsky M, Joy AA, Douglas PS. Cardiorespiratory exercise testing in clinical oncology research: systematic review and practice recommendations. Lancet Oncol 2008;9(8):757–65.

[46] Jones LW, Haykowsky MJ, Swartz JJ, Douglas PS, Mackey JR. Early breast cancer therapy and cardiovascular injury. J Am Coll Cardiol 2007;50(15):1435–41.

[47] Wagner PD. Why doesn't exercise grow the lungs when other factors do? Exerc Sport Sci Rev 2005;33(1):3–8.

[48] Koelwyn GJ, Khouri M, Mackey JR, Douglas PS, Jones LW. Running on empty: cardiovascular reserve capacity and late effects of therapy in cancer survivorship. J Clin Oncol 2012;30(36):4458–61.

[49] Ewer MS, Lippman SM. Type II chemotherapy-related cardiac dysfunction: time to recognize a new entity. J Clin Oncol 2005;23(13):2900–2.

[50] De Caro E, Fioredda F, Calevo MG, Smeraldi A, Saitta M, Hanau G, et al. Exercise capacity in apparently healthy survivors of cancer. Arch Dis Child 2006;91(1):47–51.

[51] Bolliger CT, Jordan P, Soler M, Stulz P, Tamm M, Wyser C, et al. Pulmonary function and exercise capacity after lung resection. Eur Respir J 1996;9(3):415–21.

[52] Bigger JT Jr, Hoover CA, Steinman RC, Rolnitzky LM, Fleiss JL. Autonomic nervous system activity during myocardial ischemia in man estimated by power spectral analysis of heart period variability. The multicenter study of silent myocardial ischemia investigators. Am J Cardiol 1990;66(4):497–8.

[53] Cripps TR, Malik M, Farrell TG, Camm AJ. Prognostic value of reduced heart rate variability after myocardial infarction: clinical evaluation of a new analysis method. Br Heart J 1991;65(1):14–9.

[54] Kleiger RE, Miller JP, Bigger JT Jr, Moss AJ. Decreased heart rate variability and its association with increased mortality after acute myocardial infarction. Am J Cardiol 1987;59(4):256–62.

[55] Lanza GA, Cianflone D, Rebuzzi AG, Angeloni G, Sestito A, Ciriello G, et al. Prognostic value of ventricular arrhythmias and heart rate variability in patients with unstable angina. Heart 2006;92(8):1055–63.

[56] Scott JM, Jones LW, Hornsby WE, Koelwyn GJ, Khouri MG, Joy AA, et al. Cancer therapy-induced autonomic dysfunction in early breast cancer: implications for aerobic exercise training. Int J Cardiol 2014;171(2):e50–1.

[57] Jones LW, Courneya KS, Mackey JR, Muss HB, Pituskin EN, Scott JM, et al. Cardiopulmonary function and age-related decline across the breast cancer survivorship continuum. J Clin Oncol 2012;30(20):2530–7.

[58] Amaral SL, Papanek PE, Greene AS. Angiotensin II and VEGF are involved in angiogenesis induced by short-term exercise training. Am J Physiol 2001;281(3):H1163–9.

[59] Slamon D, Eiermann W, Robert N, Pienkowski T, Martin M, Press M, et al. Adjuvant trastuzumab in HER2-positive breast cancer. New Engl J Med 2011;365(14):1273–83.

[60] Swain SM, Whaley FS, Ewer MS. Congestive heart failure in patients treated with doxorubicin: a retrospective analysis of three trials. Cancer 2003;97(11):2869–79.

[61] van Norren K, van Helvoort A, Argiles JM, van Tuijl S, Arts K, Gorselink M, et al. Direct effects of doxorubicin on skeletal muscle contribute to fatigue. Br J Cancer 2009;100(2):311–4.

[62] Von Hoff DD, Layard MW, Basa P, Davis HL Jr, Von Hoff AL, Rozencweig M, et al. Risk factors for doxorubicin-induced congestive heart failure. Ann Intern Med 1979;91(5):710–7.

[63] Genovesi-Ebert A, Marabotti C, Palombo C, Giaconi S, Rossi G, Ghione S. Echo Doppler diastolic function and exercise tolerance. Int J Cardiol 1994;43(1):67–73.

[64] Parthenakis FI, Kanoupakis EM, Kochiadakis GE, Skalidis EI, Mezilis NE, Simantirakis EN, et al. Left ventricular diastolic filling pattern predicts cardiopulmonary determinants of functional capacity in patients with congestive heart failure. Am Heart J 2000;140(2):338–44.

[65] Kang Y, Xu X, Cheng L, Li L, Sun M, Chen H, et al. Two-dimensional speckle tracking echocardiography combined with high-sensitive cardiac troponin T in early detection and prediction of cardiotoxicity during epirubicine-based chemotherapy. Eur J Heart Fail 2014;16(3):300–8.

[66] Thavendiranathan P, Poulin F, Lim KD, Plana JC, Woo A, Marwick TH. Use of myocardial strain imaging by echocardiography for the early detection of cardiotoxicity in patients during and after cancer chemotherapy: a systematic review. J Am Coll Cardiol 2014;63(25 Pt. A):2751–68.

[67] Maeda A, Honda M, Kuramochi T, Takabatake T. Doxorubicin cardiotoxicity: diastolic cardiac myocyte dysfunction as a result of impaired calcium handling in isolated cardiac myocytes. Jpn Circ J 1998;62(7):505–11.

[68] Lee BH, Goodenday LS, Muswick GJ, Yasnoff WA, Leighton RF, Skeel RT. Alterations in left ventricular diastolic function with doxorubicin therapy. J Am Coll Cardiol 1987;9(1):184–8.

[69] Stoddard MF, Seeger J, Liddell NE, Hadley TJ, Sullivan DM, Kupersmith J. Prolongation of isovolumetric relaxation time as assessed by Doppler echocardiography predicts doxorubicin-induced systolic dysfunction in humans. J Am Coll Cardiol 1992;20(1):62–9.

[70] Johnson D, Perrault H, Fournier A, Leclerc JM, Bigras JL, Davignon A. Cardiovascular responses to dynamic submaximal exercise in children previously treated with anthracycline. Am Heart J 1997;133(2):169–73.

[71] Litwin SE, Grossman W. Diastolic dysfunction as a cause of heart failure. J Am Coll Cardiol 1993;22(4 Suppl. A):49A–55A.

[72] Ludwig H, Van Belle S, Barrett-Lee P, Birgegard G, Bokemeyer C, Gascon P, et al. The European Cancer Anaemia Survey (ECAS): a large, multinational, prospective survey defining the prevalence, incidence, and treatment of anaemia in cancer patients. Eur J Cancer 2004;40(15):2293–306.

[73] Grotto HZ. Anaemia of cancer: an overview of mechanisms involved in its pathogenesis. Med Oncol 2008;25(1):12–21.

[74] Auerbach M, Ballard H, Trout JR, McIlwain M, Ackerman A, Bahrain H, et al. Intravenous iron optimizes the response to recombinant human erythropoietin in cancer patients with chemotherapy-related anemia: a multicenter, open-label, randomized trial. J Clin Oncol 2004;22(7):1301–7.

[75] Auerbach M, Silberstein PT, Webb RT, Averyanova S, Ciuleanu TE, Shao J, et al. Darbepoetin alfa 300 or 500 mug once every 3 weeks with or without intravenous iron in patients with chemotherapy-induced anemia. Am J Hematol 2010;85(9):655–63.

[76] Bastit L, Vandebroek A, Altintas S, Gaede B, Pinter T, Suto TS, et al. Randomized, multicenter, controlled trial comparing the efficacy

and safety of darbepoetin alpha administered every 3 weeks with or without intravenous iron in patients with chemotherapy-induced anemia. J Clin Oncol 2008;26(10):1611–8.

[77] Steinmetz HT. The role of intravenous iron in the treatment of anemia in cancer patients. Ther Adv Hematol 2012;3(3):177–91.

[78] Eckel RH, Jakicic JM, Ard JD, de Jesus JM, Houston Miller N, Hubbard VS, et al. 2013 AHA/ACC guideline on lifestyle management to reduce cardiovascular risk: a report of the American College of Cardiology/American Heart Association Task Force on Practice Guidelines. J Am Coll Cardiol 2014;63(25 Pt. B):2960–84.

[79] Hamer M, O'Donovan G. Cardiorespiratory fitness and metabolic risk factors in obesity. Curr Opin Lipidol 2010;21(1):1–7.

[80] Kraus WE, Houmard JA, Duscha BD, Knetzger KJ, Wharton MB, McCartney JS, et al. Effects of the amount and intensity of exercise on plasma lipoproteins. N Engl J Med 2002;347(19):1483–92.

[81] Lee DC, Sui X, Church TS, Lavie CJ, Jackson AS, Blair SN. Changes in fitness and fatness on the development of cardiovascular disease risk factors hypertension, metabolic syndrome, and hypercholesterolemia. J Am Coll Cardiol 2012;59(7):665–72.

[82] Larun L, Brurberg KG, Odgaard-Jensen J, Price JR. Exercise therapy for chronic fatigue syndrome. Cochrane Database Syst Rev 2016;(6):CD003200.

[83] Nixon S, O'Brien K, Glazier RH, Tynan AM. Aerobic exercise interventions for adults living with HIV/AIDS. Cochrane Database Syst Rev 2002;(2):CD001796.

[84] Schulz KH, Gold SM, Witte J, Bartsch K, Lang UE, Hellweg R, et al. Impact of aerobic training on immune-endocrine parameters, neurotrophic factors, quality of life and coordinative function in multiple sclerosis. J Neurol Sci 2004;225(1–2):11–8.

[85] Farrell SW, Braun L, Barlow CE, Cheng YJ, Blair SN. The relation of body mass index, cardiorespiratory fitness, and all-cause mortality in women. Obes Res 2002;10(6):417–23.

[86] Atlantis E, Chow CM, Kirby A, Singh MF. An effective exercise-based intervention for improving mental health and quality of life measures: a randomized controlled trial. Prev Med 2004;39(2):424–34.

[87] Taylor RS, Brown A, Ebrahim S, Jolliffe J, Noorani H, Rees K, et al. Exercise-based rehabilitation for patients with coronary heart disease: systematic review and meta-analysis of randomized controlled trials. Am J Med 2004;116(10):682–92.

[88] Holmes MD, Chen WY, Feskanich D, Kroenke CH, Colditz GA. Physical activity and survival after breast cancer diagnosis. JAMA 2005;293(20):2479–86.

[89] Mitchell SA. Cancer-related fatigue: state of the science. PM R. 2010;2(5):364–83.

[90] Speck RM, Courneya KS, Mâsse LC, Duval S, Schmitz KH. An update of controlled physical activity trials in cancer survivors: a systematic review and meta-analysis. J Cancer Surviv 2010;4(2):87–100.

[91] Jones LW, Liang Y, Pituskin EN, Battaglini CL, Scott JM, Hornsby WE, et al. Effect of exercise training on peak oxygen consumption in patients with cancer: a meta-analysis. Oncologist 2011;16(1):112–20.

[92] McNeely ML, Campbell KL, Rowe BH, Klassen TP, Mackey JR, Courneya KS. Effects of exercise on breast cancer patients and survivors: a systematic review and meta-analysis. CMAJ 2006;175(1):34–41.

[93] Adamsen L, Quist M, Andersen C, Møller T, Herrstedt J, Kronborg D, et al. Effect of a multimodal high intensity exercise intervention in cancer patients undergoing chemotherapy: randomised controlled trial. BMJ 2009;339:b3410.

[94] Casla S, Hojman P, Marquez-Rodas I, Lopez-Tarruella S, Jerez Y, Barakat R, et al. Running away from side effects: physical exercise as a complementary intervention for breast cancer patients. Clin Transl Oncol 2015;17(3):180–96.

[95] Segal RJ, Reid RD, Courneya KS, Sigal RJ, Kenny GP, Prud'Homme DG, et al. Randomized controlled trial of resistance or aerobic exercise in men receiving radiation therapy for prostate cancer. J Clin Oncol 2009;27(3):344–51.

[96] Courneya KS, Segal RJ, Mackey JR, Gelmon K, Reid RD, Friedenreich CM, et al. Effects of aerobic and resistance exercise in breast cancer patients receiving adjuvant chemotherapy: a multicenter randomized controlled trial. J Clin Oncol 2007;25(28):4396–404.

[97] Jones LW, Eves ND, Peterson BL, Garst J, Crawford J, West MJ, et al. Safety and feasibility of aerobic training on cardiopulmonary function and quality of life in postsurgical nonsmall cell lung cancer patients: a pilot study. Cancer 2008;113(12):3430–9.

[98] Fairey AS, Courneya KS, Field CJ, Bell GJ, Jones LW, Mackey JR. Effects of exercise training on fasting insulin, insulin resistance, insulin-like growth factors, and insulin-like growth factor binding proteins in postmenopausal breast cancer survivors: a randomized controlled trial. Cancer Epidemiol Biomarkers Prev 2003;12(8):721–7.

[99] Ligibel JA, Campbell N, Partridge A, Chen WY, Salinardi T, Chen H, et al. Impact of a mixed strength and endurance exercise intervention on insulin levels in breast cancer survivors. J Clini Oncol 2008;26(6):907–12.

[100] Dennett AM, Peiris CL, Shields N, Prendergast LA, Taylor NF. Moderate-intensity exercise reduces fatigue and improves mobility in cancer survivors: a systematic review and meta-regression. J Physiother 2016;62(2):68–82.

[101] Blaney J, Lowe-Strong A, Rankin J, Campbell A, Allen J, Gracey J. The cancer rehabilitation journey: barriers to and facilitators of exercise among patients with cancer-related fatigue. Phys Ther 2010;90(8):1135–47.

[102] Rogers LQ, Matevey C, Hopkins-Price P, Shah P, Dunnington G, Courneya KS. Exploring social cognitive theory constructs for promoting exercise among breast cancer patients. Cancer Nurs 2004;27(6):462–73.

[103] Paul K, Buschbacher R. Cancer rehabilitation: increasing awareness and removing barriers. Am J Phys Med Rehab 2011;90(5 Suppl. 1):S1–4.

[104] Courneya KS, Friedenreich CM, Quinney HA, Fields AL, Jones LW, Vallance JK, et al. A longitudinal study of exercise barriers in colorectal cancer survivors participating in a randomized controlled trial. Ann Behav Med 2005;29(2):147–53.

[105] Courneya KS, McKenzie DC, Reid RD, Mackey JR, Gelmon K, Friedenreich CM, et al. Barriers to supervised exercise training in a randomized controlled trial of breast cancer patients receiving chemotherapy. Ann Behav Med 2008;35(1):116–22.

[106] Rogers LQ, Courneya KS, Robbins KT, Malone J, Seiz A, Koch L, et al. Physical activity correlates and barriers in head and neck cancer patients. Support Care Cancer 2008;16(1):19–27.

Chapter 14

Statins in Cardio-Oncology

Z. Almuwaqqat*, O. Hung** and S. Parashar**

*Division of Hospital Medicine, Department of Medicine, Emory University, Atlanta, GA, United States;
**Division of Cardiology, Department of Medicine, Emory University, Atlanta, GA, United States

INTRODUCTION

With advancements in cancer early detection strategies and therapies, survivorship among oncology patients has improved significantly [1]. Cardiovascular health had become a major concern for cancer patients and survivors [2]. CVD risk factor profile for oncology patients might be different from the general population; they may have been exposed to chemotherapeutic or biologic agents, radiotherapy; as well as they may have some underlying traditional risk factors and comorbidities. Statins are one of the most successful agents in lowering cholesterol and reducing atherosclerotic cardiovascular disease (ASCVD) risk with a relatively well-tolerated side effect profile and pleiotropic biological potential. Statins are prescribed on a large scale for the past several years. During 2011–2012, nearly one in every four US adults aged 40 and over reported using a prescription statin medication in the past 30 days according to the National Health Center 2014 statistics. The number of US adults using prescribed statins has been steadily increasing over the past 10 years. The American College of Cardiology and American Heart Association [3] updated hypercholesterolemia guidelines in 2013 shifted the paradigm from using statins as purely lipid-lowering agents to a risk reduction modality for patients with substantially elevated ASCVD risk. The new ASCVD risk calculation is derived from large pooled cohorts representative of US population, and the calculator is easily available on-line to help clinicians determine patient's 10-year and lifetime AS-CVD risk. These guidelines recognize statins' pleiotropic effects beyond cholesterol synthesis inhibition (Table 14.1) [3]. Studies continue to investigate statin's antitumor, antiinflammatory and survival benefits. However, to date, no specific guidelines recommend using statins in oncology patients beyond the traditional lipid lowering and ASCVD risk-reduction indications. Statins have shown consistently promising results in observational studies in prevention of cancer, improvement of disease-related and overall survival,

as well as maintain optimal cardiovascular health among the oncology population (Fig. 14.1).

BACKGROUND

Mechanism of Action

Statins are widely prescribed pharmacological agents that are effective in the treatment of hypercholesterolemia as well as primary and secondary prevention of ASCVD [4]. Their role as competitive inhibitors of the hydroxy-3-methylglutaryl-coenzyme A (HMG–CoA) reductase enzyme in the mevalonate pathway was first described in 1978 [5]. In addition to inhibiting squalene and, therefore, cholesterol biosynthesis, this role is vital for the modification of cellular functions resulting in the reduction of hepatic production and secretion of lipoproteins, increased catabolism of low-density lipoprotein (LDL) and upregulation of LDL receptors. Statins are therefore effective in reducing serum LDL levels. Additionally, because the mevalonate pathway is critical to the synthesis of isoprenoids, statins have also demonstrated extensive pleiotropic effects such as reducing oxidative stress and inflammation, improving endothelial function, inhibiting vascular smooth muscle cell proliferation and decreasing platelet aggregation [6–8].

Individual Statin Characteristics and Pharmacokinetics

The first isolated statin was described in 1976 as compactin, a new antifungal metabolite from *Penicillium brevicompactum* [9]. There are eight well-studied statins, seven are still commonly prescribed in the United States. Most statins utilize the cytochrome P450 pathway (CYP) and undergo extensive first pass modification due to intestinal and hepatic metabolism [10]. Atorvastatin and rosuvastatin are considered higher potency statins and recommended in patients with established atherosclerosis or in high-risk patients

TABLE 14.1 Pleiotropic Effects of Statins

Pleiotropic Effects of Statins	
Reduce LDL cholesterol	Stimulate bone growth
Antiinflammatory effect	Immunomodulation
Improve endothelial and vascular function	Glucose Metabolism
Antioxidant effects	Antiproliferative effect
Thrombosis inhibition	Muscle, hepatic, and renal effects

Source: Abate and Chandalia, 2006. Other than potency, are all statins the same? Curr Atheroscler Rep 8(1):26–31.

such as those with diabetes. Generally, statins are classified into hydrophilic and lipophilic groups on the basis of tissue selectivity. Hydrophilic statins, such as pravastatin and rosuvastatin, have less tissue absorption, except for the liver, and fewer side effects due to lower dependence on the cytochrome p450 enzyme resulting in a lower likelihood of drug–drug interactions, and increased renal excretion [11,12].

Potential Side Effects

The most common concern about statin therapy relates to myalgia and myopathy. Myalgia and myopathy are the most common adverse reaction affecting approximately 10% of statin users [13]. A cross-sectional study that enrolled 1000 patients reported that patients with statins prescription were 1.5-fold more likely to have musculoskeletal complaints [13]. The spectrum of toxicity is broad and can range from asymptomatic creatinine kinase (CK) elevation to myalgia without CK elevation to myositis and rarely rhabdomyolysis. One observational study of more than 35,000 health maintenance organization (HMO) patients taking statins between 1997 and 2004 found that statin is associated with doubling the risk of myopathy-related event, whereas rhabdomyolysis risk was almost similar to the general population [14]. Diabetics were 1.5 more likely to have myopathic event compared to the nondiabetics taking statin [14]. In another study, statins were responsible for four excess cases of rhabdomyolysis per 10,000 person-years (or approximately 0.004% of statin users per year of therapy) [15–17]. Statin-induced necrotizing autoimmune myositis (SINAM) and anti-HMGCR antibodies are two overlapping entities that may develop in statin-exposed patients regardless of their current statin use [16]. Cerivastatin was withdrawn from the market in 2001 after a postmarketing surveillance reported that its use was associated with increased risk for rhabdomyolysis [18].

Several studies have investigated the potential hepatotoxicity of statins. The rate of liver failure in statin users is estimated at one case per million person-years of use, similar to that in the overall US population [19,20]. Only 30 cases of statin-induced liver failure were reported between 1987 and 2000 in the Western world [21,22]. A meta-analysis of 13 randomized clinical trials examined 49,275 patients who received statin or placebo therapy with a mean follow-up of 3.6 years and observed that the incidence of elevated liver transaminase levels (>3× the upper limit of normal) in patients treated with statins was not significantly different compared to those treated with placebo (1.14% vs. 1.05%) [23]. As a result, the US Food and Drug Administration revised the safety labels in 2012 to remove the need for routine periodic monitoring of liver enzymes in patients taking statins and the 2013 ACC/AHA cholesterol treatment guidelines suggest measuring hepatic function only if hepatotoxicity is suspected (IIa recommendation, level of evidence C) [3].

The debate about development of diabetes due to statins has recently received increased attention. There have been conflicting reports about the development of type-2 diabetes after receiving statin therapy [24]. For example, the

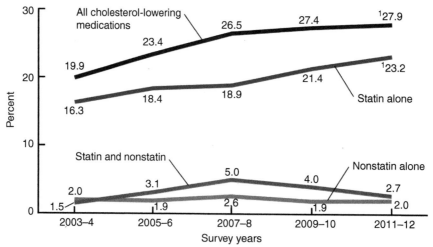

FIGURE 14.1   **Percentage of adults aged 40 and over who reported using a prescription cholesterol- lowering medication: United States, 2003–2012.** [1]Significant linear trend (*p* < 0.01). NOTE: Age-adjusted by direct method to the year 2000 projected US population. *From CDC/NCHS, National Health and Nutrition Examination Survey, 2003–2012.*

TABLE 14.2 Comparative Head-to-Head Effects of Individual Statins on Diabetes and Cancer

Atorvastatin	—	1.18 (0.71, 1.99)	1.12 (0.79, 1.62)	1.01 (0.69, 1.47)	1.06 (0.72, 1.57)
0.94 (0.59, 1.47)	Fluvastatin	—	—	—	—
0.86 (0.60, 1.20)	0.91 (0.58, 1.43)	Lovastatin	0.95 (0.62, 1.46)	0.85 (0.54, 1.33)	0.90 (0.56, 1.41)
0.90 (0.69, 1.20)	0.97 (0.65, 1.45)	1.06 (0.81, 1.42)	Pravastatin	0.90 (0.70, 1.12)	0.94 (0.72, 1.21)
0.84 (0.62, 1.16)	0.90 (0.58, 1.39)	0.99 (0.73, 1.36)	0.94 (0.73, 1.19)	Rosuvastatin	1.05 (0.80, 1.40)
0.84 (0.66, 1.08)	0.90 (0.60, 1.37)	0.98 (0.75, 1.34)	0.93 (0.77, 1.15)	0.99 (0.78, 1.30)	Simvastatin

Comparisons between drugs should be read from left to right, and the estimate is in the cell in common between the column-defining treatment and the row-defining treatment. For both outcomes, ORs.
Source: Naci H, et al. Comparative tolerability and harms of individual statins: a study-level network meta-analysis of 246,955 participants from 135 randomized, controlled trials. Circ Cardiovasc Qual Outcomes 2013;6:390–9.

JUPITER trial reported an increased incidence of diabetes in the rosuvastatin group compared to the placebo group, whereas the West of Scotland Coronary Prevention Study trial reported pravastatin to reduce the risk of diabetes [25,26]. A large meta-analysis consisting of 13 statin trials involving a total of 91,140 participants, demonstrated that statin therapy was associated with a 9% increased risk for incident diabetes (OR: 1.09; 95% CI: 1.02–1.17) with the number needed to harm of 260 [27]. However, there was a benefit in reduction of coronary heart disease (CHD) deaths, myocardial infarction (MI), and stroke. Another meta-analysis demonstrated that intensive-dose statin therapy led to a higher incidence of diabetes (OR: 1.12, 95% CI: 1.04–1.22) compared to a moderate-dose statin. However, intensive-dose statin therapy resulted in fewer major cardiovascular events (OR: 0.84, 95% CI: 0.75–0.94) compared to moderate-dose statins [17]. Although there might be a small risk for progression toward type-2 diabetes, there are significant benefits in terms of cardiovascular events' reduction by 25–45% (Table 14.2) [28]. Thus, there have been no changes in recommendations regarding statin therapy in patients with high CVD risk or existing CVD.

Other potential side effects of statin therapy are more controversial and include multiple concerns such as anemia, gastrointestinal upset, diabetes mellitus, vitamin D deficiency, sexual dysfunction, birth defects, rashes, cataracts, cognitive difficulties, memory loss, and sleep disturbances [6,7].

STATINS AND CANCER

Cancer Patients Are Also at Risk of Dying From Atherosclerotic Heart Disease

In the United States, ASCVD remains a major comorbidity of cancer patients as they frequently have one or more cardiac risk factors such as smoking, hypertension, or dyslipidemia at the time of their cancer diagnosis. About 20% of patients older than 70 years of age with newly diagnosed cancer have coexisting ASCVD [29]. In one study on 242 female breast-cancer survivors, the risk of suffering from

a major adverse cardiac event was similar or higher than developing a recurrence of their breast cancer [30]. In addition, the diagnosis of cancer may also indirectly lead to adverse lifestyle changes that further worsen hypercholesterolemia and increase cardiovascular risk [31,32].

Statin eligible patient population may be underestimated according to the Multi-Ethnic Study of Atherosclerosis (MESA) which observed a large proportion of ASCVD events occurred among adults with ASCVD risk of less than 7.5%. By adding coronary artery calcium score, high-sensitivity C-reactive protein, family history of ASCVD, and ankle–brachial index study was able to identify small subgroups of asymptomatic population with a 10-year risk of less than 7.5% but with observed ASCVD event rates greater than 7.5%. [33]. CAC score, ABI, and FH were independent predictors of ASCVD events in the MESA study [34]. Cancer survivors who may have estimated ASCVD risk of less than 7.5% according to the ACC/AHA may undergo further testing with coronary artery calcium score, high-sensitivity C-reactive protein, family history of ASCVD, and ankle–brachial index may be helpful in determining who may warrant statin therapy considerations

ASCVD may also occur as a complication of cancer therapy or as a result of accelerated progression of traditional CVD risk factors. Several special patient populations have also been identified, including Hodgkin's disease survivors, breast-cancer patients, young cancer survivors, patients receiving cardiotoxic chemotherapy treatment, and those receiving mediastinal radiation, who appear to have a higher risk of developing premature coronary artery disease [35–37]. Cancer treatment is associated with increased risk of developing coronary artery calcification [38,39]. It is unclear whether chemotherapy may accelerate atherosclerotic vascular disease and enhance the development of coronary artery calcification. Newer therapies including tyrosine kinase inhibitors (TKIs) may precipitate new or worsen preexisting hypertension. It was also observed that childhood cancer survivors are more likely to develop the combination of obesity, glucose intolerance, hyperinsulinemia, and an abnormal lipid profile than their matched control. High-risk profile for cardiovascular disease, markedly reduced spontaneous GH secretion and also additional features of the metabolic syndrome, such as higher systolic blood pressure and higher plasma glucose, and serum triglyceride levels have been observed among childhood cancer survivors [40]. Aggressive ASCVD risk reduction may therefore be especially useful in these populations.

Can Statins Treat or Prevent Cancer? Role of Statins on Cancer Development

The antitumor activities of statins have been theorized to stem from their ability to inhibit the mevalonate pathway, which plays an essential role in cancer cell proliferation and sustainability [41–44]. Several well-conducted large observational and randomized controlled trials have been performed to determine whether statins affect the treatment of specific malignancy. The results have been mixed, resulting in substantial controversy over whether statins actually have clinically significant anticancer activity (Fig. 14.2) [45–48].

Several studies have demonstrated the effectiveness of statins in the prevention and treatment of human cancers. In preclinical studies, different statins demonstrated cytotoxicity toward specific cancer cells. Compared to other statins fluvastatin, simvastatin, and lovastatin were found to be more cytotoxic against breast adenocarcinoma cells [43], whereas atorvastatin, simvastatin, lovastatin, and cerivastatin were more cytotoxic against myeloma cancer cells [42]. In addition, simvastatin and lovastatin showed higher cytotoxicity against ovarian cancer cells [44]. Lovastatin also appeared to induce apoptosis in a subset of tumors such as juvenile monomyelocytic leukemia, medulloblastoma, rhabdomyosarcoma, choriocarcinoma, and squamous cell carcinomas of the cervix, head, and neck [41]. Another study reviewed five observational studies enrolling a total of 87127 patients who received at least two different treatment strategies including rosuvastatin, atorvastatin, simvastatin, pravastatin, fluvastatin, cerivastatin, and lovastatin or observation alone. The study showed reduction in liver cancer risk among statin user as compared to observation with atorvastatin (OR 0.63, 95%CI 0.45–0.89) and fluvastatin (OR 0.58, 95%CI 0.40–0.85) [49].

There have also been numerous investigations that have demonstrated no significant reduction in cancer-specific events with use of statins. A multicenter randomized controlled trial of 20,536 patients with ASCVD found that

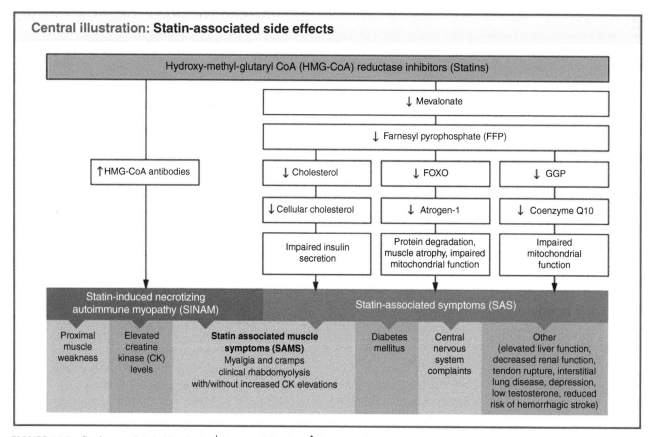

FIGURE 14.2 **Statin-associated side effects.** ↓, decreased function; ↑, increased function; CK, creatine kinase; CNS, central nervous system symptoms; DM, diabetes mellitus; FFP, farnesyl pyrophosphate; FOXO, forkhead box protein group; GGP, geranylgeranyl pyrophosphate; HMG-CoA, hydroxyl-methyl-glutaryl-coenzyme A reductase; r, rhabdomyolysis; SAMS, statin-associated muscle symptoms; SAS, statin-associated symptoms; SINAM, statin-induced necrotizing autoimmune myopathy. *From Thompson PD, et al. Statin-Associated Side Effects. J Am Coll Cardiol 2016; 67(20):2395–2410.*

allocation to simvastatin yielded a significant 23% decrease in major vascular events but no differences in cancer incidence, cancer-related mortality or nonvascular causes [50]. Additionally, a recent meta-analysis of 22 well-conducted·randomized, controlled trials with data from 66,582 patients who received statins and 66,604 who received placebo demonstrated that 5 years of statin therapy had no effect on the risk of cancer-related death [51]. The discrepancy between results of randomized controlled trials and observational studies on cancer-related mortality could be potentially explained by the presence of healthy user bias [52].

Can Statin Therapy Ameliorate Radiation-Induced Cardiovascular Toxicity?

Radiation therapy in the management of thoracic malignancies has led to a significant improvement in disease-specific survival. Among radiation-treated survivors, however, cardiovascular toxicity is now the most common cause of death besides malignancy. Toxicity typically occurs years after treatment and can manifest as premature coronary artery disease, valvular heart disease, arrhythmias, cardiomyopathy, pericarditis, or sudden cardiac death [53]. Cardiovascular mortality was shown to correlate linearly with the radiation dose received during childhood cancer treatment [54]. The risk of fatal cardiovascular events has been significantly higher for survivors and appears to increase with length of time since radiation exposure (Fig. 14.3) [55–57].

Radiation can induce atherosclerosis through the inflammatory and thrombotic cascades as well as increasing vascular permeability. Radiation-associated atherosclerotic

plaques appear to be different in both morphology and location from traditional plaque. In an autopsy study of 16 patients with radiation-associated heart disease and 10 control subjects, those who had undergone radiation tended to have more fibrous plaques rather than lipid plaques. This has led to the question whether statins can decrease risks of cardiovascular events through its pleiotropic biologic effect [55,58].

In preclinical studies, simvastatin administration has been observed to ameliorate radiation-induced intestinal injury via a protein C-independent mechanism [58]. Since the epithelium of intestines shares similarities with vascular endothelium, investigations were undertaken to determine whether statins could protect endothelium from radiation-induced injury. Age-matched rats were divided into two groups: one received total body irradiation (TBI) of 10 Gy and the other group underwent sham-irradiation to serve as controls. Compared with the controls, TBI-irradiated rats had sustained increases in total- and LDL-cholesterol, and triglycerides, as well as cellular periarterial fibrosis with cardiac mechanical dysfunction. Simvastatin was observed to ameliorate TBI-induced increases in total- and LDL-cholesterol and triglycerides, liver injury, and cardiac mechanical dysfunction. It was also concluded that simvastatin mitigated the increases in risk factors for cardiac disease and the extent of cardiac disease following TBI [55,59].

On the basis of the currently available preclinical in vitro and in vivo data, it appears statins have pleiotropic beneficial effects on radiation-induced damage [60]. A limited number of data indicate that statins, apart from alleviating deleterious nontarget effects of radiation therapy are also

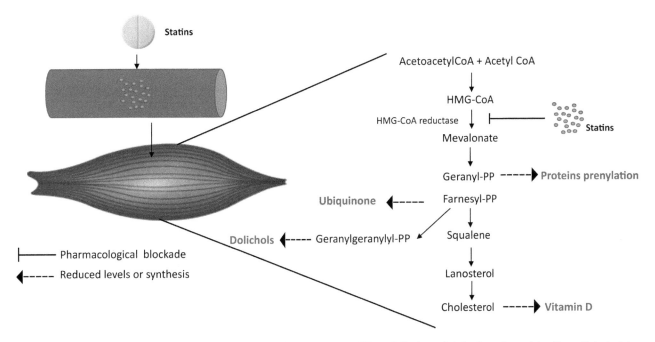

FIGURE 14.3 **Molecular mechanisms of statin induced toxicity.** *From Norata GD, et al. Statins and skeletal muscles toxicity: From clinical trials to everyday practice. Pharmacol Res 2014;88:107–113.*

radioprotective by promoting DNA repair [59]. In a clinical study, use of statin or statin + ACE inhibitor medication during radical pelvic radiotherapy significantly reduced acute gastrointestinal symptoms scores and also appeared to provide longer-term sustained protection [61]. However, this interesting aspect of statins on radiation therapy remains to be further studied. Clinical trials and meta-analysis assessing the usefulness of statin in preventing cardiovascular effects of radiation therapy in humans would be useful.

Can Statins Ameliorate Chemotherapy-Related Cardiomyopathy?

Chemotherapy-associated cardiotoxicity is one of the most limiting side effects of anthracycline use and increases both morbidity and mortality [62–64]. Vigilant surveillance throughout the administration of anthracyclines can improve outcomes, as early detection and treatment of decreased left ventricular function may limit or even reverse chemotherapy-induced cardiotoxicity [65]. Statins are commonly used to treat patients with ischemic cardiomyopathy to reduce future cardiovascular events [60]. Although statins are not recommended solely for nonischemic dilated cardiomyopathy, in a randomized trial of 63 patients with symptomatic nonischemic dilated cardiomyopathy, simvastatin compared to placebo showed improvement in cardiac function and reduction in inflammatory cytokines (tumor necrosis factor-alpha and IL-6) and brain natriuretic peptide [66].

Statins have potential protective effects in chemotherapy-related cardiomyopathy [67–69] as they have several effects other than cholesterol synthesis inhibition. Statins are implicated in reduction in neurohormonal activation and inflammatory pathways, interruption of Ras-dependent signal transduction, and suppression of matrix metalloproteinase-9 expression which may potentially inhibit cancer cells multiplication, invasion, and malignancy progression [70–72]. Animal studies have suggested that statins may attenuate anthracycline-related cardiotoxicity. Lovastatin has been shown to attenuate DNA damage in human endothelial cells [73,74], troponin I elevation, and cardiac fibrosis after exposure to doxorubicin [73–75]. In another study using fluvastatin pretreatment of doxorubicin therapy, the authors observed that compared to controls, fluvastatin-treated mice showed improved left ventricular function, reduced nitrotyrosine expression, enhanced expression of mitochondrial superoxide dismutase, attenuated mitochondrial apoptotic pathways, and reduced cardiac inflammatory response [69].

Some clinical studies have also supported the preclinical and animal studies that statin therapy initiated before and concurrent with chemotherapy is cardioprotective. In a retrospective observational study of 628 newly diagnosed relatively young women with breast cancer, uninterrupted statin therapy initiated before and concurrent with chemotherapy markedly reduced the risk for heart failure and cardiac-related mortality over average follow-up of 2.2 years (Fig. 14.4) [76]. In a randomized controlled trial

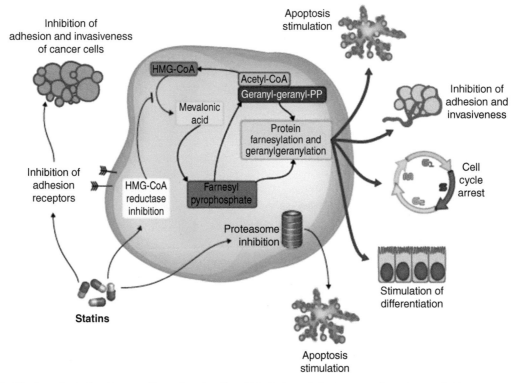

FIGURE 14.4 **The hypothesized anticancer effects of statins.** *From Kubatka P, et al. Statins in oncological research: From experimental studies to clinical practice. Crit Rev Oncol Hematol 2014;92(3):296–311.*

of atorvastatin versus placebo pretreatment, in 40 patients with various malignancies (as compared to Seicean study which included only breast cancer patients) and no cardiac history who were treated with Adriamycin or Idarubicin, the atorvastatin cohort demonstrated preservation of LVEF (61.3% vs. 62.6%, $P = 0.14$), compared to a LVEF reduction in the control group (62.9% vs. 55.0%, $P < 0.0001$). Mean reduction in left ventricular ejection fraction and mean increase in left ventricular end-diastolic diameter and left ventricular end-systolic diameter were significantly lower in the statin arm as compared with the control group ($P < 0.0001$; $P = 0.021$; $P = 0.001$, respectively) [77]. Another randomized controlled trial of 51 patients (14 receiving statins and 37 without) undergoing anthracycline chemotherapy received cardiovascular magnetic resonance imaging prior to and 6 months after chemotherapy initiation. Again, the statin cohort had less deterioration in LVEF than individuals not receiving statins [78]. Finally, a meta-analysis of 14 studies (2015 adult and pediatric patients) demonstrated that patients receiving prophylactic treatment, either with dexrazoxane, beta-blockade, angiotensin antagonists, or statins reduced cardiotoxicity, each with similar efficacy to the other [79].

STATINS AND MORTALITY AMONG CANCER PATIENTS

Do Statins Improve Disease Specific and Overall Mortality Among Cancer Patients?

Despite some trend toward positive survival benefits, the effect of statins on cancer-related mortality is mostly controversial with conflicting findings. An observational study published in the *New England Journal of Medicine* demonstrated that cancer-related mortality among statins users was reduced by 15%. The multivariable-adjusted hazard ratio for death from any cause among statin users, as compared with patients who had never used statins, was 0.85 (95% confidence interval [CI], 0.83–0.87) [80]. Although the hazard ratio difference was quite significant, the study did not prove dose–response relationship between statin and mortality nor it did have data related to the tumor-node-metastasis (TNM) stage, a major determinant of cancer-related mortality. Moreover 70% of statin users with cancer had cardiovascular disease comorbidity, as compared with 21% of patients who had never used statins before the cancer diagnosis (Fig. 14.5).

A systematic review and meta-analysis on using statins before and after cancer diagnosis on the cancer-specific mortality included 39 cohort studies and 2 case-control studies involving 990,649 participants were included. Study result was consistent with improvement in overall survival as well as cancer-specific survival among statins users before and after diagnosis of cancer. Patients who used statins after diagnosis had a HR of 0.81 (95% CI: 0.72–0.91) for all-cause mortality compared to nonusers. Those who used

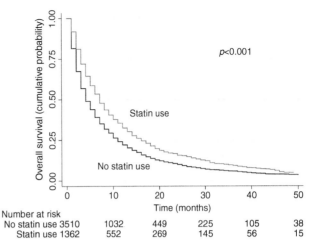

FIGURE 14.5 Kaplan-Meier Overall Survival Curves for all patients in cohort. Patients in the statin group have better overall survival compared to those in the non-statin group. *From Lin JJ, et al. The effect of statins on survival in patients with stage IV lung cancer. Lung Cancer 2016;99:137–42.*

statin after diagnosis (vs. nonusers) had an HR of 0.77 (95% CI: 0.66–0.88) for cancer-specific mortality. Prediagnostic exposure to statin was associated with both all-cause mortality (HR = 0.79, 95% CI: 0.74–0.85) and cancer-specific mortality (HR = 0.69, 95% CI: 0.60–0.79). The three largest cancer-type subgroups were colorectal, prostate, and breast cancer, and all showed a benefit from statin use. HRs per 365 defined daily doses increment were 0.80 (95% CI: 0.69–0.92) for all-cause mortality and 0.77 (95% CI: 0.67–0.89) for cancer-specific mortality [81]. Improved survival has also been described in patients with stage IV lung cancer (Fig. 14.6).

Several epidemiological studies have investigated the effects of statins on the risk of prostate cancer and survival outcomes. A recent meta-analysis of 13 studies examining the survival benefits of statins among total of 100,536 participants with prostate cancer patients, found that statin's use before and after diagnosis of prostate cancer had a significantly lower risk of both all-cause mortality and prostate cancer-related morality [82].

Using statins among heart transplantation patients and the effect on malignancy development and survival was studied in university hospital Zurich study. A total of 255 patients who underwent heart transplantation in 1985 and 2007 and survived the first year were included. During follow-up, a malignancy was diagnosed in 108 patients (42%). Statin use was associated with improved cancer-free and overall survival (both $P < 0.0001$). The cumulative incidence of tumors 8 years after transplantation was reduced in patients receiving a statin (34% vs. 13%; 95% confidence interval, 0.25–0.43 versus 0.07–0.18; $P < 0.003$). Using a regression model that analyzed the time to tumor formation with or without statin therapy, adjusted for age, male sex, type of cardiomyopathy, and immunosuppressive therapy superior survival was

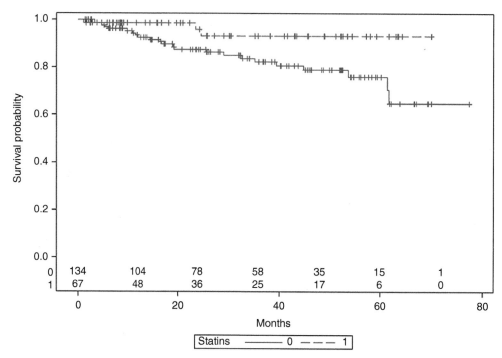

FIGURE 14.6 Incident HF and cancer-related mortality are significantly lower in the statin group, these survival curves illustrate survival in statin (red) and non-statin (blue) treated groups. *From Seicean S, et al. Effect of statin therapy on the risk for incident heart failure in patients with breast cancer receiving anthracycline chemotherapy: an observational clinical cohort study. J Am Coll Cardiol 2012;60(23):2384–90.*

demonstrated in the statin group. Statins reduced the hazard of occurrence of any malignancy by 67% (hazard ratio, 0.33; 95% confidence interval, 0.21–0.51; P < 0.0001) [83].

In contrary to the findings in the aforementioned studies a recent meta-analysis of 22 well-conducted randomized, controlled trials with data from 66,582 patients who received statins and 66,604 who received placebo demonstrated that 5 years of statin therapy had no effect on the risk of cancer-related death (relative risk, 1.00; 95% confidence interval, 0.93–1.08) [51].

The benefits of statins on cancer-related mortality remains controversial based on observational studies; future studies should investigate this relationship through well-established larger randomized clinical trials.

STATINS IN ONCOLOGY POPULATION

Should We Initiate Statin Therapy in Cancer Patients?

Cancer patients with traditional risk factors are less likely to receive aggressive statin therapy for primary and secondary prevention for several reasons. First, due to the perception of poor prognosis, statins therapy is often not initiated or is discontinued when chemotherapy is initiated. Rapid advances in oncology, however, have resulted in increasing numbers of cancer survivors who are also living longer. As a result, a diagnosis of cancer in the present day does not

necessarily indicate significantly reduced life expectancy. Additionally, these patients may continue to be at higher risk of major adverse cardiac events. CVD risk-factor modification including statin therapy when indicated, in consultation with the oncologist should therefore be aggressively pursued in these patients. Most importantly, a team-based approach with a cardio-oncologist is very useful.

Second, cancer patients are less likely to be prescribed statins due to the understandable focus on cancer therapy and complications. Chemotherapy and radiation therapy can result in a fluctuation in volume status (loss through vomiting, diarrhea or decreased oral intake, and gain through intravenous chemotherapy), diminished cardiopulmonary reserve, and development of anemia or thrombocytopenia. There is limited clinical data on statin effects during active cancer treatment, so it is reasonable to defer statin therapy during this period of management. However, as the patient improves, they should be reevaluated, in consultation with their oncologist, to determine whether statin initiation could result in long-term ASCVD risk reduction.

Finally, several antineoplastic therapies may have significant interactions with statins leading to polypharmacy concerns. Statins and some antineoplastic therapies can share common side effects such as myalgia and elevated liver enzymes that may result in the withholding of statin therapy. Systematic investigation of statin-related myalgia is straightforward to perform but can be challenging in cancer patients. Patients can be given a "statin holiday" where the offending statin is discontinued for few weeks. If the symptoms continue, then the myalgia is more likely related to chemotherapy, antibiotics, or other drugs. If the symptoms improve, then a different statin with less potential for side effects (e.g., pravastatin) can be tried at an initial low dose with slow uptitration. Typically, a hydrophilic statin (such as pravastatin) is a preferred statin due to its lower incidence of side effects including myalgias and hepatotoxicity, and lesser likelihood of interaction with oncology medications. Routine monitoring of statins for hepatotoxicity by clinicians is no longer standard of care; however, the role of statin therapy in cancer patients with already elevated liver enzymes is less clear. Risk–benefits considerations with close communication and integrated care with oncology, and monitoring of liver enzymes would be recommended.

Despite these concerns about statin therapy in cancer patients, it is important to remember that this clinical population is at higher risk for ASCVD event [31]. To date, statin therapy has shown promising results in reducing clinical events in preclinical studies, observational studies, and small clinical trials of oncology patients; however, statins may be effective ASCVD risk modifiers as opposed to having any direct antitumor activity. Future efforts could be directed at developing ASCVD risk assessment tools for oncology patients, conducting large epidemiological studies on the incidence of various types of cancers in patients on and without statin therapy, and designing large randomized controlled trials to evaluate statins as cardioprotective agents against cancer treatments.

To provide comprehensive multidisciplinary care, cardio-oncology centers may be developed to address the cardiovascular side effects of cancer therapy and improving cardiovascular outcomes for cancer survivors [84]. Such programs provide care to patients at varying stages of cancer treatment who have or are at risk for heart disease. The specialty cardio-oncology clinics provide collaborative evaluation and care of cancer patients receiving chemotherapy, radiation therapy, and neoadjuvant therapy. The objectives of these clinics are to provide expert advice and guidance for patients who are either undergoing cancer treatment, or have completed cancer treatment to aid in the prevention, monitoring, and management of cardiovascular toxicities with the goal that a cancer survivor of today does not become the cardiovascular disease patient of tomorrow [85]. Statin intolerant patients who might have an indication for cholesterol lowering due to a significant ASCVD or history of myocardial infarction may benefit from a consultation with lipidology clinic.

CONCLUSIONS

Assessment of ASCVD risk during the cancer diagnostic and prognostic work up is important because the risk of morbidity and mortality from cardiovascular events in this clinical population may be additive or multiplicative to the risk of cardiotoxicity due to chemotherapy and radiation therapy. Statins are relatively well-tolerated agents and appropriate intensity of statin therapy is used to reduce ASCVD risk in those most likely to benefit. Statin therapy, regardless of its actual antitumor activity, should be considered for adjunctive therapy to treat existing ASCVD and reduction of ASCVD risk in cancer patients in close communication and integrated care with oncology. Further studies should be directed to identifying the group of patients who are most likely to benefit from earlier statin use and investigate the effect of statin on cancer, development, survival, and cardiovascular health of cancer patients through well-established larger randomized clinical trials.

REFERENCES

[1] Jemal A, Ward E, Thun M. Declining death rates reflect progress against cancer. PLoS One 2010;5(3):e9584.

[2] Siegel R, et al. Cancer treatment and survivorship statistics 2012. CA Cancer J Clin 2012;62(4):220–41.

[3] Stone NJ, et al. 2013 ACC/AHA guideline on the treatment of blood cholesterol to reduce atherosclerotic cardiovascular risk in adults: a report of the American College of Cardiology/American Heart Association Task Force on Practice Guidelines. Circulation 2014;129(25 Suppl 2):S1–S45.

[4] Beck LH, Kumar SP. Update in preventive medicine. Ann Intern Med 1999;131(9):681–7.

[5] Brown MS, et al. Induction of 3-hydroxy-3-methylglutaryl coenzyme A reductase activity in human fibroblasts incubated with compactin (ML-236B), a competitive inhibitor of the reductase. J Biol Chem 1978;253(4):1121–8.

[6] Liao JK, Laufs U. Pleiotropic effects of statins. Annu Rev Pharmacol Toxicol 2005;45:89–118.

[7] Wagstaff LR, et al. Statin-associated memory loss: analysis of 60 case reports and review of the literature. Pharmacotherapy 2003;23(7):871–80.

[8] Abate N, Chandalia M. Other than potency, are all statins the same? Curr Atheroscler Rep 2006;8(1):26–31.

[9] Brown AG, et al. Crystal and molecular structure of compactin, a new antifungal metabolite from *Penicillium brevicompactum*. J Chem Soc Perkin 1976;1(11):1165–70.

[10] Garcia MJ, et al. Clinical pharmacokinetics of statins. Methods Find Exp Clin Pharmacol 2003;25(6):457–81.

[11] Gauthaman K, Manasi N, Bongso A. Statins inhibit the growth of variant human embryonic stem cells and cancer cells in vitro but not normal human embryonic stem cells. Br J Pharmacol 2009;157(6):962–73.

[12] Osmak M. Statins and cancer: current and future prospects. Cancer Lett 2012;324(1):1–12.

[13] Mosshammer D, et al. Statin use and its association with musculoskeletal symptoms—a cross-sectional study in primary care settings. Fam Pract 2009;26(2):88–95.

[14] Nichols GA, Koro CE. Does statin therapy initiation increase the risk for myopathy? An observational study of 32,225 diabetic and nondiabetic patients. Clin Ther 2007;29(8):1761–70.

[15] Graham DJ, et al. Incidence of hospitalized rhabdomyolysis in patients treated with lipid-lowering drugs. Jama 2004;292(21):2585–90.

[16] Mammen AL, et al. Autoantibodies against 3-hydroxy-3-methylglutaryl-coenzyme A reductase in patients with statin-associated autoimmune myopathy. Arthritis Rheum 2011;63(3):713–21.

[17] Baigent C, et al. Efficacy and safety of more intensive lowering of LDL cholesterol: a meta-analysis of data from 170,000 participants in 26 randomised trials. Lancet 2010;376(9753):1670–81.

[18] Furberg CD, Pitt B. Withdrawal of cerivastatin from the world market. Curr Control Trials Cardiovasc Med 2001;2(5):205–7.

[19] Joy TR, Hegele RA. Narrative review: statin-related myopathy. Ann Intern Med 2009;150(12):858–68.

[20] Tolman KG. Defining patient risks from expanded preventive therapies. Am J Cardiol 2000;85(12a):9e–15e.

[21] Cohen DE, Anania FA, Chalasani N. An assessment of statin safety by hepatologists. Am J Cardiol 2006;97(8a):77c–81c.

[22] Alsheikh-Ali AA, et al. Effect of the magnitude of lipid lowering on risk of elevated liver enzymes, rhabdomyolysis, and cancer: insights from large randomized statin trials. J Am Coll Cardiol 2007;50(5):409–18.

[23] de Denus S, et al. Statins and liver toxicity: a meta-analysis. Pharmacotherapy 2004;24(5):584–91.

[24] Jukema JW, et al. The controversies of statin therapy: weighing the evidence. J Am Coll Cardiol 2012;60(10):875–81.

[25] Ridker PM, et al. Rosuvastatin to prevent vascular events in men and women with elevated C-reactive protein. N Engl J Med 2008;359(21):2195–207.

[26] Freeman DJ, et al. Pravastatin and the development of diabetes mellitus: evidence for a protective treatment effect in the West of Scotland Coronary Prevention Study. Circulation 2001;103(3):357–62.

[27] Sattar N, et al. Statins and risk of incident diabetes: a collaborative meta-analysis of randomised statin trials. Lancet 2010;375(9716):735–42.

[28] Farmer JA, Torre-Amione G. Comparative tolerability of the HMG-CoA reductase inhibitors. Drug Saf 2000;23(3):197–213.

[29] Coebergh JW, et al. Serious co-morbidity among unselected cancer patients newly diagnosed in the southeastern part of The Netherlands in 1993-1996. J Clin Epidemiol 1999;52(12):1131–6.

[30] Bardia A, et al. Comparison of breast cancer recurrence risk and cardiovascular disease incidence risk among postmenopausal women with breast cancer. Breast Cancer Res Treat 2012;131(3):907–14.

[31] Jones LW, et al. Cardiovascular reserve and risk profile of postmenopausal women after chemoendocrine therapy for hormone receptor—positive operable breast cancer. Oncologist 2007;12(10):1156–64.

[32] Jones LW, et al. Early breast cancer therapy and cardiovascular injury. J Am Coll Cardiol 2007;50(15):1435–41.

[33] Yeboah J, et al. Utility of nontraditional risk markers in individuals ineligible for statin therapy according to the 2013 American College of Cardiology/American Heart Association Cholesterol Guidelines. Circulation 2015;132(10):916–22.

[34] Yeboah J, et al. Utility of nontraditional risk markers in atherosclerotic cardiovascular disease risk assessment. J Am Coll Cardiol 2016;67(2):139–47.

[35] Hooning MJ, et al. Long-term risk of cardiovascular disease in 10-year survivors of breast cancer. J Natl Cancer Inst 2007;99(5):365–75.

[36] Aleman BM, et al. Late cardiotoxicity after treatment for Hodgkin lymphoma. Blood 2007;109(5):1878–86.

[37] van den Belt-Dusebout AW, et al. Long-term risk of cardiovascular disease in 5-year survivors of testicular cancer. J Clin Oncol 2006;24(3):467–75.

[38] Pursnani A, et al. Guideline-based statin eligibility, coronary artery calcification, and cardiovascular events. JAMA 2015;314(2):134–41.

[39] Whitlock MC, et al. Cancer and its association with the development of coronary artery calcification: an assessment from the multi-ethnic study of atherosclerosis. J Am Heart Assoc 2015;4(11). pii: e002533.

[40] Talvensaari K, Knip M. Childhood cancer and later development of the metabolic syndrome. Ann Med 1997;29(5):353–5.

[41] Dimitroulakos J, et al. Differential sensitivity of various pediatric cancers and squamous cell carcinomas to lovastatin-induced apoptosis: therapeutic implications. Clin Cancer Res 2001;7(1):158–67.

[42] Cafforio P, et al. Statins activate the mitochondrial pathway of apoptosis in human lymphoblasts and myeloma cells. Carcinogenesis 2005;26(5):883–91.

[43] Campbell MJ, et al. Breast cancer growth prevention by statins. Cancer Res 2006;66(17):8707–14.

[44] Kato S, et al. Lipophilic but not hydrophilic statins selectively induce cell death in gynaecological cancers expressing high levels of HMG-CoA reductase. J Cell Mol Med 2010;14(5):1180–93.

[45] Howe K, et al. The statin class of HMG-CoA reductase inhibitors demonstrate differential activation of the nuclear receptors PXR, CAR and FXR, as well as their downstream target genes. Xenobiotica 2011;41(7):519–29.

[46] Wong WW, et al. Cerivastatin triggers tumor-specific apoptosis with higher efficacy than lovastatin. Clin Cancer Res 2001;7(7):2067–75.

[47] Novak A, et al. Cholesterol masks membrane glycosphingolipid tumor-associated antigens to reduce their immunodetection in human cancer biopsies. Glycobiology 2013;23(11):1230–9.

[48] Crick DC, et al. Geranylgeraniol overcomes the block of cell proliferation by lovastatin in C6 glioma cells. J Neurochem 1998;70(6):2397–405.

[49] Zhou YY, et al. Systematic review with network meta-analysis: statins and risk of hepatocellular carcinoma. Oncotarget 2016;7(16):21753–62.

[50] Bulbulia R, et al. Effects on 11-year mortality and morbidity of lowering LDL cholesterol with simvastatin for about 5 years in 20,536 high-risk individuals: a randomised controlled trial. Lancet 2011;378(9808):2013–20.

[51] Emberson JR, et al. Lack of effect of lowering LDL cholesterol on cancer: meta-analysis of individual data from 175,000 people in 27 randomised trials of statin therapy. PLoS One 2012;7(1):e29849.

[52] Klop C, Driessen JH, de Vries F. Statin use and reduced cancer-related mortality. N Engl J Med 2013;368(6):574.

[53] Jaworski C, et al. Cardiac complications of thoracic irradiation. J Am Coll Cardiol 2013;61(23):2319–28.

[54] Tukenova M, et al. Role of cancer treatment in long-term overall and cardiovascular mortality after childhood cancer. J Clin Oncol 2010;28(8):1308–15.

[55] Lenarczyk M, et al. Simvastatin mitigates increases in risk factors for and the occurrence of cardiac disease following 10 Gy total body irradiation. Pharmacol Res Perspect 2015;3(3):e00145.

[56] Brosius FC 3rd, Waller BF, Roberts WC. Radiation heart disease. Analysis of 16 young (aged 15 to 33 years) necropsy patients who received over 3,500 rads to the heart. Am J Med 1981;70(3):519–30.

[57] Adams MJ, et al. Radiation-associated cardiovascular disease. Crit Rev Oncol Hematol 2003;45(1):55–75.

[58] Wang J, et al. Simvastatin ameliorates radiation enteropathy development after localized, fractionated irradiation by a protein C-independent mechanism. Int J Radiat Oncol Biol Phys 2007;68(5):1483–90.

[59] Fritz G, Henninger C, Huelsenbeck J. Potential use of HMG-CoA reductase inhibitors (statins) as radioprotective agents. Br Med Bull 2011;97:17–26.

[60] Randomised trial of cholesterol lowering in 4444 patients with coronary heart disease: the Scandinavian Simvastatin Survival Study (4S). Lancet 1994;344(8934):1383–9.

[61] Wedlake LJ, et al. Evaluating the efficacy of statins and ACE-inhibitors in reducing gastrointestinal toxicity in patients receiving radiotherapy for pelvic malignancies. Eur J Cancer 2012;48(14):2117–24.

[62] Swain SM, Whaley FS, Ewer MS. Congestive heart failure in patients treated with doxorubicin: a retrospective analysis of three trials. Cancer 2003;97(11):2869–79.

[63] Shankar SM, et al. Monitoring for cardiovascular disease in survivors of childhood cancer: report from the Cardiovascular Disease Task Force of the Children's Oncology Group. Pediatrics 2008;121(2):e387–96.

[64] Carver JR, et al. American Society of Clinical Oncology clinical evidence review on the ongoing care of adult cancer survivors: cardiac and pulmonary late effects. J Clin Oncol 2007;25(25):3991–4008.

[65] Simunek T, et al. Anthracycline-induced cardiotoxicity: overview of studies examining the roles of oxidative stress and free cellular iron. Pharmacol Rep 2009;61(1):154–71.

[66] Node K, et al. Short-term statin therapy improves cardiac function and symptoms in patients with idiopathic dilated cardiomyopathy. Circulation 2003;108(7):839–43.

[67] Jensen BV. Cardiotoxic consequences of anthracycline-containing therapy in patients with breast cancer. Semin Oncol 2006;33 (3 Suppl 8):S15–21.

[68] Cardinale D, et al. Prevention of high-dose chemotherapy-induced cardiotoxicity in high-risk patients by angiotensin-converting enzyme inhibition. Circulation 2006;114(23):2474–81.

[69] Cardinale D, Colombo A, Cipolla CM. Prevention and treatment of cardiomyopathy and heart failure in patients receiving cancer chemotherapy. Curr Treat Options Cardiovasc Med 2008;10(6):486–95.

[70] Ducharme A, et al. Targeted deletion of matrix metalloproteinase-9 attenuates left ventricular enlargement and collagen accumulation after experimental myocardial infarction. J Clin Invest 2000;106(1):55–62.

[71] Bellosta S, et al. HMG-CoA reductase inhibitors reduce MMP-9 secretion by macrophages. Arterioscler Thromb Vasc Biol 1998;18(11):1671–8.

[72] Aikawa M, et al. An HMG-CoA reductase inhibitor, cerivastatin, suppresses growth of macrophages expressing matrix metalloproteinases and tissue factor in vivo and in vitro. Circulation 2001;103(2): 276–83.

[73] Huelsenbeck J, et al. Inhibition of Rac1 signaling by lovastatin protects against anthracycline-induced cardiac toxicity. Cell Death Dis 2011;2:e190.

[74] Damrot J, et al. Lovastatin protects human endothelial cells from the genotoxic and cytotoxic effects of the anticancer drugs doxorubicin and etoposide. Br J Pharmacol 2006;149(8):988–97.

[75] Iliescu C, Durand JB, Kroll M. Cardiovascular interventions in thrombocytopenic cancer patients. Tex Heart Inst J 2011;38(3): 259–60.

[76] Seicean S, et al. Effect of statin therapy on the risk for incident heart failure in patients with breast cancer receiving anthracycline chemotherapy: an observational clinical cohort study. J Am Coll Cardiol 2012;60(23):2384–90.

[77] Acar Z, et al. Efficiency of atorvastatin in the protection of anthracycline-induced cardiomyopathy. J Am Coll Cardiol 2011;58(9): 988–9.

[78] Chotenimitkhun R, et al. Chronic statin administration may attenuate early anthracycline-associated declines in left ventricular ejection function. Can J Cardiol 2015;31(3):302–7.

[79] Kalam K, Marwick TH. Role of cardioprotective therapy for prevention of cardiotoxicity with chemotherapy: a systematic review and meta-analysis. Eur J Cancer 2013;49(13):2900–9.

[80] Nielsen SF, Nordestgaard BG, Bojesen SE. Statin use and reduced cancer-related mortality. N Engl J Med 2012;367(19):1792–802.

[81] Zhong S, et al. Statin use and mortality in cancer patients: systematic review and meta-analysis of observational studies. Cancer Treat Rev 2015;41(6):554–67.

[82] Meng Y, et al. Statin use and mortality of patients with prostate cancer: a meta-analysis. Onco Targets Ther 2016;9:1689–96.

[83] Frohlich GM, et al. Statins and the risk of cancer after heart transplantation. Circulation 2012;126(4):440–7.

[84] Parashar S. Building bridges: the emerging field of cardio-oncology. Future Cardiol 2015;11(4):377–82.

[85] Dent S, et al. Cancer and cardiovascular disease: the complex labyrinth. J Oncol 2015;2015:516450.

Chapter 15

Coordinating Cardio-Oncology Care

S. Dent, A. Law, O. Aseyev, N. Ghosh and C. Johnson

Department of Medicine, Division of Medical Oncology, University of Ottawa, The Ottawa Hospital, Ottawa, ON, Canada

INTRODUCTION

Mortality rates from cancer have declined over the past 30 years largely due to early detection strategies, improved surgical approaches as well as advances in cancer therapeutics [1–3]. Improvement in survivorship, however, can come at a cost [4]. Cardiotoxicity is now the second leading cause of long-term morbidity and mortality among cancer survivors [1–3,5,6]. Conventional chemotherapy and targeted therapies are associated with an increased risk of cardiac damage including left ventricular (LV) dysfunction and heart failure (HF) [7,8], treatment-induced hypertension, vasospastic and thromboembolic ischemia, as well as rhythm disturbances and QTc prolongation that can be potentially life-threatening. While some of these cardiac adverse effects are irreversible and cause progressive cardiovascular disease (CVD), others induce only temporary dysfunction with no apparent long-term sequelae [9]. Early and late effects of chest radiation can lead to radiation-induced heart disease, including pericardial disease, myocardial fibrosis, cardiomyopathy, coronary artery disease (CAD), valvular disease, and arrhythmias in the setting of myocardial fibrosis [10]. Oncologists face the challenge of treating patients with the best cancer therapies available without adversely impacting cardiovascular (CV) health. The discipline of cardio-oncology has developed in response to the combined decision-making necessary to optimize the care of patients with cancer, whether they are receiving active treatment or are long-term survivors after successful treatment. This chapter will focus on coordination of care for cancer patients exposed to potential cardiotoxic therapy—prior to, during and following completion of their treatment—as well as discuss the roles of healthcare providers involved in this multidisciplinary approach.

CANCER AND HEART DISEASE

Cancer and heart disease are the leading causes of morbidity and mortality in the industrialized world. However, there is cause for optimism. Modern treatments have led to an improvement in the chances of surviving a diagnosis of cancer; the 5-year survival for early stage breast cancer increased from 79% in 1990 to 88% in 2012 [1,2,6,11]. Similar improvements have been seen with other solid and hematological cancers including non-Hodgkin's lymphoma and testicular cancer [3]. Long-term cancer survivors are expected to increase by approximately 30% in the next decade to an estimated 18 million by 2022 in the United States alone [6]. These improvements in survivorship can come at a cost [4]. Current anticancer therapies are associated with unique and varying degrees of direct (e.g., hypertension, arrhythmias) [12–16] as well as indirect (e.g., unfavorable lifestyle changes) sequential, and progressive CV insults.

The incidence of cancer treatment induced CV injury (cardiotoxicity) varies widely depending on the specific cancer therapy used, duration of therapy, and underlying patient comorbidities. As diagnostic techniques and treatments improve, cancer is no longer thought of as an immediate life-threatening disease but has in many cases evolved to be thought of as a chronic disease, similar to HIV or diabetes, with the expectation of long-term survival with good quality of life. Over half of adult patients diagnosed with cancer in England and Wales will survive at least 10 years, and survival rates have doubled over the past four decades [17]. In 2014, The National Health Interview Survey identified that 27.6 million adult Americans have been diagnosed with heart disease, representing 11.6% of the population [5,6,11]. While there is a paucity of data in the literature on the late effects on CV health of adult cancer survivors from cancer treatment, we can gain some insight from longitudinal studies in the pediatric population. The Childhood Cancer Survivor Study (CCSS) showed that 15–25 years after diagnosis, survivors of childhood cancer have 8.2-fold higher rate of cardiac death as compared to the age and sex matched national average. When compared to controls, long-term childhood cancer survivors had 15-fold increased rates of congestive HF, 10-fold higher rates of CVD, and 9-fold higher rates of stroke [18]. These results have significant implications for adult cancer survivors who face the

CV effects of aging compounded by the potential detrimental impact of cancer therapy on their CV health [19,20].

CARDIO-ONCOLOGY: AN EMERGING MULTIDISCIPLINARY FIELD

Recognition of the importance of CV health in adult cancer patients is paramount if we are to sustain the survivorship improvements achieved with modern cancer therapies. The important interrelationship between cardiology and oncology must be recognized along with the impact on the cancer patient from diagnosis, through treatment and survivorship. It has become increasingly common for oncologists and cardiologists to encounter patients with both cancer and heart disease, which represent the two most common causes of death worldwide [21].

Traditional cytotoxic agents and targeted therapies used to treat cancer, including chemotherapeutic agents (e.g., anthracyclines), monoclonal antibodies that target and inhibit tyrosine kinase, and antiangiogenic drugs can affect the CV system. Combination cancer therapies (e.g., anthracyclines and anti-HER2 agents) commonly used today, can amplify the risk of cardiotoxicity. Oncologists must be acutely aware of the CV risks associated with these treatments, including the presence of preexisting comorbidities (e.g., hypertension) that can increase the risk of cardiotoxicity. Cardiologists must have an understanding of the potential cardiotoxicity of cancer therapies as well as the impact of oncology treatments on cancer survival [22].

Newer targeted therapies have short-term CV toxicities (e.g., hypertension with bevacizumab) that are increasingly well understood, however, given their recent emergence in cancer care, we do not yet know the long-term cardiac consequences for patients. As new therapies continue to improve survival of cancer patients, the appropriate CV follow-up of cancer survivors at risk for cardiotoxicity will become an important public health issue.

Cardio-oncology—a new subspecialty of medicine—has emerged over the last decade, with the goal of providing cancer patients with "state of the art" cancer therapy, without compromising CV health. Cardio-oncology provides the healthcare team (oncologists, cardiologists, nurses, pharmacists) with the opportunity of improving care of cancer patients while optimizing CV health.

Why Create a Cardio-Oncology Program?

Contemporary cancer therapy has improved survival for a variety of malignancies [23]. A cancer patient's treatment plan may include one or more chemotherapy regimens, targeted therapy, radiation, and cancer surgery. While some patients need only one or two of these therapies, it is not unusual for patients to face sequential cancer treatments, each with potential cardiotoxic side effects. Cancer and CVD share common lifestyle-related risk factors, including smoking, obesity, poor dietary habits, and inactivity, such that cardiac disease and cardiac risk factors may lead to modification of cancer therapy. Risk factors (e.g., hypertension), underlying cardiac disease, and administration of potentially cardiotoxic cancer therapy can lead to CV dysfunction (Fig. 15.1), which may result in oncologists interrupting and perhaps discontinuing life-saving cancer treatment.

The growing array of targeted agents, each with potential cardiotoxicity, makes it difficult for cardiologists to keep up with the latest advances in cardio-oncology [15]. LV dysfunction resulting from anthracycline or trastuzumab based therapy, and coronary disease in patients exposed to chest radiation are familiar to most cardiologists [24,25]. However, peripheral vascular events in CML patients treated with tissue kinase inhibitors, chest pain syndromes in breast cancer patients treated with 5-fluorouracil, and severe hypertension in renal cell cancer patients receiving sunitinib are not part of the daily practice for most cardiologists [26–28]. Survey data indicate that cardiologists do not have a high level of understanding of the consequences of stopping cancer therapy due to cardiotoxicity, and are understandably uncomfortable making such clinical decisions [29].

The need to optimize cardiac health in patients undergoing cancer therapy, treat cardiotoxicity resulting from cancer therapy, and follow-up cancer survivors at long-term risk for cardiac disease are clinical needs that have driven the development of cardio-oncology [4].

ESTABLISHMENT OF A CARDIO-ONCOLOGY PROGRAM

Increasing awareness by healthcare providers of the potential detrimental impact of cancer therapies on CV health of cancer patients, during and/or following cancer therapy, has led to the establishment of increasing numbers of dedicated cardio-oncology clinics across North America, and worldwide. However, there is a paucity of literature on the essential components and infrastructure needed to support such a program.

The clinical care and support of patients during, and following their cancer therapy remains our primary goal; education is essential in order to empower patients and healthcare providers with the knowledge needed to deliver the best cancer therapies while optimizing CV health. Our understanding of the interaction between cancer therapies and CV health is limited, and mainly based on the cardiotoxicity of traditional cancer therapies (e.g., anthracyclines). As modern targeted cancer therapeutic strategies emerge, translational and clinical research is essential in order to improve our understanding of the mechanisms of cardiotoxicity as well as the potential therapeutic approaches to prevent and treat cancer therapy-related dysfunction. Thus,

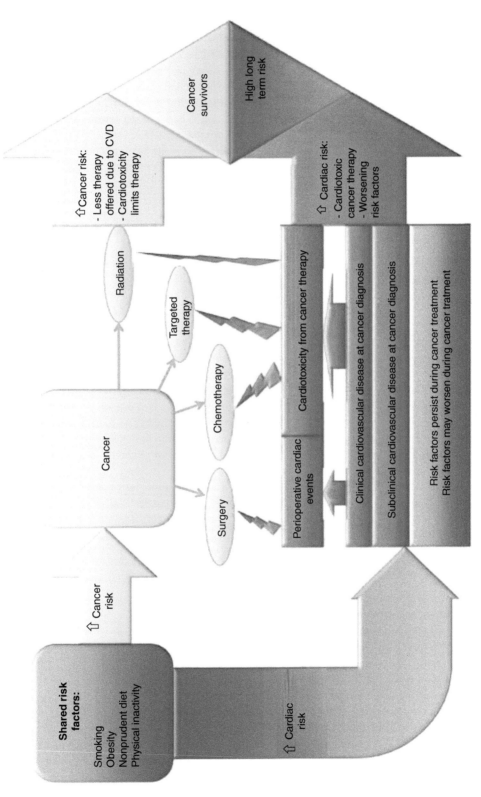

FIGURE 15.1   **Risk factors contributing to cardiotoxicity associated with cancer treatment.** *CVD, Cardiovascular disease.*

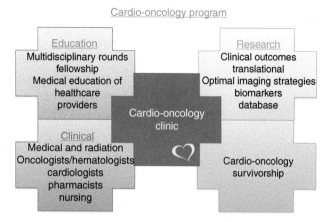

FIGURE 15.2 **Components of a cardio-oncology program.**

the essential components of a successful cardio-oncology program should include: (1) clinical care; (2) translational/clinical research; (3) patient and healthcare provider education; and (4) survivorship care (Fig. 15.2).

Cardio-Oncology Team

Collaboration between cardiologists, oncologists, and allied healthcare professionals who provide cancer care is essential.

Cardio-oncologists are medical providers who are focused on the CV health of patients who have, or had, cancer. They help ensure that optimal cancer treatment is administered by preventing, or at least mitigating, treatment-related cardiotoxicity whenever possible. They shoulder the responsibility of managing any resulting CV complications to avoid limiting effective cancer therapy. They also play a role in the management and treatment of any CV effects that either exist prior to treatment or that occur as a result of cancer therapy, or cancer itself. Cardio-oncologists also endeavor to improve clinical CV care, enhance education, and promote research for patients who have an active or prior history of malignancy [30].

Cardio-oncologists must be familiar with the cardiac risks posed by specific cancer therapies and the effects of these therapies in patients with established CVD. The recognition of the interplay of these factors is vital during the treatment planning phase. The management of various cardiac conditions may require adjustment while a patient is undergoing cancer treatment. For example, atrial fibrillation is the most commonly diagnosed arrhythmia with a prevalence of 1% in the general population, and 9% in those over age 80 [31]. Treatment of atrial fibrillation in the cancer patient can present special challenges with regards to thromboembolic prophylaxis. The cancer itself induces a hypercoagulable state putting the patient at increased risk of thromboembolism or may present a bleeding risk, such as in the case of gastric cancer, but chemotherapy can bring

on severe thrombocytopenia or an unpredictable response to anticoagulation, thus increasing the risk of significant bleeding. Familiarity with cardiac effects of less commonly used cancer therapies is required to deal with uncommon clinical scenarios, such as the management of the advanced breast cancer patient or the renal cell cancer patient who has developed severe hypercholesterolemia on everolimus and the decision whether to continue this therapy. The decision regarding the best treatment plan should be made after discussion between the cardiologist and the oncologist. This is one example where the expertise of a cardio-oncologist is required to make recommendations regarding best cardiac management when these considerations are integrated into the decision algorithm.

Outside the clinical setting, the role of the cardio-oncologist also involves the education of colleagues and trainees and to expand the knowledge base of cardio-oncologists. One of the key roles is to collaborate on research projects to answer important questions, such as: If cardiotoxicity can be predicted, can patients be stratified into low risk and high risk groups and have imaging tailored to the calculated risk? Can statins reduce the risk of transient LV dysfunction of monoclonal antibody-based tyrosine kinase inhibitors? Should all patients at risk of cardiotoxicity receive adjunctive treatment with cardiac medications prior to initiation of cancer therapy? These questions can only be answered with the creation of registries and databases that will provide evidence-based answers to guide treatment and create clinical guidelines. The field of cardio-oncology is rapidly evolving as more patients, with concomitant cancer and cardiac disease, are expected as the population ages, overall life expectancy increases, and medical treatments improve. The cardio-oncologist firmly believes and echoes the following statement from Dr. Eschenhagen, *"The cured cancer patient of today does not want to become the heart failure patient of tomorrow."* [32].

Role of Allied Healthcare Providers (Nursing, Pharmacy)

In successful cardio-oncology programs, allied healthcare providers play a key role in coordinating multidisciplinary care for cancer patients. Pharmacists are important members of the multidisciplinary team. They provide coordinated documentation of medication adjustments and dose updates, including cancer treatments, as well as patient education and engagement [33]. They can review possible drug-drug interactions that may potentiate the impact of potential cardiotoxic cancer drugs. Clinic nurses, and physician extenders (nurse practitioners/physician assistants), provide coordination of cardio-oncology appointments and other cancer care, including chemotherapy, radiology studies, oncology, and surgical appointments. They facilitate timely scheduling of serial cardiac imaging and/or laboratory studies with prompt care on the basis of results. Nurses and physician extenders can see more stable patients, freeing up time for the cardio-oncologist to incorporate more complex patients into their clinic schedule [33]. All team members assume responsibility to keep abreast of changes in cancer treatment plans (e.g., curative vs. palliative treatment) and/ or changes in a patient's CV status.

Establishing a Cardio-Oncology Clinic

The organization of a specialist cardio-oncology clinic is a complex process involving multidisciplinary collaboration, administrative support and institutional resources [34] (Fig. 15.3). In many centers, new programs must compete for clinic space, such that a new clinic location is often determined by where space is available. In a

---

Establishing a cardiac oncology clinic tips for achieving success

The organization of a specialized cardiac oncology clinic is a complex process involving multidisciplinary collaboration, administrative support, and institutional resources. Here are tips on forming your own successful COC clinic.

1. **Logistics**—COC clinics require close inter-action between oncologists and cardiologists. Choose a clinic location in close proximity to a cancer center, preferably with an electronic health record and point-of-care access to cardiac imaging.

2. **Expertise**—Cardiologists with imaging experience are well suited to this area of clinical care. Focus on recruitment of specialists who are interested in learning more about cancer therapy and prognosis.

3. **Allied Health Support**—Clinics require significant support from allied health professionals. Consider recruitment of clinic nurses with experience in both cancer treatment and cardiac disease, and who have an interest in clinical research.

4. **Resources**—Cardiac oncology is a rapidly growing field. Access to the latest medical literature and research tools is crucial for clinic success.

5. **Collaboration**—Multidisciplinary clinics work best with consistent communication between health care providers. We recommend regular case review rounds and educational sessions (with participation of clinical fellows and residents) to keep members of the clinic informed and up to date.

FIGURE 15.3 **Establishing a cardio-oncology clinic—tips for achieving success.** *COC, Cardio-Oncology Clinic. From Sulpher et al. Cardiac Oncology: Improving Cardiac Safety, Advancing Cancer Care. 2014–15 Report Card on Cancer in Canada.*

---

patient-centered healthcare system, the clinic would ideally be located in close proximity to the cancer center, in order to facilitate close interaction between oncologists and cardiologists. An electronic communication tool that is accessible and available to multiple providers involved in the patient's care is essential. All providers need access to CV test results, which may be performed at centers remote from where the cardio-oncology clinic is located. It is important that electronic health records systems integrate patient data across multiple centers and providers. Direct review of cardiac imaging, whether it is an echo-cardiogram, a nuclear study, or an angiogram, is an essential component of a clinic. This is helpful in determining the quality of imaging, which has important implications when results are suspected to be spurious, and subsequently can help determine the most suitable imaging modality for a given patient. Access to advanced cardiac imaging with newer techniques to facilitate the early detection of cardiotoxicity, and a collaborative research environment (basic and translational research) will permit the development of "best" management strategies.

Recruitment of healthcare providers with an interest and expertise in cardio-oncology is essential in establishing a successful cardio-oncology program. A cardiologist with expertise in cardiac imaging, especially advanced techniques, such as echocardiographic strain imaging, will assist the team in choosing the best imaging modality, interpretation of the results, and potential limitations of the imaging modality, as well as provide recommendations on cardiac care. An oncologist with expertise in understanding the potential cardiotoxicity associated with systemic therapies and the importance of assessing baseline cardiac risk factors and potential preventative strategies to avoid cardiotoxicity is essential. In addition, oncologists should facilitate appropriate referrals to the cardio-oncology clinic and foster discussion between members of the cardio-oncology team. Cardio-oncology clinics require significant support from allied healthcare professionals. Recruitment of clinic nurses with experience in both cancer treatment and heart disease is desirable. Pharmacists can provide important information on the potential CV complications of novel cancer therapies, particularly when these treatments are administered concurrently or with other therapeutic modalities, such as radiation (e.g., left-sided breast radiation), as well as the role of patient risk factors: diabetes, hypertension, hypercholesterolemia; smoking; and preexisting CVD, predisposing to the development of cardiotoxicity [37].

It is important that all members of the multidisciplinary cardio-oncology team be aware of the toxicity of chemotherapeutic agents and newer targeted agents to plan the optimal treatment regimens that minimize cardiotoxicity without compromising anticancer efficacy including radiotherapy.

Multidisciplinary clinics require consistent communication between healthcare providers. An efficient mechanism for such collaborative care can take the form of cardio-oncology case rounds, where cases can be discussed between oncologists, cardiologists, and allied healthcare providers, who are involved in the management of these patients. Such patient-based rounds, analogous to tumor boards, permit efficient exchange of a center's best cardiology and oncology advice for patients who may need cancer therapy that is potentially cardiotoxic, but for whom there are underlying cardiac risk factors or diseases that must be addressed. Attendees gain important insight in management strategies that may be helpful when approaching subsequent cancer patients with similar CV health issues. The discussions that surround these case conferences facilitate learning experiences for the cardio-oncology team as well as educating internal medicine, oncology, and cardiology trainees. Cardio-oncology is a rapidly developing subspecialty of medicine; access to the latest medical literature and research tools is crucial for optimization of patient care.

The majority of cardio-oncology clinics are established in large teaching hospitals, yet many cancer patients receive care in larger geographic areas including rural areas. While patients with clinical manifestations of cardiotoxicity likely need to be seen for an "in person" consultation, less significant cardiotoxicity issues, such as asymptomatic drops in LV ejection fraction, are well suited to electronic consultation. E-consults represent a promising solution to the challenge of expanding access of cardio-oncology expertise to cancer patients in rural areas [35].

While on active chemotherapy or targeted therapy, a cancer patient who needs cardio-oncology assessment and follow-up should be seen in the cardio-oncology clinic. Once cancer patients have completed their cancer therapy, however, they may transition to a survivorship clinic. Survivorship clinics, coordinated by multidisciplinary teams with expertise in the long-term management of cancer patients who have experienced cardiotoxicity, may reside in the hospital or ideally be located in the patient's community.

Who Should be Referred to a Cardio-Oncology Clinic?

Cardio-oncology clinics should develop standardized referral forms to facilitate the delivery of care for cancer patients at risk of, or who developed, cardiotoxicity from cancer therapy (Fig. 15.4). Cancer patients appropriate for referral include (1) pretreatment assessment—to assess risk of cardiotoxicity in cancer patients especially in presence of preexisting CV risk factors (e.g., CAD, stroke, peripheral vascular disease, atrial fibrillation, hypertension, diabetes, etc.), (2) patients with multiple CV risk factors which are not well controlled, (3) to prevent possible cardiotoxic effects of cancer therapy (primary or secondary prevention); or (4) for treatment of cardiotoxicity due to cancer therapy. There are currently no established benchmarks to guide

clinicians with regard to timely access and assessment of patients who experience cancer-related cardiotoxicity. Wait times to be assessed in a cardio-oncology clinic need to be balanced with the urgency of impending cancer treatments. The patient receiving active cancer treatment will generally require more urgent access (1–2 weeks), while it might be appropriate for patients not receiving active therapy (e.g., surveillance) to be seen in a less timely fashion (weeks to months) [36]. Cancer patients should be referred for an urgent consult (within 7 days) if they have symptoms of HF or their cancer treatment has been placed on hold due to cardiotoxicity (e.g., LVEF < 50%) (Fig. 15.5). All patients referred to a cardio-oncology clinic should have a clinical assessment (history and physical examination) performed with particular attention to patient's comorbidities, such as CAD and hypertension that should be aggressively managed before and during cancer treatment. CV investigations prior to and during the administration of chemotherapy known to be associated with significant cardiotoxicity will be driven by the specific cancer therapy prescribed (e.g., sunitinib and risk of hypertension) and the patient's underlying CV risk factors.

Patients receiving cancer therapy who are at high risk, or who have experienced cancer therapy related cardiac dysfunction should be discussed by the cardio-oncology team at multidisciplinary cardio-oncology rounds. The discussion should focus on the balance between the individual's potential benefits of cancer treatment versus the CV risk (Fig. 15.5). In the patients with metastatic disease receiving cancer treatment with palliative intent, the occurrence of cardiac complications and related symptoms which compromise their quality of life may not be acceptable. On the other hand, for a patient with a high probability of being cured by cancer therapy, the occurrence of symptoms due to temporary cardiotoxicity may be acceptable, if this toxicity is fully reversible.

Do Cardio-Oncology Clinics Improve Patient Care?

Evidence is accumulating to support a protocolized approach for detecting patients at high risk of cardiotoxicity from cancer therapies. Risk stratification for development of cardiotoxicity has been most extensively studied in breast cancer patients treated with anthracycline-based chemotherapy with or without trastuzumab. Clinical risk factors, cardiac biomarkers, such as troponin, and cardiac imaging either alone or in combination, can determine which patients are at highest risk for cardiotoxicity [37–40]. As we learn more about cardiotoxicity from other cancer therapies, cancer-therapy specific protocols can be implemented to risk stratify patients for cardiotoxicity from these treatments. The goal of such an approach is to identify patients at high risk for cardiotoxicity, triage them to prompt referral to a cardio-oncology clinic or a healthcare provider

Patient's name	_____
DOB	_____
MRN	_____

CARDIO-ONCOLOGY CLINIC REFERRAL FORM

Administrative assistant:

Fax to: Attn: _____
For inquiries, call

Reason for referal:	□ Urgent	□ Elective	Concerns regarding cardiotoxicity
□ New referral	□ EF < 45% during treatment	□ Baseline EF < 50%	_____
□ Re-assessment	□ Symptoms of HF	□ EF drops to < 50% or	_____
□ Follow-up	□ Cancer therapy on hold	by 10% during treatment	_____
	□ Other	□ Other	

DIAGNOSIS   _____
_____

PREVIOUS CANCER TREATMENT   □ Neoadjuvant   □ Adjuvant □ Palliative

Type of treatment	No of Cycles	Start	Stop	Known cardiotoxicity
				□
				□
				□

CANCER TREATMENT   □ Neoadjuvant   □ Adjuvant □ Palliative

Type of treatment/Planned No of Cycles		Start	Stop	Potential cardiotoxicity
	□ Current□ Planned			
	□ Current□ Planned			
	□ Current□ Planned			

KNOWN CARDIOVASCULAR RISK FACTORS:

□ CAD/Stroke/Peripheral vascular disease   □ Smoking

□ Atrial Fibrillation   □ Obesity

□ Hypertension   □ Dyslipidemia

□ Diabetes   □ Other

PREVIOUS CARDIAC INVESTIGATIONS:

Date	□ MUGA □ ECHO	LVEF ____ %
Date	□ MUGA □ ECHO	LVEF ____ %
Date	□ MUGA □ ECHO	LVEF ____ %
Date	□ MUGA □ ECHO	LVEF ____ %

COMMENTS:

REFERRING PHYSITIAN_____ Date _____

FIGURE 15.4 **Standardized referral for cardio-oncology clinic.**

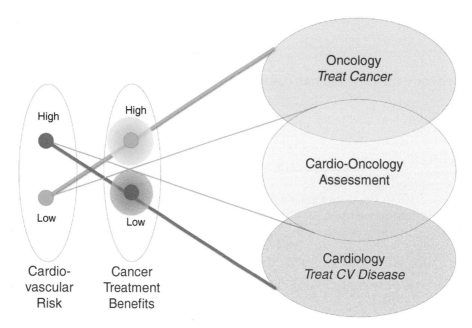

FIGURE 15.5 **Assessment of benefits of cancer treatment versus cardiovascular risk.** *CV disease, Cardiovascular disease.*

with experience in cardio-oncology, and optimize their risk factors and cardiac health. The concept is to proactively try to prevent cardiotoxicity, rather than treating it after it develops. The treatment of cardiotoxicity, including potential prevention of cardiotoxicity, is covered in other chapters.

Cardio-oncology programs need to champion patient safety in order to get institutional support for cardio-oncology protocols. Existing programs managing complications of cancer therapy may be modified to include cardiac risk monitoring, including referral of high-risk patients to a cardio-oncology clinic. Conversely, risk stratification protocols may identify patients at low risk for cardiotoxicity. If we can reliably identify patients at low risk of cardiotoxicity, we can avoid unnecessary cardiac imaging, which spares the patients from hospital visits, and reduces the costs associated with imaging. Further research is needed to confirm the safety of such an approach, and measure the economic impact of reduced CV testing in low risk cancer patients.

How Can We Measure Success of a Cardio-Oncology Program?

The importance of cardiotoxicity combined with the relative novelty of cardio-oncology as a subspecialty has led to tremendous growth in cardio-oncology research. Successful protocols that improve cardiac safety can be evaluated in a research context, and disseminated for wider adoption. Success can also be measured outside of a research setting, and is important at the local level to secure initial and ongoing support from healthcare managers. Patient testimonials indicating how cardio-oncology helped them get through cancer treatment in spite of a cardiac issue are powerful, tangible metrics that should be shared with hospital administrators.

Cancer therapy completion rates and cardiac safety, especially compared to historical controls, can indicate that a cardio-oncology program is helping deliver care that is effectively treating cancer without harming the heart. In the future, protocols that permit less testing for low risk patients with high levels of cardiac safety can reduce the high cost of cardiac imaging. Cardio-oncology programs that implement protocols that improve cancer therapy effectiveness, enhance cardiac safety, and save money will be welcomed in any healthcare system.

Community-Based Approaches for Cardiovascular Optimization in Cancer Survivors

Heart disease in cancer survivors is common, can impact quality of life, and the ability to tolerate cancer treatments. With the advent of new and refined cancer treatments, the outlook related to many cancers has improved. Improved life expectancy has resulted in the higher prevalence of unintended cardiac side effects of certain cancer treatments including some chemotherapy drugs, radiation to the chest, and other agents. Also, because many cancer patients already have risk factors for CVD when starting cancer treatments, some individuals may have a predisposition to experiencing the CV toxicities of cancer therapy [41].

CVD is the leading cause of death in cancers associated with high survival rates [42]. With the increasing number of older cancer survivors and increased rates of long-term survival, the prevalence of CVD among cancer survivors is likely to rise. For example, in 2013 *alone*, an estimated 23,800 Canadian women were diagnosed with breast cancer

[43]. These patients have an estimated 88% 5-year survival rate while breast cancer patients 50 years or older have survival rates between 80% and 90%.

Due to cardiac reserve and the activation of compensatory mechanisms, clinical manifestations may not become apparent until months to years after the initial cancer therapy exposure, well after the patient has been discharged from oncology care [15]; without adequate follow-up, the opportunity for prevention or limiting progression to significant CVD may be missed. There is evidence that the earlier cardiotoxicity is detected after completion of anthracycline-containing chemotherapy, for instance, the greater the likelihood of recovery of LV function after institution of HF therapy [44].

The long-term goal is to attenuate the long-term risks of cardiotoxic cancer therapies to ensure the best cancer and cardiac outcomes and transition from cancer patient to cancer survivor. The need for cardiac evaluation of patients once cancer treatment is completed is based on whether the treatment received poses risk of late cardiotoxicity, such as anthracyclines or mediastinal radiation, and/or the patient's estimated CV risk. Patients who are at risk for late cardiotoxicity should undergo long-term cardiac surveillance as part of the routine protocol in survivorship clinics with echocardiographic follow-up and more individualized cardiac testing based on symptoms and signs of disease.

Recent data suggest that CV risk factors are not being adequately addressed in this patient population [45]. Several factors may contribute to inadequate CVD preventative interventions [45]. Providers caring for cancer survivors may need additional education regarding how to screen and provide referrals or interventions for this patient population. Risk factor counseling may be challenging in the context of brief oncology visits after cancer treatment, especially with busy primary care encounters [45]. Finally, adequate data regarding the optimal follow-up strategy, including frequency of echocardiographic/CV screening to prevent and diagnose CV complications of cancer treatment are lacking [45]. A Clinical Practice Guideline on the prevention and monitoring of cardiac dysfunction in survivors of adult cancers will be published by the American Society of Clinical Oncology in 2016.

A New Paradigm: Community-Based Cardio-Oncology Survivorship Programs

The growing number of cancer survivors who may experience long-term cardiotoxicities as a result of cancer treatments outweighs the capacity of tertiary cancer centers and cardio-oncology programs to follow them indefinitely; therefore, there is a need to develop rational approaches for optimization of longitudinal CV care of these patients.

For all cancer survivors discharged to their community providers, cancer survivorship care plans should include the potential long-term late CV effects of cancer treatments with strategies for improving long-term CV health. However, specific subgroups of cancer survivors discharged from tertiary oncology and cardio-oncology care may benefit from long-term follow-up within specialized community-based survivorship programs dedicated to the care of these patients.

In one such model, being championed as a pilot strategy in breast cancer survivors, patients at high risk of CV complications after cancer therapy or those with CV diagnoses identified during cancer treatment are referred for long-term follow-up to a community-based program dedicated to the care of these patients [46]. The goal of such dedicated community-based programs would be twofold: to provide optimal care and surveillance of cancer survivors at risk of CV complications or who have established CVD; and to track the characteristics and outcomes of this population. Importantly, information acquired by tracking these patients over the long term could facilitate the development of more evidence-based surveillance strategies.

Objectives of a community-based cancer survivorship and CV care program:

1. To provide a common portal for longitudinal follow-up of cancer survivors at increased risk of developing long-term CV complications of cancer and cancer therapy.
   a. *Rationale:*
      i. Referral to clinicians with expertise and a vested interest in this field would facilitate evidence-based and timely institution of primary preventative measures, identification, and treatment of cancer treatment-related CV complications.
      ii. Clinicians would seek to remain current with emerging evidence in the field and in turn to implement evidence-based interventions as the field evolves.
2. To develop a registry to track interventions and outcomes in this patient population.
   a. Data collected would be analyzed to better understand the natural history of this patient population. A registry would facilitate scholarly activity to contribute to the broader field of cardio-oncology at the national and international level.
   b. Data from such a registry would serve as a vehicle to continually evaluate and improve quality of care to this patient population.
3. To provide educational resources to clinicians and the public about cancer- and cancer treatment-related CV effects.

Proposed Referral Pathway for Cancer Survivors

We envision two main categories of patients who would derive benefit from longitudinal follow-up in a community-based CV survivorship center. The first group would include patients without CV problems identified prior to or during cancer treatment, but who are, based on various factors, thought to be at increased risk of developing long-term CV complications of cancer treatment: this group will

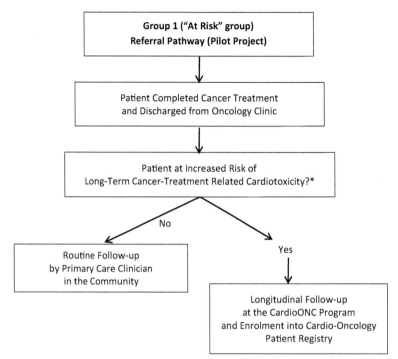

FIGURE 15.6 **Group 1 (At Risk group) referral pathway (pilot project).** *Risk assessment would be based on established treatment- and patient-related risk factors for cardiotoxicity based on cancer site.

be referred to as the "At-Risk" group. The second group would include patients with CVD diagnosed prior to or during cancer treatment: this group will be referred to as the "Established CV disease" group.

- Group 1 (At-Risk group): Patients at increased risk of long-term cancer treatment-related cardiotoxicity (Fig. 15.6).
- Group 2 (Established CV disease group): Patients who developed on-treatment cardiotoxicity (Fig. 15.7).

In summary, given that the anticipated number of cancer survivors at risk of long-term CVD related to cancer treatments outweighs the capacity of most Cancer Centres and tertiary Cardio-Oncology programs to follow them in the long-term, rational strategies to optimize the longitudinal CV care of these patients are needed. At minimum, survivorship care plans to primary care providers should include information regarding potential long-term cardiotoxicities of cancer treatment and strategies for risk factor modification. However, a more targeted strategy of surveillance of high-risk patients or those who developed CV complications during cancer treatments may allow for more timely intervention and mitigation of CV morbidity and mortality. One such approach, involving dedicated community-based cancer survivorship and CV centers would be aimed not only at optimizing care, but also at tracking patient outcomes in order to facilitate the development of more evidence-based guidelines for patient surveillance.

EDUCATION OF HEALTHCARE PROVIDERS: TRAINING AND FELLOWSHIP PROGRAMS

For the large number of patients who experience cardiac complications during their cancer treatment, or who face both cancer and heart disease, finding a trained specialist in cardio-oncology can prove to be challenging. This relatively new field is increasingly attracting early-career physicians; however, few formal training programs in cardio-oncology have been established. In addition, there is a lack of organization in the essential components of contemporary training, and expectations of trainees in cardio-oncology programs have not been well defined. Cardio-oncology training programs need to be flexible in order to accommodate the educational background of the trainee-individuals with training in oncology will have different educational goals and objectives compared to individuals with training in cardiology. In addition, it is important to offer educational opportunities to those individuals who simply wish to gain more experience in this new field—for example, medical students, internal medicine residents, and other healthcare providers.

Cardio-Oncology Training Program

The complexity of medical care of cancer patients with CVD has mandated the existence of a trained multidisciplinary team as an integral component of cancer care

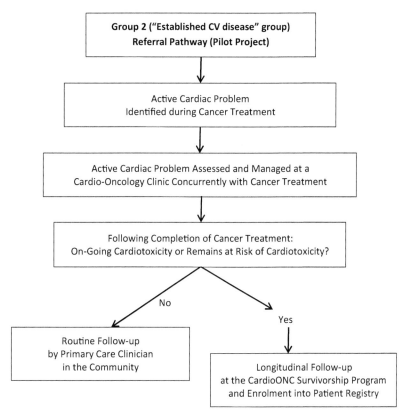

FIGURE 15.7   **Group 2 (Established CV disease group) referral pathway (pilot project).**

from diagnosis to survivorship [47]. In spite of the known complex interaction between cancer and its treatment, underlying CVD, and the CV effects of the cancer and its treatment, most cardiologists and oncologists are not trained in, or are unaware of, the multifaceted relationship between these parameters, and how to navigate them to ensure that patient management is optimized. The quality of patient care is improved when members of the healthcare team work in collaboration to share their unique patient care perspectives [48,49]. Each profession enters into practice with different skill sets, knowledge, and professional identities to enhance the care of the patient, yet many barriers exist between disciplines that can obstruct a team-based system. These barriers include a lack of interprofessional cultural competence, perceived power differentials, and profession-centric role models [50].

There is a growing need to add formal cardio-oncology modules to the basic/traditional training curriculum as well as postfellowship advanced training for those individuals who have already received formal instruction in the fields of CVD or hematology/oncology (Fig. 15.8 and Table 15.1).

Even though there are a growing number of cardio-oncology fellowship programs in North America, the content and quality vary among programs. There needs to be coherency in the provision of cardio-oncology fellowship programs so that fellows acquire competency in the subspecialty with sufficient expertise to act as independent cardio-oncology specialists. Further progress is necessary for the improvement of cardio-oncology subspecialty training.

Level 1 Training

Level 1 training in cardio-oncology should be structured as an elective rotation (2–4 weeks) with the goal of the trainee gaining a basic knowledge of cancer agents and their potential cardiotoxicity, as well as an understanding of cardiac imaging and treatment strategies for cancer patients experiencing cardiotoxicity. This level of exposure would also be suitable for allied healthcare professionals (e.g., pharmacy residents) interested in acquiring basic knowledge in cardio-oncology.

Level 2 Training
Cardiology Fellow

Those with a background in CVD should have a basic understanding of cancer pathophysiology, staging in the different malignancies, tumor growth and disease progression, prognosis of common malignancies, and common oncologic therapies, especially those that impact the CV system. These trainees should have an understanding of common cellular pathways shared by the CV system and cancer's effect on

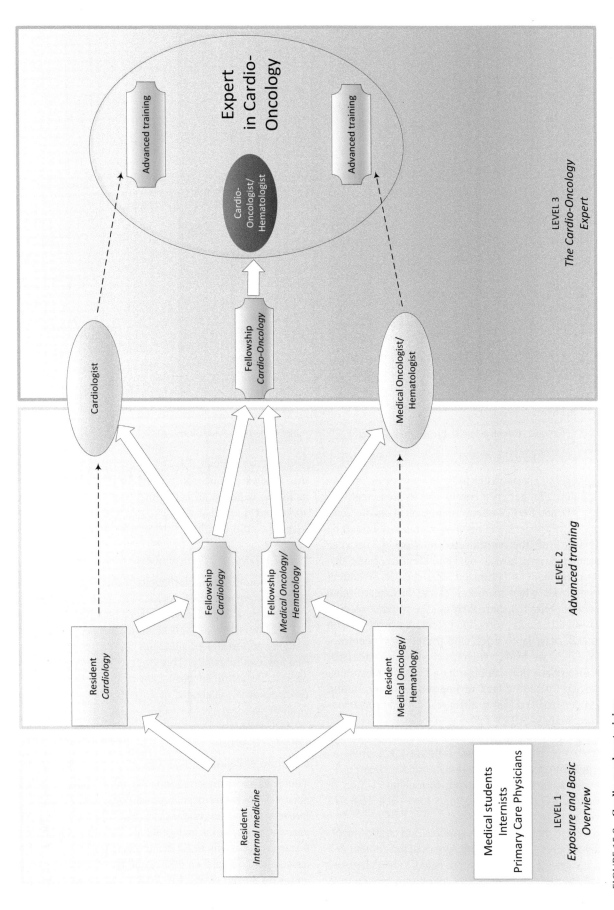

FIGURE 15.8 **Cardio-oncology training.**

TABLE 15.1 Levels of Training for Cardio-Oncology

Level of Training	Acceptable Candidate	Main Goals of Training
Level 1	Internal medicine residents	• Basic knowledge of cancer agents and their potential to cause cardiac damage • Imaging strategies—basic knowledge on cardiac imaging in oncology patients • Basic understanding of treatment strategies for cancer patients experiencing cardiac toxicities
Level 2	Medical oncology/hematology fellow or cardiology fellow	• For fellow who wish to broaden their exposure to cardiac oncology patients • More detailed assessment of patients • Intermediate knowledge base • More exposure to advanced cardiac imaging, for example, advanced echocardiography (strain/3D) • Understanding of the role of biomarkers in early detection of cardiotoxicity
Level 3	Cardio-Oncology fellow	• 12–24 months of dedicated fellowship training • Advanced knowledge of cancer agents and potential toxicities • Broad exposure to in- and outpatients • Training in biomarkers, advanced imaging • Actively involved in research and education

involved organs. They should also have an advanced understanding of systemic effects of cancer and potential oncologic emergencies affecting the CV system (e.g., tumor lysis syndrome, disseminated intravascular coagulation), as well as their management, and oncologic pharmacology that specifically affects the CV system. In addition, trainees should have an understanding of how to use and interpret cardiac imaging modalities (ECG, echocardiography, stress testing, etc.), and biomarkers to diagnose as well as monitor the cardiac effects of cancer therapy.

Medical Oncology/Hematology Fellow

Training for oncologists in cardio-oncology takes on a slightly different focus. Those with a background in hematology/oncology should have a general familiarity with the principles of CVD, especially those that are prevalent in the cardio-oncology population, such as hypertension, HF and cardiomyopathy, arrhythmias, myocardial ischemia, pericardial disease, and vascular complications, as well as their basic management and/or treatment. They should understand CV risk factors and have advanced knowledge of oncologic pharmacology, and the impact that many of the therapies used for malignancies have on the CV system. Along with a basic understanding of when and how to use pertinent CV diagnostic tools, such as ECG, echocardiograms, stress testing, and biomarkers, the trainee has to understand the benefits, indications, and limitations of these studies. Also, the fellow must have the basic ability to interpret common images and recognize the presence of more complicated disease that requires interaction with imaging experts. Exposure to cardio-oncology at this level of training might encourage residents to explore further fellowship training in cardio-oncology [50].

Level 3 Training
Cardio-Oncology Fellowships

Cardio-oncology fellowships (minimum 1 year) should provide the trainee with significant exposure to clinical cardio-oncology based patient evaluations [30,48], contributions to cardio-oncology based clinical research and education, and advanced knowledge of relevant cardio-oncology clinical trials. An expert in cardio-oncology may have different medical backgrounds (e.g., oncologist/hematologist vs. cardiologist) necessitating the need for specific goals and principles of training tailored to an individual's area of expertise (Table 15.2). A hematologist/oncologist undertaking a cardio-oncology fellowship should have a basic understanding of CV risk factors and pathophysiology of common conditions resulting from cancer therapies (e.g., hypertension) as well as be comfortable with CV diagnostic testing (e.g., ECG, echocardiograms, stress testing, biomarkers) and pharmacologic management of common CV conditions (e.g., cancer therapy-induced hypertension) [51]. The hematologist/oncologist should have an advanced knowledge of the impact of cancer treatments on CV health (e.g., tyrosine kinase inhibitors and hypertension). In contrast, the cardiologist undertaking a cardio-oncology fellowship should have an advanced understanding of CV physiology focusing on common cellular pathways shared by cancer and cardiac cells. Such individuals should have a basic understanding of cancer biology as well as common cancer therapies and molecular targets. A cardiologist training in cardio-oncology should be expected to have an advanced knowledge of cardiac imaging tools and biomarkers used to detect and monitor the cardiac effects of cancer therapy, and understand evidence-based treatment with cardio-protective drugs.

TABLE 15.2 Expert Training in Cardio-Oncology According to Primary Specialization

Cardiologist Stream	Oncologist/Hematologist Stream
• Principles of oncology care • Advanced knowledge of cancer agents and potential toxicities • Training in biomarkers, advanced cardiac imaging • Appropriate cardiac imaging techniques • Cardiotoxicity surveillance • Knowledge of cardiovascular risk assessment in cancer patients • Evidence-based treatment with cardioprotective drugs • Actively involved in research	• Understanding cardiac imaging: limitations and common techniques • Familiarity with principles of heart failure, arrhythmias, and hypertension • Familiarity with principles of echocardiography, advanced cardiac imaging, and biomarkers • Techniques of cardiac surveillance • Evidence-based treatment with cardioprotective drugs • Actively involved in research

CONCLUSIONS

Modern treatment strategies have led to an improvement in the chances of surviving a diagnosis of cancer; however, improvements in survivorship can come at a cost [4]. Current anticancer therapies, including chemotherapy, targeted agents (e.g., tyrosine kinase inhibitors) and radiation, may have short- and long-term detrimental effects on CV health. The need to optimize cardiac health in patients undergoing cancer therapy, the treatment of cardiotoxicity resulting from cancer therapy, and the follow-up of cancer survivors at long-term risk for cardiac disease are clinical needs that have driven the development of the new subspecialty of cardio-oncology [4]. The last several years has seen the establishment of an increasing number of dedicated cardio-oncology clinics across North America, and world-wide; however, there is a paucity of literature on the essential components and infrastructure needed to support such a program. The organization of cardio-oncology clinics is a complex process involving multidisciplinary collaboration, administrative support, and institutional resources [34]. Recruitment of healthcare providers with an interest and expertise in cardio-oncology is essential as are open lines of communication between healthcare providers. While there are currently no universally accepted criteria for referral to a cardio-oncology clinic it would seem reasonable to consider referrals for: pretreatment assessment (especially in presence of preexisting CV risk factors); patients at high risk for consideration of primary prevention strategies; patients with multiple CV risk factors which are not well controlled; and patients requiring treatment of cardiotoxicity due to cancer therapy. There is very limited literature on the "added value" of cardio-oncology programs. Cancer therapy completion rates and cardiac safety, especially compared to historical controls, can indicate that a cardio-oncology program is helping deliver care that is effectively treating cancer without harming the heart. The establishment of quality indicators in delivery of cardio-oncology care will facilitate support for such programs from hospital administrators and health organizations. As the number of cancer survivors at risk of long-term CVD related to cancer treatments continues to grow so will the capacity of most cancer centers and tertiary cardio-oncology programs to follow them; long-term, rational strategies to optimize the longitudinal CV care of these patients are needed. At a minimum, survivorship care plans to primary care providers should include information regarding potential long-term cardiotoxicities of cancer treatment and strategies for risk factor modification. The future of clinical care delivery in cardio-oncology is predicated on access of cancer patients to trained healthcare providers. Development of levels of training with established expectations in cardio-oncology will facilitate early exposure of trainees to this field and lead to the next generation of cardio-oncologists.

REFERENCES

[1] Howlader N, Ries LAG, Mariotto AB, Reichman ME, Ruhl J, Cronin KA. Improved estimates of cancer-specific survival rates from population-based data. J Natl Cancer Inst 2010;102(20):1584–1598. Available from: http://www.pubmedcentral.nih.gov/articlerender.fcgi?artid=2957430&tool=pmcentrez&rendertype=abstract

[2] Jemal A, Ward E, Hao Y, Thun M. Trends in the leading causes of death in the United States, 1970-2002. JAMA 2005;294(10):1255–1259. Available from: http://www.ncbi.nlm.nih.gov/pubmed/16160134

[3] Jemal A, Ward E, Thun M. Declining death rates reflect progress against cancer. PLoS One 2010;5(3):e9584. Available from: http://journals.plos.org/plosone/article?id=10.1371/journal.pone.0009584

[4] Dent S, Liu P, Brezden-masley C, Lenihan D, Dent S, Brezden-masley C. Cancer and Cardiovascular Disease: The Complex Labyrinth. J Oncol 2015;2015:516450.

[5] Bodai BI, Tuso P. Breast cancer survivorship: a comprehensive review of long-term medical issues and lifestyle recommendations. Perm J 2015;19(2):48–79. Available from: http://www.pubmedcentral.nih.gov/articlerender.fcgi?artid=4403581&tool=pmcentrez&rendertype=abstract

[6] Siegel R, DeSantis C, Virgo K, Stein K, Mariotto A, Smith T, et al. Cancer treatment and survivorship statistics, 2012. CA Cancer J Clin 2012;62(4):220–241. Available from: http://www.ncbi.nlm.nih.gov/pubmed/22700443

[7] Chen J, Long JB, Hurria A, Owusu C, Steingart RM, Gross CP. Incidence of heart failure or cardiomyopathy after adjuvant trastuzumab therapy for breast cancer. J Am Coll Cardiol 2012;60(24):2504–2512. Available from: http://www.ncbi.nlm.nih.gov/pubmed/23158536

[8] Bowles EJA, Wellman R, Feigelson HS, Onitilo AA, Freedman AN, Delate T, et al. Risk of heart failure in breast cancer patients after anthracycline and trastuzumab treatment: a retrospective cohort study. J Natl Cancer Inst 2012;104(17):1293–1305. Available from: http://www.pubmedcentral.nih.gov/articlerender.fcgi?artid=3433392&tool=pmcentrez&rendertype=abstract

[9] Aleman BMP, Moser EC, Nuver J, Suter TM, Maraldo M V., Specht L, et al. Cardiovascular disease after cancer therapy. Eur J Cancer Suppl 2014;12(1):18–28. Available from: http://linkinghub.elsevier.com/retrieve/pii/S1359634914000044

[10] Taunk NK, Haffty BG, Kostis JB, Goyal S. Radiation-induced heart disease: pathologic abnormalities and putative mechanisms. Front Oncol 2015;5:39. Available from: http://www.pubmedcentral.nih.gov/articlerender.fcgi?artid=4332338&tool=pmcentrez&rendertype=abstract

[11] Siegel RL, Miller KD, Jemal A. Cancer Statistics, 2015. CA Cancer J Clin 2015;65(1):5–29.

[12] Ewer MS, Ewer SM. Cardiotoxicity of anticancer treatments. Nat Rev Cardiol 2015;12(9):547–558. Available from: http://www.nature.com/doifinder/10.1038/nrcardio.2015.65

[13] Ali MK, Ewer MS, Gibbs HR, Swafford J, Graff KL. Late doxorubicin-associated cardiotoxicity in children. The possible role of intercurrent viral infection. Cancer 1994;74(1):182–188. Available from: http://www.ncbi.nlm.nih.gov/pubmed/8004574

[14] Hahn VS, Lenihan DJ, Ky B. Cancer therapy-induced cardiotoxicity: basic mechanisms and potential cardioprotective therapies. J Am Heart Assoc 2014;3(2):e000665. Available from: http://www.pubmedcentral.nih.gov/articlerender.fcgi?artid=4187516&tool=pmcentrez&rendertype=abstract

[15] Suter TM, Ewer MS. Cancer drugs and the heart: importance and management. Eur Heart J 2013;34(15):1102–1111. Available from: http://www.ncbi.nlm.nih.gov/pubmed/22789916

[16] Procter M, Suter TM, de Azambuja E, Dafni U, van Dooren V, Muehlbauer S, et al. Longer-term assessment of trastuzumab-related cardiac adverse events in the Herceptin Adjuvant (HERA) trial. J Clin Oncol 2010;28(21):3422–3428. Available from: http://www.ncbi.nlm.nih.gov/pubmed/20530280

[17] Henderson IC. Comparisons between different polychemotherapy regimens for early breast cancer: Meta-analyses of long-term outcome among 100 000 women in 123 randomised trials. Breast Dis 2013;24(1):76–78. Available from: http://dx.doi.org/10.1016/S0140-6736(11)61625-5

[18] Curigliano G, Cardinale D, Dent S, Criscitiello C, Aseyev O, Lenihan D, et al. Cardiotoxicity of anticancer treatments: Epidemiology, detection, and management. CA Cancer J Clin 2016;66(4):309–325. Available from: http://www.ncbi.nlm.nih.gov/pubmed/26919165

[19] Pinder MC, Duan Z, Goodwin JS, Hortobagyi GN, Giordano SH. Congestive heart failure in older women treated with adjuvant anthracycline chemotherapy for breast cancer. J Clin Oncol 2007;25(25):3808–3815. Available from: http://www.ncbi.nlm.nih.gov/pubmed/17664460

[20] Yeh ETH, Tong AT, Lenihan DJ, Yusuf SW, Swafford J, Champion C, et al. Cardiovascular complications of cancer therapy: diagnosis, pathogenesis, and management. Circulation 2004;109(25):3122–31.

[21] Xu J, Murphy SL, Kochanek KD, Bastian BA, Statistics V. National Vital Statistics Reports Deaths: Final Data for 2013. 2016;64(2);1–119.

[22] Albini A, Pennesi G, Donatelli F, Cammarota R, De Flora S, Noonan DM. Cardiotoxicity of anticancer drugs: the need for cardiooncology and cardio-oncological prevention. J Natl Cancer Inst. 2010;102(1):14–25.

[23] Dillman RO, Chico SD. Cancer patient survival improvement is correlated with the opening of a community cancer center: comparisons with intramural and extramural benchmarks. J Oncol Pract 2005;1(3):84–92. Available from: http://www.ncbi.nlm.nih.gov/pubmed/20871689

[24] Suter TM, Procter M, Van Veldhuisen DJ, Muscholl M, Bergh J, Carlomagno C, et al. Trastuzumab-associated cardiac adverse effects in the herceptin adjuvant trial. J Clin Oncol 2007;25(25):3859–65.

[25] Darby SC, Ewertz M, McGale P, Bennet AM, Blom-Goldman U, Brønnum D, et al. Risk of ischemic heart disease in women after radiotherapy for breast cancer. N Engl J Med 2013;368(11):987–998. Available from: http://www.ncbi.nlm.nih.gov/pubmed/23484825

[26] Chai-Adisaksopha C, Lam W, Hillis C. Major arterial events in patients with chronic myeloid leukemia treated with tyrosine kinase inhibitors: a meta-analysis. Leuk Lymphoma 2016;57(6):1300–1310. Available from: http://www.ncbi.nlm.nih.gov/pubmed/26373533

[27] Polk A, Vaage-Nilsen M, Vistisen K, Nielsen DL. Cardiotoxicity in cancer patients treated with 5-fluorouracil or capecitabine: a systematic review of incidence, manifestations and predisposing factors. Cancer Treat Rev 2013;39(8):974–984. Available from: http://www.ncbi.nlm.nih.gov/pubmed/23582737

[28] Maitland ML, Kasza KE, Karrison T, Moshier K, Sit L, Black HR, et al. Ambulatory monitoring detects sorafenib-induced blood pressure elevations on the first day of treatment. Clin Cancer Res 2009;15(19):6250–6257. Available from: http://www.pubmedcentral.nih.gov/articlerender.fcgi?artid=2756980&tool=pmcentrez&rendertype=abstract

[29] Sulpher J, Mathur S, Lenihan D, Johnson C, Turek M, Law A, et al. An international survey of health care providers involved in the management of cancer patients exposed to cardiotoxic therapy. J Oncol 2015;2015:391848. Available from: http://www.pubmedcentral.nih.gov/articlerender.fcgi?artid=4537762&tool=pmcentrez&rendertype=abstract

[30] Lenihan DJ, Westcott G. Cardio-oncology: a tremendous opportunity to improve patient care. Future Oncol 2015;11(14):2007–2010. Available from: http://www.ncbi.nlm.nih.gov/pubmed/26198827

[31] Go AS, Hylek EM, Phillips KA, Chang Y, Henault LE, Selby J.V., et al. Prevalence of diagnosed atrial fibrillation in adults. JAMA 2001;285(18):2370. Available from: http://jama.jamanetwork.com/article.aspx?articleid=193807

[32] Eschenhagen T, Force T, Ewer MS, de Keulenaer GW, Suter TM, Anker SD, et al. Cardiovascular side effects of cancer therapies: a position statement from the Heart Failure Association of the European Society of Cardiology. Eur J Heart Fail 2011;13(1):1–10. Available from: http://www.ncbi.nlm.nih.gov/pubmed/21169385

[33] Okwuosa TM, Barac A. Burgeoning Cardio-Oncology Programs. J Am Coll Cardiol 2015;66(10):1193–1197. Available from: http://linkinghub.elsevier.com/retrieve/pii/S0735109715045702

[34] Sulpher J, Mathur S, Graham N, Crawley F, Turek M, Johnson C, et al. Clinical experience of patients referred to a multidisciplinary cardiac oncology clinic: an observational study. J Oncol 2015;2015:671232. Available from: http://www.pubmedcentral.nih.gov/articlerender.fcgi?artid=4537752&tool=pmcentrez&rendertype=abstract

[35] Liddy C, Maranger J, Afkham A, Keely E. Ten steps to establishing an e-consultation service to improve access to specialist care.

Telemed J E Health 2013;19(12):982–990. Available from: http://www.pubmedcentral.nih.gov/articlerender.fcgi?artid=3850434&tool=pmcentrez&rendertype=abstract

[36] Virani SA, Dent S, Brezden-Masley C, Clarke B, Davis MK, Jassal DS, et al. Canadian cardiovascular society guidelines for evaluation and management of cardiovascular complications of cancer therapy. Can J Cardiol 2016;32(7):831–841. Available from: http://linkinghub.elsevier.com/retrieve/pii/S0828282X16300046

[37] Thavendiranathan P, Poulin F, Lim K-D, Plana JC, Woo A, Marwick TH. Use of myocardial strain imaging by echocardiography for the early detection of cardiotoxicity in patients during and after cancer chemotherapy: a systematic review. J Am Coll Cardiol 2014;63(25 Pt. A):2751–2768. Available from: http://www.ncbi.nlm.nih.gov/pubmed/24703918

[38] Sawaya H, Sebag IA, Plana JC, Januzzi JL, Ky B, Tan TC, et al. Assessment of echocardiography and biomarkers for the extended prediction of cardiotoxicity in patients treated with anthracyclines, taxanes, and trastuzumab. Circ Cardiovasc Imaging 2012;5(5):596–603. Available from: http://www.pubmedcentral.nih.gov/articlerender.fcgi?artid=3703313&tool=pmcentrez&rendertype=abstract

[39] Ezaz G, Long JB, Gross CP, Chen J. Risk prediction model for heart failure and cardiomyopathy after adjuvant trastuzumab therapy for breast cancer. J Am Heart Assoc 2014;3:e000472. Available from: http://jaha.ahajournals.org/cgi/doi/10.1161/JAHA.113.000472\nhttp://www.pubmedcentral.nih.gov/articlerender.fcgi?artid=3959671&tool=pmcentrez&rendertype=abstract

[40] Cardinale D, Sandri MT, Colombo A, Colombo N, Boeri M, Lamantia G, et al. Prognostic value of troponin I in cardiac risk stratification of cancer patients undergoing high-dose chemotherapy. Circulation 2004;109(22):2749–2754. Available from: http://www.ncbi.nlm.nih.gov/pubmed/15148277

[41] Ewer MS, Ewer SM. Cardiotoxicity of anticancer treatments: what the cardiologist needs to know. Nat Rev Cardiol 2010;7(10):564–575. Available from: http://www.ncbi.nlm.nih.gov/pubmed/20842180

[42] Patnaik JL, Byers T, DiGuiseppi C, Dabelea D, Denberg TD. Cardiovascular disease competes with breast cancer as the leading cause of death for older females diagnosed with breast cancer: a retrospective cohort study. Breast Cancer Res 2011;13(3):R64. Available from: http://www.pubmedcentral.nih.gov/articlerender.fcgi?artid=3218953&tool=pmcentrez&rendertype=abstract

[43] Media backgrounder 2 Canadian Cancer Statistics 2013—Canadian Cancer Society. Available from: http://www.cancer.ca/en/about-us/for-media/media-releases/national/2013/media-backgrounder-2-canadian-cancer-statistics-2013/?region=on

[44] Cardinale D, Colombo A, Sandri MT, Lamantia G, Colombo N, Civelli M, et al. Prevention of high-dose chemotherapy-induced cardiotoxicity in high-risk patients by angiotensin-converting enzyme inhibition. Circulation 2006;114(23):2474–2481. Available from: http://www.ncbi.nlm.nih.gov/pubmed/17101852

[45] Lawrence RA, McLoone JK, Wakefield CE, Cohn RJ. Primary care physicians' perspectives of their role in cancer care: a systematic review. J Gen Intern Med 2016; 31(10):1222–1236. Available from: http://www.ncbi.nlm.nih.gov/pubmed/27220499

[46] Valachis A, Nilsson C. Cardiac risk in the treatment of breast cancer: assessment and management. Breast Cancer 2015;7:21–35. Available from: http://www.ncbi.nlm.nih.gov/pubmed/25653554

[47] Gujral DM, Manisty C, Lloyd G, Bhattacharyya S. Organisation & models of cardio-oncology clinics. Int J Cardiol 2016;214:381–382.

[48] Lenihan DJ, Hartlage G, DeCara J, Blaes A, Finet JE, Lyon AR, et al. Cardio-oncology training: a proposal from the international cardioncology society and canadian cardiac oncology network for a new multidisciplinary specialty. J Card Fail 2016;22(6):465–471. Available from: http://linkinghub.elsevier.com/retrieve/pii/S1071916416300057

[49] Brown S-A. Proposing and meeting the need for interdisciplinary cardio-oncology subspecialty training. J Card Fail 2016. Available from: http://www.ncbi.nlm.nih.gov/pubmed/27150494

[50] Keller KB, Eggenberger TL, Belkowitz J, Sarsekeyeva M, Zito AR. Implementing successful interprofessional communication opportunities in health care education: a qualitative analysis. Int J Med Edu 2013;4:253–259. Available from: http://pmc/articles/PMC4205528/?report=abstract

[51] Grandin EW, Ky B, Cornell RF, Carver J, Lenihan DJ. Patterns of cardiac toxicity associated with irreversible proteasome inhibition in the treatment of multiple myeloma. J Card Fail 2015;21(2):138–144. Available from: http://www.ncbi.nlm.nih.gov/pubmed/25433360

Assessment of Cardiovascular Risk Beyond Lipid Panel in Cardio-Oncology Patients

J. Wei

Barbra Streisand Women's Heart Center, Cedars-Sinai Heart Institute, Los Angeles, CA, United States

Cardiovascular risk assessment is important for patients diagnosed with cancer, as cancer survivors experience an increased risk of cardiovascular disease (CVD)-related events [1–4]. Long-term follow-up of survivors of adolescent and young adult cancer demonstrate a more than twofold risk of developing CVD when compared to age and sex-matched patients without cancer, with the highest risk seen in survivors of leukemia and breast cancer [5]. The impact of CVD on the outcomes of cancer survivors is striking, as adolescent and young adult cancer survivors who develop CVD have an 11-fold-increased overall mortality risk compared with survivors without CVD [5]. The increased CVD events have been largely attributed to chest radiation, which accelerates the development of atherosclerosis by intimal injury, while cardiac toxicity from certain chemotherapy agents (such as anthracylines and anti-HER2-receptor antibodies) plays a role in cardiomyopathy and increased heart failure. Thus, it is essential for cancer survivors to receive CVD risk reduction strategies, including treatment of hypertension and hypercholesterolemia, as well as healthy lifestyle modifications. In this chapter, preventive risk assessment for atherosclerotic CVD in cardio-oncology patients is discussed.

Atherosclerosis is a systemic disease involving multiple vascular territories with important clinical sequelae including stroke, myocardial infarction (MI), and critical limb ischemia [6]. Childhood cancer survivors have been found to have a fivefold risk of MI compared to siblings without cancer [7]. How does a clinician predict CVD risk and determine antiatherosclerosis therapy in cancer survivors? Similar to the Framingham and Reynold CVD risk scores, the 2013 American College of Cardiology/American Heart Association (ACC/AHA) Risk Assessment Guidelines for estimating 10 year and lifetime atherosclerotic CVD event risk include traditional risk factors, such as age, cholesterol, blood pressure, and smoking, but do not include prior cancer-related cardio-toxic chemotherapy or radiation in their risk calculator (Table 16.1) [8–11]. The 2013 ACC/AHA guidelines define specific populations that are likely to benefit from statin therapy (Table 16.2) and move away from focusing on low-density lipoprotein-cholesterol (LDL-C) goals. Since the guidelines were based on randomized controlled trials and did not incorporate observational or mechanistic studies, the guidelines did not discuss cancer-related CVD risk. The 2015 National Lipid Association's Expert Panel recommendations for patient-centered management of dyslipidemia also do not mention cancer-related CVD risk, but do provide non-HDL-C and LDL-C treatment goals and also provide reassurance that lipid-lowering therapy is not associated with increased cancer risk [12,13].

Since a significant number of CVD cases occur in people without traditional risk factors, additional biomarkers may be helpful to identify those who are at increased CVD risk despite normal lipid panels. Recent studies have demonstrated that measures of atherosclerosis in vascular beds (carotid, coronary, femoral) improve prediction of CVD events over traditional risk factors [14–22]. Elevated markers of inflammation, specifically C-reactive protein (CRP), have also been found to be associated with increased CVD risk and improved risk prediction [23,24]. The 2013 ACC/AHA guidelines recommend coronary artery calcification (CAC) score, ankle-brachial index (ABI), and highly sensitive C-reactive protein (hs-CRP) as optional screening tests for further risk assessment and treatment decision making. While studies have not specifically been performed to demonstrate benefit of these additional measures in CVD risk assessment of cancer survivors, these additional measures may be considered in patients for whom a decision to initiate statin therapy is unclear. Targeted prevention strategies for cancer survivors at highest risk of developing CVD are however needed to reduce the high CVD-related morbidity and mortality in cancer survivors.

TABLE 16.1 Variables Used in Calculators for Estimating 10-year Cardiovascular Risk

Framingham	Reynolds	ACC/AHA ASCVD
Age (30–74 years)	Age (45–80 years)	Age (20–79 years)
Sex	Sex	Sex
Total cholesterol	Total cholesterol	Total cholesterol
HDL cholesterol	HDL cholesterol	HDL cholesterol
Current smoker	Current smoker	Current smoker
Systolic blood pressure	Systolic blood pressure	Systolic blood pressure
Treatment for hypertension	High sensitivity C-reactive protein (hs-CRP)	Treatment for hypertension
Diabetes	Parental history of heart attack or stroke before age 60	Diabetes
		Race (White, African American, other)

Source: D'Agostino RB, et al. General cardiovascular risk profile for use in primary care: the Framingham Heart Study. Circulation 2008;117(6):743–53; Ridker PM, et al. Development and validation of improved algorithms for the assessment of global cardiovascular risk in women: the Reynolds Risk Score. JAMA 2007;297(6):611–9; Ridker PM, et al. C-reactive protein and parental history improve global cardiovascular risk prediction: the Reynolds Risk Score for men. Circulation 2008;118:2243–51; Stone NJ, et al. 2013 ACC/AHA guideline on the treatment of blood cholesterol to reduce atherosclerotic cardiovascular risk in adults. J Am Coll Cardiol 2014;63(25_PA):2889–934.

TABLE 16.2 2013 ACC/AHA Recommendations for the Treatment of Blood Cholesterol to Reduce Atherosclerotic CVD Risk in Adults

Four Statin Benefit Groups
Clinical atherosclerotic CVD (acute coronary syndrome, history of myocardial infarction, stable or unstable angina, coronary or other arterial revascularization, stroke, transient ischemic attack, or peripheral artery disease)
Primary hypercholesterolemia (age ≥21 years and LDL-C > 190 mg/dL)
Diabetes (age 40–75 years and LDL-C 70–189 mg/dL)
Estimated 10-year atherosclerotic CVD risk ≥7.5% (using the Pooled Cohort Equations Risk Calculator) (no diabetes, age 40–75 years, LDL-C 70–189 mg/dL)

CVD, Cardiovascular disease; LDL-C, low-density lipoprotein cholesterol.
Source: Stone NJ, et al.. 2013 ACC/AHA Guideline on the Treatment of Blood Cholesterol to Reduce Atherosclerotic Cardiovascular Risk in Adults: A Report of the American College of Cardiology/American Heart Association Task Force on Practice Guidelines. J Am Coll Cardiol 2014;63(25_PA):2889–934.

CORONARY ARTERY DISEASE AND CORONARY ARTERY CALCIFICATION

Coronary Artery Disease and Chest Radiation

The relationship between chest radiation and coronary artery disease (CAD) has been established in multiple studies of various cancer survivors. Breast cancer patients who received left chest wall radiation therapy in the 1970s–80s had a ~2.5-fold increased risk for MI in 18 years compared to no radiation therapy [2]. The risk of a CAD event increased linearly with the radiation dose to the heart (7.4% per Gy) starting within the first 5 years after exposure and continuing for at least 20 years [1]. Mediastinal radiation in Hodgkin's

disease survivors prior to 1990 was related to a ~2.5-fold age-adjusted increased risk of acute MI death within 5 years, although the decrease in total radiation dose over the years appears to have decreased the risk of CAD events [25]. Risk was increased with high mediastinal doses and with young age at irradiation [26]. Nonseminomatous testicular cancer survivors who received mediastinal radiation prior to 1985 also had an increased risk of MI at young ages (~twofold increase risk in survivors <45 years), with mediastinal radiation associated with a 3.7-fold increased MI risk compared with surgery alone [4]. Contemporary radiation therapy techniques that minimize incidental cardiac irradiation appear to decrease the incidence of cardiotoxicity but there does not appear to be any radiation threshold below which there is no risk [1].

Coronary Artery Calcification

Coronary artery calcification (CAC) is a well-recognized risk factor for adverse outcomes in patients with CAD. CAC is a measure of calcification of atherosclerotic lesions in the vascular intima, which is associated with inflammatory mediators and elevated lipid content, and a measure of calcification in the vascular media, which is associated with increased arterial stiffness, advanced age, diabetes, and chronic kidney disease [27]. Although calcium regulatory mechanisms influence CAC, ingestion of a high-calcium diet has not been associated with CAC [28]. CAC is most commonly measured by computed tomography (CT), which is noninvasive, has high sensitivity and specificity for calcium detection and can quantify calcification [29] (Fig. 16.1). However, CAC does not detect luminal stenosis, or obstruction, and MI can occur in patients without CAC, especially in younger adults who smoke [30]. The most common CAC scoring method is the Agatston CAC score, which is a semiautomated score based on the extent of CAC detected by a noncontrast CT scan, using a weighted density score given to the highest attenuation value (HU) multiplied by area of the calcification speck [31]. The score of every calcified speck is summed to give the total CAC score. Higher levels of CAC correlate with increased plaque burden (both calcified and noncalcified plaque) [32,33]. The Multi-Ethnic Study of Atherosclerosis (MESA) demonstrated that although there are differences among age, sex, and race/ethnicity groups in terms of CAC distribution, the absolute CAC score has higher discrimination for CAD events than models using age-, sex-, and race/ethnicity-specific percentiles [34].

Risk Stratification With the CAC Score

As the CAC score reflects coronary artery plaque burden, the CAC score can be used as a screening tool to identify subjects with high likelihood of atherosclerosis. Studies like the MESA, which studied 6814 individuals, and the Early Identification of Subclinical Atherosclerosis by Noninvasive Imaging Research (EISNER) study, which studied 1424 individuals, have provided valuable prognostic data for CAC in patients with CVD risk factors but no known CVD. The majority of the EISNER subjects had CAC score of zero (57%) or minimal CAC score of 1–10 (21%) [35]. Subjects with CAC score 0–10 have an excellent 5-year survival of at least 99.4% [36,37], and risk-adjusted models indicate that the statistical difference between CAC score 0 versus 1–10 is not significant [38]. On the other hand, CAC score >300 has been shown to confer a 10-fold increase in the risk of a CVD event compared to adults with CAC score of zero [38,39].

As the CAC score has become an established measure for CVD risk assessment, it has also been used to guide prevention interventions, such as aspirin and statin [40,41]. A CAC score 0 predicts low risk that is unlikely to be modified by statin therapy, while presence of CAC indicates increased CVD risk. The 2013 ACC/AHA Atherosclerotic CVD Risk Assessment Guidelines indicate that CAC score >300 (or >75 percentile for age, sex, and ethnicity) is a suitable cut-off for treatment decisions [14,39,42], although CAC score >100 and CAC score >400 have also been published as appropriate cut-offs for predicting significant CVD risk and influencing treatment decisions [14,43,44]. The MESA study showed that absolute CAC score predicts events better than age-, sex-, and race/ethnicity-specific percentiles (Fig. 16.2) [34]. Studies have demonstrated that the CAC score can also promote adherence to medications [45–48]. Based on EISNER data, overall 41% of subjects with CAC score ≥1 were started on a statin and had a medication adherence rate of 90% at follow-up; statin therapy was initiated in 35% of subjects 1–99, 43% of subjects 100–399, and 65% of subjects ≥400 [49]. However, randomized control data is needed for determining whether CAC score-based interventions improve CVD outcomes.

Several studies have suggested that the CAC score is superior to other nontraditional risk markers for predicting CVD in intermediate-risk individuals and can reclassify risk in individuals [50]. In patients considered intermediate-risk from Framingham criteria, a high CAC score may indicate a higher level of risk that calls for more intensive treatment of CVD risk factors [14]. CAC scores may also shift intermediate-risk individuals to lower-risk classification.

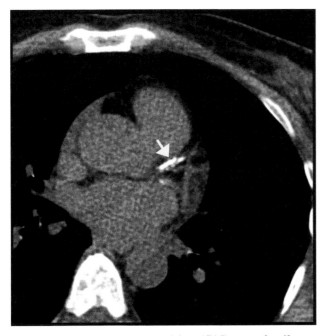

FIGURE 16.1 Coronary artery calcium (CAC) scan of a 60-year-old woman with prior history of left chest radiation for breast cancer 10 years ago and hypercholesterolemia. Total CAC score was 431.8, with the majority of calcium seen in the proximal left anterior descending artery *(arrow)*.

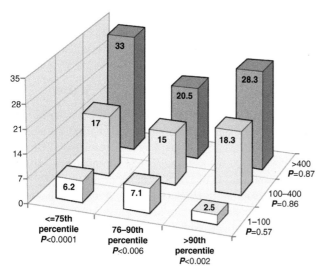

FIGURE 16.2 **Rates of incident coronary heart disease per 1000 person years at risk by categories of absolute coronary artery calcium score (CAC 1–100, 100–400, >400) and age-, sex-, and race/ethnicity-specific percentiles (≤75th, 76–90th, >90th percentiles).** While there is an increasing risk across levels of absolute CAC groups within each level of percentile, there is no increasing trend of risk across levels of percentiles once absolute CAC category is fixed. *From Budoff MJ, et al. Coronary calcium predicts events better with absolute calcium scores than age-sex-race/ethnicity percentiles: MESA (Multi-Ethnic Study of Atherosclerosis). J Am Coll Cardiol 2009;53(4):345–52.*

Recent application of the ACC/AHA CVD risk calculator to the MESA cohort found that of those qualifying for moderate or high-intensity statin therapy, 45% of patients had CAC score 0, with a 10-year event rate of 4 events per 1000 patient-years, reclassifying them at a low-risk group [51]. Similarly, evaluation of the Framingham Heart Study cohort showed that one-third of statin-eligible patients had CAC score 0, with very low 10-year event rate [52]. Although overestimation of risk by the ACC/AHA CVD risk calculator has been suggested in these studies, it is important to note that some of the MESA and Framingham participants received downstream therapy that may have prevented events and thus led to a low CVD event rate. Incorporation of CAC values has been shown be superior to incorporation of carotid intimal medial thickness (IMT) or hs-CRP for the estimation of absolute CVD risk [53]. Randomized control data is still needed for determining whether CAC scores improve CVD outcomes, and universal incorporation of CAC screening for CVD prevention is thus not recommended at this time.

Serial CAC Scores

Several studies using serial CAC scans have evaluated progression of CAC and risk of cardiovascular events. In a study of 442 individuals with CAC score 0 at baseline, about 25% developed CAC at a mean time to conversion of 4 years, with the lowest rate in the first two years of serial

scanning and then accelerating substantially [54]. In the MESA study, subjects age 45–84 years had an average annual change in CAC score of 24.9 ± 65.3 units [55]. Those with baseline CAC > 0 and annual progression of ≥300 units were 6 times more likely to suffer a MI or CAD death (HR 6.3, 95% CI 1.9–21.5) compared to those without progression. Interestingly, in MESA individuals without CAC at baseline, incidence of new CAC was independently associated with a diagnosis of cancer; however, there was no clear difference in CAC progression between cancer and noncancer individuals with CAC at baseline [56]. Despite these findings, the prognostic implications of increasing CAC scores over time have not been adequately studied, and the CAC score is not an effective tool for monitoring treatment response [57–59]. Increasing CAC score can represent progression of coronary atherosclerosis but could also represent conversion of noncalcified plaque to calcified plaque, which is considered to be more stable than noncalcified plaque [60]. Thus, routine serial CAC scans is not currently recommended in clinical practice.

Radiation Risk in CAC Scans

Radiation risk is an important concern for cancer survivors, given potential radiation–induced cancer risk. The radiation risk associated with CAC scans depends on the type of acquisition. Electron beam CT (EBCT) scanners use prospective ECG-triggering and acquire one scan at a time, while multidetector computed tomography (MDCT) scanners can acquire several parallel scans at the same time using prospective ECG-triggering or retrospective gating techniques. Retrospective gating acquires images continuously throughout the cardiac cycle, while prospective ECG-triggering only acquires images during a predetermined duration of the cardiac cycle. Thus, retrospective gating acquisitions involve higher radiation dose compared to prospective ECG-triggering acquisitions. Effective dose, a representation of the biological effect of the radiation dose received, is measured in units of sievert (Sv, SI unit) or rem (conventional unit). Due to the lower radiation risk, prospective ECG gating is recommended for all CAC scans. EBCT has an effective dose of 0.7–1.0 mSv in men and 0.9–1.3 mSv in women, while MDCT has an effective dose of 1.0–1.5 mSv in men and 1.1–1.9 mSv in women [61]. Some MDCT protocols, however, are associated with radiation doses higher than 10 mSv [62]. The average background radiation in the United States in 3.0–3.6 mSv/year [63], while a standard chest X-ray has an effective dose of 0.02 mSv [64]. While the radiation dose from CAC is low, it is not negligible and may vary widely depending on the protocol and the scanner [62]. Thus, optimization and standardization of CAC protocols and scanner selection is important for minimization of radiation dose while maintaining adequate image quality.

CAC Screening in Cancer Survivors

Universal screening should not be performed in cancer survivors, and should only be considered when the patient does not meet statin eligibility based on the ACC/AHA cholesterol guidelines (Table 16.1) [10]. Given the lack of prospective or randomized trial data to show that CAC screening reduces CVD events or improves survival, CAC screening should not be performed in low risk patients. Since some cancer survivors receive chest CTs for cancer surveillance, evaluation for coronary artery calcifications using these preexisting CT images is preferred to avoid excessive radiation exposure. Low-dose nongated CT for lung cancer screening can quantify CAC scores using Agatston methods and provide visual rating of calcium burden with good reproducibility [65], and CAC scores from low-dose nongated chest CTs have recently been shown to be predictive of CAD mortality in the National Lung Screening Trial [66].

Recently, CAC has been found to be associated with breast arterial calcifications seen on mammography (Fig. 16.3) [67,68]. The presence of breast arterial calcification predicts a CAC > 11 and is associated with other CVD risk factors, such as diabetes and chronic renal disease [67]. After adjustment for traditional risk factors, breast arterial calcification was associated with a 1.32-fold increased risk of coronary heart disease, 1.41-fold increased risk of ischemic stroke, and a 1.52-fold increased risk of heart failure [69]. Breast arterial calcification seen on mammography was determined to be superior to standard CVD risk factors and equivalent to the Framingham Risk Score and the ACC/AHA CVD risk calculator for the identification of women with high CVD risk [68]. Unlike CAC, breast arterial calcification has been shown to regress and thus appears to be a reversible process; the causes of regression and the implications of this reversible process are not yet known [70]. Since screening mammograms are recommended for women at high risk for breast cancer and also for certain breast cancer survivors, further research should determine whether serial assessment of breast arterial calcification may be useful for monitoring CVD risk.

HIGHLY SENSITIVE C-REACTIVE PROTEIN

hs-CRP is an inflammatory biomarker that is associated with increased risk of CVD events [71] and nonvascular mortality, including those from cancers [72,73]. Unlike CRPs which is reported in milligrams per deciliter and adequate

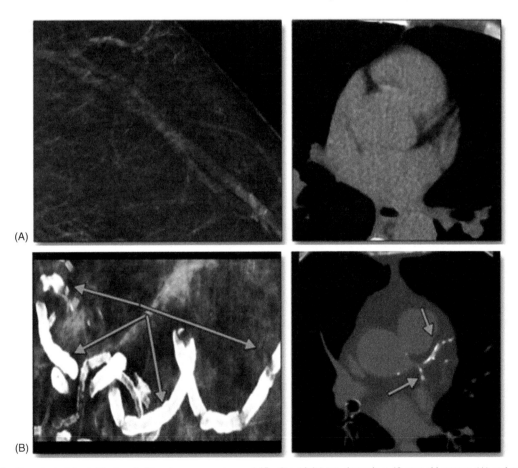

(A)

(B)

FIGURE 16.3   Breast arterial calcification (left) and coronary artery calcification (right) are absent in a 48-year old woman (A) and are present in a 61-year old woman (B) undergoing mammography and coronary artery calcium scan, respectively. *From Margolies L, et al. Digital mammography and screening for coronary artery disease. J Am Coll Cardiol Img 2016;9(4):350–60.*

for monitoring infections and systemic inflammatory disorders, hs-CRP is reported in mg/L and is more sensitive for reflecting atherosclerotic risk. hs-CRP levels < 1 mg/L reflect low CVD risk, levels between 1 and 3 mg/L reflect moderate CVD risk, and levels > 3 mg/L reflect higher CVD risk [74]. hs-CRP should not be measured in the setting of major infection or trauma as it is an acute phase reactant, and it can also be elevated by oral estrogen therapy.

According to the 2013 ACC/AHA cholesterol guidelines, hs-CRP measurement may be considered for intermediate risk individuals when clinical decisions related to the initiation of statin therapy are uncertain [10]. The JUPITER trial demonstrated that rosuvastatin 20 mg daily significantly reduced CVD events and all-cause mortality in individuals with LDL-C levels of <130 mg/dL and hs-CRP levels of >2 mg/L [75]; furthermore, those who achieved very low levels of hs-CRP and LDL-C had the greatest clinical benefits [76]. Thus, hs-CRP may be used to help determine which individuals may benefit from statin therapy. Although the ACC/AHA CVD risk calculator does not include hs-CRP, hs-CRP is included in the Reynolds Risk Score [8], which has been demonstrated to have better risk discrimination compared to the Framingham risk scores and the ACC/AHA CVD risk calculator [77]. However, the sensitivity of hs-CRP to predict CVD risk in cancer survivors has not been studied.

CAROTID ATHEROSCLEROSIS AND INTIMAL MEDIAL THICKNESS

Carotid ultrasound is capable of identifying carotid atherosclerosis, as well as predicting risk of CVD in patients with or without carotid plaques [78,79]. Common carotid artery intima-media thickness (IMT) is a surrogate marker of atherosclerosis and uses B-mode or B + M-mode ultrasonography to identify the distance between the lumen-intima and media-adventitia interfaces, which appears as a double-line pattern visualized on both walls of the common carotid artery in a longitudinal view (Fig. 16.4). Randomized control trials have demonstrated that carotid IMT measurements are reproducible and can be used to evaluate the efficacy of pharmacological interventions in carotid atherosclerosis [80]. Due to the highly variable methods for measuring carotid IMT and the various populations studied, however, published age-dependent nomograms have been limited for general application [81]. Standards for IMT measurement have recently been developed, including equipment settings, location of segments for measurement, and automated edge-detection techniques with averaging of the IMT values [81]. The 2013 ACC/AHA cholesterol guidelines did not recommend IMT measurement for routine risk assessment in clinical practice, and serial studies of IMT to assess progression or regression in individual patients are not recommended [42,82].

Since radiation-treated head and neck cancer patients are at increased risk for developing symptomatic progressive

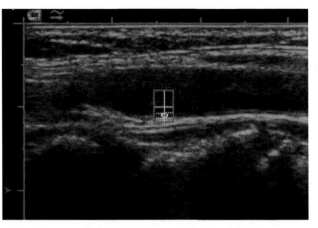

FIGURE 16.4 **Carotid intimal medial thickness (IMT) measurement of the left common carotid artery demonstrating average thickness of 0.617 mm, in a 51-year-old woman with family history of premature coronary artery disease.** This measurement is within the 50–75th percentile for a woman in her age range.

carotid stenosis and strokes [83–85], carotid screening may be useful in this population. Radiation therapy, along with other traditional CVD risk factors, appears to have a combined effect on the progression of carotid atherosclerosis [86]. Available risk calculators (Framingham risk score and ACC/AHA CVD risk calculator) may not accurately predict risk in this population. In a recent study of 134 radiation-treated head and neck cancer patients, carotid IMT demonstrated high prevalence (75%) of increased IMT in this population and changed clinical management in 50% of the patients [87]. The Framingham Risk Score and the ACC/AHA CVD risk calculator failed to detect 40–50% of cases found to be at high risk using carotid IMT [87]. Not all radiation-treated head and neck cancer patients appear to have the same CVD risk; patients with nasopharyngeal carcinoma, laryngocarcinoma, and hypopharyngeal carcinoma have a 6 times higher risk of developing carotid stenosis than patients with other tumors, potentially due to higher radiation dose [88,89]. Given the higher stroke rate in this population due to chronic radiation vasculopathy, carotid screening, and aggressive CVD risk factor reduction warrant further investigation. Unfortunately, there is currently no consensus on the frequency of screening and the time of screening initiation. Increase in carotid IMT can be observed in the first 2 years after radiation therapy [90], thus prior publications have recommended annual carotid ultrasound screening beginning 3–5 years after radiation therapy for head and neck cancers [91,92].

PERIPHERAL ATHEROSCLEROSIS AND ANKLE-BRACHIAL INDEX

Similar to the effects of radiation vasculopathy in head and neck and chest cancer patients, radiation-induced peripheral arterial disease is also a condition that is increasingly being recognized. Accelerated aortic and iliofemoral atherosclerosis has been described in patients who received radiation therapy for genitourinary cancers [93,94], while common femoral, superficial femoral, and popliteal artery atherosclerosis may occur in patients with history of lower extremity radiation therapy [95]. The average total radiation dose in these patients with symptomatic peripheral artery disease ranged from 40–65 Gy [95]. Radiation-induced peripheral artery disease may manifest as intermittent claudication or critical limb ischemia and may be treated with percutaneous or surgical revascularization. Patients with gangrene may need amputation. Given these potential serious consequences, patients with history of radiation therapy for genito-urinary cancers or lower extremity cancers may benefit from early screening for signs and symptoms of peripheral artery disease.

Routine noninvasive screening with lower extremity arterial ultrasound or ankle-brachial index (ABI) is not currently recommended but should be considered in these patients if they are showing signs or symptoms of lower extremity ischemia. ABI is the ratio of the systolic blood pressure measured at the ankle to that measured at the brachial artery and is a predictor for cardiovascular events in both symptomatic and asymptomatic individuals [96]. The 2013 ACC/AHA cholesterol guidelines consider ABI ≤ 0.9 to be a factor that might aid in CVD risk assessment, as ABI threshold ≤0.9 has >90% sensitivity and specificity to detect peripheral artery disease [10,96]. In some patients with vascular calcification due to medial calcinosis, diabetes mellitus, or end-stage renal disease, ABI may be less sensitive in detecting a stenosis, as the ankle artery may have a much higher systolic pressure than the brachial artery, leading to an ABI ≥ 1.40. Both individuals with ABI ≤ 0.90 and individuals with ABI ≥ 1.40 are at increased risk of CVD, independent of peripheral artery disease symptoms or other CVD risk factors [97,98].

CONCLUSIONS

Although the current literature is not supportive of the use of routine screening for atherosclerosis in cardio-oncology patients with prior radiation therapy, it is evident that noninvasive markers (such as CAC scans, hs-CRP, carotid IMT, or ABI) can help improve CVD risk stratification. Cancer survivors with increased CVD risk or evidence of coronary, carotid, and peripheral atherosclerosis should be aggressively treated for hypertension, diabetes, hyperlipidemia, and smoking cessation. The elevated CVD morbidity and mortality risk associated with prior radiation therapy warrants further investigation in the value of these noninvasive markers for guiding CVD prevention and interventions in these patients.

REFERENCES

[1] Darby SC, Ewertz M, McGale P, Bennet AM, Blom-Goldman U, Bronnum D, Correa C, Cutter D, Gagliardi G, Gigante B, Jensen MB, Nisbet A, Peto R, Rahimi K, Taylor C, Hall P. Risk of ischemic heart disease in women after radiotherapy for breast cancer. N Engl J Med. 2013;368:987–98.

[2] Hooning MJ, Botma A, Aleman BM, Baaijens MH, Bartelink H, Klijn JG, Taylor CW, van Leeuwen FE. Long-term risk of cardiovascular disease in 10-year survivors of breast cancer. J Natl Cancer Inst 2007;99:365–75.

[3] Aleman BM, van den Belt-Dusebout AW, De Bruin ML, van 't Veer MB, Baaijens MH, de Boer JP, Hart AA, Klokman WJ, Kuenen MA, Ouwens GM, Bartelink H, van Leeuwen FE. Late cardiotoxicity after treatment for Hodgkin lymphoma. Blood 2007;109:1878–86.

[4] van den Belt-Dusebout AW, Nuver J, de Wit R, Gietema JA, ten Bokkel Huinink WW, Rodrigus PT, Schimmel EC, Aleman BM, van Leeuwen FE. Long-term risk of cardiovascular disease in 5-year survivors of testicular cancer. J Clin Oncol 2006;24:467–75.

[5] Chao C, Xu L, Bhatia S, Cooper R, Brar S, Wong FL, Armenian SH. Cardiovascular Disease Risk Profiles in Survivors of Adolescent and Young Adult (AYA) Cancer: The Kaiser Permanente AYA Cancer Survivors Study. J Clin Oncol 2016;34:1626–33.

[6] Faxon DP, Creager MA, Smith SC Jr, Pasternak RC, Olin JW, Bettmann MA, Criqui MH, Milani RV, Loscalzo J, Kaufman JA, Jones DW, Pearce WH. Atherosclerotic Vascular Disease Conference: Executive summary: Atherosclerotic Vascular Disease Conference proceeding for healthcare professionals from a special writing group of the American Heart Association. Circulation 2004;109:2595–604.

[7] Mulrooney DA, Yeazel MW, Kawashima T, Mertens AC, Mitby P, Stovall M, Donaldson SS, Green DM, Sklar CA, Robison LL, Leisenring WM. Cardiac outcomes in a cohort of adult survivors of childhood and adolescent cancer: retrospective analysis of the Childhood Cancer Survivor Study cohort. BMJ 2009;339:b4606.

[8] Ridker PM, Buring JE, Rifai N, Cook NR. Development and validation of improved algorithms for the assessment of global cardiovascular risk in women: the Reynolds Risk Score. JAMA 2007;297:611–9.

[9] D'Agostino RB Sr, Vasan RS, Pencina MJ, Wolf PA, Cobain M, Massaro JM, Kannel WB. General cardiovascular risk profile for use in primary care: the Framingham Heart Study. Circulation 2008;117:743–53.

[10] Stone NJ, Robinson JG, Lichtenstein AH, Bairey Merz CN, Blum CB, Eckel RH, Goldberg AC, Gordon D, Levy D, Lloyd-Jones DM, McBride P, Schwartz JS, Shero ST, Smith SC, Jr, Watson K, Wilson PW, American College of Cardiology/American Heart Association Task Force on Practice Guidelines. 2013 ACC/AHA guideline on the treatment of blood cholesterol to reduce atherosclerotic cardiovascular risk in adults: a report of the American College of Cardiology/American Heart Association Task Force on Practice Guidelines. J Am Coll Cardiol 2014;63:2889–2934.

[11] Ridker PM, Paynter NP, Rifai N, Gaziano JM, Cook NR. C-reactive protein and parental history improve global cardiovascular risk prediction: the Reynolds Risk Score for men. Circulation 2008;118:2243–51. 4p. following 2251.

[12] Jacobson TA, Ito MK, Maki KC, Orringer CE, Bays HE, Jones PH, McKenney JM, Grundy SM, Gill EA, Wild RA, Wilson DP, Brown WV. National lipid association recommendations for patient-centered management of dyslipidemia: part 1—full report. J Clin Lipidol 2015;9:129–69.

[13] Jacobson TA, Maki KC, Orringer CE, Jones PH, Kris-Etherton P, Sikand G, La Forge R, Daniels SR, Wilson DP, Morris PB, Wild RA, Grundy SM, Daviglus M, Ferdinand KC, Vijayaraghavan K, Deedwania PC, Aberg JA, Liao KP, McKenney JM, Ross JL, Braun LT, Ito MK, Bays HE, Brown WV, Underberg JA, Panel NLAE. National Lipid Association Recommendations for Patient-Centered Management of Dyslipidemia: Part 2. J Clin Lipidol 2015;9. S1-122 e1.

[14] Greenland P, LaBree L, Azen SP, Doherty TM, Detrano RC. Coronary artery calcium score combined with Framingham score for risk prediction in asymptomatic individuals. JAMA 2004;291:210–5.

[15] Schiano V, Sirico G, Giugliano G, Laurenzano E, Brevetti L, Perrino C, Brevetti G, Esposito G. Femoral plaque echogenicity and cardiovascular risk in claudicants. JACC Cardiovasc Imaging 2012; 5:348–57.

[16] Hadamitzky M, Achenbach S, Al-Mallah M, Berman D, Budoff M, Cademartiri F, Callister T, Chang HJ, Cheng V, Chinnaiyan K, Chow BJ, Cury R, Delago A, Dunning A, Feuchtner G, Gomez M, Kaufmann P, Kim YJ, Leipsic J, Lin FY, Maffei E, Min JK, Raff G, Shaw LJ, Villines TC, Hausleiter J. Optimized prognostic score for coronary computed tomographic angiography: results from the CONFIRM registry (COronary CT Angiography EvaluatioN For Clinical Outcomes: An InteRnational Multicenter Registry). J Am Coll Cardiol 2013;62:468–76.

[17] Dalager S, Falk E, Kristensen IB, Paaske WP. Plaque in superficial femoral arteries indicates generalized atherosclerosis and vulnerability to coronary death: an autopsy study. J Vasc Surg 2008;47:296–302.

[18] Saam T, Hetterich H, Hoffmann V, Yuan C, Dichgans M, Poppert H, Koeppel T, Hoffmann U, Reiser MF, Bamberg F. Meta-analysis and systematic review of the predictive value of carotid plaque hemorrhage on cerebrovascular events by magnetic resonance imaging. J Am Coll Cardiol 2013;62:1081–91.

[19] Motoyama S, Kondo T, Sarai M, Sugiura A, Harigaya H, Sato T, Inoue K, Okumura M, Ishii J, Anno H, Virmani R, Ozaki Y, Hishida H, Narula J. Multislice computed tomographic characteristics of coronary lesions in acute coronary syndromes. J Am Coll Cardiol 2007;50:319–26.

[20] Wannarong T, Parraga G, Buchanan D, Fenster A, House AA, Hackam DG, Spence JD. Progression of carotid plaque volume predicts cardiovascular events. Stroke 2013;44:1859–65.

[21] Inaba Y, Chen JA, Bergmann SR. Carotid plaque, compared with carotid intima-media thickness, more accurately predicts coronary artery disease events: a meta-analysis. Atherosclerosis 2012;220:128–33.

[22] Polak JF, Szklo M, Kronmal RA, Burke GL, Shea S, Zavodni AE, O'Leary DH. The value of carotid artery plaque and intima-media thickness for incident cardiovascular disease: the multi-ethnic study of atherosclerosis. J Am Heart Assoc 2013;2:e000087.

[23] Libby P, Ridker PM, Maseri A. Inflammation and atherosclerosis. Circulation 2002;105:1135–43.

[24] Ridker PM, Rifai N, Rose L, Buring JE, Cook NR. Comparison of C-reactive protein and low-density lipoprotein cholesterol levels in the prediction of first cardiovascular events. N Engl J Med 2002;347:1557–65.

[25] Boivin JF, Hutchison GB, Lubin JH, Mauch P. Coronary artery disease mortality in patients treated for Hodgkin's disease. Cancer 1992;69:1241–7.

[26] Hancock SL, Tucker MA, Hoppe RT. Factors affecting late mortality from heart disease after treatment of Hodgkin's disease. JAMA 1993;270:1949–55.

[27] Madhavan MV, Tarigopula M, Mintz GS, Maehara A, Stone GW, Genereux P. Coronary artery calcification: pathogenesis and prognostic implications. J Am Coll Cardiol 2014;63:1703–14.

[28] Samelson EJ, Booth SL, Fox CS, Tucker KL, Wang TJ, Hoffmann U, Cupples LA, O'Donnell CJ, Kiel DP. Calcium intake is not associated with increased coronary artery calcification: the Framingham Study. Am J Clin Nutr. 2012;96:1274–80.

[29] Carr JJ, Nelson JC, Wong ND, McNitt-Gray M, Arad Y, Jacobs DR Jr, Sidney S, Bild DE, Williams OD, Detrano RC. Calcified coronary artery plaque measurement with cardiac CT in population-based studies: standardized protocol of Multi-Ethnic Study of Atherosclerosis (MESA) and Coronary Artery Risk Development in Young Adults (CARDIA) study. Radiology 2005;234:35–43.

[30] Raggi P, Callister TQ, Cooil B, He ZX, Lippolis NJ, Russo DJ, Zelinger A, Mahmarian JJ. Identification of patients at increased risk of first unheralded acute myocardial infarction by electron-beam computed tomography. Circulation 2000;101:850–5.

[31] Agatston AS, Janowitz WR, Hildner FJ, Zusmer NR, Viamonte M Jr, Detrano R. Quantification of coronary artery calcium using ultrafast computed tomography. J Am Coll Cardiol 1990;15:827–32.

[32] Rumberger JA, Simons DB, Fitzpatrick LA, Sheedy PF, Schwartz RS. Coronary artery calcium area by electron-beam computed tomography and coronary atherosclerotic plaque area. A histopathologic correlative study. Circulation 1995;92:2157–62.

[33] Sangiorgi G, Rumberger JA, Severson A, Edwards WD, Gregoire J, Fitzpatrick LA, Schwartz RS. Arterial calcification and not lumen stenosis is highly correlated with atherosclerotic plaque burden in humans: a histologic study of 723 coronary artery segments using nondecalcifying methodology. J Am Coll Cardiol 1998;31:126–33.

[34] Budoff MJ, Nasir K, McClelland RL, Detrano R, Wong N, Blumenthal RS, Kondos G, Kronmal RA. Coronary calcium predicts events better with absolute calcium scores than age-sex-race/ethnicity percentiles: MESA (Multi-Ethnic Study of Atherosclerosis). J Am Coll Cardiol 2009;53:345–52.

[35] Shaw LJ, Min JK, Budoff M, Gransar H, Rozanski A, Hayes SW, Friedman JD, Miranda R, Wong ND, Berman DS. Induced cardiovascular procedural costs and resource consumption patterns after coronary artery calcium screening: results from the EISNER (Early Identification of Subclinical Atherosclerosis by Noninvasive Imaging Research) study. J Am Coll Cardiol 2009;54:1258–67.

[36] Shaw LJ, Raggi P, Callister TQ, Berman DS. Prognostic value of coronary artery calcium screening in asymptomatic smokers and non-smokers. Eur Heart J 2006;27:968–75.

[37] Budoff MJ, McClelland RL, Nasir K, Greenland P, Kronmal RA, Kondos GT, Shea S, Lima JA, Blumenthal RS. Cardiovascular events with absent or minimal coronary calcification: the Multi-Ethnic Study of Atherosclerosis (MESA). Am Heart J 2009;158:554–61.

[38] Budoff MJ, Shaw LJ, Liu ST, Weinstein SR, Mosler TP, Tseng PH, Flores FR, Callister TQ, Raggi P, Berman DS. Long-term prognosis associated with coronary calcification: observations from a registry of 25,253 patients. J Am Coll Cardiol 2007;49:1860–70.

[39] Detrano R, Guerci AD, Carr JJ, Bild DE, Burke G, Folsom AR, Liu K, Shea S, Szklo M, Bluemke DA, O'Leary DH, Tracy R, Watson K, Wong ND, Kronmal RA. Coronary calcium as a predictor of coronary events in four racial or ethnic groups. N Engl J Med 2008;358:1336–45.

[40] Pletcher MJ, Sibley CT, Pignone M, Vittinghoff E, Greenland P. Interpretation of the coronary artery calcium score in combination with conventional cardiovascular risk factors: the Multi-Ethnic Study of Atherosclerosis (MESA). Circulation 2013;128:1076–84.

[41] Stone NJ, Robinson J, Lichtenstein AH, Bairey Merz CN, Lloyd-Jones DM, Blum CB, McBride P, Eckel RH, Schwartz JS, Goldberg AC, Shero ST, Gordon D, Smith SC Jr, Levy D, Watson K, Wilson PW. 2013 ACC/AHA Guideline on the Treatment of Blood Cholesterol to Reduce Atherosclerotic Cardiovascular Risk in Adults: A Report of the American College of Cardiology/American Heart Association Task Force on Practice Guidelines. J Am Coll Cardiol 2013;63(25):2889–934.

[42] Goff DC Jr, Lloyd-Jones DM, Bennett G, O'Donnell CJ, Coady S, Robinson J, D'Agostino RB Sr, Schwartz JS, Gibbons R, Shero ST, Greenland P, Smith SC Jr, Lackland DT, Sorlie P, Levy D, Stone NJ, Wilson PW. 2013 ACC/AHA guideline on the assessment of cardiovascular risk: a report of the American College of Cardiology/American Heart Association Task Force on Practice Guidelines. Circulation 2014;129(25 Suppl. 2):S49–73.

[43] Martin SS, Blaha MJ, Blankstein R, Agatston A, Rivera JJ, Virani SS, Ouyang P, Jones SR, Blumenthal RS, Budoff MJ, Nasir K. Dyslipidemia, coronary artery calcium, and incident atherosclerotic cardiovascular disease: implications for statin therapy from the multiethnic study of atherosclerosis. Circulation 2014;129:77–86.

[44] Hermann DM, Gronewold J, Lehmann N, Moebus S, Jockel KH, Bauer M, Erbel R. Coronary artery calcification is an independent stroke predictor in the general population. Stroke 2013;44:1008–13.

[45] Orakzai RH, Nasir K, Orakzai SH, Kalia N, Gopal A, Musunuru K, Blumenthal RS, Budoff MJ. Effect of patient visualization of coronary calcium by electron beam computed tomography on changes in beneficial lifestyle behaviors. Am J Cardiol 2008;101: 999–1002.

[46] Nasir K, McClelland RL, Blumenthal RS, Goff DC Jr, Hoffmann U, Psaty BM, Greenland P, Kronmal RA, Budoff MJ. Coronary artery calcium in relation to initiation and continuation of cardiovascular preventive medications: The Multi-Ethnic Study of Atherosclerosis (MESA). Circ Cardiovasc Qual Outcomes 2010;3:228–35.

[47] Taylor AJ, Bindeman J, Feuerstein I, Le T, Bauer K, Byrd C, Wu H, O'Malley PG. Community-based provision of statin and aspirin after the detection of coronary artery calcium within a community-based screening cohort. J Am Coll Cardiol 2008;51:1337–41.

[48] Kalia NK, Miller LG, Nasir K, Blumenthal RS, Agrawal N, Budoff MJ. Visualizing coronary calcium is associated with improvements in adherence to statin therapy. Atherosclerosis 2006;185:394–9.

[49] Rozanski A, Gransar H, Shaw LJ, Kim J, Miranda-Peats L, Wong ND, Rana JS, Orakzai R, Hayes SW, Friedman JD, Thomson LE, Polk D, Min J, Budoff MJ, Berman DS. Impact of coronary artery calcium scanning on coronary risk factors and downstream testing the EISNER (Early Identification of Subclinical Atherosclerosis by Noninvasive Imaging Research) prospective randomized trial. J Am Coll Cardiol 2011;57:1622–32.

[50] Yeboah J, McClelland RL, Polonsky TS, Burke GL, Sibley CT, O'Leary D, Carr JJ, Goff DC, Greenland P, Herrington DM. Comparison of novel risk markers for improvement in cardiovascular risk assessment in intermediate-risk individuals. JAMA 2012;308:788–95.

[51] Nasir K, Bittencourt MS, Blaha MJ, Blankstein R, Agatson AS, Rivera JJ, Miedema MD, Sibley CT, Shaw LJ, Blumenthal RS, Budoff MJ, Krumholz HM. Implications of Coronary Artery Calcium Testing Among Statin Candidates According to American College of Cardiology/American Heart Association Cholesterol Management Guidelines: MESA (Multi-Ethnic Study of Atherosclerosis). J Am Coll Cardiol 2015;66:1657–68.

[52] Pursnani A, Massaro JM, D'Agostino RB Sr, O'Donnell CJ, Hoffmann U. Guideline-Based Statin Eligibility, Coronary Artery Calcification, and Cardiovascular Events. JAMA 2015;314:134–41.

[53] deGoma EM, Dunbar RL, Jacoby D, French B. Differences in absolute risk of cardiovascular events using risk-refinement tests: a systematic analysis of four cardiovascular risk equations. Atherosclerosis 2013;227:172–7.

[54] Min JK, Lin FY, Gidseg DS, Weinsaft JW, Berman DS, Shaw LJ, Rozanski A, Callister TQ. Determinants of coronary calcium conversion among patients with a normal coronary calcium scan: what is the "warranty period" for remaining normal? J Am Coll Cardiol 2010;55:1110–7.

[55] Budoff MJ, Young R, Lopez VA, Kronmal RA, Nasir K, Blumenthal RS, Detrano RC, Bild DE, Guerci AD, Liu K, Shea S, Szklo M, Post W, Lima J, Bertoni A, Wong ND. Progression of coronary calcium and incident coronary heart disease events: MESA (Multi-Ethnic Study of Atherosclerosis). J Am Coll Cardiol 2013;61:1231–9.

[56] Whitlock MC, Yeboah J, Burke GL, Chen H, Klepin HD, Hundley WG. Cancer and Its Association With the Development of Coronary Artery Calcification: An Assessment From the Multi-Ethnic Study of Atherosclerosis. J Am Heart Assoc 2015;4:4.

[57] Youssef G, Budoff MJ. Coronary artery calcium scoring, what is answered and what questions remain. Cardiovasc Diagn Ther 2012;2:94–105.

[58] Arad Y, Spadaro LA, Roth M, Newstein D, Guerci AD. Treatment of asymptomatic adults with elevated coronary calcium scores with atorvastatin, vitamin C, and vitamin E: the St. Francis Heart Study randomized clinical trial. J Am Coll Cardiol 2005;46:166–72.

[59] Schmermund A, Achenbach S, Budde T, Buziashvili Y, Forster A, Friedrich G, Henein M, Kerkhoff G, Knollmann F, Kukharchuk V, Lahiri A, Leischik R, Moshage W, Schartl M, Siffert W, Steinhagen-Thiessen E, Sinitsyn V, Vogt A, Wiedeking B, Erbel R. Effect of intensive versus standard lipid-lowering treatment with atorvastatin on the progression of calcified coronary atherosclerosis over 12 months: a multicenter, randomized, double-blind trial. Circulation 2006;113:427–37.

[60] Criqui MH, Denenberg JO, Ix JH, McClelland RL, Wassel CL, Rifkin DE, Carr JJ, Budoff MJ, Allison MA. Calcium density of coronary artery plaque and risk of incident cardiovascular events. JAMA 2014;311:271–8.

[61] Budoff MJ, Achenbach S, Blumenthal RS, Carr JJ, Goldin JG, Greenland P, Guerci AD, Lima JA, Rader DJ, Rubin GD, Shaw LJ, Wiegers SE, American Heart Association Committee on Cardiovascular I, Intervention, American Heart Association Council on Cardiovascular R, Intervention and American Heart Association Committee on Cardiac Imaging CoCC. Assessment of coronary artery disease by cardiac computed tomography: a scientific statement from the American Heart Association Committee on Cardiovascular Imaging and Intervention, Council on Cardiovascular Radiology and Intervention, and Committee on Cardiac Imaging, Council on Clinical Cardiology. Circulation. 2006;114:1761–1791.

[62] Kim KP, Einstein AJ, Berrington de Gonzalez A. Coronary artery calcification screening: estimated radiation dose and cancer risk. Arch Int Med 2009;169:1188–94.

[63] Hunold P, Vogt FM, Schmermund A, Debatin JF, Kerkhoff G, Budde T, Erbel R, Ewen K, Barkhausen J. Radiation exposure during cardiac CT: effective doses at multi-detector row CT and electron-beam CT. Radiology 2003;226:145–52.

[64] Fazel R, Krumholz HM, Wang Y, Ross JS, Chen J, Ting HH, Shah ND, Nasir K, Einstein AJ, Nallamothu BK. Exposure to low-dose ionizing radiation from medical imaging procedures. N Engl J Med 2009;361:849–57.

[65] Jacobs PC, Isgum I, Gondrie MJ, Mali WP, van Ginneken B, Prokop M, van der Graaf Y. Coronary artery calcification scoring in low-dose ungated CT screening for lung cancer: interscan agreement. Am J Roentgenol 2010;194:1244–9.

[66] Chiles C, Duan F, Gladish GW, Ravenel JG, Baginski SG, Snyder BS, DeMello S, Desjardins SS, Munden RF, Team NS. Association of Coronary Artery Calcification and Mortality in the National Lung Screening Trial: A Comparison of Three Scoring Methods. Radiology 2015;276:82–90.

[67] Chadashvili T, Litmanovich D, Hall F, Slanetz PJ. Do breast arterial calcifications on mammography predict elevated risk of coronary artery disease? Eur J Radiol 2016;85:1121–4.

[68] Margolies L, Salvatore M, Hecht HS, Kotkin S, Yip R, Baber U, Bishay V, Narula J, Yankelevitz D, Henschke C. Digital Mammography and Screening for Coronary Artery Disease. JACC Cardiovasc Imaging 2016;9(4):350–60.

[69] Iribarren C, Go AS, Tolstykh I, Sidney S, Johnston SC, Spring DB. Breast vascular calcification and risk of coronary heart disease, stroke, and heart failure. J Womens Health 2004;13:381–9. discussion 390-392.

[70] Hendriks EJ, de Jong PA, Beulens JW, Mali WP, van der Schouw YT, Beijerinck D. Medial arterial calcification: active reversible disease in human breast arteries. JACC Cardiovasc Imaging 2015;8:984–5.

[71] Ridker PM. A test in context: high-sensitivity C-reactive protein. J Am Col Cardiol 2016;67:712–23.

[72] Kaptoge S, Di Angelantonio E, Lowe G, Pepys MB, Thompson SG, Collins R, Danesh J. Emerging Risk Factors C. C-reactive protein concentration and risk of coronary heart disease, stroke, and mortality: an individual participant meta-analysis. Lancet 2010;375:132–40.

[73] Allin KH, Bojesen SE, Nordestgaard BG. Baseline C-reactive protein is associated with incident cancer and survival in patients with cancer. J Clin Oncol 2009;27:2217–24.

[74] Pearson TA, Mensah GA, Alexander RW, Anderson JL, Cannon RO, 3rd, Criqui M, Fadl YY, Fortmann SP, Hong Y, Myers GL, Rifai N, Smith SC, Jr., Taubert K, Tracy RP, Vinicor F, Centers for Disease C, Prevention and American Heart A. Markers of inflammation and cardiovascular disease: application to clinical and public health practice: a statement for healthcare professionals from the Centers for Disease Control and Prevention and the American Heart Association. Circulation. 2003;107:499–511.

[75] Ridker PM, Danielson E, Fonseca FA, Genest J, Gotto AM Jr, Kastelein JJ, Koenig W, Libby P, Lorenzatti AJ, MacFadyen JG, Nordestgaard BG, Shepherd J, Willerson JT, Glynn RJ. Rosuvastatin to prevent vascular events in men and women with elevated C-reactive protein. N Engl J Med 2008;359:2195–207.

[76] Braunwald E. Creating controversy where none exists: the important role of C-reactive protein in the CARE, AFCAPS/TexCAPS, PROVE IT, REVERSAL, A to Z, JUPITER, HEART PROTECTION, and ASCOT trials. Eur Heart J 2012;33:430–2.

[77] DeFilippis AP, Young R, Carrubba CJ, McEvoy JW, Budoff MJ, Blumenthal RS, Kronmal RA, McClelland RL, Nasir K, Blaha MJ. An analysis of calibration and discrimination among multiple cardiovascular risk scores in a modern multiethnic cohort. Ann Int Med 2015;162:266–75.

[78] Lorenz MW, Markus HS, Bots ML, Rosvall M, Sitzer M. Prediction of clinical cardiovascular events with carotid intima-media thickness: a systematic review and meta-analysis. Circulation 2007;115:459–67.

[79] Nambi V, Chambless L, Folsom AR, He M, Hu Y, Mosley T, Volcik K, Boerwinkle E, Ballantyne CM. Carotid intima-media thickness and presence or absence of plaque improves prediction of coronary heart disease risk: the ARIC (Atherosclerosis Risk In Communities) study. J Am Col Cardiol 2010;55:1600–7.

[80] Bots ML, Evans GW, Riley WA, Grobbee DE. Carotid intima-media thickness measurements in intervention studies: design options, progression rates, and sample size considerations: a point of view. Stroke 2003;34:2985–94.

[81] Engelen L, Ferreira I, Stehouwer CD, Boutouyrie P, Laurent S and Reference Values for Arterial Measurements C. Reference intervals for common carotid intima-media thickness measured with echotracking: relation with risk factors. Eur Heart J 2013;34:2368–2380.

[82] Touboul PJ, Hennerici MG, Meairs S, Adams H, Amarenco P, Bornstein N, Csiba L, Desvarieux M, Ebrahim S, Hernandez Hernandez R, Jaff M, Kownator S, Naqvi T, Prati P, Rundek T, Sitzer M, Schminke U, Tardif JC, Taylor A, Vicaut E, Woo KS. Mannheim carotid intima-media thickness and plaque consensus (2004-2006-2011). An update on behalf of the advisory board of the 3rd, 4th and 5th watching the risk symposia, at the 13th, 15th and 20th European Stroke Conferences, Mannheim, Germany, 2004, Brussels, Belgium, 2006, and Hamburg, Germany, 2011. Cerebrovasc Dis 2012;34:290-296.

[83] Dorth JA, Patel PR, Broadwater G, Brizel DM. Incidence and risk factors of significant carotid artery stenosis in asymptomatic survivors of head and neck cancer after radiotherapy. Head Neck 2014;36:215–9.

[84] Dorresteijn LD, Kappelle AC, Boogerd W, Klokman WJ, Balm AJ, Keus RB, van Leeuwen FE, Bartelink H. Increased risk of ischemic stroke after radiotherapy on the neck in patients younger than 60 years. J Clin Oncol 2002;20:282–8.

[85] Smith GL, Smith BD, Buchholz TA, Giordano SH, Garden AS, Woodward WA, Krumholz HM, Weber RS, Ang KK, Rosenthal DI. Cerebrovascular disease risk in older head and neck cancer patients after radiotherapy. J Clin Oncol 2008;26:5119–25.

[86] Xu J, Cao Y. Radiation-induced carotid artery stenosis: a comprehensive review of the literature. Interv Neurol 2014;2:183–92.

[87] Jacoby D, Hajj J, Javaheri A, deGoma E, Lin A, Ahn P, Quon H. Carotid intima-media thickness measurement promises to improve cardiovascular risk evaluation in head and neck cancer patients. Clin Cardiol 2015;38:280–4.

[88] Cheng SW, Wu LL, Ting AC, Lau H, Lam LK, Wei WI. Irradiation-induced extracranial carotid stenosis in patients with head and neck malignancies. Am J Surg 1999;178:323–8.

[89] Chang YJ, Chang TC, Lee TH, Ryu SJ. Predictors of carotid artery stenosis after radiotherapy for head and neck cancers. J Vasc Surg 2009;50:280–5.

[90] Muzaffar K, Collins SL, Labropoulos N, Baker WH. A prospective study of the effects of irradiation on the carotid artery. Laryngoscope 2000;110:1811–4.

[91] Cheng SW, Ting AC, Lam LK, Wei WI. Carotid stenosis after radiotherapy for nasopharyngeal carcinoma. Arch Otolaryngol Head Neck Surg 2000;126:517–21.

[92] Halak M, Fajer S, Ben-Meir H, Loberman Z, Weller B, Karmeli R. Neck irradiation: a risk factor for occlusive carotid artery disease. Eur J Vasc Endovasc Surg 2002;23:299–302.

[93] Moutardier V, Christophe M, Lelong B, Houvenaeghel G, Delpero JR. Iliac atherosclerotic occlusive disease complicating radiation therapy for cervix cancer: a case series. Gynecol Oncol 2002;84:456–9.

[94] Levenback C, Burke TW, Rubin SC, Curtin JP, Wharton JT. Arterial occlusion complicating treatment of gynecologic cancer: a case series. Gynecol Oncol 1996;63:40–6.

[95] Jurado JA, Bashir R, Burket MW. Radiation-induced peripheral artery disease. Catheter Cardiovasc Interv 2008;72:563–8.

[96] Aboyans V, Criqui MH, Abraham P, Allison MA, Creager MA, Diehm C, Fowkes FG, Hiatt WR, Jonsson B, Lacroix P, Marin B, McDermott MM, Norgren L, Pande RL, Preux PM, Stoffers HE, Treat-Jacobson D, American Heart Association Council on Peripheral Vascular D, Council on E, Prevention, Council on Clinical C, Council on Cardiovascular N, Council on Cardiovascular R, Intervention, Council on Cardiovascular S and Anesthesia. Measurement and interpretation of the ankle-brachial index: a scientific statement from the American Heart Association. Circulation. 2012;126:2890–2909.

[97] Fowkes FG, Murray GD, Butcher I, Heald CL, Lee RJ, Chambless LE, Folsom AR, Hirsch AT, Dramaix M, deBacker G, Wautrecht JC, Kornitzer M, Newman AB, Cushman M, Sutton-Tyrrell K, Fowkes FG, Lee AJ, Price JF, d'Agostino RB, Murabito JM, Norman PE, Jamrozik K, Curb JD, Masaki KH, Rodriguez BL, Dekker JM, Bouter LM, Heine RJ, Nijpels G, Stehouwer CD, Ferrucci L, McDermott MM, Stoffers HE, Hooi JD, Knottnerus JA, Ogren M, Hedblad B, Witteman JC, Breteler MM, Hunink MG, Hofman A, Criqui MH, Langer RD, Fronek A, Hiatt WR, Hamman R, Resnick HE, Guralnik J, McDermott MM. Ankle Brachial Index C. Ankle brachial index combined with Framingham Risk Score to predict cardiovascular events and mortality: a meta-analysis. JAMA 2008;300:197–208.

[98] Criqui MH, McClelland RL, McDermott MM, Allison MA, Blumenthal RS, Aboyans V, Ix JH, Burke GL, Liu K, Shea S. The ankle-brachial index and incident cardiovascular events in the MESA (Multi-Ethnic Study of Atherosclerosis). J Am Coll Cardiol 2010;56:1506–12.

Chapter 17

Hypertension and Cancer

D. Geft and A. Hage
Cedars-Sinai Heart Institute, Los Angeles, CA, United States

INTRODUCTION

Cardiovascular disease remains the most common cause of death and disability in developed countries. Hypertension (HTN) is one of the most important modifiable risk factors for cardiovascular disease and it affects approximately 50 million people in the United States and approximately 1 billion people worldwide [1]. In clinical trials, antihypertensive therapy has been shown to decrease risk of stroke, myocardial infarction, and heart failure significantly [2]. The relationship between HTN and cancer is well known and it has become of greater interest and importance over time with the introduction of newer chemotherapeutic agents and their associated improved survival. HTN has been reported to be the most common comorbidity in patients with malignancy [3]. The prevalence of HTN in cancer patients is similar to that of the general population, however a much higher rate is observed once cancer therapies are initiated [4]. In addition to being affected by common factors that cause HTN, cancer patients are affected by the type of cancer, chemotherapy, and radiation therapy. A keen understanding of the mechanisms behind the development or worsening of HTN in cancer patients, whether related to the type of cancer (i.e., catecholamine secreting endocrine tumors) or type of chemotherapy, is crucial, as this helps to guide treatment of HTN. Early diagnosis and treatment of high blood pressure (BP) in cancer patients is extremely important as uncontrolled HTN can lead to cancer treatment limitation or discontinuation, chemo-induced cardiotoxicity, and even life-threatening events [5]. In this chapter we will review briefly epidemiology, pathophysiology, diagnosis, and treatment of HTN in cancer patients.

EPIDEMIOLOGY

The prevalence of HTN in cancer patients is similar to that of the general population (28–29%) [6]. The incidence and severity of new-onset HTN depends upon the type of cancer as well as the type, dose, and duration of chemotherapy.

A large retrospective cohort study demonstrated a prevalence of new-onset HTN in one-third of cancer patients with various types of solid tumors. Patients with gastric or ovarian cancer experienced the highest incidences of severe [defined as systolic blood pressure (SBP) >160–180 or diastolic blood pressure (DBP) >110–120 mmHg] or crisis level (SBP > 180 or DBP > 120 mmHg) HTN, respectively. Patients with renal cell carcinoma had the highest incidence of moderate HTN (SBP > 150–160 mmHg or DBP > 100–110 mmHg), whereas patients with breast cancer and malignant melanoma had the lowest incidences of HTN across all severity levels. Chemotherapy use appeared to be associated with a 2–3.5-fold increased risk of HTN [7].

Different classes of chemotherapeutic agents carry varying risks of developing HTN. HTN is the most common cardiovascular toxicity associated with vascular signaling pathway (VSP) inhibitors. The first clinically available VSP inhibitor, Bevacizumab, was approved in 2004 for the treatment of colon cancer. It is a monoclonal antibody targeted against soluble vascular endothelial growth factor (VEGF) protein. Clinical trials have shown an incidence of Bevacizumab-induced HTN of 28% [8]. Following Bevacizumab, several newer VSP inhibitors have been introduced such as the small receptor tyrosine kinase inhibitors (TKIs, i.e., Sunitinib, Sorafenib, Pazopanib), which are also associated with a high incidence of HTN. Meta-analysis have shown an incidence of HTN of 19–25% among VSP inhibitors overall, but there appears to be a higher incidence with the TKIs [9]. Robinson et al. demonstrated that in women treated with the TKI, Cediranib, 87% had HTN by the end of the study [10]. Almost 100% of patients treated with VSP inhibitors have an absolute increase in BP although only a subset develop true HTN [11]. BP rise is rapid in most cases, hence the need to monitor it weekly during the first cycle of chemotherapy and then every 2–3 weeks thereafter.

Alkylating agents, such as cyclophosphamide, ifosfamide, cisplatin, and busulfan are associated with a 36% incidence of HTN. There is a reported 28–80% incidence of

HTN with Mycophenolate Mofetil, depending on the dosing and an 8–9% incidence with DNA methylating agents [12]. Unpublished ongoing trials with dual mechanistic target of rapamycin (mTOR) and phosphatidyl-inositol 3 kinase (PI3K) inhibitors have been reported to elicit a rapid and significant acute rise in blood pressure during drug infusion but the incidence of HTN is not yet known.

It is likely, however, that meta-analysis of cancer trials where the incidence of HTN has been studied probably underestimate its true incidence in actual clinical practice, since patients in the general population may have comorbidities, such as diabetes, advanced age, preexisting HTN, or other cardiovascular risk factors; such patients may have been excluded from clinical trials. Dosing and drug interactions may also contribute to the development of HTN.

Interestingly, certain chemotherapeutic drugs may not directly cause HTN but the drug exposure in the setting of preexisting HTN may increase the risk of other cardiotoxicities. For example, trastuzumab therapy for HER2+ breast cancer increases the risk of developing cardiomyopathy in patients with concurrent HTN [13].

While the focus is typically on the development or exacerbation of HTN after the diagnosis of cancer and initiation of therapy, there are some reports linking the development of cancer to underlying HTN or its treatment. A large Swedish study found that HTN is associated with an increased risk for cancer death and that in men, the presence of HTN is associated with an increased risk of developing cancer [14]. A study by Li et al. showed a potential link between calcium channel blockers (CCB) and breast cancer. Their retrospective analysis showed a 2.5 times increase in invasive breast cancer among postmenopausal women who had been taking CCB for 10 or more years [15]. This relationship did not vary by type of calcium channel blocker used (short-acting vs. long-acting, dihydropyridines vs. nondihydropyridines). This study did not see an associated risk of cancer with diuretics, beta blockers (BB), or angiotensin II antagonists, which would support the notion that the cancer risk was drug-related rather than attributable to the presence of HTN or comorbidities. Other selected studies, however, have suggested an increase in cancer risk from angiotensin receptor blockers (ARB) although a meta-analysis of 15 trials did not support this [16]. Previous studies have yielded mixed findings on the association between HTN and cancer. At this point it is unknown whether the increased cancer risk in hypertensive patients is attributable to specific antihypertensive therapies, the HTN itself, or the underlying social, behavioral, and genetic characteristics that contribute to HTN which might also predispose to the development of cancer. Pending additional evidence, there are no recommendations regarding antihypertensive medications and possible cancer risk.

DIAGNOSIS

The diagnosis and threshold for medical treatment of HTN has typically followed the recommendations of the Joint National Commission 7 (JNC 7) BP cutoff for the diagnosis of HTN, which is 140/90 mmHg [1]. In diabetics or patients with chronic kidney disease (CKD), the treatment goal is a BP < 130/80 mmHg. More recently in 2014, the JNC 8 published a new set of recommendations with the primary difference being a threshold of 150/90 mmHg for the diagnosis of HTN in patients greater than 60 years old [17]. In addition, they changed the treatment goal for diabetics and patients with CKD to 140/90 mmHg. There is still a good deal of controversy regarding these new recommendations as they have not been universally accepted [18].

There are no specific guidelines addressing optimal BP cut-offs or specific antihypertensive medication use recommendations specifically in cancer patients. In general, HTN guidelines can be followed. It should be noted that to diagnose HTN, BP must be measured on three separate occasions, at least 1 week apart [1]. Baseline BP should be established prior to initiating chemotherapy and weekly BP monitoring should occur during the first cycle (followed by every 2–3 weeks if the therapy is known to be associated with developing or exacerbating HTN) [19]. Patients can be taught to measure BP at home on their own with appropriate sized BP cuff and should alert their physicians to any significant changes in BP. It is not only the absolute number that is of concern but also a sudden rise in BP after initiation of cancer therapy that must be identified and treated early.

PATHOPHYSIOLOGY

Multiple mechanisms have been implicated in the development of HTN in cancer patients. Some are related to cancer treatment and some related to the cancers themselves. These include endothelial dysfunction associated with reduced nitric oxide bioavailability, increased endothelin production, increased sympathetic nervous system activity, increased vascular sensitivity to circulating vasoactive compounds, overproduction of sodium-retaining hormones, and vasoconstrictors, such as endothelin-1 and angiotensin II, psychosocial stress, renal thrombotic microangiopathy with secondary glomerular structural and functional changes, vascular rarefaction, and alterations in expression of kallikrein–kinin system [12,20].

CHEMOTHERAPY-INDUCED HTN

Although HTN is associated with many chemotherapeutic agents, much emphasis has been placed on VSP inhibitors. A number of mechanisms have been proposed to explain VSP inhibitor-induced HTN. Activation of the VEGFR-2 by

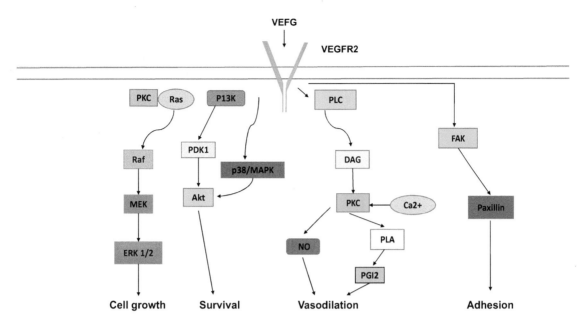

FIGURE 17.1 **VEGF Signaling in Endothelial Cells.** VEGF signaling in vascular endothelium is implicated in various pathways related to cell growth/ hypertrophy, survival, vasodilation, migration, and adhesion. Akt, serine/threonine kinase or protein kinase B; DAG, diacylglycerol; ERK, extracellular signal regulated kinases; FAK, focal adhesion kinase; MEK, mitogen activated protein kinase; NO, nitric oxide; PI3K, Phosphatidylinositol 3-kinase; PKC, protein kinase C; PLA, phospholipase A2; PGI2, prostaglandin I2; PLC, phospholipase C; p38/MAPK, mitogen activated protein kinase.

VEGF induces expression of nitric oxide synthase in endothelial cells, which promotes vascular permeability and vasodilation [21]. Inhibiting this pathway, therefore, decreases nitric oxide production and vasodilation, leading to HTN (Fig. 17.1). In support this concept, the use of VEGF agonists to promote angiogenesis in models of ischemic cardiomyopathy were associated with hypotension [22]. In addition, Endothelin-1, a potent vasoconstrictor, is also implicated in the mechanism of VSP-mediated HTN [23]. VEGF signaling also plays an important role in maintaining endothelial cell viability and structure. Inhibition of VEGF leads to endothelial cell apoptosis and chronic remodeling of the capillary beds, a process known as rarefaction [24]. Mourad et al. demonstrated a significant decrease in dermal capillary density as well as a decreased capillary dilatory response in human subjects receiving VSP inhibitor therapy, implicating both a functional and anatomic effect on blood vessels [25]. Importantly, decreased capillary density was reversible, along with the associated HTN, after cessation of VSP inhibitor treatment [26]. Capillary rarefaction occurs in the heart as well and may be a contributor to VSP-associated cardiomyopathy.

HTN can occur within the first 24 h of VSP inhibitor administration but more commonly will develop over the first few weeks. BP usually returns to normal after cessation of the chemotherapeutic agent. Interestingly, HTN has even been used as a biologic marker of clinical efficacy of these cancer drugs. A retrospective analysis by Rini et al. of 5000 renal cell carcinoma patients showed that sunitinib-associated HTN was significantly and independently associated with improved survival (30.9 vs. 7.2 months median survival). Importantly, treating the high BP in those patients to normotensive levels did not detract from these positive outcomes [27].

Alkylating agents, such as cyclophosphamide and ifosfamide are also associated with a relatively high rate of HTN as well as other cardiotoxicities. The mechanism is believed to be related to disruption of endothelial function and chronic toxicity causing renal endothelial damage leading to HTN and microalbuminemia [28].

Several mechanisms have been suggested through which calcineurin inhibitors (such as cyclosporine and tacrolimus) cause HTN including increased sympathetic activity, increased renal proximal tubular resorption, altered synthesis of vasodilating prostaglandins, direct vascular effects, and nephrotoxicity leading to fluid retention [29]. Cyclosporine-induced new-onset HTN incidence is between 11% and 80% depending on the dose and duration of therapy [30]; preexisting HTN, creatinine >2, and maintenance therapy with steroids increase the risk of cyclosporine-induced HTN [31]. The incidence of cyclosporine-induced HTN is particularly elevated in patients undergoing bone marrow transplantation (57%) [32], and is unrelated to age, sex, or race [33]. Tacrolimus, a related calcineurin inhibitor, causes HTN less often than cyclosporine and in some cases, switching from cyclosporine to tacrolimus can resolve the HTN, at least initially [29]. In addition, tacrolimus-induced HTN can often be successfully treated with only a single antihypertensive agent.

STEROID-INDUCED HTN

Steroids are commonly used as part of chemotherapeutic regimens for many different malignancies. The incidence of steroid-induced HTN is about 20% [34]. It is also dose-dependent and occurs more frequently in the elderly and in patients with a family history of HTN. Several mechanisms are involved including increased vascular sensitivity to vasoconstrictors, such as catecholamines, vasopressin or angiotensin II, suppression of vasodilatory systems such as nitric oxide synthase, prostacyclin and kinin–kallikrein systems, activation of mineralcorticoid receptors, increased conversion of glucocorticoids to mineralcorticoids (i.e., licorice candy), and volume and sodium retention [35].

ERYTHROPOIETIN-INDUCED HTN

Anemia is very common in cancer patients, especially with chronic renal insufficiency, and recombinant human erythropoietin (Epo) is often used for treatment of anemia. HTN is the most common side effect of Epo, occurring in 20–30% of patients. The mechanisms involved in Epo-induced HTN are not clear. Vaziri et al. suggest a number of potential mechanisms including alterations in the production of endogenous vasopressors, decreased responsiveness to vasodilatory agents, arterial remodeling by the stimulatory effects of vascular cell growth, and increased viscosity [36]. HTN associated with Epo is usually mild but case reports of hypertensive crisis, including encephalopathy, have been reported [37]. HTN appears to be dose dependent and may become evident 2 weeks to 4 months after initiation of treatment. Risk factors for Epo-induced HTN include preexisting HTN, a low baseline hematocrit with rapid rise, and intravenous administration of Epo [38].

As mentioned earlier, ongoing clinical trials of dual mTOR kinase/PI3K inhibitors have identified HTN as a possible side effect (Not yet published, personal communication with principal investigator Monica Mita, M.D.). The mechanism of HTN caused by these agents is not yet clear. Patients should have controlled BP prior to starting the medication and routine BP surveillance while taking the medication as some patients have experienced rapid and sharp rises in BP with symptoms even after the first dose.

NONPHARMACOLOGIC THERAPY INDUCED HTN

In addition to chemotherapy, surgery, or radiation therapy involving the head and neck can lead to baroreflex failure causing difficult-to-treat and labile HTN [39]. Volatile HTN is the most common presentation of baroreflex failure. It can develop insidiously or present as hypertensive crises in which BP surges occur lasting minutes to hours, accompanied by tachycardia, diffuse sweating, palpitations, lightheadedness,

and severe headaches. SBP is often > 250 mmHg and can exceed 300 mmHg. BP surges are often triggered by mental or physical stress. These emergencies must be treated immediately. Labile HTN can be extremely difficult to manage and medications, such as clonidine, which are not typically first-line agents for routine HTN, are recommended in this case. Referring the patient to a specialist can help with complicated HTN management.

TUMOR-RELATED HTN

As mentioned earlier, certain types of tumors may be associated with developing HTN. This may in part be related to the type of cancer, its associated risk factors (i.e., kidney disease) and rate of progression but it appears to primarily relate to the specific type and dosing of chemotherapy used. There are a few tumors however, namely, endocrine tumors, that directly lead to HTN through production of vasoactive compounds. Pheochromocytomas and sympathetic/parasympathetic paragangliomas are tumors that synthesize and secrete epinephrine (Epi), norepinephrine (NE), and dopamine (DA) [40]. They are found in 0.2–0.6% of people with HTN [41]. HTN is the most common sign of pheochromocytoma, occurring in approximately 90% of patients [42]. It can occur in a sustained (50%) or paroxysmal (45%) pattern. Sustained HTN occurs more in predominantly NE producing tumors while paroxysmal HTN with Epi producing tumors, which are highly typical for MEN2-related pheochromocytomas. Tumors predominantly producing dopamine often are normotensive [43].

Another well-known endocrine tumor causing HTN is Cushing's syndrome, a syndrome of glucocorticoid excess from either corticotropin-releasing hormone (CRH)/adrenocorticotropic hormone (ACTH) producing tumors or cortisol producing tumors. HTN occurs in approximately 80% of Cushing's patients and 95% of patients with ectopic Cushing's [44]. Interestingly, it is often associated with a loss of the normal sleep-related decrease in blood pressure. The mechanisms of hypercortisolemia-induced HTN include mineralcorticoid effects of cortisol (decreased conversion of cortisol to cortisone), activation of the renin angiotensin system, RAS (upregulation of central and peripheral angiotensin II receptors), and action of cortisol on peripheral and systemic vasculature (decreased production of nitric oxide synthase and increased vascular sensitivity to catecholamines) [45].

Primary hyperaldosteronism is another tumor-related cause of HTN due to excess production of aldosterone, typically from adrenal adenomas but other causes exist as well. The BP is often substantially elevated (160–180 mmHg systolic) and hypokalemia may or may not be present [46]. These patients also tend to have greater left ventricular mass measurements compared with age matched hypertensive patients [47]. One retrospective study showed they may also have significantly higher rates of stroke, myocardial infarction, and atrial fibrillation [48].

MANAGEMENT AND TREATMENT

In the past eras, when life expectancy from cancer was short and prognosis poor, there was little concern for controlling risk factors, such as HTN. Nowadays, with the evolution of newer therapies improving survival and overall prognosis, there is an emphasis on treating HTN as it has been shown that controlling comorbidities like HTN can improve survival and reduce chemotherapy-related complications. It has also been shown that the burden of comorbidities may be as important as tumor stage to overall prognosis [49]. The goal, therefore, of controlling HTN in cancer patients is to reduce morbidity, end-organ damage and mortality, and to improve their ability to tolerate intended doses and duration of cancer therapy. In general, BP should be optimally controlled prior to starting a chemotherapeutic agent and close monitoring should be implemented along with appropriate antihypertensive medication adjustments for adequate BP control. If done properly, it is very unlikely that a cancer therapy will need to be discontinued due to HTN.

In 2010, a panel of experts from the Investigational Drug Steering Committee of the National Cancer Institute published its recommendations to optimize risk stratification, BP monitoring, and safe administration of new chemotherapeutic agents. In general, treatment of HTN in cancer patients should follow the same recommendations as for the general public as guided by the JNC 7 or 8. The choice of antihypertensive, however, should take into account the mechanism of HTN, the possibility of drug–drug interactions and any other comorbidities that would carry a compelling indication to use a specific BP medication. When patients are already on an antihypertensive prior to chemotherapy, it should be noted that the dose may require an adjustment due to weight loss that can occur during chemotherapy. Furthermore, patients who are on medications, such as ACE-I prior to chemotherapy should have their renal function and potassium monitored due to fluid and electrolyte shifts that can occur due to cancer treatment.

There are no randomized trials comparing various antihypertensive medications specifically in cancer patients. There is published data, however, suggesting that CCB and ACE inhibitors (ACEI) or ARB are effective in controlling VEGF inhibitor-induced HTN [50]. BB and diuretics appear to be safe as well. Nondihydropyridine CCBs (diltiazem and verapamil) should be avoided in patients taking TKIs, such as sunitinib and sorafenib because of the formers' inhibition of the CYP3A4 system, by which the TKIs are metabolized. Caution is also advised for the use of one of the dihydropyridine CCBs—nifedipine—which can induce VEGF secretion [51]. It is important to remember that HTN induced by VSP inhibitors can be reversible once the chemotherapy is stopped and the return to baseline BP is usually within the same time frame as it took to develop HTN from the chemotherapy [52]. Calcineurin inhibitors (cyclosporine and tacrolimus) affect intracellular calcium and therefore CCBs have been used successfully to treat cyclosporine-induced HTN [53]. One must be cautious, however, because CCBs, such as diltiazem can elevate calcineurin inhibitor levels. Isradipine (a CCB) has been shown to prevent cyclosporine-induced HTN when administered prior to initiating cyclosporine. ACEIs have also proven effective at controlling BP in patients on calcineurin inhibitors, however there is some reluctance given the potential nephrotoxic effects of calcineurin inhibitors [54]. One must also watch closely for hyperkalemia when using ACEI, ARB, or potassium-sparing diuretics in these patients. ARBs, such as losartan have been shown to be effective at treating HTN caused by Mycophenolate Mofetil [55]. Treating steroid-induced HTN involves fluid and sodium restriction. Diuretics appear to be the antihypertensives of choice but ACEI or mineralcorticoid receptor antagonists have also been shown to be beneficial. Ofcourse, discontinuation of steroids is the best treatment. For baroreflex failure, clonidine should be considered. In management and treatment of HTN, race, ethnicity, and comorbidities should be taken into account as with noncancer patients. For example, BB and ACEI in patients with heart failure, ACEI, or ARB in diabetics or patients with CKD, and thiazide diuretics or CCB in African Americans [17].

For endocrine tumors causing HTN, treatment is often a combination of both medical and surgical approaches. In pheochromocytomas, the ultimate treatment is surgical removal of the tumor; however, it is essential that good BP control is achieved prior to surgery. Phenoxybenzamine is a nonselective alpha-1 and alpha-2 blocker that reduces BP fluctuations, easing vasoconstriction, and helping to prevent intraoperative hypertensive crises in cases where large amounts of catecholamines can be released into circulation with tumor manipulation [56]. Alpha-1 blockers, such as prazosin or terazosin have been used as well and are shorter-acting which may help lessen postoperative hypotension. CCBs and BBs can be helpful to help prevent reflex tachycardia caused by phenoxybenzamine [57]. It is crucial, however, that beta-blockade only be used subsequent to alpha-blockade because unopposed beta-blockade can result in a significant rise in BP.

Definitive therapy for a Cushing's tumor-related HTN is surgical excision of the ACTH- or cortisol-secreting tumor. Postoperative levels of cortisol provide good prognostic information regarding surgical outcomes. BP control is difficult without control of hypercortisolemia. ACEI or ARBs are preferred drugs given the upregulation of RAS, and addition of CCB or BB may be helpful for optimal BP control. Nearly one-third, however, have persistent HTN requiring long term antihypertensive medications even after achieving eucortisolemia [58].

For primary hyperaldosteronism secondary to unilateral adrenal adenoma or hyperplasia, unilateral adrenalectomy is the treatment of choice over medical therapy. For bilateral disease, medical therapy is recommended and the treatment of choice for HTN is a mineralcorticoid receptor antagonist (spironolactone or eplerenone) [59]. One randomized trial, however, did show a more profound antihypertensive effect in DBP with spironolactone compared to eplerenone [60]. For those who do not tolerate these medications, a potassium-sparing diuretic, such as Amiloride is recommended. If HTN still persists, a thiazide diuretic or ACEI can be used.

CONCLUSIONS

The prevalence of new-onset HTN or worsening underlying HTN is quite high in cancer patients, primarily due to the highly effective chemotherapeutic agents used today. Timely diagnosis and initiation of appropriate therapy for HTN in cancer patients is extremely important to avoid premature discontinuation of much needed chemotherapy and serious adverse cardiovascular events.

REFERENCES

[1] Chobanian AV, Bakris GL, Black HR, et al. Seventh report of the Joint National Committee on Prevention, Detection, Evaluation, and Treatment of High Blood Pressure. Hypertension 2003;42:1206–52.

[2] Neal B, MacMahon S, Chapman N. Effects of ACE inhibitors, calcium antagonists, and other blood-pressure-lowering drugs: Results of prospectively designed overviews of randomized trials. Blood Pressure Lowering Treatment Trialists' Collaboration. Lancet 2000;356:1955–64.

[3] Piccirillo JF, Tierney RM, Costas I, Grove L, Spitznagel EL Jr. Prognostic importance of comorbidity in a hospital-based cancer registry. JAMA 2004;291(20):2441–7.

[4] Maitland ML, Bakris GL, Black HR, Chen HX, Durand J-B, Elliott WJ, et al. Cardiovascular Toxicities Panel, convened by the Angiogenesis Task Force of the National Cancer Institute Investigational Drug Steering Committee. Initial assessment, surveillance, and management of blood pressure in patients receiving vascular endothelial growth factor signaling pathway inhibitors. J Natl Cancer Inst 2010;102(9):596–604.

[5] Chu TF, Rupnick MA, Kerkela R, et al. Cardiotoxicity associated with tyrosine kinase inhibitor sunitinib. Lancet 2007;370:2011–9.

[6] Brookes L. National Health and Nutrition Examination Survey(NHANES) data on hypertension. In: American Society of Hypertension 18th Annual Scientific Session. 2003.

[7] Fraeman K, Nordstrom B, Luo W, Landis S, Shantakumar S. Incidence of New-Onset Hypertension in Cancer Patients: A Retrospective Cohort Study. Int J Hypertens 2013;2013:10.

[8] Kabbinavar F, et al. Phase II randomized trial comparing bevacizumab plus fluorouracil (FU)/leucovorin (LV) with FU/LV alone in patients with metastatic colorectal cancer. J Clin Oncol 2003;21:60–5.

[9] Wu S, et al. Incidence and risk of hypertension with sorafenib in patients with cancer: a systematic review and meta-analysis. Lancet Oncol 2008;9:117–23.

[10] Robinson, et al. Hypertension induced by vascular endothelial growth factor signaling pathway inhibition: mechanisms and potential use as a biomarker. Semin Nephrol 2010;30:591–601.

[11] Maitland ML, et al. Ambulatory monitoring detects sorafenib-induced blood pressure elevations on the first day of treatment. Clin Cancer Res 2009;15:6250–7.

[12] ABi Aad S, Pierce M, Barmaimon G, Farhat F, Benjo A, Mouhayar E. Hypertension induced by chemotherapeutic and immunosuppressive agents: A new challenge. Crit Rev Oncol Hematol 2015;93: 28–35.

[13] Jahanzeb M. Adjuvant Trastuzumab therapy for HER2-positive breast cancer. Clin Breast Cancer 2008;8(4):324–33.

[14] Stocks T, Van Hemelrijck M, Manjer J, Bjørge T, Ulmer H, Hallmans G, Lindkvist B, Selmer R, Nagel G, Tretli S, Concin H, Engeland A, Jonsson H, Stattin P. Blood pressure and risk of cancer incidence and mortality in the metabolic syndrome and cancer project. Hypertension 2012;59:802–10.

[15] Li CI, Daling JR, Tang M-TC, Haugen KL, Parter PL, Malone KE. Use of antihypertensive medications and breast cancer risk among women aged 55 to 74 years. JAMA Intern Med 2013;173(17): 1629–37.

[16] ARB Trialists Collaboration. Effects of telmisartan, irbesartan, valsartan, candesartan, and losartan on cancers in 15 trials enrolling 138,769 individuals. J Hypertens 2011;29(4):623–35.

[17] James PA, Oparil S, Carter BL, et al. 2014 evidence-based guideline for the management of high blood pressure in adults: report from the panel members appointed to the Eighth Joint National Committee (JNC 8). JAMA 2013;311:507–20.

[18] Krakoff, et al. 2014 Hypertension recommendations from the eighth Joint National Committee Panel Members raise concerns for elderly black and female populations. J Am Coll Cardiol 2014;64: 394–402.

[19] Maitland ML, Bakris GL, Black HR, et al. Initial assessment, surveillance, and management of blood pressure in patients receiving vascular endothelial growth factor signaling pathway inhibitors. J Natl Cancer Inst 2010;102:596–604.

[20] Oparil S, Zaman MA, Calhoun DA. Pathogenesis of hypertension. Ann Intern Med 2003;139:761–76.

[21] Olsson AK, et al. VEGF receptor signaling in control of vascular function. Nat Rev Mol Cell Biol 2006;7:359–71.

[22] Henry TD, et al. The VIVA trial: vascular endothelial growth factor in ischemia for vascular angiogenesis. Circulation 2003;107:1359–65.

[23] Kappers MH, et al. Hypertension induced by the tyrosine kinase inhibitor sunitinib is associated with increased circulating endothelin-1 levels. Hypertension 2010;56:675–81.

[24] Baffert F, et al. Cellular changes in normal blood capillaries undergoing regression after inhibition of VEGF signaling. Am J Physiol Heart Circ Physiol 2006;290:H547–59.

[25] Mourad J-J, et al. Blood pressure rise following angiogenesis inhibition by bevacizumab. A crucial role for microcirculation. Ann Oncol 2008;19:927–34.

[26] Steeghs N, et al. Reversibility of capillary density after discontinuation of bevacizumab treatment. Ann Oncol 2010;21:1100–5.

[27] Rini BI, Cohen DP, Lu DR, et al. Hypertension as a biomarker of efficacy in patients with metastatic renal cell carcinoma treated with sunitinib. J Natl Cancer Inst 2011;103:763–73.

[28] Daher IN, Yeh ET. Vascular complications of selected cancer therapies. Nat Clin Pract Cardiovasc Med 2008;5:797–805.

[29] Morales JM, Andres A, Rengel M, Rodicio JL. Influence of cyclosporin, tacrolimus and rapamycin on renal function and arterial hypertension after renal transplantation. Nephrol Dial Transplant 2001;16(Suppl. 1):121–4.

[30] Deray G, Benhmida M, Le Hoang P, et al. Renal function and blood pressure in patients receiving long-term, low-dose cyclosporine therapy for idiopathic autoimmune uveitis. Ann Intern Med 1992;117:578–83.

[31] Ponticelli C, Montagnino G, Aroldi A, Angelini C, Braga M, Tarantino A. Hypertension after renal transplantation. Am J Kidney Dis 1993;21:73–8.

[32] Loughran TP Jr, Deeg HJ, Dahlberg S, Kennedy MS, Storb R, Thomas ED. Incidence of hypertension after marrow transplantation among 112 patients randomized to either cyclosporine or methotrexate as graft-versus-host disease prophylaxis. Br J Haematol 1985;59:547–53.

[33] Grossman E, Messerli FH. Secondary hypertension: interfering substances. J Clin Hypertens (Greenwich) 2008;10:556–66.

[34] Grossman EMF. Management of drug-induced and iatrogenic hypertension. 3rd ed. Hypertension primer. Dallas, TX: Lippincott Williams & Wilkins; 2003. p. 516–519.

[35] Kelly JJ, Tam SH, Williamson PM, et al. The nitric oxide system and cortisol induced hypertension in humans. Clin Exp Pharmacol Physiol 1988;25:945–6.

[36] Vaziri ND. Mechanism of erythropoietin-induced hypertension. Am J Kidney Dis 1999;33:821–8.

[37] Novak BL, Force RW, Mumford BT, Solbrig RM. Erythropoietin-induced hypertensive urgency in a patient with chronic renalinsufficiency: case report and review of the literature. Pharmacotherapy 2003;23:265–9.

[38] Luft FC. Erythropoietin and arterial hypertension. Clin Nephrol 2000;53:S61–4.

[39] Ketch T, Biaggioni I, Robertson R, Robertson D. Four faces of baroreflex failure: hypertensive crisis, volatile hypertension, orthostatic tachycardia, and malignant vagotonia. Circulation 2002;105(21):2518–23.

[40] Zuber S, Kantorovich V, Pacak K. Hypertension in pheochromocytoma: characteristics and treatment. Endocrinol Metab Clin North Am. 2011;40(2):295–311.

[41] Omura M, Saito J, Yamaguchi K, et al. Prospective study on the prevalence of secondary hypertension among hypertensive patients visiting a general outpatient clinic in Japan. Hypertens Res 2004;27(3):193–202.

[42] Calhoun DA, Jones D, Textor S, et al. Resistant hypertension: diagnosis, evaluation, and treatment: a scientific statement from the American Heart Association Professional Education Committee of the Council for High Blood Pressure Research. Hypertension 2008;51(6):1403–19.

[43] Manger WM. An overview of pheochromocytoma. Ann N Y Acad Sci 2006;1073:1–20. Pheochromocytoma First International Symposium.

[44] Stewart PM, Walker BR, Holder F. II beta-hydroxysteroid dehydrogenase activity in Cushing's syndrome: explaining the mineralocorticoid excess state of the ectopic adrenocorticotropin syndrome. J Clin Endocrinol Metab 1995;80:3617–20.

[45] Singh Y, Narendra K, Menon AS. Endocrine hypertension—Cushing's syndrome. Indian J Endocrinol Metab 2011;15(Suppl. 4):S313–6.

[46] Zarifis J, Lip GY, Leatherdale B, Beevers G. Malignant hypertension in association with primary aldosteronism. Blood Press 1996;5(4):250.

[47] Shigematsu Y, Hamada M, Okayama H, Hara Y, Hayashi Y, Kodama K, Kohara K, Hiwada K. Left ventricular hypertrophy precedes other target-organ damage in primary aldosteronism. Hypertension 1997;29(3):723.

[48] Milliez P, Girerd X, Plouin PF, Blacher J, Safar ME, Mourad JJ. Evidence for an increased rate of cardiovascular events in patients with primary aldosteronism. J Am Coll Cardiol 2005;45(8):1243.

[49] Piccirillo JF, Tierney RM, Costas I, Grove L, Spitznagel EL Jr. Prognostic importance of comorbidity in a hospital-based cancer registry. JAMA 2004;291:2441–7.

[50] Copur MS, Obermiller A. An algorithm for the management of hypertension in the setting of vascular endothelial growth factor signaling inhibition. Clin Colorectal Cancer 2011;10:151–6.

[51] Izzedine H, Ederhy S, Goldwasser F, et al. Management of hypertension in angiogenesis inhibitor-treated patients. Ann Oncol 2009;20:807–15.

[52] Azizi, et al. Home blood pressure monitoring in patients receiving sunitinib. N Engl J Med 2008;358:95–7.

[53] Rodicio JL. Calcium antagonists and renal protection from cyclosporinenephrotoxicity: long-term trial in renal transplantation patients. J Cardiovasc Pharmacol 2000;35:S7–S11.

[54] Mourad G, Ribstein J, Mimran A. Converting-enzyme inhibitor versus calcium antagonist in cyclosporine-treated renal transplants. Kidney Int 1993;43:419–25.

[55] Fujihara CK, Noronha IL, Malheiros Antunes GR, de Oliveira IB, Zatz R. Combined mycophenolate mofetil and losartan therapy arrests established injury in the remnant kidney. J Am Soc Nephrol 2000;11:283–90.

[56] Ross E, Prichard B, Kaufman L, et al. Preoperative and operative management of patients with phaeochromocytoma. Br Med J 1967;1(5534):191–8.

[57] Tokioka H, Takahashi T, Kosogabe Y, et al. Use of diltiazem to control circulatory fluctuations during resection of a phaeochromocytoma. Br J Anaesth 1988;60(5):582–7.

[58] Sharma ST, Niemen LK. Cushing's syndrome: all variants, detection, and treatment. Endocrinol Metab Clin N Am 2011;40:379–91.

[59] Karagiannis A, Tziomalos K, Papageorgiou A, Kakafika AI, Pagourelias ED, Anagnostis P, Athyros VG, Mikhailidis DP. Spironolactone versus eplerenone for the treatment of idiopathic hyperaldosteronism. Expert Opin Pharmacother 2008;9(4):509.

[60] Parthasarathy HK, Ménard J, White WB, Young WF Jr, Williams GH, Williams B, Ruilope LM, McInnes GT, Connell JM, MacDonald TM. A double-blind, randomized study comparing the antihypertensive effect of eplerenone and spironolactone in patients with hypertension and evidence of primary aldosteronism. J Hypertens 2011;29(5):980–90.

Chapter 18

Pulmonary Hypertension and Cancer

D. Geft and A. Hage

Cedars-Sinai Heart Institute, Los Angeles, CA, United States

INTRODUCTION

Pulmonary hypertension (PH) can occur in the cancer patient for a variety of cardio-pulmonary reasons. While heart failure and parenchymal lung disease constitute the majority of the abnormalities which can lead to PH, pulmonary vascular disease (PVD), or pulmonary arterial hypertension (PAH) can be the main reason why the cancer patient develops PH.

PAH is characterized by an increased resistance of the distal vascular walls of the pulmonary arteries leading to vascular lumen narrowing, right ventricular failure, and death.

PH of any cause, whether related to PVD, pulmonary toxicity from chemotherapeutic agents or radiation therapy, infectious or neoplastic pulmonary etiologies or left heart disease, will in the long-term negatively affect the prognosis of the patient and needs to be rapidly diagnosed and appropriately treated.

For years PAH has been compared to cancer in view of its multiple clinical and anatomical similarities [1]. For example, they both have self-sufficiency in growth signals, insensitivity to growth inhibitors, evasion of apoptosis, limitless replicative potential, sustained angiogenesis, metabolic energetic modifications, and similar inflammatory responses [2]. It has been noted that PAH also shares many pathophysiological and molecular pathways with cancer including excess proliferation of smooth muscle cells (SMC) [3] and endothelial cells (EC) [4], impaired apoptosis similar to neoplasia, and many predisposing and disease-modifying abnormalities, including endothelial injury/dysfunction, bone morphogenetic protein receptor-2 gene mutations, decreased expression of the K^+ channel (Kv1.5), transcription factor activation [hypoxia-inducible factor-1 (HIF-1)], expression of surviving, and increased expression/activity of both serotonin transporters and platelet-derived growth factor receptors [2]. Together, these abnormalities create a cancer-like, proliferative, apoptosis-resistant phenotype.

In this chapter, we will not elaborate on the similarities between cancer and PAH, but rather on the definition, classification, mechanisms, diagnosis, and therapy of PH in the cancer patient.

DEFINITION OF PH

PH is defined as an increase in mean pulmonary arterial pressure (mPAP) ≥ 25 mmHg at rest as assessed by right heart catheterization (RHC) [5]. PAH refers to a group of PH patients characterized hemodynamically by the presence of precapillary PH, defined by a pulmonary artery wedge pressure (PAWP) ≤ 15 mmHg and a pulmonary vascular resistance (PVR) > 3 Wood units (WU) in the absence of other causes of precapillary PH, such as PH due to lung diseases, chronic thromboembolic PH (CTEPH) or other rare diseases [6]. A PAWP > 15 implies at least some component of PH related to post capillary processes, most commonly left heart disease. One of the most common problems in the diagnostic workup of patients with PH is the distinction between PAH and PH due to left heart failure with preserved ejection fraction (HFpEF). A normal PAWP at rest does not rule out the presence of HFpEF, a common confounding etiology of PH. Volume or exercise challenge during right heart catheterization may be useful to unmask the presence of left heart disease [5]. While the normal mPAP at rest is 14 ± 3 mmHg with an upper limit of normal of approximately 20 mmHg [7], the clinical significance of a mPAP between 21 and 24 mmHg is unclear.

CLASSIFICATION OF PULMONARY HYPERTENSION

The classification of PH was recently updated at the fifth world symposium held in Nice, France, and summarized in Table 18.1. Patients with cancer can have PH from any cause and may fit into any of the five groups. Multiple mechanisms are implicated in the development of PH in cancer patients and a single patient can have overlap between various mechanisms and PH groups. For example, a patient may have PAH (group 1) and develop cancer, or they may have cancer and be treated with chemotherapeutic agents, such as alkylating agents, radiation therapy, or undergo autologous or allogeneic hematopoietic stem cell transplantation and develop PVOD (pulmonary veno-occlusive disease) (WHO

TABLE 18.1 Comprehensive Clinical Classification of Pulmonary Hypertension

1. Pulmonary arterial hypertension

  1.1. Idiopathic
  1.2. Heritable
      1.2.1. BMPR2 mutation
      1.2.2. Other mutations
  1.3. Drugs and toxins induced
  1.4. Associated with:
      1.4.1. Connective tissue disease
      1.4.2. Human immunodeficiency virus (HIV) infection
      1.4.3. Portal hypertension
      1.4.4. Congenital heart disease
      1.4.5. Schistosomiasis

1′. Pulmonary veno-occlusive disease and/or pulmonary capillary haemangiomatosis

  1′.1. Idiopathic
  1′.2. Heritable
      1′.2.1. EIF2AK4 mutation
      1′.2.2. Other mutations
  1′.3. Drugs, toxins and radiation induced
  1′.4. Associated with:
      1′.4.1. Connective tissue disease
      1′.4.2. HIV infection

1″. Persistent pulmonary hypertension of the newborn

2. Pulmonary hypertension due to left heart disease

  2.1. Left ventricular systolic dysfunction
  2.2. Left ventricular diastolic dysfunction
  2.3. Valvular disease
  2.4. Congenital /acquired left heart inflow/outflow tract obstruction and congenital cardiomyopathies
  2.5. Congenital /acquired pulmonary veins stenosis

3. Pulmonary hypertension due to lung diseases and/or hypoxia

  3.1. Chronic obstructive pulmonary disease
  3.2. Interstitial lung disease
  3.3. Other pulmonary diseases with mixed restrictive and obstructive pattern
  3.4. Sleep-disordered breathing
  3.5. Alveolar hypoventilation disorders
  3.6. Chronic exposure to high altitude
  3.7. Developmental lung diseases

4. Chronic thromboembolic pulmonary hypertension and other pulmonary artery obstructions

  4.1. Chronic thromboembolic pulmonary hypertension
  4.2. Other pulmonary artery obstructions
      4.2.1. Angiosarcoma
      4.2.2. Other intravascular tumors
      4.2.3. Arteritis
      4.2.4. Congenital pulmonary arteries stenoses
      4.2.5. Parasites (hydatidosis)

5. Pulmonary hypertension with unclear and/or multifactorial mechanisms

  5.1. Haematological disorders: chronic haemolytic anaemia, myeloproliferative disorders, splenectomy
  5.2. Systemic disorders: sarcoidosis, pulmonary histiocytosis, lymphangioleiomyomatosis, neurofibromatosis
  5.3. Metabolic disorders: glycogen storage disease, Gaucher disease, thyroid disorders
  5.4. Others: pulmonary tumoral thrombothic microangiopathy, osing mediastinitis, chronic renal failure (with/without dialysis), segmental pulmonary hypertension

BMPR2 ¼ bone morphogenetic protein receptor, type 2; EIF2AK4 ¼ eukaryotic.translation initiation factor 2 alpha kinase 4; HIV ¼ human immunodeficiency virus.

Source: 2015 ESC/ERS Guidelines for the diagnosis and treatment of pulmonary hypertension. European Heart Journal 2016; 37(1), 67–119.

group 1). A patient may have diastolic dysfunction, coronary artery disease (CAD) or valvular heart disease and PH secondary to left heart disease (WHO group 2), then develop cancer which can worsen the PH via chemotherapy or even by local compression or obstruction of the pulmonary arteries (WHO group V), pulmonary veins (often referred to as pulmonary venous hypertension) or metastases to the lungs. They may also have lung disease, such as chronic obstructive pulmonary disease (COPD) related to smoking and develop PH (WHO group 3) as well as a lung cancer. Cancer patients may develop Group IV PH related to chronic thromboembolic disease either from true thrombi forming (prothrombotic state) or emboli of the tumors themselves. Patients with chronic myeloproliferative disorders, a heterogeneous group of diseases, may have precapillary PH mimicking group 1 PAH [8] (particularly in presence of hemolytic anemia).

Several reports in the literature have highlighted the development of PH in conditions, such as drug- or stem cell transplantation-related PVOD, portal hypertension, splenectomy, extramedullary hematopoiesis, or pulmonary leukemic infiltration [8]. Furthermore, increased levels of circulating megakaryocytes and thrombocytosis, which can be found in patients with myeloproliferative disorders, might cause pulmonary capillary obstruction and microthrombosis [8]. Interestingly, one patient with PH associated with myeloid metaplasia with concomitant thrombocytosis has been reported; correction of thrombocytosis by hydroxyurea led to improvement of PH in this patient [9]. Generally, however, PH developed in advanced stages of myeloproliferative disorders and chemotherapeutic treatment did not affect the course of PH [8].

Regarding extramedullary lymphoproliferative diseases, four cases of pulmonary intravascular lymphoma mimicking PAH have been reported [10]. However, these cases showed either abnormal radiological or laboratory findings at the time of PH diagnosis. Furthermore, tumor-related PH may also develop from heart and lung diseases due to paraneoplastic mechanisms or therapy (WHO group 2 or 3). With underlying neoplastic disease, development of PAH alongside PVOD has also been associated with administration of anti-neoplastic agents (WHO group 1). A well-recognized example documents treatment with the tyrosine kinase inhibitor dasatinib in patients with chronic myeloid leukemia, which may cause development of PAH in rare cases [11]. PAH has also been described after childhood cancer and leukemia [12]

CANCER AND PAH

Pulmonary arterial hypertension can develop acutely or insidiously as result of metastatic cancer or its complications, such as [13] pulmonary tumor thrombotic microangiopathy (PTTM). PTTM occurs in 1.4% of patients who die of cancer, and death is due to right heart strain and cardiorespiratory arrest. Unfortunately, PTTM is difficult to diagnose in

patients, as the rate of clinical decline is rapid, and patients typically die within hours to days of the first signs of pulmonary arterial hypertension. A number of proteins have been implicated as mediators in the development of PTTM. Vascular endothelial growth factor [14,15] and tissue factor [16] are expressed more frequently in cancer cells leading to PTTM than those with traditional tumor emboli. Platelet-derived growth factor (PDGF) is also expressed more frequently in PTTM-associated cancer cells [14] although the association may be more complex with PDGF overexpression also present in alveolar macrophages and PDGF receptor expression in the proliferating fibromuscular intimal cells [17]. Osteopontin has also been implicated, but the overexpression of these factors falls short of accounting fully for the pathogenesis of PTTM which remains to be elucidated.

Genetic mutations described both in cancer and PAH have been described, such as in Cowden syndrome [18], a difficult-to-recognize heritable cancer syndrome caused by a germline mutation in the phosphatase-and-tensin homolog deleted on the chromosome 10 (*PTEN*) gene. Heterozygous mutations in bone morphogenetic protein (BMP) receptor type 2 (BMPR2), a growth factor belonging to the transforming growth factor β superfamily, have been reported in ~70% of patients with hereditary PAH and in ~25% of patients with sporadic idiopathic PAH [19]. BMPs and their receptors play a role in cell growth control, even in cancers [18].

Downstream signaling of BMPR2 includes the PI3K-AKT-mTOR pathway, which, when activated, leads to cellular proliferation. This pathway is negatively regulated by *PTEN*, a major tumor-suppressor gene. *PTEN* mutations are responsible for many of the sporadic cancer syndromes, including CS [20]. They lead to uncontrolled cell growth and are associated with endothelial cell hyperproliferation and impaired vascular remodeling [21]. Recently, data from animal studies show a relationship between PTEN and cardiopulmonary vascular remodeling, as PTEN activation was shown to regulate cardiomyocyte hypertrophy and survival as well as pulmonary smooth muscle cell proliferation and survival [22].

Inactivation of PTEN, on the other hand, was associated with AKT-dependent upregulation of HIF-1α. It promoted medial smooth muscle cell hyperplasia, vascular remodeling, and histopathology consistent with PH through increased HIF-1α-mediated production of SDF-1α and recruitment of hematopoietic progenitor cells to the vasculature [20,21].

PH can also be caused by direct compression from tumor or tumor invasion of the pulmonary artery. Tapson et al. described a very interesting case of 60 year old female with abdominal bloating and dyspnea who was ultimately found to have a high grade intimal sarcoma of the pulmonary artery. PA pressures were confirmed to be 79/21 mmHg by right heart catheterization. The patient was treated with surgery and pulmonary artery stenting (With permission from Tapson V, personal communication, unpublished.) (Fig. 18.1).

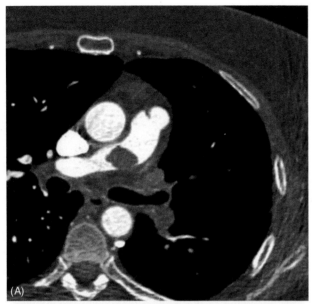

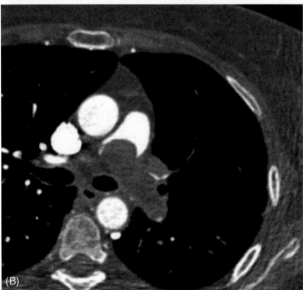

FIGURE 18.1 High grade intimal sarcoma of the pulmonary artery causing local compression and invasion of the pulmonary artery leading to severe pulmonary hypertension. *Courtesy of Victor Tapson, MD, Cedars-Sinai Medical Center.*

CHEMOTHERAPEUTIC AGENTS AND PAH

It has been noted for years that chemotherapeutic agents occasionally caused PH either by involving the lung parenchyma (i.e., pulmonary fibrosis), or the pulmonary vasculature (i.e., dasatinib causing distal pulmonary arterial obstruction or alkylating agents causing pulmonary veno-occlusive disease (PVOD), characterized by progressive obstruction of small pulmonary veins, and a dismal prognosis). In three different animal models, cyclophosphamide was able to induce PH on the basis of hemodynamic, morphological, and biological parameters. In these models, histopathological assessment confirmed significant pulmonary venous

involvement highly suggestive of PVOD. Together, clinical data and animal models demonstrated a plausible cause-effect relationship between alkylating agents and PVOD [23].

Although a definite diagnosis of PVOD requires histological confirmation, [24] lung biopsy is often considered to be a high-risk procedure in cancer patients with PH, who are considered critically ill patients. A noninvasive approach on the basis of compatible clinical, functional, radiological and hemodynamic assessment can be sufficient to support a confident diagnosis of PVOD [25]. Several chemotherapeutic agents, including alkylating agents, plant alkaloid and naturally occurring molecules, antimetabolites, and cytotoxic antibiotics agents have been incriminated and suggested from the French PH Network to induce PVOD [23], and, in particular, among the alkylating or alkylating-like chemotherapeutic agents, drugs, such as cyclophosphamide, mitomycin, cisplatin, carmustine, and procarbazine, and from the cytotoxic antibiotics, doxorubicin, daunorubicin and bleomycin, and from the plant alkaloids, Vincristine, etoposide, and docetaxel. From the antimetabolites, the most common are Cytarabine, and methotrexate [26–28].

Radiation therapy and bone marrow transplantation (BMT) have also been noted to be risk factors for the development of PVOD [29–31]. The pathophysiological mechanisms of PVOD remain poorly understood [32].

The similarity of endothelial cell response to different bifunctional alkylating agents suggests that DNA cross-linking may inhibit cell proliferation and thereby limit the repair capacity of endothelial monolayers. This might contribute to the progressive pulmonary vascular injury that occurs after administration of certain DNA cross-linking agents in vivo [33]. The pattern of pulmonary endothelial cell injury induced by chemotherapy agents is reminiscent of that seen after treatment with another well-known bifunctional alkylating agent, monocrotaline pyrrole (the active metabolite of monocrotaline), which is commonly used to trigger experimental PH in rats [32].

Cyclophosphamide

Cyclophosphamide (CP) is a common component of multi-drug regimens, with a high potential for pulmonary toxicity, and has been reported to cause acute and chronic pulmonary injury in both humans and animals. The activities of the enzymes involved in the metabolism of CP show significant tissue selectivity, and the lack of detoxifying enzymes, such as aldehyde oxidase and aldehyde dehydrogenase, in the lungs accounts for selective cyclophosphamide toxicity in lung tissue [34]. Furthermore, it has been demonstrated that endothelial cells are more susceptible to the effects of CP than other cell types [35,36]. Previous in vitro studies with cyclophosphamide, busulfan, azathioprine, monocrotaline, and dacarbazine suggest that these drugs can cause hepatic veno-occlusive disease by targeting sinusoidal endothelial cells via glutathione (GSH) depletion [37,38]. Rats exposed to cyclophosphamide show reduced pulmonary GSH content, glucose-6-phosphate dehydrogenase, GSH reductase, GSH peroxidase, and superoxide dismutase activities. Therefore, one mechanism of pulmonary toxicity of CP could be mediated by oxidative damage (With permission from Tapson V, personal communication, unpublished).

In experimental models, cyclophosphamide exposure induced PH in a dose dependent manner in three different animal models: mouse, rat, and rabbit. In rats, the severity of PH and vascular remodeling was sex dependent (females were more susceptible than males), time dependent, and dose dependent. At high dose, cyclophosphamide led to a significant pathological pulmonary serotonin accumulation, a known pathway in the pathophysiology of PH (With permission from Tapson V, personal communication, unpublished).

Cyclophosphamide at high dose led to slightly different histological changes in rats and rabbits. In other experimental models of cyclophosphamide exposure, the development of PH was frequently associated with pulmonary venous remodeling. Lung injury leading to interstitial fibrosis is another well-documented complication of cyclophosphamide and various other chemotherapeutic agents (With permission from Tapson V, personal communication, unpublished).

As mentioned earlier, the pathophysiological features of PVOD in the setting of chemotherapy and the mechanisms leading to pulmonary venous remodeling and capillary proliferation are largely unknown [39]. Recently, it has been demonstrated that a heritable form of PVOD is due to biallelic mutation of the EIF2AK4 gene [40]. EIF2AK4 gene codes for GCN2, a serinethreonine kinase that can induce changes in gene expression in response to amino acid deprivation. The role and expression of GCN2 in the pulmonary vasculature are largely unknown; however, a decrease of GCN2 activity may lead to an increase in vulnerability to oxidative stress and an increase in inflammation. EIF2AK4 (−/−) knockout mice have been shown to display increased susceptibility to both acute or chronic liver damage induced by carbon tetrachloride, which is accompanied by increased necrosis and greater inflammatory infiltrates compared to wild-type mice. Interestingly, there was a pronounced vasculitis of small pulmonary veins in CP-exposed animals. Because only a minority of patients treated with alkylating agents will develop PVOD, further studies on genetic susceptibility and the role of GCN2 in human chemotherapy induced PVOD are required.

It has recently been shown that heritable pulmonary arterial hypertension can be related to missense mutations in KCNK3 (the gene encoding KCNK3), resulting in loss of function, and the reduction in the potassium channel current [41]. Accordingly, CP-induced pulmonary vascular dysfunction was associated with decreased expression of KCNK3 protein in the lungs (With permission from Tapson V, personal communication, unpublished). Mesna and amifostine are cytoprotective agents given in combination with chemotherapy to reduce normal tissue toxicity. In rats tamifostine, but not mesna, ameliorated CP-induced PH, with a notable improvement in

survival and pulmonary hemodynamics (With permission from Tapson V, personal communication, unpublished).

The tyrosine kinase inhibitor Dasatinib, a broad inhibitor of PDGFR, BCR/ABL, c-Kit, and Srckinases, potently inhibited the mitogenic and motogenic responses to growth factors in PASMCs and inhibited vascular remodeling in experimental models of PH . Initial clinical trials with dasatinib suggested that a percentage of patients are susceptible to pericardial and pleural effusions [42]. More concerning, however, and despite the enthusiasm of initial efficacy profile, it was noted on recent data from a French registry that chronic treatment with dasatinib for chronic myeloid leukemia was associated with the onset of severe PAH in humans, marked by severe symptoms and marked hemodynamic compromise [43].

CANCER CHEMOTHERAPEUTIC AGENTS WITH POTENTIAL TO TREAT OR PREVENT PAH

While several chemotherapeutic agents have been implicated in the development of PH, there are other chemotherapeutic agents that appear to have a protective or even curative effect against PH. Strangely, even the same agent can sometimes do both, depending on the underlying condition. As described earlier, CP can lead to PH by various mechanisms (i.e., PVOD), however, in clinical practice, it has been shown to have significant therapeutic success for the treatment of PAH in the setting of inflammatory conditions, such as systemic lupus erythematosus and mixed connective tissue disease [44]. Paradoxically, CP might reverse PAH when associated with inflammatory conditions, but it may induce PVOD in subjects with underlying susceptibility.

ROLE OF TYROSINE KINASE INHIBITORS (TKI'S) IN PAH

Imatinib

The small-molecule TKI imatinib was initially developed as an inhibitor of PDGF receptor (PDGFR). Its clinical utility was subsequently developed by rationally using the inhibitory activity against ABL1 kinase, which becomes constitutively active in CML, and against the mutationally activated KIT and PDGFRA kinases in GIST [45]. Among the receptor tyrosine kinases, platelet-derived growth factor receptor (PDGFR) has a pivotal role in the "pseudomalignant" inward remodeling of PAH vessels. Imatinib, an orally available inhibitor of BCR/ABL, c-Kit, and PDGFR, reverses the pathological remodeling in experimental PH [46]. Long-term observations from phase 3 studies have revealed a lower incidence of cardiovascular events in patients treated with imatinib compared with patients not treated with TKI or patients treated with newer TKIs, such as nilotinib, [47] suggesting that perhaps imatinib itself may be inherently protective against vascular events. However, appropriately powered, prospective, controlled comparisons are lacking. Further evidence of a beneficial vascular effect of imatinib came from a case report of a patient with familial idiopathic pulmonary arterial hypertension who was deteriorating on maximal existing medical therapy but who had improved exercise capacity and hemodynamics after treatment with imatinib [48]. The presumed mechanism for this benefit was inhibition of PDGFR signaling in the pulmonary vasculature; PDGF can cause increased proliferation and migration of pulmonary vascular smooth muscle cells. Indeed, imatinib reversed experimentally induced PH and had favorable pulmonary vasodilatory effects in animal models of PH, [49] prompting several prospective clinical trials of imatinib for patients with PAH. In a prospective clinical trial of imatinib as an add-on drug to conventional pulmonary arterial hypertension therapy, imatinib improved exercise capacity, and hemodynamics [50].

In a multicenter phase III trial in PAH [the Imatinib in Pulmonary Arterial Hypertension (IMPRES) trial], imatinib significantly improved the 6-min walk distance, cardiac output, pulmonary vascular resistance, and N-terminal brain natriuretic peptide levels. However, the severity of adverse effects was higher in the imatinib group, and unexpected subdural hematoma occurred, representing a major obstacle to its further clinical use for PAH [46].

Nilotinib

Nilotinib, formerly known as AMN107, is a second-generation TKI that is 30 times more potent than imatinib and is used as an oral treatment for chronic myeloid leukemia. In experimental PH models, nilotinib treatment caused a nearly complete reversal of pulmonary vascular remodeling [51].

Epidermal Growth Factor Receptor Blockers

Serine elastase activates epidermal growth factor receptor (EGFR) signaling, which has been implicated in the pathobiology of PAH. EGFR TKIs gefitinib, erlotinib, and lapatinib significantly attenuate monocrotaline-induced PH in rats [52].

Fibroblast Growth Factor Receptor Inhibitors

Endothelial FGF2 is overproduced in IPAH and contributes to PASMC hyperplasia [53]. Furthermore, administration of short interfering RNAs that target FGF2 or pharmacological fibroblast growth factor receptor 1 inhibition (with SU5402) reverses established PH in experimental models [53].

Multikinase Inhibitors—Sorafenib and Sunitinib

Sorafenib is a multikinase inhibitor against Raf, PDGFR, vascular EGFR, c-Kit, and Flt-3. Sorafenib attenuates both hypoxia- and monocrotaline-induced PH in rats [54]. Similarly, sunitinib, another multikinase inhibitor, has potent antiremodeling effects in experimental models of PH [55]. A monocentric open label

clinical trial indicated that sorafenib treatment increases exercise capacity and right ventricular (RV) ejection fraction [56]. However, the substantial side-effect profile limits the suitability of broad multikinase inhibition for PAH treatment.

In essence, there is a need to identify methods to harness the powerful antiproliferative potency of TKIs to achieve reverse remodeling and improved survival in PH while avoiding severe adverse effects. This may include local delivery of TKIs by using inhalative application technologies, evaluation of the reverse-remodeling potential, and selectivity of new generation TKIs, and targeting a restricted subset of tyrosine kinases relevant (or even exclusive) for PAH to increase the selectivity of this approach.

Diagnosis of PH

The diagnosis of PH in the cancer patient, like in other patients, requires a high index of suspicion, relying on signs and symptoms, and confirming it with the necessary imaging and hemodynamic testing to confirm the diagnosis and design appropriate therapy. The symptoms of PH are often non specific and often include dyspnea on exertion, fatigue, and occasionally angina or even syncope. Ultimately, the patient may have signs related to progressive RV dysfunction and failure, such as edema and ascites. The physical signs of PH include left parasternal lift, an accentuated pulmonary component of the second heart sound, an RV third heart sound, a pansystolic murmur of tricuspid regurgitation and a diastolic murmur of pulmonary regurgitation. Elevated jugular venous pressure, hepatomegaly, ascites, peripheral edema, and cool extremities characterize patients with advanced disease and right heart failure.

The ECG may show abnormalities, such as, P pulmonale, right axis deviation, RV hypertrophy, RV strain, and various degrees of right bundle branch block. The chest X-ray may show abnormalities, such as central pulmonary arterial dilatation and "pruning" (loss) of peripheral blood vessels. Enlargement of the right atrium (RA) and RV may be seen in more advanced cases. A chest X-ray may assist in the differential diagnosis of PH by showing signs suggesting lung disease, WHO group 3, or pulmonary venous congestion due to left heart disease or WHO group 2.

Echocardiography is the screening tool of choice in determining whether PH is present, particularly if tricuspid regurgitation (TR) is present, in which case it is relatively easy to estimate the systolic pulmonary artery pressure. In the absence of TR, the presence of pulmonic regurgitation (PR) is also helpful to estimate the mean and diastolic pulmonary artery pressures. The pulmonary valve (PV) /right ventricular outflow tract (RVOT) acceleration time is often helpful in the absence of TR or PR. Assessment of right sided cardiac chambers is also important in suspecting the presence of and estimating the severity of PH, as well as the presence of pericardial effusion, a poor prognostic sign. It is important to note that if the treatment of PH with PAH specific therapy (such as phosphodiesterase inhibitors, endothelin receptor antagonists or prostaglandins) is being considered, echocardiography alone is not sufficient to support a treatment decision and a right (and sometimes left) cardiac catheterization is required [57]. The gold standard for confirming pulmonary arterial pressure is right heart catheterization with a Swan-Ganz catheter.

Pulmonary function tests and arterial blood gases can sometimes help differentiate between pulmonary vascular and underlying airway or parenchymal lung disease. Lung volumes are usually only mildly impaired in PAH and an abnormally low DLCO, defined as <45% of predicted, is associated with a poor outcome [58]. On arterial blood gas analysis, due to alveolar hyperventilation at rest, the arterial oxygen pressure (PaO_2) remains normal or is only slightly lower than normal and arterial carbon dioxide pressure ($PaCO_2$) is mildly decreased [59].

A ventilation/perfusion (V/Q) lung scan should be performed in patients with PH to look for chronic thromboembolic pulmonary hypertension (CTEPH). Obtaining a V/Q scan cannot be emphasized enough, particularly in cancer patients as they may be prothrombotic. The V/Q scan has been the screening method of choice for CTEPH because of its higher sensitivity compared with CT pulmonary angiogram (CTPA), especially in inexperienced centers. A normal- or low-probability V/Q scan effectively excludes CTEPH with a sensitivity of 90–100% and a specificity of 94–100%; however, many V/Q scans are not diagnostic. While in PAH the V/Q lung scan may be normal, it may also show small peripheral unmatched and nonsegmental defects in perfusion. A caveat is that unmatched perfusion defects may also be seen in other pulmonary vascular disease, such as PVOD. While a V/Q scan is still recommended as the screening test of choice, ventilation scans are often replaced with either a recent chest radiograph or a recent high-resolution CT of the lungs, but such practices are not really evidence-based. Also, CT is preferred in many centers since it is more readily available. A few studies suggest that single photon emission CT (SPECT), also a nuclear medicine technique, could be superior to V/Q planar scan and CTPA, but these results need more extensive evaluation. More recently, newer techniques, such as three-dimensional magnetic resonance (MR) perfusion mapping, have been demonstrated to be as sensitive as traditional perfusion scintigraphy in screening for CTEPH. MR can also be used as a radiation-free modality to assess both ventilation and perfusion in CTEPH.

CONCLUSIONS

PH can occur in cancer patients for a number of reasons and via a variety of different mechanisms. Whether related to the cancer itself, effects of chemotherapy or radiation, cardiopulmonary toxicities or embolic phenomena, timely diagnosis and appropriate treatment are essential. Quite interestingly, several chemotherapeutic agents have been shown to cause PH while others, such as Imatinib, have demonstrated beneficial and potentially curative effects on PH. Unfortunately, those chemotherapeutic medications that have shown some benefit in the treatment or prevention of PH thus far have been limited by other adverse side effects. Hopefully with ongoing research and clinical trials, we will continue to gain more insight into the relationship between cancer and PH.

REFERENCES

[1] Rai PR, et al. The Cancer Paradigm of Severe Pulmonary Arterial Hypertension. Am J Respir Crit Care Med 2008;178:558–64.

[2] Delom F, et al. Pulmonary Arterial Hypertension and Cancer: An update on Their Similarities. Ann Res Rev Biol 2014;4(1):20–37.

[3] Eddahibi S, Humbert M, Fadel E, Raffestin B, Darmon M, Capron F, et al. Serotonin transporter overexpression is responsible for pulmonary artery smooth muscle hyperplasia in primary pulmonary hypertension. J Clin Invest 2001;108:1141–50.

[4] Teichert-Kuliszewska K, Kutryk MJ, Kuliszewski MA, Karoubi G, Courtman DW, Zucco L, et al. Bone morphogenetic protein receptor-2 signaling promotes pulmonary arterial endothelial cell survival: implications for loss-of-function mutations in the pathogenesis of pulmonary hypertension. Circ Res 2006;98:209–17.

[5] Hoeper MM, Bogaard HJ, Condliffe R, Frantz R, Khanna D, Kurzyna M, Langleben D, Manes A, Satoh T, Torres F, Wilkins MR, Badesch DB. Definitions and diagnosis of pulmonary hypertension. J Am Coll Cardiol 2013;62(Suppl):D42–50.

[6] 2015 ESC/ERS Guidelines for the diagnosis and treatment of pulmonary hypertension.

[7] Kovacs G, Berghold A, Scheidl S, Olschewski H. Pulmonary arterial pressure during rest and exercise in healthy subjects: a systematic review. Eur Respir J 2009;34:888–94.

[8] Adir Y, Humbert M. Pulmonary hypertension in patients with chronic myeloproliferative disorders. Eur Respir J 2010;35:1396–406.

[9] Marvin KS, Spellberg RD. Pulmonary hypertension secondary to thrombocytosis in a patient with myeloid metaplasia. Chest 1993;103:642–4.

[10] Kotake T, Kosugi S, Takimoto T, et al. Intravascular large B-cell lymphoma presenting pulmonary arterial hypertension as an initial manifestation. Intern Med 2010;49:51–4.

[11] Hennigs JK, Keller G, Baumann HJ, et al. Multi tyrosine kinase inhibitor dasatinib as novel cause of severe pre-capillary pulmonary hypertension? BMC Pulm Med 2011;11:30.

[12] Limsuwan A, et al. Pulmonary arterial hypertension after childhood cancer therapy and bone marrow transplantation. Cardiology 2006;105:188–94.

[13] Ho AL, et al. The diagnostic challenge of pulmonary tumour thrombotic microangiopathy as a presentation for metastatic gastric cancer: a case report and review of the literature. BMC Cancer 2015;15:450.

[14] Uruga H, Fujii T, Kurosaki A, Hanada S, Takaya H, Miyamoto A, et al. Pulmonary tumor thrombotic microangiopathy: a clinical analysis of 30 autopsy cases. Intern Med 2013;52(12):1317–23.

[15] Abe H, Hino R, Fukayama M. Platelet-derived growth factor-A and vascular endothelial growth factor-C contribute to the development of pulmonary tumor thrombotic microangiopathy in gastric cancer. Virchows Arch 2013;462(5):523–31.

[16] Okubo Y, Wakayama M, Kitahara K, Nemoto T, Yokose T, Abe F, et al. Pulmonary tumor thrombotic microangiopathy induced by gastric carcinoma: morphometric and immunohistochemical analysis of six autopsy cases. Diagn Pathol 2011;6(1):27.

[17] Yokomine T, Hirakawa H, Ozawa E, Shibata K, Nakayama T. Pulmonary thrombotic microangiopathy caused by gastric carcinoma. J Clin Pathol 2010;63(4):367–9.

[18] Ha D, et al. Pulmonary arterial hypertension in a patient with Cowden syndrome and the PTEN mutation. Pulm Circ 2014;4(4):728–31.

[19] Rabinovitch M. Molecular pathogenesis of pulmonary arterial hypertension. J Clin Invest 2012;122:4306–13.

[20] Zbuk KM, Eng C. Cancer phenomics: RET and PTEN as illustrative models. Nat Rev Cancer 2007;7:35–45.

[21] Nemenoff RA, Simpson PA, Furgeson SB, Kaplan-Albuquerque N, Crossno J, Garl PJ, Cooper J, Weiser-Evans MC. Targeted deletion of PTEN in smooth muscle cells results in vascular remodeling and recruitment of progenitor cells through induction of stromal cell–derived factor-1α. Circ Res 2008;102:1036–45.

[22] Oudit GY, Penninger JM. Cardiac regulation by phosphoinositide 3-kinases and PTEN. Cardiovasc Res 2009;82:250–60.

[23] Ranchoux B, et al. Chemotherapy-induced pulmonary hypertension: role of alkylating agents. Am J Pathol 2015;185:356–71.

[24] Nicod P, Moser KM. Primary pulmonary hypertension: the risk and benefit of lung biopsy. Circulation 1989;80:1486–8.

[25] Montani D, Achouh L, Dorfmüller P, Le Pavec J, Sztrymf B, Tchérakian C, Rabiller A, Haque R, Sitbon O, Jaïs X, Dartevelle P, Maître S, Capron F, Musset D, Simonneau G, Humbert M. Pulmonary veno-occlusive disease: clinical, functional, radiologic, and hemodynamic characteristics and outcome of 24 cases confirmed by histology. Medicine (Baltimore) 2008;87:220–33.

[26] Joselson R, Warnock M. Pulmonary veno-occlusive disease after chemotherapy. Hum Pathol 1983;14:88–91.

[27] Knight BK, Rose AG. Pulmonary veno-occlusive disease after chemotherapy. Thorax 1985;40:874–5.

[28] Swift GL, Gibbs A, Campbell IA, Wagenvoort CA, Tuthill D. Pulmonary veno-occlusive disease and Hodgkin's lymphoma. Eur Respir J. 1993;6:596–8.

[29] Salzman D, Adkins DR, Craig F, Freytes C, LeMaistre CF. Malignancy-associated pulmonary veno-occlusive disease: report of a case following autologous bone marrow transplantation and review. Bone Marrow Transplant 1996;18:755–60.

[30] Kuga T, Kohda K, Hirayama Y, Matsumoto S, Nakazawa O, Ando M, Ezoe A, Nobuoka A, Mochizuki C. Pulmonary veno-occlusive disease accompanied by microangiopathic hemolytic anemia 1 year after a second bone marrow transplantation for acute lymphoblastic leukemia. Int J Hematol 1996;64:143–50.

[31] Troussard X, Bernaudin JF, Cordonnier C, Fleury J, Payen D, Briere J, Vernant JP. Pulmonary veno-occlusive disease after bone marrow transplantation. Thorax 1984;39:956–7.

[32] Perros F, Cohen-Kaminsky S, Gambaryan N, Girerd B, Raymond N, Klingelschmitt I, Huertas A, Mercier O, Fadel E, Simonneau G, Humbert M, Dorfmüller P, Montani D. Cytotoxic cells and granulysin in pulmonary arterial hypertension and pulmonary veno-occlusive disease. Am J Respir Crit Care Med 2013;187:189–96.

[33] Hoorn CM, Wagner JG, Petry TW, Roth RA. Toxicity of mitomycin C toward cultured pulmonary artery endothelium. Toxicol Appl Pharmacol 1995;130:87–94.

[34] Cooper JA Jr, Merrill WW, Reynolds HY. Cyclophosphamide modulation of bronchoalveolar cellular populations and macrophage

[35] Hamano Y, Sugimoto H, Soubasakos MA, Kieran M, Olsen BR, Lawler J, Sudhakar A, Kalluri R. Thrombospondin-1 associated with tumor microenvironment contributes to low-dose cyclophosphamidemediated endothelial cell apoptosis and tumor growth suppression. Cancer Res 2004;64:1570–4.

[36] Ohtani T, Nakamura T, Toda K-I, Furukawa F. Cyclophosphamide enhances TNF-alpha-induced apoptotic cell death in murine vascular endothelial cell. FEBS Lett 2006;580:1597–600.

[37] DeLeve LD. Cellular target of cyclophosphamide toxicity in the murine liver: role of glutathione and site of metabolic activation. Hepatology 1996;24:830–7.

[38] Srivastava A, Poonkuzhali B, Shaji RV, George B, Mathews V, Chandy M, Krishnamoorthy R. Glutathione S-transferase M1 polymorphism: a risk factor for hepatic venooclusive disease in bone marrow transplantation. Blood 2004;104:1574–7.

[39] Montani D, Price LC, Dorfmuller P, Achouh L, Jaïs X, Yaïci A, Sitbon O, Musset D, Simonneau G, Humbert M. Pulmonary venooclusive disease. Eur Respir J 2009;33:189–200.

[40] Eyries M, Montani D, Girerd B, Perret C, Leroy A, Lonjou C, Chelghoum N, Coulet F, Bonnet D, Dorfmüller P, Fadel E, Sitbon O, Simonneau G, Tregouët D-A, Humbert M, Soubrier F. EIF2AK4 mutations cause pulmonary veno-occlusive disease, a recessive form of pulmonary hypertension. Nat Genet 2014;46:65–9.

[41] Ma L, Roman-Campos D, Austin ED, Eyries M, Sampson KS, Soubrier F, Germain M, Trégouët D-A, Borczuk A, Rosenzweig EB, Girerd B, Montani D, Humbert M, Loyd JE, Kass RS, Chung WK. A novel channelopathy in pulmonary arterial hypertension. N Engl J Med 2013;369:351–61.

[42] Kelly K, Swords R, Mahalingam D, Padmanabhan S, Giles FJ. Serosal inflammation (pleural and pericardial effusions) related to tyrosine kinase inhibitors. Target Oncol 2009;4:99–105.

[43] Montani D, Bergot E, Günther S, Savale L, Bergeron A, Bourdin A, Bouvaist H, Canuet M, Pison C, Macro M, et al. Pulmonary arterial hypertension in patients treated by dasatinib. Circulation 2012;125:2128–37.

[44] Jais X, et al. Immunosuppressive therapy in lupus- and mixed connective tissue disease-associated pulmonary arterial hypertension: a retrospective analysis of twenty-three cases. Arthritis Rheum 2008;58(2):521–31.

[45] Savage DG, Antman KH. Imatinib mesylate: a new oral targeted therapy. N Engl J Med 2002;346:683–93.

[46] Schermuly RT, Dony E, Ghofrani HA, Pullamsetti S, Savai R, Roth M, Sydykov A, Lai YJ, Weissmann N, Seeger W, et al. Reversal of experimental pulmonary hypertension by PDGF inhibition. J Clin Invest 2005;115:2811–21.

[47] Giles FJ, Mauro MJ, Hong F, Ortmann CE, McNeill C, Woodman RC, Hochhaus A, le Coutre PD, Saglio G. Rates of peripheral arterial occlusive disease in patients with chronic myeloid leukemia in the chronic phase treated with imatinib, nilotinib, or non-tyrosine kinase therapy: a retrospective cohort analysis. Leukemia 2013;27:1310–5.

[48] Ghofrani HA, Seeger W, Grimminger F. Imatinib for the treatment of pulmonary arterial hypertension. N Engl J Med 2005;353:1412–3.

[49] Schermuly RT, Dony E, Ghofrani HA, Pullamsetti S, Savai R, Roth M, Sydykov A, Lai YJ, Weissmann N, Seeger W, Grimminger F. Reversal of experimental pulmonary hypertension by PDGF inhibition. J Clin Invest 2005;115:2811–21.

[50] Hoeper MM, Barst RJ, Bourge RC, Feldman J, Frost AE, Galié N, Gómez-Sánchez MA, Grimminger F, Grünig E, Hassoun PM,

Morrell NW, Peacock AJ, Satoh T, Simonneau G, Tapson VF, Torres F, Lawrence D, Quinn DA, Ghofrani HA. Imatinib mesylate as add-on therapy for pulmonary arterial hypertension: results of the randomized IMPRES study. Circulation 2013;127:1128–38.

[51] Pullamsetti SS, Berghausen EM, Dabral S, Tretyn A, Butrous E, Savai R, Butrous G, Dahal BK, Brandes RP, Ghofrani HA, et al. Role of Src tyrosine kinases in experimental pulmonary hypertension. Arterioscler Thromb Vasc Biol 2012;32:1354–65.

[52] Dahal BK, Cornitescu T, Tretyn A, Pullamsetti SS, Kosanovic D, Dumitrascu R, Ghofrani HA, Weissmann N, Voswinckel R, Banat GA, et al. Role of epidermal growth factor inhibition in experimental pulmonary hypertension. Am J Respir Crit Care Med 2010;181:158–67.

[53] Izikki M, Guignabert C, Fadel E, Humbert M, Tu L, Zadigue P, Dartevelle P, Simonneau G, Adnot S, Maitre B, et al. Endothelial-derived FGF2 contributes to the progression of pulmonary hypertension in humans and rodents. J Clin Invest 2009;119:512–23.

[54] Klein M, Schermuly RT, Ellinghaus P, Milting H, Riedl B, Nikolova S, Pullamsetti SS, Weissmann N, Dony E, Savai R, et al. Combined tyrosine and serine/threonine kinase inhibition by sorafenib prevents progression of experimental pulmonary hypertension and myocardial remodeling. Circulation 2008;118:2081–90.

[55] Kojonazarov B, Sydykov A, Pullamsetti SS, Luitel H, Dahal BK, Kosanovic D, Tian X, Majewski M, Baumann C, Evans S, et al. Effects of multikinase inhibitors on pressure overload-induced right ventricular remodeling. Int J Cardiol 2013;167:2630–7.

[56] Gomberg-Maitland M, Maitland ML, Barst RJ, Sugeng L, Coslet S, Perrino TJ, Bond L, Lacouture ME, Archer SL, Ratain MJ. A dosing/cross-development study of the multikinase inhibitor sorafenib in patients with pulmonary arterial hypertension. Clin Pharmacol Ther 2010;87:303–10.

[57] Galie N, et al. ESC/ERS guidelines for the diagnosis and treatment of pulmonary hypertension. Eur Heart J 2016;37(1):67–119.

[58] Sun XG, Hansen JE, Oudiz RJ, Wasserman K. Pulmonary function in primary pulmonary hypertension. J Am Coll Cardiol 2003;41:1028–35.

[59] Hoeper MM, Pletz MW, Golpon H, Welte T. Prognostic value of blood gas analyses in patients with idiopathic pulmonary arterial hypertension. Eur Respir J 2007;29:944–50.

Chapter 19

The Role of Echocardiography in the Detection of Chemotherapy-Induced Cardiotoxicities

P.T. Gleason, J.C. Lisko and S. Lerakis

Division of Cardiology, Emory University School of Medicine, Atlanta, GA, United States

INTRODUCTION

Advances in chemotherapeutics have greatly improved the prognoses of numerous malignancies; however, cancer survivors face considerable morbidity and mortality due to the long term effects of their treatment. Survivors of childhood cancer, breast cancer, and lymphoma are most likely to experience significant cardiotoxicities as a result of treatment [1]. There are a range of effects, from subclinical changes in myocardial function to overt heart failure, a late manifestation of cardiotoxicity that conveys a poor prognosis. Cardiotoxicty is defined as a symptomatic decrease in left ventricular ejection fraction (LVEF) of 5% or an asymptomatic decrease of 10% to an ejection fraction (EF) of <55% [2]. Given the significant mortality in these patients, cardiac dysfunction needs to be detected prior to symptomatic heart failure. Echocardiography is a widely available and radiation-free method of noninvasively evaluating cardiac structure and function. Specifically, it allows for a comprehensive evaluation of global systolic and diastolic function, regional wall motion abnormalities, valvular function, and the assessment of the pericardium.

STANDARD ECHOCARDIOGRAPHIC VIEWING PLANES

The standard echocardiographic examination begins with an assessment of the heart in the parasternal long axis view (PLAX) (Fig. 19.1). These images are obtained with the transducer between the third or fourth intercostal space and adjacent to the sternum. In this plane the long axis of the heart bisects the aortic valve and mitral valve. From this viewing plane, inferomedial positioning of the transducer allows for visualization of the right ventricular inflow and outflow tracts. Returning to the PLAX view, clockwise rotation of the transducer between 70 and 110° generates the parasternal short axis view. This plane allows for short axis cardiac assessment from base to apex. By placing the transducer at the cardiac apex, all four chambers of the heart are visualized in one viewing plane. In this plane the LV appears to be an ellipse and the interventricular septum, apex, LV free wall, and RV free wall are all visualized. The apical five-chamber view is generated from this view by positioning the transducer anteriorly and clockwise and includes the LV outflow tract, right and left aortic valve leaflets, and ascending aorta. Counterclockwise transducer rotation and anterior angulation from this plane bring the left-ventricular outflow tract, anterior septum, aortic valve leaflets, and ascending aorta into view.

In a patient that is able to lay in supine position and perform a breath hold at full inspiration, the transducer can be placed below the xiphoid process in the subcostal four chamber view. This view allows for assessment of the right ventricle (RV) from base to apex, inferior inter ventricular septum, and LV free wall. The subcostal four-chamber view is also useful for the assessment of the pericardium, pericardial effusions, and the inferior vena cava entering the right atrium. Finally, placing the transducer in the suprasternal notch allows for assessment of the great vessels and aorta [3].

EVALUATING LEFT VENTRICULAR EJECTION FRACTION

LVEF is defined as the ratio of stroke volume to end-diastolic volume, and is the most used metric in the assessment of LV function. Given the complex anatomic shape of the left ventricle (LV), exact LV volume is difficult to quantify. Numerous methods have been determined to best approximate this value [4].

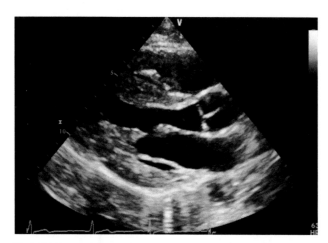

FIGURE 19.1 **Standard parasternal long axis (PLAX) view.**

The prolate ellipsoid is commonly used to geometrically define the LV and to make calculations of ventricular volumes. Simpson's rule is a theoretical method of estimating left ventricular volume by dividing the LV into multiple smaller geometric shapes [5]. During an echo study, multiple short-axis slices can be acquired at known distances from the LV apex to base. As the height of the slice is then known, the area of the theoretical cylinder can be acquired by planimetry or directly measured using the slice minor diameters. The accuracy of LV volume estimation using this method would increase with the number of slices measured during the echo study; however, inherent limitations in echo windows do not allow for accurate assessment of the entire LV.

The principles underlying Simpson's method are simplified and applied clinically using only two views 90° apart from a predefined long axis. The height of the theoretical cylinder is determined by dividing the LV into an even number of slices, and the orthogonal diameters are measured as the distance between two orthogonal lines from the long axis to the endocardium.

This modified Simpson's method accounts for anatomic variation in LV shape, provided an adequate number of slices are used in the calculation [6]. A further simplification of Simpson's rule divides the LV into a series of discs with a known height H and planimiterized area and considers the LV apex to be a separate ellipse. The sum of these values correlates well with measured LV volume (Fig. 19.2).

EF can be determined after quantifying ventricular volumes during systole and diastole as detailed earlier. Less laborious methods for determining LVEF have also been developed and validated. Clinically, the LVEF is often visually estimated as a percentage with a subjective description of the degree of impairment. Unlike the Simpson's method, visual estimation of EF allows the interpreter to evaluate the LV in multiple viewing planes. While studies have suggested that visual estimation of EF correlates well with the modified Simpson's rule estimation of EF, there is significant in-

trareader variability. This variability is increased in studies limited by suboptimal viewing windows [7].

Inherent limitations of Simpson's method are poor quality imaging windows, >20% nonvisualized endocardium, and severe LV cavity geometric distortion. Given the inherent complexity of the Simpson's method, it is recommended that if the EF appears to be normal on visual assessment no quantified techniques need to be performed.

3D ECHO

A significant advancement in echocardiographic technology is the advent of 3D imaging. This technique acquires pyramidal datasets during a single heart beat. A major advance over 2D echocardiography is the elimination of geometric modeling in calculation of LV volumes [8]. Given this advantage, numerous studies have shown 3D echo to be superior to 2D echo for assessment of LVEF and test retest variability—essential principles for detecting clinical or subclinical cardiotoxicity [8,9]. The American Society of Echocardiography (ASE) and European Association of Cardiovascular Imaging (EACI) recommend 3D echo as the "test of choice" for cardio-oncology patients; however, lack of wide spread availability and the need for advanced training limit its application in clinical practice [10].

CALCULATING EJECTION FRACTION

LVEF is the most common echocardiographic parameter used to evaluate LV systolic function. The ASE/EACI recommend the modified biplane Simpson's method for quantification of LV volumes and calculation of EF. While fractional shortening was previously used to estimate EF, the technique does not adequately assess the global LV, posing inherent errors in volume assessment, especially in patients with regional wall motion abnormalities. An EF 53–73% is considered to be within normal limits. The addition of a 16 segment resting wall motion score index has been identified as a sensitive marker of anthracycline-induced cardiotoxicity [10]. Unfortunately, a major limitation of current research on cardiotoxicity from oncologic agents is the use of inconsistent methods of quantifying EF. Visual estimation of EF should always be compared to prior studies in an effort to minimize intrareader variability and to readily identify changes suggestive of myocardial damage.

DIASTOLIC DYSFUNCTION

Echocardiography is well suited for the noninvasive assessment of LV diastolic function. Multiple indicators are incorporated into the assessment of diastolic function including LV wall thickness, left atrial volume, pulmonary artery pressures, transmitral Doppler inflow velocities, and pulmonary venous Doppler flow patterns. Measurement of

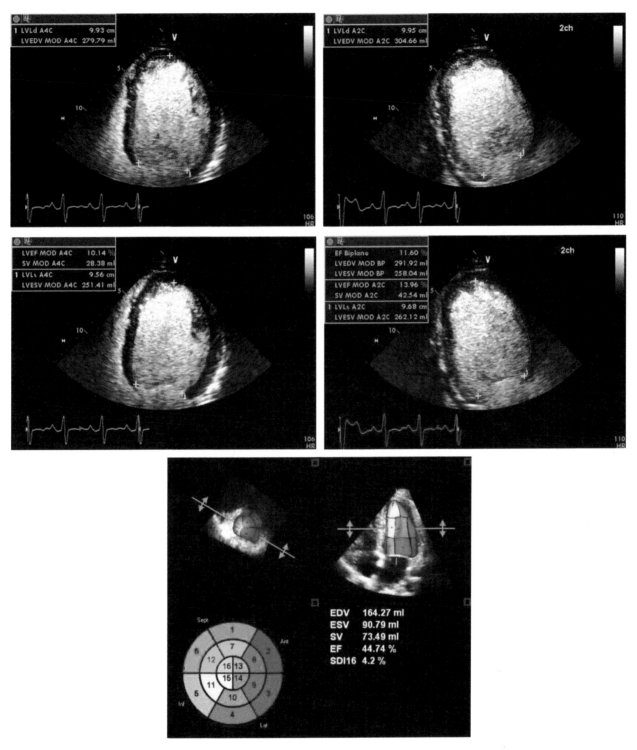

FIGURE 19.2   Modified Simpson's method to evaluate LVEF using contrast.

diastolic function is an important aspect of echocardiography and has been shown to have significant prognostic implications [11].

Transmitral Doppler flow is evaluated by pulse wave Doppler across the tips of the mitral valve leaflets. Two waves occur—an early (E) wave generated by rapid ventricular filling and a later (A) wave generated from atrial contraction. As atrial contraction is required, atrial fibrillation precludes assessment of diastology. In patients without diastolic dysfunction, the E wave rapidly rises (acceleration time—AT) and falls (deceleration time—DT). As patients first start to develop diastolic dysfunction, LV filling becomes increasing dependent on atrial contraction, which can effect isovolumetric relaxation time (IVRT), AT, and DT. These changes cause three alterations to the pattern of mitral inflow. Patients with impaired relaxation demonstrate a decreased E velocity, an E/A ratio <1, and a prolongation of both the isovolumetric relaxation time, and deceleration time.

With worsening diastolic dysfunction, left atrial pressure increases and the E/A ratio reverts to >1. This "pseudo-normal pattern" will change to an impaired relaxation pattern with Valsalva. As left atrial pressure continues to rise, the E/A ratio increases to >2 as the isovolumetric and DT shorten [12,13].

Using the apical four chamber view, the right upper pulmonary vein can often be visualized on a standard transthoracic echo. In normal individuals, the major flow direction during diastole is forward. Reversal of this pattern suggests elevated left atrial pressure and diastolic dysfunction.

The role of diastology to predict early LV dysfunction remains unclear. Work by Stoddard et al determined that a >37% increase in isovolumetric relaxation time was 78% sensitive and 88% specific for predicting the development of doxorubicin-induced systolic dysfunction at 3 months post the final dose of doxorubicin [14]. Conversely, work by Lange et al. did not find any significant changes in diastolic parameters in a cohort of patients treated with Trastuzmab [15]. These discordant findings may be partially explained by the variable cardiac loading conditions. Given the uncertainty surrounding diastolic dysfunction in cancer survivors, it is currently not used to predict progression to overt LV dysfunction.

RIGHT VENTRICULAR FUNCTION

The cardiotoxic effects of chemotherapeutic agents and radiation on the RV has not been adequately studied. Like the LV, the RV can be affected by a primary malignancy, neoplastic spread, or by treatment agents. While one study of 37 patients reported a subclinical decline in both RV systolic and diastolic function following the administration of regimens consisting of cyclophosphamide + adriamycin or cyclophoshamide + adriamycin + 5-fluorouracil, most of the subjects indices remained within normal range [16].

Current guidelines recommend a comprehensive assessment of the RV during echocardiography. A standard examination should include assessment of right atrial size, right ventricular size, tricuspid annular plane systolic excursion (TAPSE), pulsed DTI-derived systolic peak velocity of the tricuspid annulus, RV fractional area shortening and an estimation of the pulmonary artery pressure [10].

ECHOCARDIOGRAPHIC EVALUATION OF PULMONARY PRESSURES

The tyrosine kinase inhibitors imatinib, dasatinib, and nilotinib are used in the treatment of CML. Dasatinib has a less specific target profile compared to the other agents. One study reviewing the French PH registry describes an increased incidence of pulmonary hypertension in patients treated with dasatinib. Of the patients identified in the study, no other causes or risk factors for PH were identified and clinical improvement was observed in the majority of patients after withdrawal of the agent [17].

Echocardiography is an essential modality for the noninvasive assessment of right heart pressures. The pulmonary artery systolic pressure is calculated by using the commonly visualized tricuspid regurgitant (TR) jet and estimating the right atrial pressure from respiratory flow variation of the inferior vena cava. Additional echocardiographic signs of PH are bulging of the interventricular septum into the LV during systole and RV hypertrophy. Prolonged elevation of RV pressures leads to progressive RV failure evidenced by ventricular dilation, flattening of the interventricular septum, worsening TR, and increased right atrial size. Based on TTE, PH is classified as likely if PASP is >50 and TR peak velocity (TRV) is >3.4. The condition is unlikely when PASP is <36, TRV is <2.8, and none of the findings detailed earlier are present [18].

Major limitations of TTE in evaluating RV function are the irregular shape of the ventricle, limited definition of the endocardium, preload dependence, and overestimation of TR jet.

Tissue Doppler, strain, and real-time three-dimensional echocardiography are all useful techniques in overcoming these limitations. By Tissue Doppler, basal RV free wall S' <10 cm/s is a marker of RV dysfunction and lateral mitral annular velocities correlate with PCWP—allowing for the noninvasive evaluation of a left heart etiology [19].

Two-dimensional strain imaging has shown to be useful prognostically in patients with PH. Work by Haeck et al demonstrated that RV longitudinal peak systolic strain ≥ −19% was a risk for worse New York Heart Association Functional Class, lower TAPSE, and all cause mortality [20].

Three-dimensional echocardiography eliminates the need for geometric assumptions in determining RV volume. This modality has been shown to comprehensively assess RV remodeling and function in patients with PH [21].

STRAIN ECHO FOR CARDIOTOXICITY

Strain echocardiography (SE) has emerged as a critically important tool for the clinician in assessing and monitoring LV function in patients undergoing cancer treatment [22,23].

Strain or strain rate echocardiography is a method for evaluating myocardial mechanics by measuring the relationship between points in the myocardium. This can be achieved using either tissue Doppler imaging (TDI) or speckle tracking in 2- or 3- dimensional (D) echocardiography, and can be measured in longitudinal, radial, and circumferential axes [22,23]. Using these methods, two points within the myocardium are measured in relation to one another throughout the cardiac cycle. Myocardial deformation causing points to move toward each other, as they do in systole, decrease strain and render negative strain values. Conversely, points that move away from each other, as in diastole, increase strain and generate positive strain values. Thus strain values can be assigned for both systolic as well as diastolic function and offers the clinician valuable information about global and regional wall motion function. Conventionally, strain has most often referred to in terms of systolic assessment [19,22–24].

TDI is a form of pulse Doppler and enables the measurement of strain rate. As with other Doppler measurements, TDI strain rate measurements have limitations. It uses a fixed Doppler sampling signal, which may not sample myocardium as the heart moves during the cardiac cycle. Furthermore, TDI derived strain rate is an angle-dependent measurement, so structures that are perpendicular to the ultrasonic beam, such as the apex in the apical four chamber view, will not be measured well. Lastly, TDI is a semiquantitative measurement and can be subject to noise from the blood pool making it difficult to interpret, and therefore limiting its clinical utility [22,25,26].

Speckle tracking uses the raw acoustic signals, which are arranged in unique patterns and create echocardiographic images. By identifying these patterns, or speckle tracking, specific points can be used to calculate and display strain. Strain values can be overlaid on a polar map for ease of interpreting results, giving the clinician a useful global and regional assessment of LV function (Figs. 19.3 and 19.4). Normal values are negative, in the high teens and 20s [24]. Advantages of speckle tracking derived strain or strain rate include some of the limitations of visual wall motion analysis used with 2D echocardiography. Tethering, off-axis views, and difficulties in analyzing subtle wall

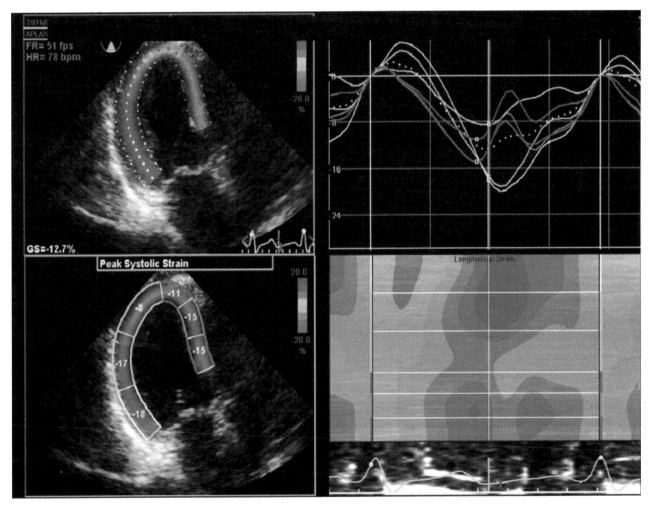

FIGURE 19.3   Three Chamber view demonstrating abnormal strain with normal EF in a patient post chemotherapy.

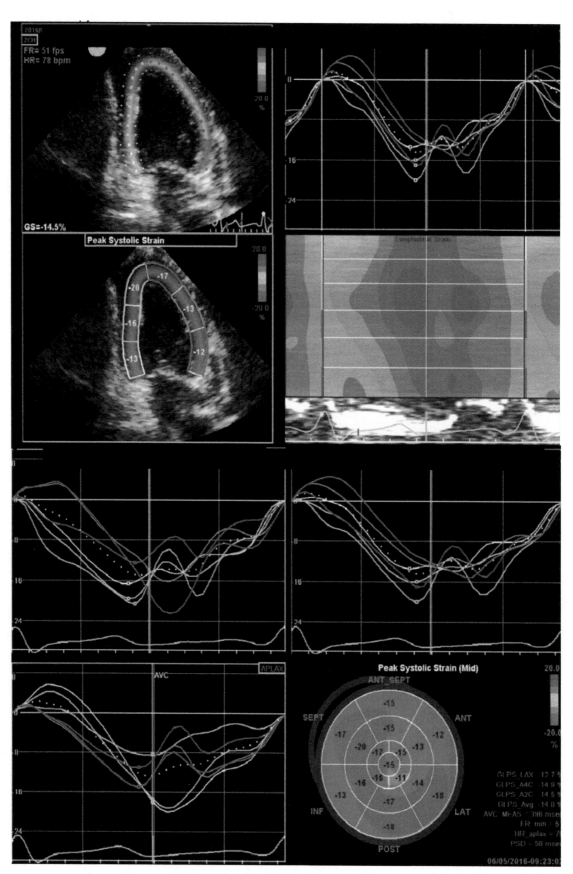

FIGURE 19.4 **Two-chamber view demonstrating abnormal strain with normal EF in a patient post chemotherapy.**

motion, are areas that strain offers advantages over 2D echo, thus providing the clinician with a better assessment of LV mechanics [22].

Generally, speckle tracking strain echocardiography (STSE) is easy to obtain, more reliable, and easier to interpret than strain rate obtained from TDI [22,25,27]. Going forward, STSE will likely be the predominant method used for strain assessment of LV function during and after cancer therapy. Likewise, measuring strain in the radial and circumferential axes has been studied and can be effective in assessing myocardial mechanics. However, global longitudinal systolic strain (GLS) is the most often studied and is readily reproducible in most labs [22,28–30]. GLS has also been compared to other imaging modalities, such as MRI and found to be accurate in assessing regional and global function [30].

With regard to cardiotoxicity monitoring, STSE has been shown to be superior to biomarkers and conventional 2D echocardiography techniques at detecting early, subclinical myocardial dysfunction during and after cancer treatment. Strain has been shown to have superior prognostic value over LVEF in observational studies in heart failure patients as well [26,29,31–37]. There is also evidence that abnormal strain before chemotherapy initiation is highly predictive of future cardiac events after treatment [38]. To date, there are few studies that demonstrate the prognostic value of strain prior to the development of cardiotoxicity. The largest of these studies by Mornos et al. examined 74 patients and 37 controls with breast, lymphoma, ALL, AML, and osteosarcoma. Over a 52 ± 2 week follow-up period the combined index GLS $\times$ LVEF was found to be the best predictor of late cardiotoxicity (area under the curve = 0.93) [39]. At 6 weeks of follow-up a change of GLS of 2.8% was determined to be 79% sensitive and 73% specific for the development of cardiotoxicity at 52 weeks.

To date, there are no randomized prospective trials evaluating the role of early initiation of heart failure medications to patients with abnormal GLS. Work be Seicean et al. evaluated the cardioprotective effect of beta-blockade in breast cancer patients undergoing chemotherapy. In this matched study of 920 breast cancer patients with a normal EF at baseline were, 106 patients on continuous beta-blockade during treatment were matched with 212 similar patients not maintained on beta-blockers. Over a median 3.2 ± 2.0 year follow-up, continuous use of beta-blockers was associated with a lower risk of new heart failure events [40]. This work further emphasizes the need for prospective trials to evaluate early initiation of therapy based on GSL given the benefit in patients with normal LVEF.

The prevention of cardiac dysfunction during adjuvant breast cancer therapy (PRADA) trial studied concomitant therapy with either candesartan-metoprolol, candesartan-placebo, placebo-metoprolol, or placebo-placebo in addition to anthracycline-containing regimens with or without trastuzumab and radiation. Of the 130 women studied, the baseline LVEF was >60%, determined by cardiac MRI, and the baseline peak GLS, determined by TTE, was >20 in each group. The candesartan group experienced a statistically significant 0.8% LVEF decline compared to the 2.6% decline in the placebo group. Notably, there was no changed in GLS throughout the follow-up [41]. While this study suggests a slight numerical EF benefit to treatment with candesartan the clinical significance remains uncertain. Long-term follow-up of this cohort may further delineate the role of early treatment initiation based on changes in GLS.

RECOMMENDED DIAGNOSTIC ALGORITHM

These considerations guide clinicians about the appropriate time initiation of cardiac medications to preserve cardiac function and decrease cardiovascular events. The exact timing of initiating heart failure therapy remains an area of research and debate.

Current recommendations from the ASE/EACI state that in general, patients receiving therapies with known cardiotoxic side effects should undergo an echocardiogram before initiation of therapy and every 3 months during treatment or if heart failure symptoms develop. After finishing therapy, a follow-up echocardiogram should be performed at 6 months or with the development of symptoms [10].

In patients beginning a chemotherapeutic regimen with any agent associated with Type I toxicity a baseline echo with GLS imaging is recommended to assess LVEF in addition to troponin I. In addition to baseline LVEF, previously undiagnosed abnormalities in cardiac anatomy also needs to be assessed prior to initiation of chemotherapy. For patients with an LVEF <53% or GLS less than the lower limit of normal or positive troponin I cardiology consultation is recommended and cardiac MRI is to be considered for further assessment of LVEF. For patients with a LVEF >54%, GLS greater than the lower limit of normal, or negative troponin I, a follow-up echo is recommended at the completion of chemotherapy and again at 6 months postconclusion of therapy for anthracycline doses less than 240 mg/m^2. If this dose is exceeded a repeat echo with GLS and troponin should be checked prior to each 50 mg/m^2 anthracycline dose. The diagnostic algorithm is similar for patients undergoing therapy with trastuzumab; however, patients with a LVEF > 53%, GLS greater than the lower limit of normal, and negative troponin I require these studies to be repeated every 3 months during therapy. If a patient is receiving trastuzumab after receiving a regimen associated with Type I toxicity, the screening algorithm remains the same with the notable exception of repeating the studies 6 months following the completion of treatment.

A biomarker-based algorithm for detecting subclinical LV dysfunction also begins with a baseline echocardiographic evaluation of LVEF followed by a Troponin I following each cycle. Patients with positive Troponin I are referred to cardiology while those that remain troponin negative undergo repeat echocardiography 6 months following the completion of chemotherapy [10]. Negishi et al. found that a difference in GLS of <8% is unlikely to be clinically meaningful, while changes of >15% are very likely to be significant [33]. A reduction in LVEF on medications, such as trastuzamab can often reverse and improve once the therapy is discontinued and standard heart failure treatment is initiated [42]. However, it should be noted that the true incidence and reversibility of cardiotoxic therapies is not well established. Furthermore, no treatments have been studied in a randomized trial to prevent injury, and none have been studied with regard to reversal of abnormalities in strain imaging [10,43–45]. Given the prognostic capabilities of strain in this population, it is important to continue to research treatment options oriented at prevention of cardiac dysfunction in this population in hopes of improving survival.

TRANSESOPHAGEAL ECHOCARDIOGRAPHY

Compared to transthoracic echocardiography, transesophageal echocardiography (TEE) allows for superior visualization of posterior cardiac structures given the close anatomic proximity of the esophagus to the posteromedial heart. Currently, TEE has not been shown to provide incremental value over TTE in a standard examination for cardio-toxicity.

While standard TEE imaging planes visualize the majority of the LV, the apex is often foreshortened. This truncation may lead to underestimation of LV volume and EF using Simpson's method. Additionally, inadequate visualization of the apex decreases the sensitivity of TEE for wall motion abnormalities and apical thrombi [46].

Both tissue Doppler and speckle tracking are applied in TEE; however, normal values have yet to be established. Given the value of TTE strain imaging, the role of TEE in the detection of cardio-toxicity will likely remain limited until these values are determined and validated.

Patients actively undergoing or postchemotherapy are at an increased risk of immunosuppression, health care acquired infections, and often have indwelling catheters. In these patients with clinical signs or symptoms of endocarditis, TEE is indicated for further evaluation of valvular pathology [47]. Additionally, TEE is indicated in for evaluation of the left atrial appendage, acute aortic pathology, prosthetic valve dysfunction, or in patients less than 50 years of age with an embolism of unknown etiology [48].

Disadvantages of a TEE exam compared to a TTE exam include the requirement for patients to be fasting, the need for multiple medical personnel, and the requirement for sedation.

STRESS ECHOCARDIOGRAPHY

Stress echocardiography allows for the addition of a stress agent, exercise, or dobutamine, to a standard echocardiographic examination in order to assess cardiac function and contractile reserve. A stress echo can detect both new stress-induced wall motion abnormalities or worsening of a resting wall motion abnormality suggestive of myocardial ischemia. Additionally, dobutamine stress echocardiography allows for visualization of abnormal but viable myocardium. In segments that are dysfunctional but viable, the addition of low-dose dobutamine increases contractility. Currently, stress echocardiography is recommended prior to the administration of a chemotherapeutic agent associated with ischemia in patients at moderate to high risk of coronary atherosclerotic disease [10]. Studies suggest that a fall in contractile reserve is predictive of an eventual LVEF reduction to <50 [49]. Conversely, in patients with known reduced systolic function due to cardiotoxicity, an improvement in contractile reserve may predict an overall better outcome [50].

VALVULAR DYSFUNCTION

Echocardiography is well suited to assess valvular dysfunction, a complication of chemotherapeutics and radiation therapy. Pathophysiologically, valvular dysfunction has been shown to occur slowly from fibrosis, valve retraction, and calcification following radiation therapy [51]. Mitral regurgitation may also be secondary to LV dysfunction and remodeling. Additionally, patients undergoing chemotherapy are often immunosuppressed and at an increased risk of infections that can lead to valve seeding. The risk of developing endocarditis is further increased in patients requiring indwelling catheters for chemotherapeutic agent infusions or patients with preexisting valve lesions.

The prevalence and risk factors associated with valvular dysfunction have been studied in lymphoma survivors (Figs. 19.5 and 19.6). Regurgitant lesions were the most common lesions observed in the study cohort, with dysfunction risk proportionately rising with cardiotoxic burden. Of those with regurgitant lesions the prevalence of aortic regurgitation and TR was significantly increased compared to controls while the prevalence of mitral regurgitation was similar in treatment and control groups. The majority of valvular disease was graded moderate severity. Additional risk factors for valvular dysfunction included: female sex, age >50 at the time of diagnosis, >3 lines of chemotherapy before auto-HCT, and cardiac radiation >30 Gy [51].

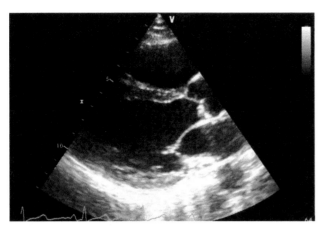

FIGURE 19.5   Parasternal long axis view showing radiation induced thickening of the aortic valve.

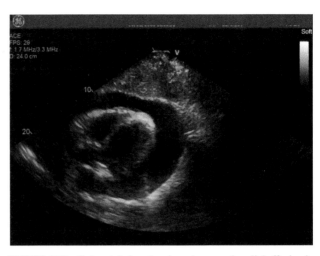

FIGURE 19.7   Subcostal view showing a large pericardial effusion in a patient post chemotherapy and radiation.

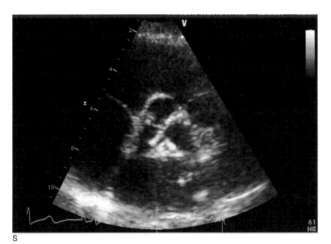

FIGURE 19.6   Short axis view showing radiation induced thickening of the aortic valve.

PERICARDIAL DISEASE

Pericardial disease routinely manifests in oncology patients as either metastatic spread of a primary malignancy or as an unintended side effect of treatment (Fig. 19.7). The most common metastatic tumors to the pericardium include lung carcinoma, breast carcinoma, melanoma, leukemia, and lymphoma [52]. Chemotherapeutic agents and radiation therapy can also induce pericarditis with or without an effusion causing hemodynamic instability.

Echocardiography is the first line imaging modality to evaluate the pericardium. In patients with pericarditis, echocardiography can show a pericardial effusion, hyper-echoic pericardium, or pericardial thickening along with other structural and Doppler features suggestive of constrictive pericarditis.

In a normal individual, the pericardium and epicardium are nearly in contrast, which echocardiographically appears as a reflective band surrounding the heart. The normal pericardial cavity contains between 20 and 30 mL of fluid; however, this may increase following neoplastic spread to the pericardium, mediastinal radiation, or in inflammatory conditions. A pericardial effusion is identified by evidence of separation of the visceral and parietal surfaces, decreased movement of the parietal pericardium, or movement of the heart within the pericardium when a large effusion is present. As pericardial effusions and invasive neoplastic processes typically begin to collect behind the posterior wall of the LV, the parasternal long axis view is the primary imaging plane employed. Areas on neoplastic invasion appear to be more reflective than surrounding regions and distort the otherwise smooth pericardium.

CONTRAST USE DURING ECHOCARDIOGRAPHIC EXAMINATIONS

An inherent limitation of echocardiography is the ability to define the endocardial borders in approximately 20% of the patient population. Contrast echocardiography is commonly performed to better delineate the left ventricular endocardium, which allows for better evaluation of wall motion. Current American Society of Echocardiography guidelines recommend contrast echocardiography to assess segmental wall motion abnormalities, increase the proportion of diagnostic studies, and increase reader confidence in interpretation [53]. Contrast administration may be especially useful in breast cancer survivors who have undergone mastectomy or breast implantation.

Approved contrast agents for echocardiography include Levovist, Optison, Definity, SonoVue, CARDIOsphere, and Imagify. These agents share a common structure of a microbubble filled with a high-molecular weight gas. These intravenous agents opacify cardiac chambers without impacting LV function, systemic hemodynamics, or gas exchange [53].

Numerous studies have evaluated the safety of these contrast agents. Uncommon but mild intolerances to these agents include headache, weakness, and fatigue. Allergic reaction to the contrast agent is a serious rare adverse event occurring during 1/10,000 studies [53].

Of note, contrast echocardiography is contraindicated in patients with a known shunt. A bubble study utilizes agitated saline to identify a cardiac shunt in patients with a suspected atrial septal defect or patent foramen ovale prior to the administration of contrast. As patients with active malignancies are at an increased risk of thrombosis early identification of a shunt may guide management of anticoagulation.

LIMITATIONS

2D echocardiography derived EF is subject to intrareader variability.

Additionally, the smallest visual change in EF that can be detected is an 11% change [54]. Echo image quality is both operator and patient dependent. The technical quality and interpretability decreases with inexperienced operators who are unable to achieve good imaging plane while patient factors including obesity and chronic obstructive pulmonary disease can interfere with the echo windows.

CONCLUSIONS

Given the significant morbidity and mortality associated with cardiovascular complications of cancer therapy, strategies for early detection, and prevention of cardiotoxicity are needed. While echocardiography has its limitations, it is the standard imaging modality for detection of chemotherapy-induced cardiac dysfunction. It is widely available, noninvasive, radiation-free, and a relatively inexpensive technique to assess cardiac structure and function. While 2D Doppler echocardiographic imaging is standard, many specialized centers offer speckle tracking strain imaging to detect subclinical LV dysfunction prior to overt reduction in EF. While randomized studies demonstrating improved cardiovascular outcomes based on GLS-guided initiation of therapy are lacking, it is increasingly recognized that GLS is a marker of LV dysfunction that is better than EF at predicting cardiotoxicity. Whether wide-spread use of these novel echocardiographic techniques will impact morbidity and mortality in cardiovascular cancer survivorship is uncertain at this time.

CONFLICTS

Gleason: None, Lisko: None, Lerakis: Research grant from GE Healthcare.

REFERENCES

[1] Chen MH, Colan SD, Diller L. Cardiovascular disease: cause of morbidity and mortality in adult survivors of childhood cancers. Circ Res 2011;108(5):619–28.

[2] Villarraga HR, Herrmann J, Nkomo VT. Cardio-oncology: role of echocardiography. Prog Cardiovasc Dis 2014;57(1):10–8.

[3] Weyman AE. Standard plane positions-standard imaging planes. In: Weyman AE, editor. Principles and Practice of Echocardiography. 2nd ed. Media, PA: Williams & Wilkins; 1994. p. 98–122.

[4] Vuille CaWA. Left ventricle I: general considerations, assessment of chamber size and function. In: Weyman AE, editor. Principles and Practice of Echocardiography. Media, PA: Williams & Wilkins; 1994. p. 576–84.

[5] Georke RJCE. Calculation of right and left ventricular volumes: methods using standard computer equiptment and biplane angiograms. Invest Radiol 1967;2(153).

[6] Wyatt HL, Heng MK, Meerbaum S, Gueret P, Hestenes J, Dula E, Corday E. Cross-sectional echocardiography. Analysis of mathematical models for quantifying mass of the left ventricle in dogs. Circulation. 1979;60(5):1104–13.

[7] Thavendiranathan P, Grant AD, Negishi T, Plana JC, Popovic ZB, Marwick TH. Reproducibility of echocardiographic techniques for sequential assessment of left ventricular ejection fraction and volumes: application to patients undergoing cancer chemotherapy. J Am Coll Cardiol 2013;61(1):77–84.

[8] Jenkins C, Bricknell K, Hanekom L, Marwick TH. Reproducibility and accuracy of echocardiographic measurements of left ventricular parameters using real-time three-dimensional echocardiography. J Am Coll Cardiol 2004;44(4):878–86.

[9] Gutierrez-Chico JL, Zamorano JL, Perez de Isla L, Orejas M, Almeria C, Rodrigo JL, et al. Comparison of left ventricular volumes and ejection fractions measured by three-dimensional echocardiography versus by two-dimensional echocardiography and cardiac magnetic resonance in patients with various cardiomyopathies. Am J Cardiol 2005;95(6):809–13.

[10] Plana JC, Galderisi M, Barac A, Ewer MS, Ky B, Scherrer-Crosbie M, et al. Expert consensus for multimodality imaging evaluation of adult patients during and after cancer therapy: a report from the American Society of Echocardiography and the European Association of Cardiovascular Imaging. J Am Soc Echocardiogr 2014;27(9):911–39.

[11] Nagueh SF, Appleton CP, Gillebert TC, Marino PN, Oh JK, Smiseth OA, et al. Recommendations for the evaluation of left ventricular diastolic function by echocardiography. J Am Soc Echocardiogr 2009;22(2):107–33.

[12] Arai K, Hozumi T, Matsumura Y, Sugioka K, Takemoto Y, Yamagishi H, et al. Accuracy of measurement of left ventricular volume and ejection fraction by new real-time three-dimensional echocardiography in patients with wall motion abnormalities secondary to myocardial infarction. Am J Cardiol 2004;94(5):552–8.

[13] Moller JE, Søndergaard E, Poulsen S, Egstrup K. Pseudonormal and restricive filling patterns predict left ventricular dilation and cardiac death after a first myocardial infarction: a serial color M-mode doppler echocardiographic study. J Am Coll Cardiol 2000;36(15):1841–6.

[14] Stoddard M, Seeger J, Liddell N, Haldey T, Sullivan D, Kupersmith J. Prolongation of isovolumetric relaxation time as assessed by Doppler echocardiography predicts doxorubicin-induced systolic dysfunction in humans. J Am Coll Cardiol 1992;20(1):62–9.

[15] Lange SA, Ebner B, Wess A, Kogel M, Gajda M, Hitschold T, et al. Echocardiography signs of early cardiac impairment in patients with breast cancer and trastuzumab therapy. Clin Res Cardiol 2012;101(6):415–26.

[16] Tanindi A, Demirci U, Tacoy G, Buyukberber S, Alsancak Y, Coskun U, et al. Assessment of right ventricular functions during cancer chemothcrapy. Eur J Echocardiogr 2011;12(11):834–40.

[17] Montani D, Bergot E, Gunther S, Savale L, Bergeron A, Bourdin A, et al. Pulmonary arterial hypertension in patients treated by dasatinib. Circulation 2012;125(17):2128–37.

[18] Galie N, Task Force for Diagnosis and Treatment of Pulmonary Hypertension of European Society of Cardiology, European Respiratory Society, International Society of Heart and Lung Transplantation. et al. Guidelines for the diagnosis and treatment of pulmonary hypertension. Eur Respir J 2009;34(6):1219–63.

[19] Marwick TH, Leano RL, Brown J, Sun JP, Hoffmann R, Lysyansky P, et al. Myocardial strain measurement with 2-dimensional speckletracking echocardiography: definition of normal range. JACC Cardiovasc Imaging 2009;2(1):80–4.

[20] Haeck ML, Scherptong RW, Marsan NA, Holman ER, Schalij MJ, Bax JJ, et al. Prognostic value of right ventricular longitudinal peak systolic strain in patients with pulmonary hypertension. Circ Cardiovasc Imaging 2012;5(5):628–36.

[21] Bossone E, D'Andrea A, D'Alto M, Citro R, Argiento P, Ferrara F, et al. Echocardiography in pulmonary arterial hypertension: from diagnosis to prognosis. J Am Soc Echocardiogr 2013;26(1):1–14.

[22] Feigenbaum H, Mastouri R, Sawada S. A practical approach to using strain echocardiography to evaluate the left ventricle. Circ J 2012;76(7):1550–5.

[23] Thavendiranathan P, Poulin F, Lim KD, Plana JC, Woo A, Marwick TH. Use of myocardial strain imaging by echocardiography for the early detection of cardiotoxicity in patients during and after cancer chemotherapy: a systematic review. J Am Coll Cardiol 2014;63(25 Pt. A):2751–68.

[24] Amundsen BH, Helle-Valle T, Edvardsen T, Torp H, Crosby J, Lyseggen E, et al. Noninvasive myocardial strain measurement by speckle tracking echocardiography: validation against sonomicrometry and tagged magnetic resonance imaging. J Am Coll Cardiol 2006;47(4):789–93.

[25] Kalogeropoulos AP, Georgiopoulou VV, Gheorghiade M, Butler J. Echocardiographic evaluation of left ventricular structure and function: new modalities and potential applications in clinical trials. J Card Fail 2012;18(2):159–72.

[26] Mastouri R, Rehman S, Sawada S, Feigenbaum H. Prognostic value of strain echocardiography in patients undergoing chemotherapy. J Am Coll Cardiol 2012;59(13):E1122.

[27] Leitman M, Lysyansky P, Sidenko S, Shir V, Peleg E, Binenbaum M, et al. Two-dimensional strain-a novel software for real-time quantitative echocardiographic assessment of myocardial function. J Am Soc Echocardiogr 2004;17(10):1021–9.

[28] Armstrong GT, Joshi VM, Ness KK, Marwick TH, Zhang N, Srivastava D, et al. Comprehensive echocardiographic detection of treatment-related cardiac dysfunction in adult survivors of childhood cancer: results from the St. Jude Lifetime Cohort Study. J Am Coll Cardiol 2015;65(23):2511–22.

[29] Nahum J, Bensaid A, Dussault C, Macron L, Clemence D, Bouhemad B, et al. Impact of longitudinal myocardial deformation on the prognosis of chronic heart failure patients. Circ Cardiovasc Imaging 2010;3(3):249–56.

[30] Toro-Salazar OH, Ferranti J, Lorenzoni R, Walling S, Mazur W, Raman SV, et al. Feasibility of echocardiographic techniques to detect subclinical cancer therapeutics-related cardiac dysfunction among high-dose patients when compared with cardiac magnetic resonance imaging. J Am Soc Echocardiogr 2016;29(2):119–31.

[31] Fallah-Rad N, Walker JR, Wassef A, Lytwyn M, Bohonis S, Fang T, et al. The utility of cardiac biomarkers, tissue velocity and strain imaging, and cardiac magnetic resonance imaging in predicting early left ventricular dysfunction in patients with human epidermal growth factor receptor II-positive breast cancer treated with adjuvant trastuzumab therapy. J Am Coll Cardiol 2011;57(22):2263–70.

[32] Hare JL, Brown JK, Leano R, Jenkins C, Woodward N, Marwick TH. Use of myocardial deformation imaging to detect preclinical myocardial dysfunction before conventional measures in patients undergoing breast cancer treatment with trastuzumab. Am Heart J 2009;158(2):294–301.

[33] Negishi K, Negishi T, Hare JL, Haluska BA, Plana JC, Marwick TH. Independent and incremental value of deformation indices for prediction of trastuzumab-induced cardiotoxicity. J Am Soc Echocardiogr 2013;26(5):493–8.

[34] Rhea IB, Uppuluri S, Sawada S, Schneider BP, Feigenbaum H. Incremental prognostic value of echocardiographic strain and its association with mortality in cancer patients. J Am Soc Echocardiogr 2015;28(6):667–73.

[35] Saito M, Negishi K, Eskandari M, Huynh Q, Hawson J, Moore A, et al. Association of left ventricular strain with 30-day mortality and readmission in patients with heart failure. J Am Soc Echocardiogr 2015;28(6):652–66.

[36] Sawaya H, Sebag IA, Plana JC, Januzzi JL, Ky B, Cohen V, et al. Early detection and prediction of cardiotoxicity in chemotherapytreated patients. Am J Cardiol 2011;107(9):1375–80.

[37] Shah AM, Claggett B, Sweitzer NK, Shah SJ, Anand IS, Liu L, et al. Prognostic importance of impaired systolic function in heart failure with preserved ejection fraction and the impact of spironolactone. Circulation 2015;132(5):402–14.

[38] Ali MT, Yucel E, Bouras S, Wang L, Fei HW, Halpern EF, et al. Myocardial strain is associated with adverse clinical cardiac events in patients treated with anthracyclines. J Am Soc Echocardiogr 2016;29(6):522–7.

[39] Mornos C, Petrescu L. Early detection of anthracycline-mediated cardiotoxicity: the value of considering both global longitudinal left ventricular strain and twist. Can J Physiol Pharmacol 2013;91(8):601–7.

[40] Seicean S, Seicean A, Alan N, Plana JC, Budd GT, Marwick TH. Cardioprotective effect of beta-adrenoceptor blockade in patients with breast cancer undergoing chemotherapy: follow-up study of heart failure. Circ Heart Fail 2013;6(3):420–6.

[41] Gulati G, Heck SL, Ree AH, Hoffmann P, Schulz-Menger J, Fagerland MW, et al. Prevention of cardiac dysfunction during adjuvant breast cancer therapy (PRADA): a 2 x 2 factorial, randomized, placebo-controlled, double-blind clinical trial of candesartan and metoprolol. Eur Heart J 2016;37(21):1671–80.

[42] Martin M, Esteva FJ, Alba E, Khandheria B, Perez-Isla L, GarciaSaenz JA, et al. Minimizing cardiotoxicity while optimizing treatment efficacy with trastuzumab: review and expert recommendations. Oncologist 2009;14(1):1–11.

[43] Cardinale D, Colombo A, Bacchiani G, Tedeschi I, Meroni CA, Veglia F, et al. Early detection of anthracycline cardiotoxicity and improvement with heart failure therapy. Circulation 2015;131(22):1981–8.

[44] Writing Committee M, Yancy CW, Jessup M, Bozkurt B, Butler J, Casey DE Jr, et al. 2013 ACCF/AHA guideline for the management of heart failure: a report of the American College of Cardiology Foundation/American Heart Association Task Force on practice guidelines. Circulation 2013;128(16):e240–327.

[45] Yeh ET, Vejpongsa P. Subclinical cardiotoxicity associated with cancer therapy: early detection and future directions. J Am Coll Cardiol 2015;65(23):2523–5.

[46] Smith M, MacPhail B, Harrison M, Lenhoff S, DeMaria A. Value and limitations of transesophageal echocardiography in determinaton of left ventricular volumes and ejection fraction. J Am Coll Cardiol 1992;19(6):1213–22.

[47] Mugge A, Daniel W, Frank G, Lichtlen P. Echocardiography in infective endocarditis: reassessment of prognositc implications of vegatation size determined by the transthoracic and the transesophagel approach. J Am Coll Cardiol 1989;14(3):631–8.

[48] Hahn RT, Abraham T, Adams MS, Bruce CJ, Glas KE, Lang RM, et al. Guidelines for performing a comprehensive transesophageal echocardiographic examination: recommendations from the American Society of Echocardiography and the Society of Cardiovascular Anesthesiologists. J Am Soc Echocardiogr 2013;26(9):921–64.

[49] Civelli M, Cardinale D, Martinoni A, Lamantia G, Colombo N, Colombo A, et al. Early reduction in left ventricular contractile reserve detected by dobutamine stress echo predicts high-dose chemotherapy-induced cardiac toxicity. Int J Cardiol 2006;111(1):120–6.

[50] Grosu A, Bombardini T, Senni M, Duino V, Gori M, Picano E. End-systolic pressure/volume relationship during dobutamine stress echo: a prognostically useful non-invasive index of left ventricular contractility. Eur Heart J 2005;26(22):2404–12.

[51] Murbraech K, Wethal T, Smeland KB, Holte H, Loge JH, Holte E, et al. Valvular dysfunction in lymphoma survivors treated with autologous stem cell transplantation: a national cross-sectional study. JACC Cardiovasc Imaging 2016;9(3):230–9.

[52] Bussani R, De-Giorgio F, Abbate A, Silvestri F. Cardiac metastases. J Clin Pathol 2007;60(1):27–34.

[53] Mulvagh SL, Rakowski H, Vannan MA, Abdelmoneim SS, Becher H, Bierig SM, et al. American Society of Echocardiography Consensus Statement on the clinical applications of ultrasonic contrast agents in echocardiography. J Am Soc Echocardiogr 2008;21(11):1179–201. quiz 281.

[54] Marwick TH, Narula J. Why, when, and how often?: The next steps after defining the right tools for noninvasive imaging of cardiotoxicity. JACC Cardiovasc Imaging 2014;7(8):851–3.

Chapter 20

Principles of Cancer Rehabilitation

A. Asher*, A. Ng** and J. Engle**

*Cedars Sinai Medical Center, Los Angeles, CA, United States; **University of Texas MD Anderson Cancer Center, Houston, TX, United States

INTRODUCTION/HISTORY OF CANCER REHABILITATION

Americans afflicted with cancer are living longer and the outlook continues to get better for people with cancer. On the strength of public awareness, early detection, and improved multimodal cancer treatment, for many patients cancer has evolved from an often fatal disease to a chronic, treatable condition. Cancer survivors have increased in number by more than threefold over the last 30 years. Today there are over 14 million survivors, with the expectation of this number doubling over the next 30 years [1]. Among patients diagnosed today, nearly two-thirds are expected to survive at least 5 or more years [2]. A significant cohort of these survivors will live 10, 15, 20, or more years after a cancer diagnosis. With the burgeoning number of survivors of cancer today comes increasing attention to issues related to rehabilitation and QoL, as survival in isolation is no longer an adequate measure of wellness.

Although many cancer survivors may be disease free, many are not "free of their disease." They may face a vast scope of issues including, but not limited to, fatigue, pain, lymphedema, anxiety, and functional impairments as a result of their cancer or its treatment (Table 20.1). Therefore, for many cancer patients, returning to "normal" life can be a very difficult transition. Many cancer survivors live with considerable disability due to effects of treatment. For example, a population-based cohort study of 975 Australian working adults with colorectal cancer, 33% of men and 40% of women were not able to return to work 12 months after their diagnosis [3]. In 2005, the Institute of Medicine published a seminal report, *From Cancer Patient to Cancer Survivor: Lost in Transition*, which also began to address the increasingly important role that rehabilitation plays in the lives of cancer survivors [4].

The central tenet of cancer rehabilitation is to help cancer patients and survivors regain and improve their physical, psychosocial, and vocational functioning *within the limitations* imposed by the disease and its treatment [5].

The multidisciplinary-team approach central to comprehensive cancer rehabilitation is ideal for meeting the needs of survivors of cancer. Many of the toxicities and complications of cancer and its treatment can be mitigated by rehabilitation interventions. For example, cancer-related fatigue (CRF), depression, anxiety, cognitive dysfunction, pain syndromes, peripheral neuropathy, balance and gait problems, dysphagia, and lymphedema can all be potentially managed by the rehabilitation team [6].

Despite the known benefits, a number of major challenges exist toward the delivery of quality and comprehensive cancer rehabilitation. The patient may be experiencing frequent changes in medical, functional, and psychological status through the course of oncologic treatment, from diagnosis to treatment through survivorship. Therefore, functional and rehabilitation goals may change often which requires more routine assessment. From a rehabilitation professional perspective, oncologic treatment options are continually changing which requires maintenance of current knowledge for a large array of cancers, treatments, and associated side effects and disability. Cancer rehabilitation is a relatively new subspecialty within the arena of rehabilitation medicine. Many providers of rehabilitation generally have not received adequate training in the special needs of cancer patients and survivors [7]. Other barriers include a nonexistent or weak interface between oncology and rehabilitation professionals, even when available within the same institution. Furthermore, despite the potential benefits of outpatient cancer rehabilitation services, accessing this care through insurance barriers can be challenging. The diversity in health-care plans with complicated authorization and reimbursements, limited coverage schedules, funding caps, and strict guidelines for continuation of therapy may result in inadequate services for some survivors of cancer [8].

Despite the real barriers in providing high-quality cancer rehabilitation service to the rapidly growing cancer survivorship community, the comprehensive rehabilitation model evaluates the sum total of problems that a survivor

TABLE 20.1 Potential Issues Faced By Cancer Survivors

Cancer-related fatigue and sleep disturbances

Peripheral neuropathy and balance disorders

Osteoporosis

Secondary malignancies

Existential and spiritual issues

Vocational and financial issues

Functional decline

Poor quality of life

Family and caregiver distress

Psychosocial distress and coping after cancer treatment

Sexuality and body image

Lymphedema

Pain and neuropathy

Cognitive changes

Cardiorespiratory effects

faces and coordinates interdisciplinary treatment. In addition to improving QoL, some recent evidence also suggests that higher functional levels from rehabilitation interventions are also associated with higher survival rates [9,10]. The goal of this chapter is to provide an overview of some of the most common clinical problems faced in the cancer rehabilitation arena and rehabilitation approaches toward its management, including:

- CRF and the role of therapeutic exercise
- Cancer-related cognitive dysfunction
- Rehabilitation approach to pain
- Lymphedema
- Rehabilitation principles in the patient with breast cancer
- Radiation fibrosis syndrome
- Management of peripheral neuropathy and balance impairment

CANCER-RELATED FATIGUE AND ROLE OF THERAPEUTIC EXERCISE

Fatigue is the most common, and one of the most devastating symptoms among patients with cancer [11]. According to the National Comprehensive Cancer Network, CRF is defined as a "persistent, subjective sense of physical, emotional, and/or cognitive exhaustion related to cancer or its treatment that is not proportional to recent activity" [12]. Although it is generally believed to affect over 80–90% of patients who are going through active cancer treatment, about one-third of survivors continue to experience persistent fatigue well into survivorship [13–15]. Fatigue has been

rated as having a greater negative impact on QoL than other cancer-related symptoms such as pain, depression, and nausea [13]. It is important to distinguish so-called "healthy" fatigue from CRF. Healthy fatigue is fatigue that is eventually relieved by rest and sleep. CRF is not proportional to recent activity and interferes with usual functioning. For example, patients with CRF will complain of difficulty with doing routine activities that previously did not cause any distress, such as laundry, running errands, or cooking. In fact, CRF has a negative impact on all areas of function, including mood, physical function, work performance, social interaction, family care, cognitive performance, school work, and community activities [16–18].

The etiology of CRF is not entirely clear, although many potential factors may contribute to this symptom or may be a consequence of this syndrome. Potential factors include: direct toxicity from chemotherapy and radiation therapy [19], the cancer itself [20], genetic vulnerability [21], hormonal changes [22], medication side effects [23], poor sleep [24], depression and anxiety [25], chronic stress, poor nutrition [12], loss of muscle mass and inactivity [26], and other chronic medical problems [27]. Other proposed mechanisms include hypothalamic-pituitary-adrenal axis dysregulation, circadian rhythm desynchronization, and cardiovascular deconditioning. Inflammation related to cytokines is increasingly being recognized as playing a key role in the genesis of CRF. Basic research on neural–immune interactions has shown that proinflammatory cytokines can cause potent changes in behavior including reduced activity, fatigue, decreased social behavior, and cognitive dysfunction [19]. More debilitating levels of CRF have been associated with increased serum measurements of proinflammatory cytokines [28]. Furthermore, these inflammatory mediators are also being associated with a higher risk of cancer risk or recurrence [29,30].

Evaluation of Cancer-Related Fatigue

The National Comprehensive Cancer Network guidelines recommend that every cancer patient should be screened for fatigue [31]. Unfortunately, CRF is often underreported and overlooked by health care professionals [32–35]. The use of screening assessments can help clinicians to key into symptoms such as fatigue. Fatigue is often included in many multisymptom screening assessments including the Edmonton Symptom and Assessment Scale and the MD Anderson Symptom Inventory. On a 1–10 scale, fatigue severity of more than 4 should be evaluated by further history and physical. Over 20 detailed fatigue measurement tools have been used to better delineate patient fatigue symptoms including the Brief Fatigue Inventory [36], Functional Assessment of Cancer Therapy: Fatigue or FACT-F [37], Revised Piper Fatigue Scale [38], and Multidimensional Fatigue Inventory [39].

In addition to fatigue measurement tools, a thorough history and physical evaluation are essential in the evaluation of CRF patients. Clinicians should discern the patient's cancer history including treatments and time since treatment. Current and past medications should be reviewed. Questions regarding confounding factors including sleep quality, stress, mood, etc. could be helpful. A physical examination should include a cardiac, pulmonary, neurologic, cognitive, and functional evaluation. A fatigue laboratory panel is among the initial screening tools for CRF. Elements of the fatigue laboratory panel may include a cell blood count, electrolytes, folate, vitamin B12, thyroid-stimulating hormone, testosterone level (in males), erythrocyte sedimentation rate or c-reactive protein, and urinalysis.

Treatment of Cancer-Related Fatigue

All patients and their families should be offered specific information about fatigue during and following treatment, including education about the difference between normal and CRF, persistence beyond treatment, and causes and contributory factors. The NCCN also recommends counseling for patients about general strategies such as energy conservation techniques and distraction which can be useful in coping with fatigue [31]. Energy conservation is defined as the deliberately planned management of one's personal energy resources to prevent their depletion. This involves setting realistic expectation of what may be accomplished in a given day, pacing activities, and delegating nonessential tasks. Distraction may involve activities such as reading, music, and games which also may help the perception of fatigue.

Because of the interplay of cancer symptoms, treating symptoms or conditions that could contribute to fatigue is one strategy. For patients with sleep disorder, specific measures to improve sleep hygiene and cognitive behavioral therapy may be helpful. If fatigue is accompanied by significant symptoms of depression, a trial of an antidepressant may be warranted [40–42]. A nutrition evaluation and perhaps appetite stimulation for malnourished patients could be considered for those with cachexia and associated fatigue. Other contributing factors such as anemia, pain, and other medical comorbidities need to be considered. A trial of testosterone supplementation is sometimes provided for men with fatigue who are found to have hypogonadism [43]. Neurostimulants, in particular methylphenidate, have also been studied in multiple placebo controlled trials. The scientific evidence supporting the use of neurostimulants for CRF is generally mixed. However, the evidence to date seems to support its role among patients with advanced disease and severe fatigue or in active treatment [44]. Mind–body programs such as yoga have also emerged as a viable treatment to reduce fatigue and improve sleep quality among cancer survivors [45].

Exercise as a Treatment for Fatigue

Exercise has been shown in multiple randomized control trials to be an effective treatment for CRF [46–48]. Indeed, a recent Cochrane Database Systemic review concluded that exercise may be regarded as beneficial for individuals with CRF, particularly during postcancer therapy [49]. Further research is required to determine the optimal type, intensity, and timing of exercise intervention for mitigating CRF. The mechanism by which fatigue is reduced with exercise is likely multifactorial. Exercise and physical activity in cancer patients has been shown to improve aerobic capacity, minimize muscle loss, improve body composition, and improve conditioning, in addition to psychological benefits [50,51]. One possible mechanism that has been gaining increased attention is the antiinflammatory effects of exercise. Hyperinflammation is likely associated with a number of cancer-related symptoms include fatigue, cachexia, and some pain syndromes. Exercise, based on studies primarily conducted in the general population, reduces inflammation through a number of factors:

1. *Exercise reduces visceral fat (i.e., "bad" fat).* An increase in visceral fat is correlated with a higher production of proinflammatory cytokines such as TNF, IL-6, and leptin. For this reason, visceral fat is associated with increased all-cause mortality and the development of diabetes, cardiovascular disease, and dementia as well as several cancers [52,53]. Regular exercise can reduce waist circumference and reduce visceral fat—even in the absence of body weight reduction [54].

2. *Exercise releases IL-6 from contracting muscle.* Typically, IL-6 is associated as being a proinflammatory cytokine. However, the role of IL-6 may depend on the source where it is being produced. With exercise, the transient rise in IL-6 from muscle during exercise then leads to a subsequent rise in antiinflammatory cytokines, such as IL-10 and IL-1 receptor antagonist [55].

3. *Exercise increases the secretion of adrenal hormones,* such as cortisol, epinephrine, and norepinephrine, which have potent antiinflammatory effects [56].

4. *Exercise changes the phenotype of fat cells to produce less inflammation.* M1-type macrophages are associated with the production of inflammatory cytokines and obesity [57]. With consistent exercise, there is a phenotypic switch of adipose tissue macrophages toward M2-type macrophages which produce antiinflammatory cytokines.

5. *Exercise may reduce inflammation via downregulation of toll-like receptors on monocytes and macrophages* [58]. Activation of toll-like receptors results in increased production of proinflammatory cytokines. Other mechanisms are also believed to play a role in the antiinflammatory effects of exercise.

In addition to the aforementioned benefits of exercise on CRF, emerging evidence also indicates that regular aerobic exercise is associated with significant reductions in cancer recurrence and cancer-specific mortality in patients with early stage breast, prostate, and colorectal cancers [59]. Accumulating and more compelling evidence suggests that higher levels of fitness are associated with higher survival rates in the oncology setting [60]. Adequate education and support are needed to help the patient exercise adequately and safely.

However, despite the multitude of described benefits of exercise in the oncology setting, fewer than half of cancer survivors reach their prediagnosis level of activity [61]. Moreover, only 21.5% of cancer survivors can recall a discussion of exercise with their health-care professional [61]. This is important to note because physical activity is a *modifiable* lifestyle factor that can potentially play a major role in the health of the patient with cancer.

Major national organizations have adopted similar recommendations for exercise behavior among cancer survivors. The American Cancer Society, American Society of Clinical Oncology, and the American College of Sports Medicine, all recommend that cancer patients and survivors adhere to exercise guidelines for the general population [62]. That recommendation consists of 150 min per week of moderate intensity aerobic activity or 75 min of vigorous-intensity exercise or an equivalent combination. For strength training, 2–3 weekly sessions that include exercises for major muscle groups is recommended. However, these guidelines are still fairly nonspecific. Individualized treatment programs that are patient tailored by a rehabilitation professional may be optimal. Cancer patients can suffer from a wide array of musculoskeletal and medical issues that need to be considered individually. Brown et al. found that exercise programs that were too intense actually led to worsening cancer fatigue [63]. There are concerns that very intense, long-duration exercises can actually impede optimal immune function. For example, runners who ran more than 866 miles/year have been found to have an increased rate of viral infection. These findings led to the proposal of a "J-shaped" curve to define the relationship of exercise and susceptibility to infection [64]. Other considerations include cardiac history, pulmonary history, and the effects of pancytopenia. Some patients suffer from cardiomyopathy from chemotherapy or prior cardiovascular disease that needs to be accounted for. Neuropathy and other musculoskeletal disorders should be considered as impaired proprioception from chemotherapy-induced peripheral neuropathy (CIPN) as they may put patients at higher risk for falls. Orthopedic concerns such as existing or impending pathologic fractures need to be considered when creating an exercise prescription. Weight bearing or range of motion limitations may need to be prescribed. Neutropenic patients may need to take extra precautions to prevent becoming infected including wearing a mask and gloves. Communications with exercise professionals and physical therapists is vital to ensure safety concerns are being managed appropriately [65].

CANCER-RELATED COGNITIVE IMPAIRMENT

Cancer treatments are aggressive and often include multimodal strategies such as surgery, radiation, chemotherapy, and immunotherapy. These multimodal strategies are often attributed to improve survival rates; unfortunately, most are not highly specific and may place normal cells and organs at risk, including the central nervous system. Moreover, many of the adjunctive medications that cancer patients receive, such as corticosteroids, antiepileptic medications, immunosuppressive agents, opioids, hypnotics, and antiemetics, may also contribute to impaired cognition. Therefore, cognitive dysfunction may be a consequence of the cancer, its treatment, or both.

The term "chemobrain" was coined after breast cancer patients started to notice mental fogginess around the same time they were being treated with chemotherapy. This term has its limitations since many other causes may contribute for cognitive dysfunction among cancer patients, such as depression, hormonal changes, insomnia, and even the cancer itself [66]. Nevertheless, the term "chemobrain" has increasingly become more publicized, particularly among the breast cancer community [67]. Although "chemobrain" was first identified and named by breast cancer survivors, the same constellation of symptoms also affects other cancer patients. A typical patient with "chemobrain" may report some or all of the concerns listed in Table 20.2.

No single symptom or set of symptoms is pathognomonic for cognitive dysfunction due to cancer and its treatment. Moreover, cognitive complaints often are associated with persistent fatigue and depressive symptoms that historically have complicated evaluation and research. Over the last decade, the literature on cognitive changes after cancer

TABLE 20.2 Typical Concerns Reported by Patients With "Chemobrain"

Memory lapses
Difficulty concentrating or staying focused on a task
Trouble remembering details such as names, dates, or phone numbers
Difficulty multitasking such as carrying a conversation and following a cooking recipe
Slower processing speeds
Difficulty with word retrieval

treatment has rapidly expanded and been subjected to much more rigorous study. The research, in general, has demonstrated that cognitive concerns can negatively and sometimes dramatically impact function, QoL, and community integration [68,69]. Fortunately, long-term memory and syndromes suggestive of cortical dysfunction, such as aphasia, agnosia, and apraxia, are generally not affected [70].

Most studies suggest that up to 75% of patients with cancer experience cognitive impairment during treatment, and 15–35% of cancer survivors experience cognitive problems months to years following treatment [71,72]. However, the prevalence of cognitive dysfunction varies widely in the literature, and multiple challenges impede the accurate assessment of the incidence of cognitive dysfunction, including the lack of prechemotherapy assessment of cognitive function, differences in the populations being studied, and the lack of standardized assessment tools and neuropsychological batteries. Measurement of cancer-related cognitive dysfunction in the literature is hampered further by differences in inclusion criteria, timing of cognitive assessments, and varying comparison groups (i.e., published normative data, healthy matched controls, patients with cancer not treated with chemotherapy, etc.). Furthermore, patients differ with respect to tumor type, stage of disease, concomitant treatment (nausea regimens, hormonal treatments, and multimodality treatments), and medical comorbidities—all of which could impact cognitive function [73]. Some researchers have reported that cognitive changes associated with cancer treatment often resolve within 1 year, whereas others have documented long-term changes that last for more than 20 years [74–76].

Multiple studies using prechemotherapy cognitive assessments have demonstrated that some patients have cognitive dysfunction *prior* to receiving any treatment. For example, several studies have noted that approximately 20–35% of patients with breast cancer have lower than expected cognitive performance on the basis of age and education at the pretreatment assessment [71,77–79]. Pretreatment cognitive dysfunction also has been found in other populations, including patients with acute myelogenous leukemia and lung cancer [80,81]. In addition, because cancer is generally an illness that affects older populations, it is not surprising that age is a confounding factor for cognitive challenges. One-fifth of geriatric patients with cancer screen positively for cognitive disorders [82].

The majority of studies in this area have been conducted using women with breast cancer. Cross-sectional data suggest that 16–75% of patients with breast cancer experience cognitive impairment during chemotherapy, compared with 4–11% of healthy controls [72]. Jim et al. reported meta-analysis findings on cognitive function obtained from 17 studies of 807 survivors of breast cancer treated with standard-dose chemotherapy at least 6 months previously. Cognitive deficits were limited to verbal and visuospatial

ability and were generally small in magnitude [83]. However, many experts purport that a subset of cancer survivors may be particularly vulnerable to more significant cognitive changes [84]. For example, one recent study used neuropsychological tests to demonstrate that a subgroup of breast cancer survivors continued to experience a decline in cognitive function over time after treatment [85]. Another recent report evaluating cognitive function among survivors of allogeneic stem cell transplantation found that, after 5 years, survivors continued to recover within some cognitive domains (e.g., verbal fluency and executive function) but deficits remained for more than 40% of patients [86].

Hypotheses for Causal Mechanisms

Many mechanisms have been suggested to explain cognitive dysfunction in patients with cancer, including direct neurotoxic effects of therapy (e.g., inhibition of hippocampal neurogenesis), genetic predisposition, oxidative damage, and immune dysregulation. Definitive evidence to support a single mechanism is absent, and discovering a final common mechanistic pathway may be unrealistic.

Direct neurotoxicity from chemotherapy is one obvious hypothesis for the etiology of cognitive dysfunction in this setting (hence the term chemobrain). However, determining the biggest offender in the various classes of chemotherapeutic agents is problematic. Because multiple classes of drugs often are used in combination, it is difficult to isolate the effects of chemotherapy from other aspects of treatment, such as radiation therapy and surgery. Nevertheless, we know that certain agents (e.g., methotrexate and 5-fluorouracil) are particularly neurotoxic and cause diffuse white matter changes on neuroimaging [70,87,88]. Animal studies have suggested that certain chemotherapeutic agents (e.g., carmustine, cisplatin, and cytarabine) may be more toxic to white matter progenitor cells and hippocampal stem cells than they are to actual cancer cells [89,90]. Anemia is also a well-known side effect of myelosuppressive chemotherapies. Anemia may cause cerebral hypoxia due to a decrease in hemoglobin concentration, and has been associated with fatigue and cognitive dysfunction [91].

Genetic factors also may predispose some patients with cancer to cognitive dysfunction. Variants of genes encoding apolipoprotein E (*APOE*) and catechol-O-methyltransferase (*COMT*) have both been associated with age-related cognitive decline in the general population [92]. ApoE plays a role in neuronal repair and plasticity after injury, and one study suggested that long-term cancer survivors with at least 1 ApoE4 allele who were previously treated with chemotherapy had poorer cognitive function [93]. COMT plays a role in the breakdown of catecholamines. Small et al. found that patients with breast cancer who had the COMT-Val allele performed worse on tests of attention, verbal fluency, and motor speed [94].

The appreciation that some patients with cancer have cognitive problems prior to receiving any chemotherapy has changed our understanding of the mechanisms behind this syndrome. One hypothesis to explain this phenomenon is that risk factors may be shared for cognitive dysfunction and certain cancers. For example, poor DNA repair mechanisms have been linked to both problems [95]. Another potential mechanism is known as the "accelerated aging hypothesis," which proposes that cancer treatment accelerates the aging process through a variety of mechanisms, including increased DNA damage, shortened telomeres, inflammation, and oxidative stress [71]. Different patients may be vulnerable to different mechanisms, which can account for the observations that older breast cancer survivors may be at elevated risk for cognitive dysfunction [96].

The field of psychoneuroimmunology has shed light on the mechanisms of cognitive change after cancer treatment. Tissue trauma and inflammation from surgery, radiation, chemotherapy, biologic therapy, and targeted therapy can trigger systemic inflammation that can cross the blood–brain barrier and have deleterious effects on the CNS [20,97]. Circulating proinflammatory cytokines have been shown to impair learning and memory in animals [98]. In these studies, administration of proinflammatory cytokines to the brain increases the metabolism of key neurotransmitters, including noradrenaline, dopamine, and serotonin [99]. These neurotransmitters are central to the regulation of memory, learning, sleep, and mood. Moreover, administration of innate immune cytokines to laboratory animals has been shown to disrupt long-term potentiation in the hippocampus and thereby disrupt memory consolidation [100]. Once cytokines reach the brain, they stimulate the resident immune cells (i.e., microglia) to produce other proinflammatory cytokines and inflammatory mediators [101,102]. This may explain why cognitive dysfunction is not limited to patients with brain tumors (primary or metastatic) or to treatment directly targeting the brain.

Psychological and emotional stress can alter the hypothalamic pituitary adrenal axis and sympathetic nervous system, which then can alter the immune system in a similar way [103]. In this light, some investigators have argued that chemobrain can be viewed in the same way as other somatoform illnesses, such as fibromyalgia or chronic fatigue syndrome. This hypothesis purports that the physical and psychological distress of cancer treatment triggers biologic alterations (such as acute shifts in cytokines) that result in epigenetic alterations. These epigenetic modifications may create long-term homeostatic changes that are responsible for the neuroplastic alterations in cancer-related cognitive dysfunction [104]. Recent evidence also has pointed to certain single nucleotide polymorphisms (e.g., in *IL1R1*) that may significantly increase the chance for cytokine-induced changes in cognition after treatment [105]. This evidence supports the International Cognition and Cancer Task Force report, highlighting a consistent finding in the literature that subgroups of patients are more vulnerable to cognitive changes [106].

Assessment Techniques

A gold standard for subjective or objective assessment of cancer treatment–related cognitive changes has yet to be established. Many challenges have been noted, including inconsistent correlation between objective and subjective measures, the lack of objective instruments sensitive enough to capture the subtle cognitive changes perceived by some survivors, and the lack of instruments that accurately simulate the real-world environment in which cancer survivors must function. Objective neuropsychological testing requires special training and significant time to administer, thus adding to survivors' burden. Neuroimaging has been used in the clinical trial setting to document cancer treatment–related changes in brain structure and function. Researchers continue to search for accessible, cost-effective measures of intervention efficacy.

The National Comprehensive Cancer Network (NCCN) Guidelines for Survivorship do not yet recommend any one brief screening tool for assessing cognitive function, but suggest screening survivors with questions regarding their ability to pay attention, find words, remember things, think clearly, and perform functions [107]. They also suggest ascertaining the time of onset for cognitive complaints and assessing the trajectory over time. Additionally, survivors should be assessed for concomitant conditions that may contribute to cognitive issues such as anxiety, depression, fatigue, sleep disturbance, and pain. These conditions should be appropriately addressed. Likewise, survivors' medications should be reviewed, because many medications can contribute to alterations in cognition.

Interventions

The treatment of cognitive impairment in the cancer setting is not well established. Research results thus far have been equivocal regarding the use of neurostimulants (e.g., methylphenidate and modafinil) as interventions for cancer-related cognitive changes. More recent studies for methylphenidate have been negative for efficacy [108,109] or the results have been mixed [110]. Modafinil studies also have been equivocal because of small sample sizes, uncontrolled designs, differences in dose and duration of therapy, and variations in which cognitive domains show improvement. Additionally, many of these studies do not use cognition as the primary endpoint [111]. At this time, neither drug has sufficient evidence of efficacy to move forward with an approved indication [111]. However, some clinicians do use these agents off-label on a case-by-case basis.

Cognitive rehabilitation encompasses a number of interventions with different (or different combinations of) foci. In very general terms, cognitive training typically involves a series of exercises to enhance attention, concentration, and memory skills. These exercises may be computerized, and repetition and practice are important to the success of the intervention. Cognitive behavioral training is focused more on adaptive strategies to compensate for deficits in the various cognitive domains, and may also focus on confounding factors such as anxiety, depression, and fatigue. Some recent evidence has been promising in supporting the role of cognitive rehabilitation programs in reducing cognitive impairment among breast cancer survivors [112,113]. Evidence also continues to build in support of aerobic, resistance, and mindfulness-based exercise as potential interventions for cancer and cancer treatment–related cognitive changes. The primary rationales proposed for the success of physical activity and exercise are: (1) a reduction in markers of inflammation that accompany cancer and cancer treatments and (2) an increase in brain-derived neurotrophic factor levels and hippocampal volume [114–116]. Exercise is known to combat fatigue and sleep disturbances [117,118] and has been shown to improve cognitive performance in a variety of patient populations, such as the elderly [119], those with Alzheimer's disease[120], Parkinson's disease [121], and preliminarily those with various types of cancer [117,122–126]. Exercise intervention studies thus far have been preliminary in nature and many questions remain regarding the most effective type(s) of exercise regimens, timing, duration, frequency, and intensity (i.e., dosage).

REHABILITATION APPROACH TO PAIN IN THE PATIENT WITH CANCER

Cancer pain can be complex as it can be due to the cancer itself, the cancer treatment, or possibly unrelated causes. Whatever its cause, pain can affect many aspect of a person's life including physical functioning, ability to think clearly, emotional outlook, and ability to socialize. About 30–50% of cancer patients experience pain. The prevalence is much higher with advanced disease (over 80%). Given that pain is frequently associated with cancer, *all* cancer patients should be routinely screened for pain. Cancer patients and survivors can face a wide range of pain syndromes including the following: oral mucositis (i.e., from chemotherapy, radiation therapy, etc.), bone pain (bone metastasis, pathological fractures), visceral pain (such as with gastrointestinal or gynecologic tumors), soft-tissue pain (such as with sarcomas, cramps from nerve injuries related to treatment, or inflammation from radiation), neuropathic pain (leptomeningeal disease, cranial neuralgias, radiculopathy and plexopathy, CIPN), postsurgical pain syndrome (such as postthoractomy pain, phantom limb pain, and post radical neck dissection), and paraneoplastic pain syndromes (such

as hypertrophic osteoarthropathy associated with lung cancer) [127]. A discussion of the pathophysiology and management of the various cancer pain syndromes is beyond the scope of this chapter. It is imperative to emphasize that cancer pain is best managed in the context of palliative care which focuses on a broad array of other symptoms (such as fatigue, appetite, anxiety, sleep, depression, etc.) and also integration of social, emotional, physical, and existential needs as part of the comprehensive, individualized plan. What follows is a brief overview of rehabilitation interventions that may be useful as an *adjunct,* rather than replacements for, conventional cancer-pain management.

Rehabilitation medicine and physical agents for pain management for the management of cancer-related pain has been conceptualized into four broad categories: those that (1) modulate nociception, (2) stabilize or unload painful structures, (3) influence physiological processes that indirectly influence nociception, or (4) alleviate pain arising from excess strain on muscles and soft tissues [128]. Table 20.3 provides an overview of these different treatment options. These types of interventions may be particularly useful for patients with cancer who cannot tolerate the side effects of opioid and adjuvant medications or those patients who are reluctant to use pharmacologic treatment.

LYMPHEDEMA

Lymphedema is an abnormal accumulation of protein-rich lymphatic fluid in soft tissues due to disruptions or blockage of vessels by tumor, fibrosis, or inflammation. Primary lymphedema is a result of a rare development abnormality of the lymphatic system, whereas secondary lymphedema occurs as a result of cancer, surgical resection of lymphatic systems, lymph nodes, mastectomy or breast surgery, radiation-induced fibrosis or as a result of obstruction from metastatic tumors. Breast cancer and treatment are a common cause of upper extremity lymphedema.

Breast cancer patients have a 15–20% chance of developing lymphedema after treatment. The risk of developing lymphedema is highest in women who have axillary lymph-node dissection followed by radiation treatments. Sagen et al. observed more adverse effects in women treated with anterior lymph-node dissection than with sentinel lymph-node biopsy after 2.5 years follow-up, with arm lymphedema in 17% of those with anterior lymph-node dissection versus 3% in the sentinel lymph-node biopsy group [135].

There are no standardized tests for measuring or testing lymphedema, however, the most widely used is measuring around the affected limb. Clinical practice guidelines that discuss assessment, diagnosis, and treatment are shown (Table 20.4). Redness, warmth, open wounds, or fever should warrant further workup and diagnosis for cellulitis. Although the treatment for lymphedema is preventive with education, hygiene, and elevation, therapy including complex

TABLE 20.3 Rehabilitation and Physical Interventions For Cancer Pain

Modulation of Nociceptive Activity	Example of Clinical Application
Heat and cold	Myalgia related to chemotherapy
Electrical stimulation (transcutaneous electronic nerve stimulation)	Postthoracotomy pain syndrome [129]
Desensitization techniques	CIPN [130]
Stabilization and Unloading Strategies	**Example of Clinical Application**
Assistive devices (single point canes, walkers, wheelchair)	Unload painful lytic bone lesion
Therapeutic exercise	Stabilize bony structures using isometric strengthening of the hip abductor muscles to unload painful hip joints
Orthotics	Thoracolumbosacral corset for vertebral compression fracture
Modalities with Physiologic Effects	**Example of Clinical Application**
Light and laser therapies	Low level laser therapy for mucositis related to stem cell transplantation [131]
Complex decongestive therapy	Lymphedema of arm after breast cancer [132]
Rehabilitation Approaches to Pain	**Example of Clinical Application**
Injections	Subacromial bursa injection for rotator cuff tendonitis after breast cancer treatment [133]
Myofascial release	Manual release of trigger point in scapular muscle after breast cancer surgery [134]

decongestive therapy (CDT) with an experienced therapist, manual lymph drainage and compressive garments are also helpful.

There is no cure for lymphedema but treatments will often prevent worsening of the disease and impact QoL. Breast cancer patients going through anterior lymph-node dissection surgery and radiation treatments may benefit from further postoperative physical therapy, including resistance and strength exercise, focusing on pain management. Harris et al. identified, summarized, and synthesized recommendations from recent practice guidelines (2001–2011) on upper extremity rehabilitation (as listed in Table 20.4).

REHABILITATION PRINCIPLES IN THE PATIENT WITH BREAST CANCER

Breast cancer is the second most common malignancy among women, exceeded only by lung cancer. There are currently more than 2.8 million breast cancer survivors in the United States [137]. The current model of care for individuals with breast cancer focuses on treatment of the disease, followed by ongoing surveillance to detect recurrence. Treatment may include chemotherapy, radiation, and resection either by lumpectomy or mastectomy. In the immediate postoperative period, medical issues can also arise including wound issues such as cellulitis, flap necrosis, abscess, nonclosure of wound, dehiscence, hematoma, and seroma development [138]. Surgical breast cancer patients may not only have functional limitations of range of motion,

lymphedema, and weakness of the ipsilateral upper extremity but they also suffer with emotional distress of depression, pain, and self-image. These dysfunctions may persist for many years and have repercussions on the performance of daily living activities [139].

Pain

Approximately 35% of women experience persistent levels of moderate arm/shoulder pain in the first 6 months following breast cancer surgery [140]. Ewertz et al. found that persistent pain in the breast area, arm, and shoulder were reported by 30–50% of patients up to 3–5 years after surgery, lymphedema in 15–25% of patients, and restrictions of arm and shoulder movement in 35% [141].

Range of Motion

Evidence suggests that survivors who undergo breast reconstruction may be at higher risk for development of upper quarter dysfunction (UQD), defined as restricted upper quarter mobility, pain, lymphedema, and impaired sensation and strength [138]. Levy et. al found characteristics significantly associated with early ROM impairment (but not later impairment) included axillary lymph-node dissection, removal of more than 15 nodes, mastectomy surgery, and stage-II breast cancer. The presence of positive nodes, being of older age, and having a body mass index (BMI) > 25 were significantly associated with reduced shoulder ROM after 1 year [142].

TABLE 20.4 Assessment and Diagnosis of Lymphedema

Assessment and Diagnosis of Lymphedema

- Evidence supports early lymphedema diagnosis and referral for therapies to reduce patient burden.
- Clinicians should elicit symptoms of heaviness, tightness, or swelling in the affected arm.
- Pre- and postoperative measurements of both arms are useful in the assessment and diagnosis of lymphedema.
- Circumferential measurements should be taken at following four points:
  - At the metacarpal–phalangeal joints
  - At the wrists
  - 10 cm distal to the lateral epicondyles
  - 12 cm proximal to the lateral epicondyles.
- A difference of more than 2 cm at any of the four measurement points may warrant treatment of the lymphedema, provided that tumor involvement of the axilla or brachial plexus, infection, and axillary vein thrombosis have been ruled out
- Additional efforts to define relevant clinical outcomes for the assessment or patients with lymphedema would be valuable.

Interventions for Lymphedema

- Practitioners may want to encourage long-term and consistent use of compression garments by women with lymphedema.
- Compression garments should be worn from morning to night and be removed at bedtime.
- Patients should be informed that lymphedema is a lifelong condition and that compression garments must be worn on a daily basis.
- Patients can expect stabilization and/or modest improvement of lymphedema with the use of the garment in the prescribed fashion.
- Complex physical therapy, manual lymph drainage, and compression and massage therapy are associated with volume reductions.
- One randomized trial has demonstrated a trend in favor of pneumatic compression pumps compared with no treatment.
- Further randomized trials are required to determine whether pneumatic compression provides additional benefits over compression garments alone.
- Complete decongestive therapy, also known as complex decongestive physiotherapy and complex physical therapy, is the recommended treatment for lymphedema.
- There is some evidence that compression therapy and manual lymph drainage may improve established lymphedema, but further studies are needed.
- There is no current evidence to support the use of medical therapies, including diuretics, benzopyrones, and selenium compounds.

Other Considerations for Lymphedema Management

- Clinical experience supports encouraging patients to consider some practical advice regarding skin care, exercise, and body weight.
- Evidence exists that a BMI >30 is a risk factor for lymphedema. Although there is no clear relationship between high BMI and development of secondary lymphedema following treatment for cancer, maintenance of a healthy body weight in cancer survivors should be encouraged because of the other associated health benefits.
- Immediate attention to signs of infection and prompt initiation of antibiotic therapy are critical to preventing sepsis.
- Infection risk is essential to reduce the risk of developing or exacerbating lymphedema.
- Conservative surgical and radiation treatment for cancer should be used to reduce the risk of secondary lymphedema.
- Surgical techniques may be useful for a small subset of secondary lymphedema sufferers who have failed to obtain relief from less invasive measures.

Source: Adapted from Harris SR, et al. Clinical practice guidelines for breast cancer rehabilitation: syntheses of guideline recommendations and qualitative appraisals. Cancer 2012;118(8 Suppl.):2312–24.

Cancer-Related Fatigue

Physical activity for breast cancer patients has been reported to decrease fatigue, to improve emotional well-being, and to increase physical strength. Although the exact pathophysiologic and molecular mechanisms of CRF are not well known, current studies are underway to learn more about the effects of exercise and strength training and the effect on fatigue, QoL, and changes in molecular, immunological, and inflammatory changes in breast cancer patients during adjuvant radiotherapy [143].

Psychological Health

Findings suggest that moderate arm/shoulder pain is associated with clinically meaningful decrements in functional status and QoL. In addition, patients with more pain reported higher levels of depression, anxiety, and sleep disturbance than patients who did not experience pain [140].

Physical functional disabilities that were present late in postoperative period of breast cancer survivors with limitations of shoulder range of motion negatively influenced functional capacity and QoL [139]. Evidence supports prospective surveillance for early identification and treatment as a means to prevent or mitigate many of these concerns to prevent decline of QoL [144].

Musculoskeletal health

Musculoskeletal health can be compromised by breast cancer treatment. In particular, bone loss and arthralgias are prevalent side effects experienced by women treated with chemotherapy and/or adjuvant endocrine therapy. Bone loss leads to osteoporosis and related fractures, whereas arthralgias threaten QoL and compliance to treatment [145].

Benefits to Exercise

Evidence suggests that rehabilitation and exercise are effective in preventing and managing many physical side effects of breast cancer treatment. Nevertheless, few women are referred to rehabilitation during or after treatment, and fewer receive baseline assessments of impairment and function to facilitate early detection of impairment and functional limitations [146]. Overall, current research evidence indicates that regular participation in physical activity after breast cancer diagnosis may mitigate common side effects of breast cancer adjuvant therapy, including fatigue, depression, impaired QoL, decreased muscular strength, decreased aerobic capacity, and weight gain [147]. Physical activity may help address future impairments; slowing bone loss, and improving joint pain [145]. Observational evidence suggests that women who are physically active after breast cancer diagnosis have a 30–50% lower risk of breast cancer recurrence, breast cancer death, and overall death compared with sedentary individuals [148]. Participating in regular exercise after breast cancer treatment has been also reported a positive effect on QoL, anxiety and self-esteem with improvement in body image and feelings of sexual attractiveness [149]. Although more research is needed to fully define the role of exercise in breast cancer survivors, the many proven benefits of physical activity have led the American Cancer Society and American College of Sports Medicine to encourage regular participation in moderate-intensity recreational activity for most breast cancer survivors [148].

Exercise Prescription

The American Cancer Society and National Comprehensive Cancer Network (NCCN) survivorship guidelines recommend that cancer survivors engage in at least 150 min per week of ≥moderate intensity physical activity. As the majority of BCS are not meeting these aerobic physical activity guidelines, behavior change interventions aimed at increasing physical activity in this population are warranted [150]. The most commonly reported exercise parameters were three sessions per week, at moderate intensity being equivalent to 50–80% of the maximum heart rate for greater than 30 min [151].

Early ROM

Early assisted mobilization (beginning on the first postoperative day) and home rehabilitation, in conjunction with written information on precautionary hygienic measures to observe, play a crucial role in reducing the occurrence of postoperative side effects of the upper limb [152]. Harris et al. identified, summarized, and synthesized recommendations from recent practice guidelines (2001–2011) on upper extremity rehabilitation (as listed in Table 20.5).

Prehabilitation

Although traditionally rehabilitation starts after surgical intervention, new studies are showing benefit to adding an exercise program, prior to acute treatment. Prehabilitation is a part of the continuum of care, starting from the time of diagnosis to the beginning of acute treatment. Prehabilitation can be useful, as impairments are identified at beginning of treatment and plans made for future targeted interventions to reduce incidence or severity of future impairments [153]. In surgical patients, studies show that a poor preoperative

---

TABLE 20.5 Upper Extremity Rehabilitation

Upper Extremity Rehabilitation

- Preoperative, bilateral upper extremity function should be assessed to provide a baseline before treatments.
- Postoperative physical therapy should begin the first day following surgery.
- Gentle range of motion exercises should be encouraged after the first week of surgery.
- Active stretching exercises can begin after 1 week of surgery, or when the drain is removed, and should be continued for 6–8 weeks or until full range of motion is achieved in the affected upper extremity.
- Women should be instructed also in scar-tissue massage.
- Postoperative assessments should occur regularly up to 1 year after surgery.
- Progressive resistive exercises, that is strengthening, can begin with light weights (1–2 pounds) within 4–6 weeks after surgery.

Electrotherapy Modalities

- Laser treatment, electrical stimulation, microwave, and thermal therapy are not recommended at this time due to insufficient evidence to support their use, and there are published precautions and contraindications for their use in persons with neoplasms.
- Therapeutic ultrasound is contraindicated over sites of possible metastasis in women with histories of breast cancer.

Source: Adapted from Harris SR, et al. Clinical practice guidelines for breast cancer rehabilitation: syntheses of guideline recommendations and qualitative appraisals. Cancer 2012;118(8 Suppl.):2312–24.

performance results in greater morbidity including postoperative complications, and prolonged functional recovery period as well as increased mortality [154]. Although clinical trials in prehabilitation of breast cancer patients are limited at this time, studies of colorectal cancer patients show that patients who participated in a prehabilitation program were able to walk further in 6 min walk test 2 months postsurgery [154]. In lung cancer patients, a short-term exercise program prior to surgery resulted in a shorter length of stay, and physiological improvements including improved gas exchange and better lung perfusion [155]. Introduction of prehabilitation exercises and exercise program to breast cancer patients may facilitate adherence to exercise posttreatment, improving outcomes including QoL and decreasing morbidity and mortality.

Integrative Therapies

Yoga, Tai Chi, and Qigong

Yoga has demonstrated improvements in fatigue, psychosocial functioning, and emotional distress [156]. Tai Chi studies with cancer patients and survivors have produced similar findings, and more, including improvements in physical functioning, QoL, self-esteem, improved insulin metabolism, cardiovascular health, and some markers of inflammation [156].

Research has shown there may be benefits of Qigong for cancer patients (across cancer diagnosis sites) during and after treatment, including reductions in fatigue, lowered C-reactive protein, and improved mood, cognitive function, and QoL. Specific to breast cancer patients undergoing treatment, Qigong has been found to reduce fatigue for women with depressive symptoms at baseline. In a randomized control trial of Qigong and Tai Chi, researchers showed improvement for two prevalent symptoms among breast cancer survivors, depression and sleep dysfunction [156].

Music Therapy

Music therapy has also been found to have positive effects on improving depression of female patients with breast cancer, and shortening the duration of hospital stay after radical mastectomy. Music therapy could be considered in breast cancer patients to aid in their recovery process [157].

RADIATION FIBROSIS SYNDROME

Radiation therapy is given to almost two-thirds of cancer patients with the goal to cure, or for palliation to provide symptom management, and/or control growth. The top three cancers that receive radiation therapy include lung cancer, prostate cancer, and lung cancer [158]. Radiation therapy is aimed at destroying cancer cells, and varying doses of radiation are required for different types of cancer cells. Radiation works on the cancer cells through direct and indirect mechanisms via ionization. Internal radiation is delivered within the body and is known as brachytherapy. External delivery of radiation may be given through external beam modalities including image-guided radiotherapy and intensity-modulated radiotherapy [159–161].

Breast cancer has a long history of comprehensive treatment strategies that include the use of radiation therapy. Recently, radiation therapy has been seen as an integral component of breast conservation surgery. Survival advantage in patients that receive radiation therapy and breast conservation surgery was demonstrated in a meta-analysis. Cost effectiveness and local control were also noted when radiation therapy was combined with breast conservation surgery [162].

During radiation therapy, attempts are made to spare normal cells they may be damaged in the process. Side effects including fibrosis may result [158]. Radiation fibrosis is a complex multifactorial process, which causes tissues to accumulate extracellular matrix (ECM) components including collagen disrupting the usual ECM synthesis and breakdown. Only minutes after radiation, increased vessel permeability and vessel dilation have been documented. Inflammatory mechanisms, reactive oxygen species, and microvascular injury have been attributed as a contributory factor to radiation fibrosis. Radiation fibrosis is an irreversible late side effect of radiation therapy that may occur years after treatment. Interstitial fibrin deposition, increased collagen formation, and continued microvascular injury may be noted on a microscopic level years after receiving radiation therapy [163].

Disability may occur as a cumulative effect of radiation, chemotherapy, and/or surgery. Radiation complications may be seen in any tissue type and signs/symptoms may arise during treatment or even years after the completion of treatment. Several unintended side effects of radiation may be caused by tissue remodeling, epithelial regeneration, cytokines, and/or activation of coagulation system. Thrombin's abnormal deposition is characteristic in radiation fibrosis. It is important to note that radiation can alter any structure in the radiation field including nerve, muscle, bone, tendon, ligaments, etc. Side effects of radiation include fatigue, pain, lymphedema, focal myopathy, osteonecrosis, muscle spasms, radiation-induced plexopathy, contractures, radiculopathies, mononeuropathies, peripheral nervous system dysfunction (and subsequent neuropathic pain), viscera, brittle bones with susceptibility to fracture, and various other issues [159–161]. Breast cancer patients may experience shoulder dysfunction after treatment. Acute adhesive capsulitis is most commonly seen and may be a result of axillary radiation. Patients may be hesitant to move the affected arm secondary to pain and inflammation of the tissues [161]. The radiation field may include muscle fibers that undergo progressive fibrosis leading to a focal myopathy. Pain and spasms occur in the myopathic muscles, which are weaker compared to the normal muscles [160].

Research on risk factors for radiation fibrosis is ongoing. Breast cancer patients with larger body habitus and/or breast may experience a larger burden of acute increased toxicity after receiving radiation therapy [162]. The risk of radiation fibrosis may be dose dependent and location dependent. Radiation side effects are cumulative and patients who are treated more than once in the same region may develop increased radiation fibrosis. Pre-existing medical conditions and other yet-to-be-determined risk factors probably contribute to the development of radiation fibrosis [160]. Cardiac and lung side effects from radiation may occur even if the patient received lose dose radiation. "Hotspots" within breast tissue where a larger amount of radiation (possibly due to 2D "classic" techniques of radiation administration) may have been given and can cause increased toxicity and poor cosmetic appearance. Over the past several decades, care has been taken to improve the planning and administration of radiation. Dosing is can be calculated in 3D and CT planning scans are utilized for strategic targeting of tumor tissue and decreased dosing to cardiac and lung tissue [162].

Various interventions are available to mitigate the side effects of radiation fibrosis and radiation in breast cancer patients. Pain and fatigue may be lessened by nonpharmacologic means. Referral should be considered to physiatry, physical therapy, and/or occupational therapy. Additional interventions of benefit include use of acupuncture, ergonomics, modalities, energy conservation and activity pacing. Patients should engage in physical activities at a moderate activity level 30 min a day on most days on the week and maintaining this level of activity during and after treatment [136]. First-line medications include nerve stabilizers to treat spasms and pain. If needed, opioid medications as a second-line treatment [159–161]. Patients may achieve temporary relief from trigger point injections by experienced practitioners [161].

Referral may be made to a cancer rehabilitation specialist who treats patients with radiation fibrosis and is experienced in Botulinum toxin administration. Botulinum toxin serves as an intervention to treat issues including migraines, spasticity, cervical dystonia, musculoskeletal pain, neuropathic pain, and muscle spasms. Neuropathic pain may be mitigated by Botulinum toxin; however, this relationship is not well understood. Botulinum toxin may be considered in patients who have postmastectomy syndrome; yet, should not be considered without the use of range of motion exercises in patients with fixed contractures. The practitioner must remember that Botulinum toxin may cause side effects including dysphagia and muscle weakness. Great care must be taken to avoid injections close to hardware and/or tumors due to an increased likelihood of infection and/or

bleeding. Prior to injection, the practitioner must perform full history and physical evaluation including evaluation of proper imaging, laboratory evaluation, and monitoring for liver dysfunction and/or anticogulation. EMG localization may further assist in accurate Botulinum administration in the appropriate patients [160].

MANAGEMENT OF PERIPHERAL NEUROPATHY AND BALANCE IMPAIRMENT

Peripheral neuropathy is commonly seen in the cancer population. The toxic and dose-dependent side effects of potentially curative chemotherapy can cause injury to muscle and peripheral nerves. Peripheral neuropathy can also be caused by several sources including tumors compressing the nerves, paraneoplastic syndromes, underlying medical conditions, vitamin deficiency, and toxicity. Patients may experience a variety of symptoms that can decrease QoL such as loss of sensation, burning sensations, and/or loss of proprioception. Diagnosis may be further elucidated with the assistance of electromyography analysis [161].

CIPN is a frequent chemotherapy-related treatment side effect. It is estimated that 38% of patients who are treated with multiple chemotherapy agents experience CIPN [159]. There are several chemotherapy agents that have been found to cause CIPN including vincristine, bortezomib, taxoids, platins, thalidomide, suramin, epothilones, and misonidazole [158]. Sensory CIPN occurs more commonly than motor CIPN. Symptoms are described as distal, symmetric, and "stocking and glove" (foot and hand) distributions. Sensations can be described at allodynia, dysethesia, lacinating, cold intolerance, and/or burning. Toxicity may cause discontinuation of treatment with a particular agent or decrease in dose [164]. Autonomic, motor, and sensory nerves can be involved in CIPN. Patients may have difficulty maintaining functional independence and activities of daily living secondary to CIPN [165]. Patients may continue to have painful symptoms after chemotherapy is discontinued, this is known as "coasting" [166].

Various mechanisms contribute to CIPN. The dorsal root ganglion (DRG), efferent and afferent axons are located outside the central nervous system and therefore lack protective barriers allowing susceptibility to neurotoxic chemotherapy. CIPN may result due to distal axonal degeneration, direct damage to sensory nerve root bodies of the DRG, and microtubule-mediated transport disturbance of the axon [167]. Mitochondrial structures and function that have been compromised may contribute to the pathogenesis of cancer and CIPN mechanisms and subsequent pain behavior. Reactive oxygen species, associated with specific chemotherapies and demonstrated in multiple models, may increase inflammation and contribute to CIPN [161].

The diagnosis of CIPN typically occurs after a period of gradually progressing symptoms. Peripheral neuropathy due to diabetes, paraneoplastic sensory neuropathy, and/or peripheral neuropathy caused by metabolism/toxins should be eliminated. The most common clinical presentation of CIPN is distal axonpathy. A patient with CIPN may have an abnormal neurologic exam, such as an absence of reflexes, decreased proprioception, abnormal Rhomberg, decreased 2-point discrimination, etc. An extensive baseline neurologic exam should be conducted prior to initiation of potentially neurotoxic chemotherapy. History should include pre-existing conditions (including hereditary, endocrine, and neurologic conditions) and caution should be made regarding potentially neurotoxic medications. The symptoms associated with CIPN are graded 1–5. Patients may require additional diagnostic modalities including EMG studies (Table 20.6) [161].

There are a variety of treatment options available for breast cancer patients with peripheral neuropathy. Early diagnosis of CIPN is the first step. Patients may develop irreversible symptoms at a rapid rate. Care should be made to assist with activities of daily living, and prevent falls. Education should be provided about home safety, skin care and checks, and balance strategies (vision compensation). Weakness and/or numbness can lessen with physical therapy, occupational therapy, modalities, and/or time [160].

Clinical practice guidelines on Breast Cancer Rehabilitation published in *Cancer* in 2012 recommend that CIPN patients with functional deficits be referred to physical or occupational therapy. Transcutaneous electrical nerve stimulation may be helpful to treat CIPN. In medication-resistant patients, acupuncture may be used as an adjunct treatment. "Therapeutic intervention, education, and practical advice provided by these rehabilitation specialists can prove invaluable in helping patients to both correct CIPN-induced functional deficits and to cope with the difficulties and challenges these deficits cause in their everyday life" [136]. Assistive devices, orthotics, and durable medical equipment should be provided to patients with CIPN to improve safety and QoL. Therapy program should focus on improving functional deficits, maintaining and improving balance, range of motion (active and passive exercises), and strengthening [160].

TABLE 20.6 A Grading Scale: CIPN Symptoms

Adverse Event	Definition	Grade 1	Grade 2	Grade 3	Grade 4	Grade 5
Dysesthesia	A disorder characterized by distortion of sensory perception, resulting in an abnormal and unpleasant sensation	Mild sensory alteration	Moderate sensory alteration; limiting instrumental ADL	Severe sensory alteration; limiting self-care ADL	—	—
Neuralgia	A disorder characterized by intense painful sensation along a nerve or group of nerves	Mild pain	Moderate symptoms; limiting instrumental ADL	Severe symptoms; limiting self-care ADL	—	—
Peripheral motor neuropathy	A disorder characterized by inflammation or degeneration of the peripheral motor nerves	Asymptomatic; clinical or diagnostic observations only; intervention not indicated	Moderate sensory alteration; limiting instrumental ADL	Severe symptoms; limiting self-care ADL; assistive device indicated	Life-threatening consequences; urgent intervention indicated	Death
Peripheral sensory neuropathy	A disorder characterized by inflammation or degeneration of the peripheral sensory nerves	Asymptomatic; loss of deep tendon reflexes or paresthesia	Moderate pain; limiting instrumental ADL	Severe pain; limiting self-care ADL	Life-threatening consequences; urgent intervention indicated	Death
Paresthesia	A disorder characterized by functional disturbances of sensory neurons resulting in abnormal cutaneous sensations of tingling, numbness, pressure, cold, and warmth that are experienced in the absence of a stimulus	Mild symptoms	Moderate symptoms; limiting instrumental ADL	Severe symptoms; limiting self-care ADL	—	—

Source: Adapted from the CTACE v4.03 (Common Terminology Criteria for Adverse Events (CTCAE). Version 4.03.National Cancer Institute; 2010).

Many medications have been tried to treat CIPN. Duloxetine, after extensive review of literature, was the only medication that could be recommended for treatment of CIPN if prescribed by a practitioner well-versed in the treatment of CIPN. Gabapentin, tricyclic antidepressants, or compounded cream (ketamine, baclofen, and amitriptyline) may be considered for select patients after extensive discussion of risks and benefits and lack of treatment options. Despite many clinical trials, no medication or supplement has been found to prevent CIPN [164]. At this time, there is no medication that can reverse CIPN [160].

CIPN is an underreported and underdiagnosed problem in cancer patients [162]. Symptoms can be treated through a multifaceted approach including education, balance compensation, physical and occupational therapy, modalities, acupuncture, assistive device prescriptions, and medications. Additional research is needed to find additional treatments that can benefit patients who have CIPN.

CONCLUSIONS

The ultimate goal of cancer rehabilitation is to support the patient with cancer to achieve optimal physical, social, physiological, and vocational functioning *within the limits* imposed by the disease and its treatment. Cancer survivors and their families have increasingly advocated for the importance of QoL as a desired outcome of treatment. This requires the need to provide continuity of care and the recognition that independence in daily function is a high priority for many cancer survivors. Recent evidence suggests that more cancer survivors have a reduced health-related QoL as a result of physical impairments than due to psychological ones [169]. Moreover, research has also demonstrated that the majority of cancer survivors have significant impairments that often go undetected and/or untreated [170]. On the other hand, accumulated evidence has shown that rehabilitation can improve pain, function, and QoL in cancer survivors at every stage along the course of treatment [171]. Where chemotherapy, surgery, and radiation are often passive interventions from the perspective of the patient, rehabilitation is an active process that has the capacity to engage and empower the cancer survivor. Achieving capacity to meet the complex rehabilitation needs of a growing population of cancer survivors and identifying the most cost-effective and beneficial programs represents a significant challenge for the oncologic rehabilitation community.

ACKNOWLEDGMENT

The authors wish to thank Ms. Charlotte Bailey for her assistance in the preparation of this chapter.

REFERENCES

[1] American Cancer Society. Cancer Facts and Figures 2008. Atlanta: American Cancer Society; 2008.

[2] SEER Cancer Statistics Review, 1975–2006, Bethesda, MD: N.C. Institute; 2008.

[3] Gordon L, Lynch BM, Newman B. Transitions in work participation after a diagnosis of colorectal cancer. Aust N Z J Public Health 2008;32(6):569–74.

[4] Hewitt M, Greenfiled S, Stovall E. From cancer patient to cancer survivor: lost in transition. Washington DC: Institue of Medicine; 2005.

[5] Cole RP, Scialla SJ, Bednarz L. Functional recovery in cancer rehabilitation. Arch Phys Med Rehabil 2000;81(5):623–7.

[6] Gamble GL, et al. The future of cancer rehabilitation: emerging subspecialty. Am J Phys Med Rehabil 2011;90(5 Suppl. 1):S76–87.

[7] Silver JK, Gilchrist LS. Cancer rehabilitation with a focus on evidence-based outpatient physical and occupational therapy interventions. Am J Phys Med Rehabil 2011;90(5 Suppl. 1):S5–S15.

[8] Alfano CM, et al. Cancer survivorship and cancer rehabilitation: revitalizing the link. J Clin Oncol 2012;30(9):904–6.

[9] Roberts PS, et al. The impact of inpatient rehabilitation on function and survival of newly diagnosed patients with glioblastoma. PM R 2014;6(6):514–21.

[10] Saotome T, Klein L, Faux S. Cancer rehabilitation: a barometer for survival? Support Care Cancer 2015;23(10):3033–41.

[11] Bruera E, Yennurajalingam S. Challenge of managing cancer-related fatigue. J Clin Oncol 2010;28(23):3671–2.

[12] Mock V, et al. Cancer-related fatigue. Clinical Practice Guidelines in Oncology. J Natl Compr Canc Netw 2007;5(10):1054–78.

[13] Hofman M, et al. Cancer-related fatigue: the scale of the problem. Oncologist 2007;12(Suppl. 1):4–10.

[14] Kim SH, et al. Fatigue and depression in disease-free breast cancer survivors: prevalence, correlates, and association with quality of life. J Pain Symptom Manage 2008;35(6):644–55.

[15] Kuhnt S, et al. Fatigue in cancer survivors—prevalence and correlates. Onkologie 2009;32(6):312–7.

[16] Berger AM, Gerber LH, Mayer DK. Cancer-related fatigue: implications for breast cancer survivors. Cancer 2012;118(8 Suppl.):2261–9.

[17] Bower JE. Management of cancer-related fatigue. Clin Adv Hematol Oncol 2006;4(11):828–9.

[18] Horneber M, et al. Cancer-related fatigue: epidemiology, pathogenesis, diagnosis, and treatment. Dtsch Arztebl Int 2012;109(9):161–71. quiz 172.

[19] Miller AH, et al. Neuroendocrine-immune mechanisms of behavioral comorbidities in patients with cancer. J Clin Oncol 2008;26(6):971–82.

[20] Seruga B, et al. Cytokines and their relationship to the symptoms and outcome of cancer. Nat Rev Cancer 2008;8(11):887–99.

[21] Bower JE, et al. Cytokine genetic variations and fatigue among patients with breast cancer. J Clin Oncol 2013;31(13):1656–61.

[22] Kumar RJ, Barqawi A, Crawford ED. Adverse events associated with hormonal therapy for prostate cancer. Rev Urol 2005;7(Suppl. 5): S37–43.

[23] Mitchell SA. Cancer-related fatigue: state of the science. PM R 2010;2(5):364–83.

[24] Ray M, et al. Fatigue and sleep during cancer and chemotherapy: translational rodent models. Comp Med 2008;58(3):234–45.

[25] Reuter K, Harter M. The concepts of fatigue and depression in cancer. Eur J Cancer Care (Engl) 2004;13(2):127–34.

[26] Neil SE, et al. Cardiorespiratory and neuromuscular deconditioning in fatigued and non-fatigued breast cancer survivors. Support Care Cancer 2013;21(3):873–81.

[27] Bower JE. Cancer-related fatigue—mechanisms, risk factors, and treatments. Nat Rev Clin Oncol 2014;11(10):597–609.

[28] Bower JE, et al. Fatigue and gene expression in human leukocytes: increased NF-kappaB and decreased glucocorticoid signaling in breast cancer survivors with persistent fatigue. Brain Behav Immun 2011;25(1):147–50.

[29] Hong DS, Angelo LS, Kurzrock R. Interleukin-6 and its receptor in cancer: implications for translational therapeutics. Cancer 2007;110(9):1911–28.

[30] Knupfer H, Preiss R. Significance of interleukin-6 (IL-6) in breast cancer (review). Breast Cancer Res Treatment 2007;102(2):129–35.

[31] NCCN Clinical Practice Guidelines in Oncology- Cancer-Related Fatigue (2015). 2015, National Comprehensive Cancer Network.

[32] Collins S, et al. Presence, communication and treatment of fatigue and pain complaints in incurable cancer patients. Patient Educ Couns 2008;72(1):102–8.

[33] Knowles G, et al. Survey of nurses' assessment of cancer-related fatigue. Eur J Cancer Care (Engl) 2000;9(2):105–13.

[34] Shun SC, Lai YH, Hsiao FH. Patient-related barriers to fatigue communication in cancer patients receiving active treatment. Oncologist 2009;14(9):936–43.

[35] Vogelzang NJ, et al. Patient, caregiver, and oncologist perceptions of cancer-related fatigue: results of a tripart assessment survey. The Fatigue Coalition. Semin Hematol 1997;34(3 Suppl. 2):4–12.

[36] Mendoza TR, et al. The rapid assessment of fatigue severity in cancer patients: use of the Brief Fatigue Inventory. Cancer 1999;85(5):1186–96.

[37] Yellen SB, et al. Measuring fatigue and other anemia-related symptoms with the Functional Assessment of Cancer Therapy (FACT) measurement system. J Pain Symptom Manage 1997;13(2):63–74.

[38] Piper BF, et al. The revised Piper Fatigue Scale: psychometric evaluation in women with breast cancer. Oncol Nurs Forum 1998;25(4):677–84.

[39] Smets EMA, et al. The multidimensional fatigue inventory (Mfi) psychometric qualities of an instrument to assess fatigue. J Psychosom Res 1995;39(3):315–25.

[40] Levesque M, et al. Efficacy of cognitive therapy for depression among women with metastatic cancer: a single-case experimental study. J Behav Ther Exp Psychiatry 2004;35(4):287–305.

[41] Savard J, et al. Randomized clinical trial on cognitive therapy for depression in women with metastatic breast cancer: psychological and immunological effects. Palliat Support Care 2006;4(3):219–37.

[42] Strong V, et al. Management of depression for people with cancer (SMaRT oncology 1): a randomised trial. Lancet 2008;372(9632):40–8.

[43] Del Fabbro E, et al. Testosterone replacement for fatigue in hypogonadal ambulatory males with advanced cancer: a preliminary double-blind placebo-controlled trial. Support Care Cancer 2013;21(9):2599–607.

[44] Moraska AR, et al. Phase III, randomized, double-blind, placebo-controlled study of long-acting methylphenidate for cancer-related fatigue: North Central Cancer Treatment Group NCCTG-N05C7 trial. J Clin Oncol 2010;28(23):3673–9.

[45] Mustian KM, et al. Multicenter, randomized controlled trial of yoga for sleep quality among cancer survivors. J Clin Oncol 2013;31(26):3233–41.

[46] Courneya KS, et al. The group psychotherapy and home-based physical exercise (group-hope) trial in cancer survivors: physical fitness and quality of life outcomes. Psychooncology 2003;12(4):357–74.

[47] Milne HM, et al. Impact of a combined resistance and aerobic exercise program on motivational variables in breast cancer survivors: a randomized controlled trial. Ann Behav Med 2008;36(2):158–66.

[48] Segal R, et al. Structured exercise improves physical functioning in women with stages I and II breast cancer: results of a randomized controlled trial. J Clin Oncol 2001;19(3):657–65.

[49] Cramp F, Daniel J. Exercise for the management of cancer-related fatigue in adults. Cochrane Database Syst Rev 2008;(2). CD006145.

[50] Klika RJ, Callahan KE, Drum SN. Individualized 12-week exercise training programs enhance aerobic capacity of cancer survivors. Phys Sportsmed 2009;37(3):68–77.

[51] McAuley E, et al. Physical activity and fatigue in breast cancer and multiple sclerosis: psychosocial mechanisms. Psychosom Med 2010;72(1):88–96.

[52] Ross R, Bradshaw AJ. The future of obesity reduction: beyond weight loss. Nat Rev Endocrinol 2009;5(6):319–25.

[53] Xue F, Michels KB. Diabetes, metabolic syndrome, and breast cancer: a review of the current evidence. Am J Clin Nutr 2007;86(3):ps823–35.

[54] Steensberg A, et al. IL-6 enhances plasma IL-1ra, IL-10, and cortisol in humans. Am J Physiol Endocrinol Metab 2003;285(2):E433–7.

[55] Pedersen BK, Edward F. Adolph distinguished lecture: muscle as an endocrine organ: IL-6 and other myokines. J Appl Physiol (1985) 2009;107(4):1006–14.

[56] Lumeng CN, Bodzin JL, Saltiel AR. Obesity induces a phenotypic switch in adipose tissue macrophage polarization. J Clin Invest 2007;117(1):175–84.

[57] Pedersen BK, Febbraio MA. Muscle as an endocrine organ: focus on muscle-derived interleukin-6. Physiol Rev 2008;88(4):1379–406.

[58] Gleeson M, et al. The anti-inflammatory effects of exercise: mechanisms and implications for the prevention and treatment of disease. Nat Rev Immunol 2011;11(9):607–15.

[59] Betof AS, Dewhirst MW, Jones LW. Effects and potential mechanisms of exercise training on cancer progression: a translational perspective. Brain Behav Immun 2013;30(Suppl.):S75–87.

[60] Schmid D, Leitzmann MF. Cardiorespiratory fitness as predictor of cancer mortality: a systematic review and meta-analysis. Ann Oncol 2015;26(2):272–8.

[61] Sabatino SA, et al. Provider counseling about health behaviors among cancer survivors in the United States. J Clin Oncol 2007;25(15):2100–6.

[62] Runowicz CD, et al. American Cancer Society/American Society of Clinical Oncology Breast Cancer Survivorship Care Guideline. J Clin Oncol 2016;34(6):611–35.

[63] Brown P, et al. Will improvement in quality of life (QOL) impact fatigue in patients receiving radiation therapy for advanced cancer? Am J Clin Oncol 2006;29(1):52–8.

[64] Nieman DC. Exercise, infection, and immunity. Int J Sports Med 1994;15(Suppl. 3):S131–41.

[65] Cristian A, Tran A, Patel K. Patient safety in cancer rehabilitation. Phys Med Rehabil Clin N Am 2012;23(2):441–56.

[66] Ferguson RJ, et al. Brain structure and function differences in monozygotic twins: possible effects of breast cancer chemotherapy. J Clin Oncol 2007;25(25):3866–70.

[67] Hurria A, Somlo G, Ahles T. Renaming "chemobrain". Cancer Invest 2007;25(6):373–7.

[68] Argyriou AA, et al. Either called "chemobrain" or "chemofog," the long-term chemotherapy-induced cognitive decline in cancer survivors is real. J Pain Symptom Manage 2011;41(1):126–39.

[69] Vardy J, et al. Cancer and cancer-therapy related cognitive dysfunction: an international perspective from the Venice cognitive workshop. Ann Oncol 2008;19(4):623–9.

[70] Wefel JS, Witgert ME, Meyers CA. Neuropsychological sequelae of non-central nervous system cancer and cancer therapy. Neuropsychol Rev 2008;18(2):121–31.

[71] Ahles TA, Root JC, Ryan EL. Cancer- and cancer treatment-associated cognitive change: an update on the state of the science. J Clin Oncol 2012;30(30):3675–86.

[72] Janelsins MC, et al. An update on cancer- and chemotherapy-related cognitive dysfunction: current status. Semin Oncol 2011;38(3):431–8.

[73] Nelson WL, Suls J. New approaches to understand cognitive changes associated with chemotherapy for non-central nervous system tumors. J Pain Symptom Manage 2013;46(5):707–21.

[74] Collins B, et al. Cognitive effects of chemotherapy in post-menopausal breast cancer patients 1 year after treatment. Psychooncology 2009;18(2):134–43.

[75] Ahles TA, et al. Neuropsychologic impact of standard-dose systemic chemotherapy in long-term survivors of breast cancer and lymphoma. J Clin Oncol 2002;20(2):485–93.

[76] Koppelmans V, et al. Neuropsychological performance in survivors of breast cancer more than 20 years after adjuvant chemotherapy. J Clin Oncol 2012;30(10):1080–6.

[77] Ahles TA, et al. Cognitive function in breast cancer patients prior to adjuvant treatment. Breast Cancer Res Treat 2008;110(1):143–52.

[78] Wefel JS, et al. 'Chemobrain' in breast carcinoma?: a prologue. Cancer 2004;101(3):466–75.

[79] Hermelink K, et al. Cognitive function during neoadjuvant chemotherapy for breast cancer: results of a prospective, multicenter, longitudinal study. Cancer 2007;109(9):1905–13.

[80] Meyers CA, Albitar M, Estey E. Cognitive impairment, fatigue, and cytokine levels in patients with acute myelogenous leukemia or myelodysplastic syndrome. Cancer 2005;104(4):788–93.

[81] Meyers CA, Byrne KS, Komaki R. Cognitive deficits in patients with small cell lung cancer before and after chemotherapy. Lung Cancer 1995;12(3):231–5.

[82] Rodin MB, Mohile SG. A practical approach to geriatric assessment in oncology. J Clin Oncol 2007;25(14):1936–44.

[83] Jim HS, et al. Meta-analysis of cognitive functioning in breast cancer survivors previously treated with standard-dose chemotherapy. J Clin Oncol 2012;30(29):3578–87.

[84] Rodin G, Ahles TA. Accumulating evidence for the effect of chemotherapy on cognition. J Clin Oncol 2012;30(29):3568–9.

[85] Wefel JS, et al. Acute and late onset cognitive dysfunction associated with chemotherapy in women with breast cancer. Cancer 2010;116(14):3348–56.

[86] Syrjala KL, et al. Prospective neurocognitive function over 5 years after allogeneic hematopoietic cell transplantation for cancer survivors compared with matched controls at 5 years. J Clin Oncol 2011;29(17):2397–404.

[87] Schagen SB, et al. Late effects of adjuvant chemotherapy on cognitive function: a follow-up study in breast cancer patients. Ann Oncol 2002;13(9):1387–97.

[88] Winocur G, et al. The effects of the anti-cancer drugs, methotrexate and 5-fluorouracil, on cognitive function in mice. Pharmacol Biochem Behav 2006;85(1):66–75.

[89] Dietrich J, et al. CNS progenitor cells and oligodendrocytes are targets of chemotherapeutic agents in vitro and in vivo. J Biol 2006;5(7):22.

[90] Seigers R, Fardell JE. Neurobiological basis of chemotherapy-induced cognitive impairment: a review of rodent research. Neurosci Biobehav Rev 2011;35(3):729–41.

[91] O'Shaughnessy JA, et al. Feasibility of quantifying the effects of epoetin alfa therapy on cognitive function in women with breast cancer undergoing adjuvant or neoadjuvant chemotherapy. Clin Breast Cancer 2005;5(6):439–46.

[92] Harris SE, Deary IJ. The genetics of cognitive ability and cognitive ageing in healthy older people. Trends Cogn Sci 2011;15(9):388–94.

[93] Ahles TA, et al. The relationship of APOE genotype to neuropsychological performance in long-term cancer survivors treated with standard dose chemotherapy. Psychooncology 2003;12(6):612–9.

[94] Small BJ, et al. Catechol-O-methyltransferase genotype modulates cancer treatment-related cognitive deficits in breast cancer survivors. Cancer 2011;117(7):1369–76.

[95] Ahles TA, Saykin AJ. Candidate mechanisms for chemotherapy-induced cognitive changes. Nat Rev Cancer 2007;7(3):192–201.

[96] Yamada TH, et al. Neuropsychological outcomes of older breast cancer survivors: cognitive features ten or more years after chemotherapy. J Neuropsychiatry Clin Neurosci 2010;22(1):48–54.

[97] Ganz PA. Doctor, will the treatment you are recommending cause chemobrain?". J Clin Oncol 2012;30(3):229–31.

[98] Holden JM, et al. Effects of lipopolysaccharide on consolidation of partial learning in the Y-maze. Integr Physiol Behav Sci 2004;39(4):334–40.

[99] Shintani F, et al. Interleukin-1 beta augments release of norepinephrine, dopamine, and serotonin in the rat anterior hypothalamus. J Neurosci 1993;13(8):3574–81.

[100] Maier SF, Watkins LR. Immune-to-central nervous system communication and its role in modulating pain and cognition: Implications for cancer and cancer treatment. Brain Behav Immun 2003;17(Suppl. 1):S125–31.

[101] Vitkovic L, et al. Cytokine signals propagate through the brain. Mol Psychiatry 2000;5(6):604–15.

[102] Banks WA. The blood-brain barrier in psychoneuroimmunology. Neurol Clin 2006;24(3):413–9.

[103] Irwin MR, Cole SW. Reciprocal regulation of the neural and innate immune systems. Nat Rev Immunol 2011;11(9):625–32.

[104] Wang XM, et al. Chemobrain: a critical review and causal hypothesis of link between cytokines and epigenetic reprogramming associated with chemotherapy. Cytokine 2015;72(1):86–96.

[105] Merriman JD, et al. Association between an interleukin 1 receptor, type I promoter polymorphism and self-reported attentional function in women with breast cancer. Cytokine 2014;65(2):192–201.

[106] Wefel J, et al. International cognition and cancer task force reommendations to harmonise studies of cognitive function in patients with cancer. Lancet Oncol 2011;12:703–8.

[107] NCCN Clinical Practice Guidelines in Oncology—Distress Management. National Comprehensive Cancer Network; 2014. p. 66.

[108] Lower EE, et al. Efficacy of dexmethylphenidate for the treatment of fatigue after cancer chemotherapy: a randomized clinical trial. J Pain Symptom Manage 2009;38:650–62.

[109] Mar Fan HG, et al. A randomised, placebo-controlled, double-blind trial of the effects of d-methylphenidate on fatigue and cognitive dysfunction in women undergoing adjuvant chemotherapy for breast cancer. Support Care Cancer 2008;16:577–83.

[110] Escalante CP, et al. A randomized, double-blind, 2-period, placebo-controlled crossover trial of a sustained-release methylphenidate in the treatment of fatigue in cancer patients. Cancer J 2014;20: 8–14.

[111] Von Ah D, Jansen C, Allen DH. Evidence-based interventions for cancer- and treatment-related cognitive impairment. Clin J Oncol Nurs 2014;18:17–25.

[112] Ercoli LM, et al. Cognitive rehabilitation group intervention for breast cancer survivors: results of a randomized clinical trial. Psychooncology 2015;24(11):1360–7.

[113] Von Ah D, et al. Putting evidence into practice: evidence-based interventions for cancer and cancer treatment-related cognitive impairment. Clin J Oncol Nurs 2011;15(6):607–15.

[114] Erickson KI, et al. Exercise training increases size of hippocampus and improves memory. PNAS 2011;108:30.

[115] Fairey AS, et al. Effect of exercise training on C-reactive protein in postmenopausal breast cancer survivors: A randomized controlled trial. Brain Behav Immun 2005;19:381–8.

[116] Szuhany KL, Bugatti M, Otto MW. A meta-analytic review of the effects of exercise on brain-derived neurotrophic factor. J Psychiatr Res 2014;60:56–64.

[117] Knobf MT, et al. The effect of a community-based exercise intervention on symtoms and quality of life. Cancer Nursing 2013;37:E43–50.

[118] Mustian KM. Yoga as treatment for insomnia among cancer patients and survivors: a systematic review. Eur Med J Oncol 2013;1:106–15.

[119] Erickson KI, Kramer AF. Aerobic exercise effects on cognitive and neural plasticity in older adults. Br J Sports Med 2009;43(1):22–4.

[120] de Andrade L, et al. Benefits of multimodal exercise intervention for postural control and frontal cognitive functions in individuals with Alzheimer's disease: a controlled trial. J Am Geriatr Soc 2013;61:1919–26.

[121] Murray D, et al. The effects of exercise on cognition in Parkinson's disease: a systematic review. Transl Neurodegener 2014;3(1):5.

[122] Baumann FT, et al. 12-Week resistance training with breast cancer patients during chemotherapy: effects on cognitive abilities. Breast Care 2011;6:142–3.

[123] Crowgey T, et al. Relationship between exercise behavior, cardiorespiratory fitness, and cognitive function in early breast cancer patients treated with doxoubicin-containing chemotherapy: a pilot study. Appl Physiol Nutr Metab 2014;39:724–9.

[124] Derry HM, et al. Yoga and self-reported cognitive problems in breast cancer survivors: a randomized controlled trial. Psychooncology 2014;24(8):958–66.

[125] Oh B, et al. Effect of medical qigong on cognitive function, quality of life, and a biomarker of inflammation in cancer patients: a randomized controlled trial. Support Care Cancer 2012;20:1235–42.

[126] Sprod LK, et al. Exercise and cancer treatment symptoms in 408 newly diagnosed older cancer patients. J Geriatr Oncol 2012;3:90–7.

[127] Glare PA, et al. Pain in cancer survivors. J Clin Oncol 2014;32(16): 1739–47.

[128] Cheville AL, Basford JR. Role of rehabilitation medicine and physical agents in the treatment of cancer-associated pain. J Clin Oncol 2014;32(16):1691–702.

[129] DeSantana JM, et al. Effectiveness of transcutaneous electrical nerve stimulation for treatment of hyperalgesia and pain. Curr Rheumatol Rep 2008;10(6):492–9.

[130] Stanton-Hicks M, et al. Complex regional pain syndromes: guidelines for therapy. Clin J Pain 1998;14(2):155–66.

[131] Ferreira B, da Motta Silveira FM, de Orange FA. Low-level laser therapy prevents severe oral mucositis in patients submitted to hematopoietic stem cell transplantation: a randomized clinical trial. Support Care Cancer 2016;24(3):1035–42.

[132] Rodrick JR, et al. Complementary, alternative, and other non-complete decongestive therapy treatment methods in the management of lymphedema: a systematic search and review. PM R 2014;6(3):250–74. quiz 274.

[133] Stubblefield MD, Keole N. Upper body pain and functional disorders in patients with breast cancer. PM R 2014;6(2):170–83.

[134] Cheville AL, Tchou J. Barriers to rehabilitation following surgery for primary breast cancer. J Surg Oncol 2007;95(5):409–18.

[135] Sagen A, et al. Upper limb physical function and adverse effects after breast cancer surgery: a prospective 2.5-year follow-up study and preoperative measures. Arch Phys Med Rehabil 2014;95(5):875–81.

[136] Harris SR, et al. Clinical practice guidelines for breast cancer rehabilitation: syntheses of guideline recommendations and qualitative appraisals. Cancer 2012;118(8 Suppl.):2312–24.

[137] American Cancer Society. Breast Cancer Facts & Figures 2015–2016, I. Atlanta: American Cancer Society; 2015.

[138] McNeely ML, et al. A prospective model of care for breast cancer rehabilitation: postoperative and postreconstructive issues. Cancer 2012;118(8 Suppl.):2226–36.

[139] Martins da Silva RC, Rezende LF. Assessment of impact of late postoperative physical functional disabilities on quality of life in breast cancer survivors. Tumori 2014;100(1):87–90.

[140] Miaskowski C, et al. Identification of patient subgroups and risk factors for persistent arm/shoulder pain following breast cancer surgery. Eur J Oncol Nurs 2014;18(3):242–53.

[141] Ewertz M, Jensen AB. Late effects of breast cancer treatment and potentials for rehabilitation. Acta Oncol 2011;50(2):187–93.

[142] Levy EW, et al. Predictors of functional shoulder recovery at 1 and 12 months after breast cancer surgery. Breast Cancer Res Treat 2012;134(1):315–24.

[143] Potthoff K, et al. Randomized controlled trial to evaluate the effects of progressive resistance training compared to progressive muscle relaxation in breast cancer patients undergoing adjuvant radiotherapy: the BEST study. BMC Cancer 2013;13:162.

[144] Stout NL, et al. A prospective surveillance model for rehabilitation for women with breast cancer. Cancer 2012;118(8 Suppl.):2191–200.

[145] Winters-Stone KM, et al. Impact + resistance training improves bone health and body composition in prematurely menopausal breast cancer survivors: a randomized controlled trial. Osteoporos Int 2013;24(5):1637–46.

[146] Binkley JM, et al. Patient perspectives on breast cancer treatment side effects and the prospective surveillance model for physical rehabilitation for women with breast cancer. Cancer 2012;118(8 Suppl.):2207–16.

[147] Loprinzi PD, Cardinal BJ. Effects of physical activity on common side effects of breast cancer treatment. Breast Cancer 2012;19(1):4–10.

[148] Ligibel JA. Role of adjuvant and posttreatment exercise programs in breast health. J Natl Compr Canc Netw 2011;9(2):251–6.

[149] Luoma ML, et al. Experiences of breast cancer survivors participating in a tailored exercise intervention—a qualitative study. Anticancer Res 2014;34(3):1193–9.

[150] Rogers LQ, et al. Effects of the BEAT Cancer physical activity behavior change intervention on physical activity, aerobic fitness, and quality of life in breast cancer survivors: a multicenter randomized controlled trial. Breast Cancer Res Treat 2015;149(1):109–19.

[151] Pastakia K, Kumar S. Exercise parameters in the management of breast cancer: a systematic review of randomized controlled trials. Physiother Res Int 2011;16(4):237–44.

[152] Scaffidi M, et al. Early rehabilitation reduces the onset of complications in the upper limb following breast cancer surgery. Eur J Phys Rehabil Med 2012;48(4):601–11.

[153] Silver JK, Baima J. Cancer prehabilitation: an opportunity to decrease treatment-related morbidity, increase cancer treatment options, and improve physical and psychological health outcomes. Am J Phys Med Rehabil 2013;92(8):715–27.

[154] Gillis C, et al. Prehabilitation versus rehabilitation: a randomized control trial in patients undergoing colorectal resection for cancer. Anesthesiology 2014;121(5):937–47.

[155] Pehlivan E, et al. The effects of preoperative short-term intense physical therapy in lung cancer patients: a randomized controlled trial. Ann Thorac Cardiovasc Surg 2011;17(5):461–8.

[156] Larkey LK, et al. Randomized controlled trial of Qigong/Tai Chi Easy on cancer-related fatigue in breast cancer survivors. Ann Behav Med 2015;49(2):165–76.

[157] Zhou K, et al. A clinical randomized controlled trial of music therapy and progressive muscle relaxation training in female breast cancer patients after radical mastectomy: results on depression, anxiety and length of hospital stay. Eur J Oncol Nurs 2015;19(1):54–9.

[158] Radiation Therapy for Cancer. National Cancer Institute; 2010.

[159] Stubblefield MD. Radiation fibrosis syndrome: neuromuscular and musculoskeletal complications in cancer survivors. PM R 2011;3(11):1041–54.

[160] Stubblefied MD. Radiation fibrosis syndrome. In: Cooper G, editor. Therapeutic uses of botulinum toxin. Totowa, NJ: Humana Press; 2007. p. 19–38.

[161] O'Dell M, Stubblefield M. Cancer rehabilitation: principles and practice. New York, NY: Demos Medical Publishing; 2009.

[162] Currey AD, et al. Reducing the human burden of breast cancer: advanced radiation therapy yields improved treatment outcomes. Breast J 2015;21(6):610–20.

[163] Yarnold J, Brotons MC. Pathogenetic mechanisms in radiation fibrosis. Radiother Oncol 2010;97(1):149–61.

[164] Hershman DL, et al. Prevention and management of chemotherapy-induced peripheral neuropathy in survivors of adult cancers: American Society of Clinical Oncology clinical practice guideline. J Clin Oncol 2014;32(18):1941–67.

[165] Stubblefield MD, et al. A prospective surveillance model for physical rehabilitation of women with breast cancer: chemotherapy-induced peripheral neuropathy. Cancer 2012;118(8 Suppl.):2250–60.

[166] Han Y, Smith MT. Pathobiology of cancer chemotherapy-induced peripheral neuropathy (CIPN). Front Pharmacol 2013;4:156.

[167] Hausheer FH, et al. Diagnosis, management, and evaluation of chemotherapy-induced peripheral neuropathy. Semin Oncol 2006;33(1):15–49.

[169] Weaver KE, et al. Mental and physical health-related quality of life among U.S. cancer survivors: population estimates from the 2010 National Health Interview Survey. Cancer Epidemiol Biomarkers Prev 2012;21(11):2108–17.

[170] Ugolini D, et al. Scientific production in cancer rehabilitation grows higher: a bibliometric analysis. Support Care Cancer 2012;20(8):1629–38.

[171] Silver JK, Baima J, Mayer RS. Impairment-driven cancer rehabilitation: an essential component of quality care and survivorship. CA Cancer J Clin 2013;63(5):295–317.

Chapter 21

Management of Advanced Heart Failure in a Cancer Patient

A. Lajoie, J. Dunhill and M.A. Hamilton

Cedars-Sinai Medical Center, Los Angeles, CA, United States

In addition to chemotherapy-induced cardiomyopathy (CCMP), evidence suggests that patients with heart failure from other etiologies have a 60% greater incidence of cancer compared to matched controls (Fig. 21.1). Furthermore, patients with heart failure and cancer have higher 5-year mortality compared to controls with cancer alone or heart-failure patients who do not develop malignancies [1]. Careful management of patients with both diagnoses is therefore crucial, and in this chapter we explore the decisions involved in providing advanced heart-failure therapies for patients with prior or active cancer diagnoses.

CASE

A 50-year-old woman presents to her primary care doctor with progressive dyspnea on exertion and lower extremity edema. She is short of breath climbing one flight of stairs and describes four-pillow orthopnea. The patient is referred for an echocardiogram and is also due for preventative screening so a mammogram is scheduled. Echo reveals an ejection fraction (EF) of 30% with global hypokinesis. Subsequent angiogram reveals no significant coronary artery disease and evaluation for etiology of heart failure is unrevealing. She is started on guideline-directed medical therapy for idiopathic nonischemic cardiomyopathy (NICM). Shortly afterward, mammography is performed and results are suggestive of a mass in the upper outer left breast. MRI confirms a 2.5 cm suspicious focus in the left breast and slightly prominent left axillary lymph nodes. Core biopsy is consistent with infiltrating ductal carcinoma, estrogen receptor positive, progesterone receptor negative, her-2 indeterminate, and with a high proliferation rate (Ki-67 35%).

Medical Management of Patients With Both Advanced Heart Failure and Cancer

At the time of publication, there are no guidelines for heart-failure management that are specific to cancer patients. European Society of Cardiology (ESC) heart failure guidelines advise that patients who develop CCMP should receive standard heart-failure therapy [2]. Therefore, general heart-failure recommendations from the ESC, American College of Cardiology and American Heart Association should be used to guide management [3]. Care should be provided through collaboration between the patient's oncologist and cardiologist, and when possible, a cardiologist specializing in cardio-oncology.

Current heart-failure guidelines for patients with reduced EF recommend treatment with a beta blocker and an angiotensin converting enzyme (ACE) inhibitor or angiotensin receptor blocker (ARB). Some patients with symptomatic heart failure also benefit from aldosterone antagonists (if renal function and potassium levels permit their use), and combination therapy of nitrates with hydralazine is recommended for African-American patients and all heart-failure patients who are not able to take ACE inhibitors or ARBs [4,5].

In patients with NYHA symptom class II–III on goal directed medical therapy with an EF less than 35%, placement of an implantable cardioverter defibrillator (ICD) is recommended to prevent sudden cardiac death. However, ICD is only recommended for those with a life expectancy of at least 12 months, so should not be placed in patients who have an expected mortality from their cancer in less than a year [6]. If patients require MRIs as part of their oncologic evaluation, this should be performed prior to ICD placement, or an MRI compatible ICD should be considered (Table 21.1) [7].

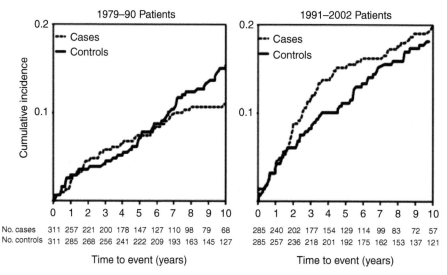

FIGURE 21.1 **In recent years, patients with heart failure have had a greater incidence of cancer diagnoses compared to people without heart failure.** *From Hasin T, et al. Patients with heart failure have an increased risk of incident cancer. J Am Coll Cardiol 2013;62:881–6.*

TABLE 21.1 Demonstrated Benefits of Guideline-Recommended HF Therapies

Guideline Recommended Therapy	Relative Risk Reductions in Pivotal Randomized Clinical Trial(s) (%)	Number Needed to Treat for Mortality (m)	Number Needed to Treat for Mortality (Standardized to 12 m)	Relative Risk Reduction in Meta-analysis
ACEI/ARB [4–6]	17	22 over 42	77	20%
β-Blocker [7–10]	34	28 over 12	28	31%
Aldosterone antagonist [11–13]	30	9 over 24	18	25%
Hydralazine/nitrate [14]	43	25 over 10	21	NA
CRT [15–18]	36	12 over 24	24	29/22%
ICD [19–22]	23	14 over 60	70	26%

NA, Not available.
Source: Fonarow GC, et al. Potential impact of optimal implementation of evidence-based heart failure therapies on mortality. Am Heart J 2011;161:30. e3–1024.e3.

There is little evidence on therapies to improve mortality in heart failure with preserved ejection fraction (HFpEF). Management includes focus on controlling hypertension, fluid status, and treatment of ischemia [4]. Use of echo to measure longitudinal strain in HFpEF may provide useful prognostic information as impaired strain has been shown to predict HF hospitalization and cardiac death [8].

Heart failure can have a graver prognosis than certain cancers including nonmelanoma skin cancers and early stages of bowel and breast cancer (Fig. 21.2) [9], making risk of exacerbation of heart failure from cardiotoxic chemotherapy agents potentially greater than the therapeutic

benefits of certain cancer treatments. The type of cardiomyopathy influences prognosis and should be considered when determining eligibility for and timing of cancer therapy [10]. For example, in a patient with NYHA functional class-IV heart failure from ischemic cardiomyopathy and early stage prostate cancer, it would be reasonable to delay cancer therapy that would interfere with heart-failure management until the patient has been stabilized on goal directed medical therapy. For patients with acutely life-threatening malignancies such as leukemia in blast crisis, chemotherapy must take priority over chronic management of heart failure. In our case patient, diuresis to a euvolemic

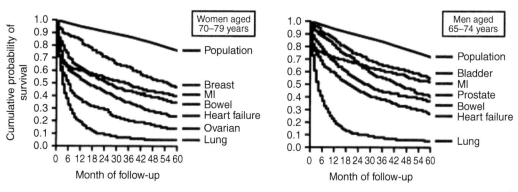

FIGURE 21.2   Age-specific probability of survival following a first admission for heart failure, myocardial infarction, and the four most common types of cancer specific to men and women relative to the overall population. Data for women aged 70–79 years (28% of the total cohort) are based on the following number of patients: heart failure ($n = 1167$), myocardial infarction ($n = 1600$) and cancer of the lung ($n = 475$), breast ($n = 441$), bowel ($n = 369$), and ovary ($n = 108$). Similarly data for men aged 65–74 years (26% of the total cohort) are based on the following numbers of patients: heart failure ($n = 1063$), myocardial infarction ($n = 2083$) and cancer of the lung ($n = 1064$), bowel ($n = 485$), prostate ($n = 452$), and bladder ($n = 264$). *From Stewart S, et al. More 'malignant' than cancer? Five-year survival following a first admission for heart failure. Eur J Heart Failure 2001;3:315–22.*

state and at minimum initiating guideline-directed medical therapy for heart failure would be reasonable prior to initiating cancer therapy.

When caring for unstable patients with heart failure it is important to consider potential noncardiac causes of hemodynamic compromise. Development of lower extremity edema could be secondary to heart failure, or alternatively due to lymphatic obstruction with tumor progression. Anemia may result in dyspnea on exertion similar to symptoms of increased cardiac pressures. Hypotension and tachycardia may be due to heart-failure exacerbation, but the possibility of pericardial involvement of the tumor resulting in tamponade must also be evaluated with an echocardiogram. The leukemia therapies imatinib and dasatinib can have side effects of dyspnea and peripheral edema independent of cardiac function, though they have been reported to possibly also cause ventricular dysfunction [11–13].

The patient has some functional improvement after treatment with a diuretic, beta blocker, and ACE inhibitor. Her surgeon requests cardiac risk assessment prior to breast surgery.

EFFECT OF ADVANCED HEART FAILURE ON CARDIAC RISK OF ONCOLOGIC SURGERIES

History of heart failure is an independent predictor of cardiac complications of noncardiac surgery [14,19]. Surgical risk of cardiac complications is further increased in patients with signs of acute heart failure preoperatively [14,20]. Therefore, heart-failure patients should be optimally clinically managed prior to oncologic surgery when possible, and nonemergent surgeries delayed for decompensated patients.

As in management of all patients with heart failure, continuation of medical therapy in the perioperative period is generally advised. It is a class-I recommendation that beta blockers be continued in patients who have been taking them chronically, but quick titration should not be done in the preoperative period and beta blockers should not be initiated in the setting of decompensated heart failure or on the day of surgery. ACE inhibitors may be continued preoperatively, but given that their benefit is from chronic use in heart-failure patients with reduced EF, it is appropriate to stop them perioperatively if there are concerns for hypotension or large fluid shifts [21].

Patients with ICDs should have tachycardia therapies turned off to avoid oversensing from intraoperative electromagnetic interference. While therapies are suspended, patients should be on a continuous cardiac monitor with external defibrillators available. The ICD must be turned back on with programming checked prior to removing the patient from external cardiac monitors [21].

Fluid status must be managed closely by the patient's cardiologists and anesthesiologists in the setting of volume administration during anesthesia and operative fluid shifts. Patients are often placed on maintenance intravenous fluids while not permitted to eat or drink around the time of surgery, which can lead to fluid overload in heart-failure patients if not monitored closely. Similarly, blood transfusions to treat perioperative blood loss often need to be administered with a diuretic to accommodate for relatively rapid increases in intravascular volume. In select patients, placement of a pulmonary artery catheter may be useful to guide fluid and inotrope therapy perioperatively. Routine use of invasive hemodynamic monitoring is not recommended given no evidence of benefit on outcomes and possible increase in catheter-related complications [22].

In patients on QT prolonging cardiac medications such as amiodarone or sotalol, perioperative therapies that also affect the QT interval must be used cautiously. These include certain antiemetics such as ondansetron, delirium treatments including haloperidol, and multiple antiarrhythmics. Certain cancer treatments including tyrosine kinase inhibitors may also prolong QT intervals [11,15]. Electrolyte levels should be carefully repleted perioperatively.

The patient is referred to surgery and undergoes a left lumpectomy and sentinel node dissection. Final pathology has a 2.2 cm tumor with no involvement of axillary nodes. Oncotype diagnosis is sent and is in the high-risk range with a score of 32, so chemotherapy is recommended given the high risk of recurrence without treatment beyond surgery.

Choice of Chemotherapy Regimen

In patients who have underlying heart failure at the time of cancer treatment, the use of cardiotoxic chemotherapy regimens should be restricted. Myocardial toxicity from anthracyclines needs to be avoided in patients with systolic heart failure, especially when alternative less cadiotoxic regimens are thought to be at least equally effective [16]. Anthracyclines are thought to inhibit topoisomerase II, resulting in dose-dependent cardiac myocyte death with typically permanent systolic dysfunction [17,18]. They are contraindicated in patients with an EF less than 30%. If anthracyclines are necessary for patients with an EF less than 50%, regular monitoring for deterioration of cardiac function must be performed [23]. In patients requiring anthracycline therapy for survival, total dose should be limited in addition to use of extended infusions instead of bolus doses in order to minimize peak plasma levels [24].

Trastuzumab and pertuzumab are monoclonal antibodies that block the HER2 receptor that is expressed in some breast cancers and is also part of a myocyte signaling pathway. The pathophysiology of cardiotoxicity from HER2-targeted agents is not well understood, but HER2 knockout mice develop dilated cardiomyopathy and have increased susceptibility to anthracycline-induced myocyte toxicity [25,26]. Cardiac function usually recovers after cessation of use as it does not directly damage myocytes, but there is higher risk when used in patients with prior anthracycline exposure or underlying cardiac dysfunction and therefore is contraindicated in the setting of heart failure [27–29].

The antimetabolite 5-fluorouracil has a low but significant incidence of cardiotoxicity including coronary vasospasm, so should be avoided in patients with ischemic heart disease and those prone to arrhythmias [30,31]. Taxanes cause histamine release which could exacerbate conduction disorders and arrhythmias [32]. Patients on tyrosine kinase inhibitors should have electrocardiogram (EKG) assessment for QT prolongation. Hypertension secondary to vascular endothelial growth factor (VEGF) ligands and

tyrosine kinase inhibitors needs to be closely monitored, especially in patients with heart failure with preserved EF, and antihypertensive regimens should be vigilantly adjusted to prevent heart-failure exacerbations [11,15,33–35]. On the other hand, patients may become hypovolemic from nausea and emesis during chemotherapy, necessitating dosage decrease of afterload reducing agents and diuretics.

Multiple randomized trials evaluating the use of ACE inhibitors or beta blockers during chemotherapy have failed to find significant protective effect to prevent chronic decline in cardiac function [36,37]. However, in one recent study of patients who developed anthracycline-related cardiotoxicity, those who were able to tolerate combination therapy of ACE inhibitors and beta blockers had greater improvement in EF compared to patients who were on only one of the two heart-failure medications [38]. It is reasonable to assume that continuing goal-directed medical therapy for heart failure during cancer therapy is beneficial for the underlying cardiomyopathy, and may possibly help limit acute deterioration of systolic function due to chemotherapy [39–42].

Statins have been evaluated for their potential antioxidant effects to protect patients from anthracycline-induced cardiomyopathy. Animal studies have shown that pretreatment with statins can minimize extent of anthracycline-related cardiotoxicity [43], and one human study suggested atorvastatin may help to maintain EF in patients treated with anthracyclines [44].

Current practice to monitor for cardiotoxicity involves use of imaging to detect decline in cardiac function after chemotherapy administration. Although this approach attempts to minimize the extent of myocardial damage, it does not allow for treatment modification before measurable decline in cardiac function occurs. Recent research has shown promise for the use of serum biomarkers to detect subclinical cardiotoxicity, before decrease in EF develops [45,46]. In patients with HER2-positive breast cancer and baseline EF $\geq$ 50%, increases in ultrasensitive troponin I and myeloperoxidase levels after treatment with an anthracycline and trastuzumab were associated with subsequent decline in EF, suggesting that chemotherapy adjustments triggered by elevated biomarkers could possibly reduce the risk of subsequent cardiac dysfunction [47].

Although troponin level may provide prognostic information, it has not been consistently shown to detect cardiac dysfunction in studies involving CCMP [48].

Serum levels of brain natriuretic peptide (BNP) may be predictive of subsequent anthracycline cardiotoxicity [49,50]. BNP, however, should not be relied upon in place of cardiac imaging as not all cases of CCMP result in measurements above 100 (the level traditionally is used as a cutoff to indicate heart failure) [51]. In a patient population with baseline cardiomyopathy prior to chemotherapy, the significance of BNP levels is even more uncertain.

A chemotherapy regimen with low risk of cardiotoxic effect (docetaxel/cyclophosphamide) is chosen and she completes six cycles of treatment. Following this she is referred to radiation oncology.

Radiation therapy is known to have cardiotoxic effects. These effects are dose dependent, and the heart receives a higher-radiation dose during treatment of left-sided chest cancers compared to right-sided tumors [52–54]. Radiation administered for esophageal cancer may result in pericardial effusions given the proximity of the esophagus to the pericardium [55,56].

Radiation dose should be limited as much as possible in all patients, but for patients with underlying heart disease, the risk of further insult from radiation therapy should be considered when weighing oncologic benefits of radiation protocols. Treatment decisions must be made through collaboration between the patient's radiation oncologist, medical oncologist, and cardiologist. All patients who receive chest radiation therapy should be monitored for subsequent valvular, pericardial, myocardial, and coronary heart disease with an annual history and physical exam. Patients should be evaluated for development of coronary artery disease with a stress test 5–10 years after chest radiation therapy is completed, and reassessment every 5 years [57]. In patients without baseline coronary atherosclerosis, such as those with NICM, evaluation for radiation-induced coronary artery disease could be performed with a coronary artery calcium scan in place of stress testing. Echocardiography should be performed 5–10 years after radiation exposure to evaluate for development of valvular disease, myocardial restriction, or pericardial constriction [57].

Despite the increased risk of having a left-sided breast tumor, the patient and her doctors decide to undergo radiation therapy, which she completes without complication. She is continued on guideline-directed medical therapy for heart failure, but experiences a decline in functional status over the following years. After being in remission from her breast cancer for 3 years, her EF is now less than 20% and she is NYHA functional class IV. She has an ICD, but does not meet criteria for chronic resynchronization therapy. Advanced heart-failure therapies are considered.

Heart Transplantation in Cancer Patients

End-stage heart failure is reported to occur in 2–4% of patients with CCMP [3], and a greater number of patients with other etiologies of advanced heart failure will have past and current cancer diagnoses. Treatment for advanced heart failure depends in part on the etiology of the cardiomyopathy. Stress-induced cardiomyopathy, peripartum cardiomyopathy, and cardiotoxicity from HER2–targeted chemotherapy are examples of often reversible heart failure [58–64]. For these cases, patients should be supported medically, with withdrawal of cardiotoxic agents when possible, and if needed, with temporary mechanical circulatory support (MCS). The majority of patients with end-stage heart failure have irreversible etiologies, including nonrevascularizable ischemic cardiomyopathy, idiopathic dilated cardiomyopathy, and anthracycline-induced cardiomyopathy [18]. For these patients, more permanent advanced heart-failure therapies should be considered, including cardiac transplantation.

Multiple case series have shown no significant difference in posttransplant survival when comparing cancer patients and patients without a history of malignancy [65–67]. The caveat here is that these are retrospective observational studies and patients with better prognoses are selected for transplant. Type of malignancy affects posttransplant prognosis, as was shown in a retrospective review of heart transplant patients in the United Network for Organ Sharing (UNOS) database. Between 2000 and 2011, 5.6% of orthotopic heart transplant (OHT) patients had pretransplant malignancies. Compared to heart transplant patients without a history of malignancy, patients with a history of leukemia, lymphoma, or myeloma had increased 30 day (HR 1.82; $P = 0.04$), 1 year (HR 1.93; $P < 0.001$), and 5-year mortality (HR 1.54; $P = 0.01$) [68].

Given the scarcity of donor hearts, from an ethical standpoint, organs should be allocated with priority to patients with the best posttransplant prognosis, necessitating exclusion of patients with a high mortality risk from cancer. Heart transplantation can now provide an expectation of excellent survival and quality of life, with a greater than 50% 10-year survival [69]. Therefore, for all comorbidities, an anticipated 5-year survival of at least 80% independent of a patient's cardiac disease is generally advised for heart transplant listing. In the past, current neoplasms aside from nonmelanoma skin cancer were considered absolute contraindications to heart transplantation. Though the most recent European Society of Cardiology guidelines for heart-failure management list treated cancer within the last 5 years as a contraindication to heart transplant, the current International Society for Heart and Lung Guidelines on listing requirements for heart transplantation recognize the importance of evaluating varying prognoses of different malignancies when allotting limited organ resources. The guidelines include the following:

"Pre-existing neoplasms are diverse and many are treatable with excision, radiotherapy or chemotherapy to induce cure or remission. In these patients needing cardiac transplantation, collaboration with oncology specialists should occur to stratify each patient as to their risk of tumor recurrence. Cardiac transplantation should be considered when tumor recurrence is low based on tumor type, response to therapy and negative metastatic work-up. The specific amount of time to wait to transplant after neoplasm

remission will depend on the aforementioned factors and no arbitrary time period for observation should be used (Level of Evidence: C) [70]."

For cancer survivors, a remission period of at least 5 years is usually recommended prior to listing for OHT, though guidelines indicate an exception for low-grade malignancies such as prostate cancer, with guidance from an oncologist [70]. The 5-year remission criteria for heart transplant listing is based in part on kidney transplant registry data that reported a 21% rate of recurrence or new malignancy in 1258 patients with pretransplant malignancy; 87% of these recurrences occurred in patients whose initial malignancy was treated within 5 years prior to transplantation [71].

Risk of recurrence was described for different types of malignancies in this cohort. Incidentally diagnosed and early stage tumors were less likely to recur, as expected given an overall greater cure rate of low-grade malignancy. Of the patients in this population, 8% had cancers for which treatment was delayed until after kidney transplant, many of which were nonmelanoma skin cancers and prostate cancer. Authors concluded on the basis of the observational data that a 5-year cancer-free period should be required prior to transplant listing for patients with lymphoma, and most breast, colon, prostate, and large symptomatic renal carcinomas. A 2-year period was recommended for stage-I breast cancers, Dukes A or B I colon cancer, low Gleason score prostate cancers, small asymptomatic renal carcinomas, and Clark's level-II melanoma. They further suggest that a remission period is not necessary in certain small focal malignancies of the prostate and uterus, as well as nonmelanoma skin cancers due to more favorable prognoses.

In patients with a history of cancer prior to OHT, case reports suggest recurrence rates ranging from 0% during 2-year follow-up to 33%, all occurring within 5 years [65–67,72]. In these referenced studies, nonmelanoma skin cancers, which have a favorable prognosis, were the most frequent to recur. A series from a single center in Germany of oncology patients from 1989 to 1995 with a cancer-free period prior to heart transplantation of zero days to 20 years included two patients with bladder and prostate adenocarcinomas that were resected posttransplant. Of these patients, 60% were long-term survivors [72].

Assessment of recurrence risk is improving with the use of cancer gene expression profiles, which is not addressed in the current guidelines on transplant candidacy. For breast cancer, the 21-gene Recurrence Score [73,74], PAM50 Risk of Recurrence score [75–77], and Amsterdam 70-gene profile [78–80] can help to guide treatment and predict a patient's likelihood of recurrence at 10 years. Therefore, some stage-I breast cancers may have higher recurrence risk than stage-II breast cancers, and the previous recommendations should only be used for guidance with informed assessment of individual risk made by an oncologist.

Hereditary cancers are related to genetic mutations that dramatically increase the lifetime risk for malignancy, such as the BRCA gene which is associated with higher rates of breast and ovarian cancer. Family history should be obtained in transplant candidates and genetic screening performed when indicated. Patients who are positive for these genes require adjusted screening schedules both pre- and posttransplant, and often prophylactic interventions such as mastectomy need to be considered. Timing of prophylactic surgeries should be based on individual characteristics as intraoperative risk may be greater pretransplant, but risk of infection and impaired wound healing is greater on immunosuppressive therapy.

The additional factor of age is not discussed in the guidelines but significantly affects patient risk. Patients are being transplanted at increasingly older ages, and this advanced age is associated with higher risks of cancer occurrence after transplant, especially prostate cancer and primary bone-marrow disorders. Therefore, it is especially important to increase cancer screening in older patients being listed for transplant.

Based on the available data, oncologists should guide decisions for transplant listing based on each individual's expected prognosis and risk of recurrence. When necessary, delaying cancer treatment until after transplant is reasonable for easily treated low-grade malignancies such as basal-cell carcinoma or ductal carcinoma in situ. As advances are made in oncologic treatment and cancer gene profiling, shorter cancer remission periods may be considered for a greater number of diagnoses. Once a patient is determined to be a candidate for listing, guideline-based cancer screening should continue, including more frequent screening for virus-related malignancies (e.g., human papilloma virus associated cervical cancer) which have the potential to progress aggressively in the setting of future immunosuppression [81,82].

Mechanical Circulatory Support in Cancer Patients

Patients with end-stage heart failure who are not candidates for transplant or are too unwell to wait the anticipated time for a donor organ to become available may benefit from MCS, currently including ventricular support devices as well as the total artificial heart. Multiple factors are considered when determining candidacy for MCS. Bleeding or thrombosis risk, especially related to hematologic malignancies, must be assessed given the thrombogenic internal hardware components of MCS and required anticoagulation. Patients with history of chest radiation therapy are at increased risk for operative complications due to chest wall fibrosis. This increases the risk of any MCS or OHT surgery, and even more so in patients who will have one surgery for MCS implanted as a bridge to transplant and a subsequent transplant surgery.

There are multiple forms of MCS from which devices are selected on the basis of patient's characteristics. Extracorporeal membrane oxygenation (ECMO) is a temporary form of MCS typically used in acute situations to stabilize patients until recovery of cardiac pathology or as a bridge to more permanent treatment. Blood is exchanged through arterial and venous cannulas and circulated through an external machine. Left ventricular assist devices (LVADs) come in varying forms and are implanted to increase left ventricular output. LVADs are durable and allow patients to be ambulatory with limited external hardware. For patients who also have right ventricular failure, a right ventricular assist device may be added, or more often the heart is entirely replaced with a total artificial heart.

The 2013 International Society for Heart and Lung Transplantation Guidelines for MCS state that patients with a history of cancer who are determined to be free of malignancy may be candidates for MCS as a bridge to transplant provided that an oncologist has assessed their risk for recurrence (class I, level of evidence C) [83]. MCS may further be used as a bridge to transplant for patients with advanced heart failure who have not completed the recommended 5-year remission period prior to transplant but are likely to be cured of cancer and become future transplant candidates [84].

Given the advanced age of many patients on MCS as destination therapy, it is expected that some of these patients will be diagnosed with cancer after MCS implantation. Bridging of anticoagulation is required during surgical interventions and resection of intrathoracic tumors may be anatomically complicated, but standard oncologic care can be provided for most diagnoses in patients with implanted MCS [85]. Risk of device thrombosis may be greater in these patients given the prothrombotic state often induced by malignancy. Certain cancer therapies may also increase risk of clot formation, such as certain antiangiogenic agents (anti-VEGF), which increases risk for arterial thromboembolic events [86].

Patients with current malignancy who are determined by an oncologist to have a life expectancy of at least 2 years are considered candidates for MCS as destination therapy (class IIa, level of evidence C). It is recommended that patients with a life expectancy of less than 2 years should not receive MCS (class III, level of evidence C) [83]. Temporary MCS (ECMO and ventricular assist devices) may be used to support patients through the hemodynamic challenges of life-saving chemotherapy with expected recoverable conditions including stress-induced cardiomyopathy [87,88].

Heart Transplantation and Mechanical Circulatory Support for Chemotherapy-Induced Cardiomyopathy

OHT appears to be an effective option for patients with CCMP, with similar outcomes to patients with other types of NICM. Retrospective analysis of CCMP patients who underwent OHT between 2000 and 2008 showed that survival at 1, 3, and 5 years post-OHT was not different between patients with NICM and CCMP [89].

In one series of patients with anthracycline-related CCMP who required MCS, there was no difference in survival compared to patients with MCS for other causes of heart failure [90]. Need for concomitant right ventricular support is greater in patients with CCMP compared to patients with other causes of cardiomyopathy [89,90]. Therefore, this patient population should be carefully evaluated for the need for biventricular support when MCS treatment decisions are being made.

The patient has VAD placement as a bridge to transplant. She remains in remission for an additional 2 years (total of 5 years from her breast cancer treatment), and is listed for transplant. Although listed for transplant, she continues to undergo appropriate cancer screening. At transplantation she is started on an immunosuppression regimen including use of sirolimus instead of azathioprine. She is monitored closely for recurrence and de novo malignancy.

Posttransplant Considerations

OHT requires chronic immunosuppression of the recipient patient, making the susceptibility of malignancies to recur in this setting a critical consideration. Nonmelanoma skin cancer appears to be the most likely to occur in the setting of decreased immune surveillance. Therapies should be adjusted to potentially minimize risk of malignancy recurrence, such as using sirolimus which may have a lower risk of malignancy [91], and minimizing cyclosporine and azathioprine which are associated with increased rates of skin cancer [92–94].

Most cancer screening guidelines do not differ for transplant patients in comparison to the general population. Some malignancies do, however, warrant more frequent screening in the setting of immunosuppression due to potentially more rapid progression. Transplant patients should be vigilant about sun protection given their increased risk of skin cancers and more aggressive course compared to the general population [95,96]. Patients should perform monthly self-exams and have annual dermatologic exams [97].

Cervical cancer develops more rapidly in immunosuppressed patients because it is secondary to viral infection. It is therefore recommended that pelvic exams and Pap smears be performed annually in adult transplant patients

[81]. Similarly, patients with risk factors for anal intraepithelial cancers should also be screened regularly [82,98].

Male transplant recipients over age 50 are screened annually for prostate cancer [99,100], differing from the United States Preventative Services Task Force guidelines that PSA screening is not recommended for the general population [101]. Screening for urologic cancers with urinalysis to detect hematuria is recommended for patients with risk factors including cumulative doses of cyclophosphamide greater than 20 g or history of analgesic nephropathy [81,102].

Some studies have shown an increased risk of colorectal cancer in transplant recipients, though the incidence varies across demographics [103–105]. Currently there are not specific colon-cancer screening recommendations for immunosuppressed patients. Breast cancer does not appear to occur at increased rates in transplant patients, therefore, guidelines do not differ from those for the general population [106].

In conclusion, due to the prevalence of both conditions, a concurrent diagnosis of malignancy in heart-failure patients is not uncommon. In addition, since cancer therapies can acutely result in heart-failure exacerbations and may also cause chronic deterioration of cardiac function, all patients undergoing potentially cardiotoxic chemotherapy should undergo cardiac evaluation. Patients with baseline heart failure should be closely managed jointly by their oncologist and cardiologist throughout all aspects of their cancer treatment. When end-stage heart failure occurs, a prior history of malignancy does not preclude all patients from successful cardiac transplant or MCS, depending on individual risk of recurrence.

REFERENCES

[1] Hasin T, et al. Patients with heart failure have an increased risk of incident cancer. J Am Coll Cardiol 2013;62:881–6.

[2] Authors/Task Force Members, et al. ESC Guidelines for the diagnosis and treatment of acute and chronic heart failure 2012: The Task Force for the Diagnosis and Treatment of Acute and Chronic Heart Failure 2012 of the European Society of Cardiology. Developed in collaboration with the Heart Failure Association (HFA) of the ESC. Eur Heart J 2012;33:1787–847.

[3] Yeh ETH, Bickford CL. Cardiovascular complications of cancer therapy: incidence, pathogenesis, diagnosis, and management. J Am Coll Cardiol 2009;53:2231–47.

[4] Yancy CW, et al. 2013 ACCF/AHA Guideline for the Management of Heart Failure A Report of the American College of Cardiology Foundation/American Heart Association Task Force on Practice Guidelines. Circulation 2013;128:e240–327.

[5] Taylor AL, et al. Combination of isosorbide dinitrate and hydralazine in blacks with heart failure. N Engl J Med 2004;351:2049–57.

[6] Russo AM, et al. ACCF/HRS/AHA/ASE/HFSA/SCAI/SCCT/SCMR 2013 appropriate use criteria for implantable cardioverter-defibrillators and cardiac resynchronization therapy: a report of the American College of Cardiology Foundation appropriate use criteria task force, Heart Rhythm Society, American Heart Association, American Society of Echocardiography, Heart Failure Society of America, Society for Cardiovascular Angiography and Interventions, Society of Cardiovascular Computed Tomography, and Society for Cardiovascular Magnetic Resonance. Heart Rhythm 2013;10:e11–58.

[7] Fonarow GC, et al. Potential impact of optimal implementation of evidence-based heart failure therapies on mortality. Am Heart J 2011;161:1024e3–30e3.

[8] Shah AM, et al. Prognostic importance of impaired systolic function in heart failure with preserved ejection fraction and the impact of spironolactone. Circulation 2015;132:402–14.

[9] Stewart S, MacIntyre K, Hole DJ, Capewell S, McMurray JJV. More 'malignant' than cancer? Five-year survival following a first admission for heart failure. Eur J Heart Failure 2001;3:315–22.

[10] Felker GM, et al. Underlying causes and long-term survival in patients with initially unexplained cardiomyopathy. N Engl J Med 2000;342:1077–84.

[11] Orphanos GS, Ioannidis GN, Ardavanis AG. Cardiotoxicity induced by tyrosine kinase inhibitors. Acta Oncologica 2009;48:964–70.

[12] Kantarjian H, et al. Dasatinib or high-dose imatinib for chronic-phase chronic myeloid leukemia after failure of first-line imatinib: a randomized phase 2 trial. Blood 2007;109:5143–50.

[13] Kerkelä R, et al. Cardiotoxicity of the cancer therapeutic agent imatinib mesylate. Nat Med 2006;12:908–16.

[14] Lee TH, et al. Derivation and prospective validation of a simple index for prediction of cardiac risk of major noncardiac surgery. Circulation 1999;100:1043–9.

[15] Chu TF, et al. Cardiotoxicity associated with tyrosine kinase inhibitor sunitinib. Lancet 2007;370:2011–9.

[16] Eschenhagen T, et al. Cardiovascular side effects of cancer therapies: a position statement from the Heart Failure Association of the European Society of Cardiology. Eur J Heart Fail 2011;13:1–10.

[17] Lyu YL, et al. Topoisomerase IIbeta mediated DNA double-strand breaks: implications in doxorubicin cardiotoxicity and prevention by dexrazoxane. Cancer Res 2007;67:8839–46.

[18] Ewer MS, Lippman SM. Type II chemotherapy-related cardiac dysfunction: time to recognize a new entity. JCO 2005;23:2900–2.

[19] Goldman L, et al. Multifactorial index of cardiac risk in noncardiac surgical procedures. N Engl J Med 1977;297:845–50.

[20] Detsky AS, Abrams HB, Forbath N, Scott JG, Hilliard JR. Cardiac assessment for patients undergoing noncardiac surgery. A multifactorial clinical risk index. Arch Intern Med 1986;146:2131–4.

[21] Fleisher LA, et al. 2014 ACC/AHA guideline on perioperative cardiovascular evaluation and management of patients undergoing noncardiac surgery: a report of the American College of Cardiology/American Heart Association Task Force on practice guidelines. J Am Coll Cardiol 2014;64:e77–137.

[22] Sandham JD, et al. A randomized, controlled trial of the use of pulmonary-artery catheters in high-risk surgical patients. N Engl J Med 2003;348:5–14.

[23] Schwartz RG, et al. Congestive heart failure and left ventricular dysfunction complicating doxorubicin therapy. Seven-year experience using serial radionuclide angiocardiography. Am J Med 1987;82:1109–18.

[24] van Dalen EC, van der Pal HJH, Caron HN, Kremer LC. Different dosage schedules for reducing cardiotoxicity in cancer patients receiving anthracycline chemotherapy. Cochrane Database Syst Rev 2009;CD005008.

[25] Ozcelik C, et al. Conditional mutation of the ErbB2 (HER2) receptor in cardiomyocytes leads to dilated cardiomyopathy. Proc Natl Acad Sci USA 2002;99:8880–5.

[26] Liu F-F, et al. Heterozygous knockout of neuregulin-1 gene in mice exacerbates doxorubicin-induced heart failure. Am J Physiol Heart Circ Physiol 2005;289:H660–666.

[27] Martín M, et al. Minimizing cardiotoxicity while optimizing treatment efficacy with trastuzumab: review and expert recommendations. Oncologist 2009;14:1–11.

[28] Sandoo A, Kitas G, Carmichael A. Breast cancer therapy and cardiovascular risk: focus on trastuzumab. Vasc Health Risk Manag 2015;11:223–8.

[29] Di Cosimo S. Heart to heart with trastuzumab: a review on cardiac toxicity. Target Oncol 2011;6:189–95.

[30] Monsuez J-J, Charniot J-C, Vignat N, Artigou J-Y. Cardiac side-effects of cancer chemotherapy. Int J Cardiol 2010;144:3–15.

[31] Sorrentino MF, Kim J, Foderaro AE, Truesdell AG. 5-fluorouracil induced cardiotoxicity: review of the literature. Cardiol J 2012; 19:453–8.

[32] Albini A, et al. Cardiotoxicity of anticancer drugs: the need for cardio-oncology and cardio-oncological prevention. JNCI J Natl Cancer Inst 2010;102:14–25.

[33] Escudier B, et al. Sorafenib in advanced clear-cell renal-cell carcinoma. N Engl J Med 2007;356:125–34.

[34] Sica DA. Angiogenesis inhibitors and hypertension: an emerging issue. J Clin Oncol 2006;24:1329–31.

[35] Izzedine H, et al. Management of hypertension in angiogenesis inhibitor-treated patients. Ann Oncol 2009;20:807–15.

[36] Bosch X, et al. Enalapril and carvedilol for preventing chemotherapy-induced left ventricular systolic dysfunction in patients with malignant hemopathies: The OVERCOME Trial (preventiOn of left Ventricular dysfunction with Enalapril and caRvedilol in patients submitted to intensive ChemOtherapy for the treatment of Malignant hEmopathies). J Am Coll Cardiol 2013;61:2355–62.

[37] Georgakopoulos P. et al. Cardioprotective effect of metoprolol and enalapril in doxorubicin-treated lymphoma patients: A prospective, parallel-group, randomized, controlled study with 36-month follow-up. Am J Hematol 2010;85:894–6.

[38] Cardinale D, et al. Early detection of anthracycline cardiotoxicity and improvement with heart failure therapy. Circulation 2016;133(4):e363.

[39] Cardinale D, et al. Anthracycline-induced cardiomyopathy: clinical relevance and response to pharmacologic therapy. J Am Coll Cardiol 2010;55:213–20.

[40] Lotrionte M, et al. Review and meta-analysis of incidence and clinical predictors of anthracycline cardiotoxicity. Am J Cardiol 2013;112:1980–4.

[41] Kaya MG, et al. Protective effects of nebivolol against anthracycline-induced cardiomyopathy: a randomized control study. Int J Cardiol 2013;167:2306–10.

[42] Kalay N, et al. Protective effects of carvedilol against anthracycline-induced cardiomyopathy. J Am Coll Cardiol 2006;48:2258–62.

[43] Riad A, et al. Pretreatment with statin attenuates the cardiotoxicity of doxorubicin in mice. Cancer Res 2009;69:695–9.

[44] Acar Z, et al. Efficiency of atorvastatin in the protection of anthracycline-induced cardiomyopathy. J Am Coll Cardiol 2011;58:988–9.

[45] Cardinale D, et al. Trastuzumab-induced cardiotoxicity: clinical and prognostic implications of troponin I evaluation. J Clin Oncol 2010;28:3910–6.

[46] Daniela Cardinale MTS, Cardinale D, Sandri MT, Colombo A, Colombo N, Boeri M, Lamantia G, et al. Prognostic value of troponin I in cardiac risk stratification of cancer patients undergoing high-dose chemotherapy. Circulation 2004;109(22):2749–54.

[47] Ky B, et al. Early increases in multiple biomarkers predict subsequent cardiotoxicity in patients with breast cancer treated with doxorubicin, taxanes, and trastuzumab. J Am Coll Cardiol 2014;63:809–16.

[48] Germanakis I, Anagnostatou N, Kalmanti M. Troponins and natriuretic peptides in the monitoring of anthracycline cardiotoxicity. Pediatr Blood Cancer 2008;51:327–33.

[49] Sandri MT, et al. N-terminal pro-B-type natriuretic peptide after high-dose chemotherapy: a marker predictive of cardiac dysfunction? Clin Chem 2005;51:1405–10.

[50] Meinardi MT, et al. Prospective evaluation of early cardiac damage induced by epirubicin-containing adjuvant chemotherapy and locoregional radiotherapy in breast cancer patients. J Clin Oncol 2001;19:2746–53.

[51] Vogelsang TW, Jensen RJ, Hesse B, Kjaer A. BNP cannot replace gated equilibrium radionuclide ventriculography in monitoring of anthracycline-induced cardiotoxity. Int J Cardiol 2008;124:193–7.

[52] Darby SC, et al. Risk of ischemic heart disease in women after radiotherapy for breast cancer. N Engl J Med 2013;368:987–98.

[53] Clarke M, et al. Effects of radiotherapy and of differences in the extent of surgery for early breast cancer on local recurrence and 15-year survival: an overview of the randomised trials. Lancet 2005;366:2087–106.

[54] Favourable and unfavourable effects on long-term survival of radiotherapy for early breast cancer: an overview of the randomised trials. Early Breast Cancer Trialists' Collaborative Group. Lancet 2000;355:1757–70.

[55] Fukada J, et al. Symptomatic pericardial effusion after chemoradiation therapy in esophageal cancer patients. Int J Radiat Oncol Biol Phys 2013;87:487–93.

[56] Martel MK, Sahijdak WM, Haken RK, Ten, Kessler ML, Turrisi AT. Fraction size and dose parameters related to the incidence of pericardial effusions. Int J Radiat Oncol Biol Phys 1998;40:155–61.

[57] Lancellotti P, et al. Expert consensus for multi-modality imaging evaluation of cardiovascular complications of radiotherapy in adults: a report from the European Association of Cardiovascular Imaging and the American Society of Echocardiography. J Am Soc Echocardiogr 2013;26:1013–32.

[58] Bybee KA, et al. Systematic review: transient left ventricular apical ballooning: a syndrome that mimics ST-segment elevation myocardial infarction. Ann Intern Med 2004;141:858–65.

[59] Akashi YJ, Goldstein DS, Barbaro G, Ueyama T. Takotsubo cardiomyopathy: a new form of acute, reversible heart failure. Circulation 2008;118:2754–62.

[60] Cooper LT, et al. Myocardial recovery in peripartum cardiomyopathy: prospective comparison with recent onset cardiomyopathy in men and nonperipartum women. J Card Fail 2012;18:28–33.

[61] Perez EA, Rodeheffer R. Clinical cardiac tolerability of trastuzumab. J Clin Oncol 2004;22:322–9.

[62] Slamon DJ, et al. Use of chemotherapy plus a monoclonal antibody against HER2 for metastatic breast cancer that overexpresses HER2. N Engl J Med 2001;344:783–92.

[63] Ewer MS, et al. Reversibility of trastuzumab-related cardiotoxicity: new insights based on clinical course and response to medical treatment. J Clin Oncol 2005;23:7820–6.

[64] Guarneri V, et al. Long-term cardiac tolerability of trastuzumab in metastatic breast cancer: the M.D. Anderson Cancer Center experience. J Clin Oncol 2006;24:4107–15.

[65] Dillon TA, et al. Cardiac transplantation in patients with preexisting malignancies. Transplantation 1991;52:82–5.

[66] Goldstein DJ, et al. Orthotopic heart transplantation in patients with treated malignancies. Am J Cardiol 1995;75:968–71.

[67] Edwards BS, et al. Cardiac transplantation in patients with preexisting neoplastic diseases. Am J Cardiol 1990;65:501–4.

[68] Beaty CA, George TJ, Kilic A, Conte JV, Shah AS. Pre-transplant malignancy: an analysis of outcomes after thoracic organ transplantation. J Heart Lung Transplant 2013;32:202–11.

[69] Lund LH, et al. The registry of the International Society for Heart and Lung Transplantation: thirty-first official adult heart transplant report—2014; focus theme: retransplantation. J Heart Lung Transplant 2014;33:996–1008.

[70] Mehra MR, et al. Listing criteria for heart transplantation: International Society for Heart and Lung Transplantation Guidelines for the Care of Cardiac Transplant Candidates—2006. J Heart Lung Transplant 2006;25:1024–42.

[71] Penn I. Evaluation of transplant candidates with pre-existing malignancies. Ann Transplant 1997;2:14–7.

[72] Koerner MM, et al. Results of heart transplantation in patients with preexisting malignancies. Am J Cardiol 1997;79:988–91.

[73] Paik S, et al. A multigene assay to predict recurrence of tamoxifen-treated, node-negative breast cancer. N Engl J Med 2004;351:2817–26.

[74] Mamounas EP, et al. Association between the 21-gene recurrence score assay and risk of locoregional recurrence in node-negative, estrogen receptor-positive breast cancer: results from NSABP B-14 and NSABP B-20. J Clin Oncol 2010;28:1677–83.

[75] Parker JS, et al. Supervised risk predictor of breast cancer based on intrinsic subtypes. J Clin Oncol 2009;27:1160–7.

[76] Dowsett M, et al. Comparison of PAM50 risk of recurrence score with oncotype DX and IHC4 for predicting risk of distant recurrence after endocrine therapy. J Clin Oncol 2013;31:2783–90.

[77] Gnant M, et al. Predicting distant recurrence in receptor-positive breast cancer patients with limited clinicopathological risk: using the PAM50 Risk of Recurrence score in 1478 postmenopausal patients of the ABCSG-8 trial treated with adjuvant endocrine therapy alone. Ann Oncol 2014;25:339–45.

[78] van de Vijver MJ, et al. A gene-expression signature as a predictor of survival in breast cancer. N Engl J Med 2002;347:1999–2009.

[79] van 't Veer LJ, et al. Gene expression profiling predicts clinical outcome of breast cancer. Nature 2002;415:530–6.

[80] Buyse M, et al. Validation and clinical utility of a 70-gene prognostic signature for women with node-negative breast cancer. J Natl Cancer Inst 2006;98:1183–92.

[81] Morath C, et al. Malignancy in Renal Transplantation. JASN 2004;15:1582–8.

[82] Ogunbiyi OA, et al. Prevalence of anal human papillomavirus infection and intraepithelial neoplasia in renal allograft recipients. Br J Surg 1994;81:365–7.

[83] Feldman D, et al. The 2013 International Society for Heart and Lung Transplantation Guidelines for mechanical circulatory support: executive summary. J Heart Lung Transplant 2013;32:157–87.

[84] Sundbom P, et al. Young woman with breast cancer and cardiotoxicity with severe heart failure treated with a HeartMate IITM for nearly 6 years before heart transplantation. ASAIO J 2014;60:e3–4.

[85] Loyaga-Rendon RY, Inampudi C, Tallaj JA, Acharya D, Pamboukian SV. Cancer in end-stage heart failure patients supported by left ventricular assist devices. ASAIO J 2014;60:609–12.

[86] Zangari M, et al. Thrombotic events in patients with cancer receiving antiangiogenesis agents. J Clin Oncol 2009;27:4865–73.

[87] Zeballos C, Moraca RJ, Bailey SH, Magovern GJ. Temporary mechanical circulatory support for takotsubo cardiomyopathy secondary to primary mediastinal B-cell lymphoma. J Card Surg 2012;27:119–21.

[88] Rateesh S, Shekar K, Naidoo R, Mittal D, Bhaskar B. Use of extracorporeal membrane oxygenation for mechanical circulatory support in a patient with 5-fluorouracil induced acute heart failure. Circ Heart Fail 2015;8:381–3.

[89] Oliveira GH, et al. Characteristics and survival of patients with chemotherapy-induced cardiomyopathy undergoing heart transplantation. J Heart Lung Transplant 2012;31:805–10.

[90] Oliveira GH, et al. increased need for right ventricular support in patients with chemotherapy-induced cardiomyopathy undergoing mechanical circulatory support: outcomes from the INTERMACS Registry (Interagency Registry for Mechanically Assisted Circulatory Support). J Am Coll Cardiol 2014;63:240–8.

[91] Salgo R, et al. Switch to a sirolimus-based immunosuppression in long-term renal transplant recipients: reduced rate of (pre-)malignancies and nonmelanoma skin cancer in a prospective, randomized, assessor-blinded, controlled clinical trial: switch to sirolimus in long-term RTR. Am J Transplant 2010;10:1385–93.

[92] Dantal J, et al. Effect of long-term immunosuppression in kidney-graft recipients on cancer incidence: randomised comparison of two cyclosporin regimens. Lancet 1998;351:623–8.

[93] Wisgerhof HC, et al. Subsequent squamous- and basal-cell carcinomas in kidney-transplant recipients after the first skin cancer: cumulative incidence and risk factors. Transplantation 2010;89:1231–8.

[94] O'Donovan P, et al. Azathioprine and UVA light generate mutagenic oxidative DNA damage. Science 2005;309:1871–4.

[95] Ulrich C, et al. Prevention of non-melanoma skin cancer in organ transplant patients by regular use of a sunscreen: a 24 months, prospective, case-control study. Br J Dermatol 2009;161(Suppl 3):78–84.

[96] Feuerstein I, Geller AC. Skin cancer education in transplant recipients. Prog Transplant 2008;18:232–41. quiz 242.

[97] Mudigonda T, et al. Incidence, risk factors, and preventative management of skin cancers in organ transplant recipients: a review of single- and multicenter retrospective studies from 2006 to 2010. Dermatol Surg 2013;39:345–64.

[98] Tramujas da Costa e Silva I, et al. High-resolution anoscopy in the diagnosis of anal cancer precursor lesions in renal graft recipients. Ann Surg Oncol 2008;15:1470–5.

[99] Kasiske BL, et al. The evaluation of renal transplantation candidates: clinical practice guidelines. Am J Transplant 2001;1(Suppl 2):3–95.

[100] EBPG Expert Group on Renal Transplantation. European best practice guidelines for renal transplantation. Section IV: long-term

management of the transplant recipient. Nephrol Dial Transplant 2002;17(Suppl 4):1–67.

[101] Moyer VA. U.S. Preventive Services Task Force. Screening for prostate cancer: U. S. Preventive Services Task Force recommendation statement. Ann Intern Med 2012;157:120–34.

[102] Vlaovic P, Jewett MAS. Cyclophosphamide-induced bladder F cancer. Can J Urol 1999;6:745–8.

[103] Park JM, et al. Increased incidence of colorectal malignancies in renal transplant recipients: a case control study. Am J Transplant 2010;10:2043–50.

[104] Webster AC, Craig JC, Simpson JM, Jones MP, Chapman JR. Identifying high risk groups and quantifying absolute risk of cancer after kidney transplantation: a cohort study of 15,183 recipients. Am J Transplant 2007;7:2140–51.

[105] Kwon JH, et al. Prevalence of advanced colorectal neoplasm after kidney transplantation: surveillance based on the results of screening colonoscopy. Dig Dis Sci 2015;60:1761–9.

[106] Engels EA, Pfeiffer RM, Fraumeni JF, et al. SPectrum of cancer risk among us solid organ transplant recipients. JAMA 2011;306:1891–901.

Chapter 22

Heart Transplantation and Left Ventricular Assist Devices in Cancer Survivors

E.P. Kransdorf and M.M. Kittleson

Cedars-Sinai Heart Institute, Los Angeles, CA, United States

INTRODUCTION

Every year, between 5 and 10 new pharmacotherapies are approved by the United States Food and Drug Administration (FDA) for treatment of cancer [1]. A small number of these agents will be associated with cardiotoxic effects that may not have been identified during the agent's initial safety assessment. In addition, certain established pharmacotherapies are well known to have cardiotoxic effects, but effective alternatives are lacking. The field of cardio-oncology has developed to diagnose, manage, and treat patients affected by the acute or chronic cardiotoxic effects of cancer therapies.

As a young medical discipline, cardio-oncology faces several barriers to widespread implementation. First, oncologists and cardiologists each utilize distinct terminology to describe the adverse effects of cancer therapies. For example, an oncologist may describe a patient who develops a drop in the left ventricular ejection fraction (LVEF) without symptoms of heart failure after chemotherapy as having "congestive heart failure (CHF)." In contrast, the term used by the cardiologist, "asymptomatic left ventricular dysfunction," may not be meaningful to the oncologist. In addition, there is often a prolonged interval between a patient's cancer treatment and the development of cardiotoxic effects, making diagnosis and management more difficult.

There are two main groups of cancer survivors that are encountered within the population of patients with advanced heart failure: those who developed cardiomyopathy as a consequence of their cancer therapy (i.e., therapy-induced cardiomyopathy) and those who have advanced heart failure independent of a prior history of malignancy. The archetype of the first group is a woman with breast cancer and a subsequent anthracycline-induced cardiomyopathy. The archetype of the second group is a man with ischemic cardiomyopathy who presents for heart transplant evaluation with a history of prostate adenocarcinoma. In this chapter, we will review the epidemiology and clinical features of the two main therapy-induced cardiomyopathies, anthracycline- and radiation-induced cardiomyopathies. We will then discuss the role of mechanical circulatory support and heart transplantation as treatment for these cardiomyopathies. Finally, we will highlight the increased risk of malignancy after transplantation and discuss potential interventions to mitigate this risk.

EPIDEMIOLOGY AND CLINICAL FEATURES OF THERAPY-INDUCED CARDIOMYOPATHIES

The oncologist's arsenal includes hundreds of anticancer pharmacotherapies. Luckily, only a small number of these agents are associated with cardiotoxic effects, and in most cases these cardiotoxic effects do not lead to permanent cardiac dysfunction. The pharmacotherapies that are most frequently associated with left ventricular dysfunction have been discussed elsewhere in this textbook, but are summarized in Table 22.1 [2].

The two cancer therapies most commonly associated with cardiomyopathy are anthracyclines and thoracic radiation. The anthracyclines are discussed elsewhere in this textbook but will be briefly reviewed here. In adults, doxorubicin is the most commonly used anthracycline, which is used to treat breast adenocarcinoma, ovarian adenocarcinoma, Hodgkin and non-Hodgkin lymphoma, and acute myeloid leukemia. Anthracyclines are also used in conjunction with thoracic radiation to treat breast adenocarcinoma and Hodgkin lymphoma, which are known to potentiate cardiotoxicity as compared to chemotherapy alone [3–5].

TABLE 22.1 Incidence of Left Ventricular Systolic Dysfunction With Various Chemotherapeutic Agents

Chemotherapy Agent	Incidence (%)	Frequency of Use
Anthracyclines		
Doxorubicin	3–26	+ + +
Epirubicin	1–3	+ +
Idarubicin	5–18	+
Alkylating agents		
Cyclophosphamide	7–28	+ + +
Ifosfamide	17	+ + +
Antimetabolites		
Clofarabine	27	+
Antimicrotubule agents		
Docetaxel	2–8	+ +
Monoclonal antibody-based tyrosine kinase inhibitors		
Bevacizumab	2–3	+ +
Trastuzumab	2–28	+ +
Proteasome inhibitor		
Velcade	2–5	+ +
Small molecule tyrosine kinase inhibitors		
Dasatinib	2–4	+ +
Imatinib mesylate	1–2	+
Lapatinib	2	+
Sunitinib	3–11	+ + +

Source: Yeh ET, Bickford CL. Cardiovascular complications of cancer therapy. J Am Coll Cardiol 2009;53:2231–47.

Chemotherapy-Induced Cardiomyopathy

By convention, chemotherapy-induced cardiomyopathy generally refers to anthracycline-induced cardiomyopathy. Such cardiomyopathy has been traditionally described to present in three distinct patterns: an acute form affecting less than 1% of patients immediately after drug administration, a chronic but early-onset form affecting 1–2% of patients during therapy or during the first year after treatment, and a chronic late-onset form affecting 1–5% of patients at least 1 year after completing therapy [2]. Interestingly, recent data question the validity of this classification. In a study of 2625 patients receiving anthracycline-containing chemotherapy regimens followed by serial echocardiography at baseline, during, and after chemotherapy, a reduction in ejection fraction (EF) of greater than 10% occurred in 9% of patients [6]. The median time between the last dose of chemotherapy and the development of the reduced EF was 3.5 months, and this drop occurred within the first year after treatment in 98% of patients. Additional studies performed using cardiac magnetic resonance imaging (CMRI), which is extremely sensitive for changes in myocardial function, show similar results [7,8]—that the end-systolic volume increases and the EF decreases to a small degree within 3–6 months after anthracycline therapy.

The paradigm emerging from these recent data (Fig. 22.1) is that anthracycline therapy induces variable degrees of subclinical myocardial damage, that is detectable using sensitive myocardial biomarkers [9,10]. The degree of myocardial damage is related to the dose of anthracycline used, among other factors. Subsequent to this initial insult, myocardial contractility decreases, which is detectable by echocardiography as a drop in EF [9]. Over time, especially

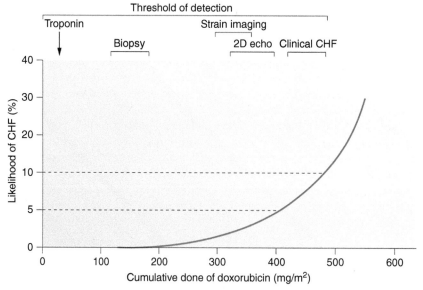

FIGURE 22.1 **Relationship between the cumulative administered anthracycline dose (*x*-axis) and the likelihood of developing heart failure, as indicated by the percent of patients within the treated population who develop symptomatic heart failure (*y*-axis).** Several sensitive techniques, such as myocardial biomarker testing (e.g., troponin), endomyocardial biopsy, and myocardial strain imaging, can detect myocardial damage prior to the development of symptomatic heart failure. *From Ewer MS, Ewer SM. Cardiotoxicity of anticancer treatments. Nat Rev Cardiol 2015;12(9):547–58.*

in the context of additional cardiovascular comorbidities, such as hypertension or diabetes mellitus [12], these patients with left ventricular dysfunction will have progressive decline in cardiac function and will eventually present with symptomatic heart failure.

Early on, studies using endomyocardial biopsies to detect myocardial injury showed that the most critical risk factor for the development of chemotherapy-induced cardiomyopathy was the cumulative dose of the anthracycline administered [13]. At a cumulative doxorubicin dose of 400 mg/m^2, 3% of patients developed cardiomyopathy, whereas at a cumulative doxorubicin dose of 550 mg/m^2, 7% of patients developed cardiomyopathy [14]. More recent data suggested that the cardiotoxic dose of doxorubicin was lower than initially realized, with 5% of patients developing cardiomyopathy at a dose of 400 mg/m^2 and 26% of patients developing cardiomyopathy at a dose of 550 mg/m^2 [15]. In a large study of 2625 patients receiving anthracycline-containing chemotherapy, multivariable analysis of risk factors for the development of cardiotoxicity showed that EF at the completion of chemotherapy (hazard ratio 1.37), age (hazard ratio 1.07), female sex (hazard ratio 1.61), family history of coronary artery disease (hazard ratio 1.67), and cumulative anthracycline dose (hazard ratio 1.09 for each 50 mg/m^2 increase in dose) were independent predictors of cardiotoxicity [6].

Recent investigations have focused on the potential benefits of guideline-directed heart failure therapy in chemotherapy-induced cardiomyopathy. Indeed, after initiation of beta-adrenergic blockers and angiotensin converting enzyme inhibitors, many patients with chemotherapy-induced cardiomyopathy will have normalization of LVEF [6]. Small trials have also shown that treatment with these agents during chemotherapy may prevent the development of cardiotoxicity [16].

Hospitalizations for acute exacerbations of heart failure are common in patients with cardiomyopathies [17]. In a recent study of 156,013 patients hospitalized with acute heart failure in the Get With the Guidelines Registry between 2005 and 2013, 721 patients or 1.2% had chemotherapy-induced cardiomyopathy [18]. Patients hospitalized for chemotherapy-induced cardiomyopathy had an average age of 66 years and were predominantly women (68%). Neither in-hospital mortality nor median length of stay greater than 4 days were significantly higher for chemotherapy-induced cardiomyopathy as compared to other etiologies of nonischemic cardiomyopathy.

Radiation-Induced Cardiomyopathy

Thoracic radiation is commonly used as a component of multimodality therapy for adults with breast adenocarcinoma and Hodgkin lymphoma. In general, the cardiotoxic effects of thoracic radiation include cardiomyopathy as well as coronary artery disease and valvular dysfunction

[19]. Radiation-induced coronary artery disease and valvular dysfunction are discussed elsewhere in this textbook. Radiation-induced cardiomyopathy is pathophysiologically and clinically distinct from chemotherapy-induced cardiomyopathy, and most often results in a restrictive cardiomyopathy; the left ventricular size and EF are normal to mildly reduced, and diastolic filling is impaired as indicated by an elevated E to A ratio [20].

In a study of 2524 Dutch survivors of Hodgkin lymphoma treated between 1965 and 1995 with a median follow-up time of 20.3 years, of whom 81% were treated with mediastinal radiation, the standardized incidence ratio (SIR) for heart failure was 6.8 compared with the general population [21]. The 40-year cumulative incidence of heart failure was 24.8%. In a second Dutch study of 4414 survivors of breast adenocarcinoma, radiation to the internal mammary chain plus the breast was associated with a 2.7-fold increased risk of heart failure [22]. Thus, cancer survivors treated with thoracic radiation are at a substantially increased risk of heart failure after treatment.

Unlike chemotherapy-induced cardiomyopathy, radiation-induced cardiomyopathy is an irreversible process that is unlikely to respond to guideline-directed medical therapy for heart failure, such as beta-adrenergic blockers and angiotensin converting enzyme inhibitors [23]. Heart transplantation is indicated for severe cases.

ROLE OF MECHANICAL CIRCULATORY SUPPORT IN CANCER SURVIVORS

The use of mechanical circulatory support (MCS) in patients with advanced heart failure has dramatically increased in the United States since the FDA approval of continuous-flow left ventricular assist devices (LVAD) [24]. The most widely used device, the Thoratec HeartMate II LVAD, was approved by the FDA as a bridge-to-transplantation in 2008, and has been implanted in over 10,000 patients worldwide. The HeartMate II was subsequently FDA-approved for use in patients ineligible for heart transplantation (destination therapy) in 2010. In 2012, the HeartWare HVAD LVAD was approved for use as a bridge-to-transplantation. The use of the HVAD LVAD for destination therapy is still under investigation as part of the ENDURANCE clinical trial [25], but preliminary results suggest that the use of the HVAD results in comparable 2-year survival to the HeartMate II. A smaller number of patients with advanced biventricular heart failure, who are candidates for heart transplantation, will receive biventricular assist devices, such as the SynCardia Total Artificial Heart (TAH).

According to the Heart Failure Society of America Comprehensive Heart Failure Practice Guideline, MCS is indicated for: (1) patients awaiting heart transplantation who have become refractory to maximal medical circulatory support, and (2) patients with severe heart failure refractory to conventional therapy who are not candidates for heart transplantation, particularly those who cannot be weaned from intravenous inotropic support [26]. The International Society for Heart and Lung Transplantation Guidelines for Mechanical Circulatory Support indicate that patients with a history of treated cancer who are in long-term remission may be candidates for MCS as a bridge-to-heart transplantation, whereas patients with a history of recently treated or active cancer who have a reasonable life expectancy (greater than 2 years) may be candidates for MCS as destination therapy [27]. Thus, MCS is not recommended for patients with active cancer who have a life expectancy less than 2 years. In patients with cancer at high risk of relapse undergoing MCS implantation as destination therapy, implantation of the Thoratec HeartMate II LVAD is currently the only option, as the HeartWare HVAD LVAD and the SynCardia TAH are approved for use only as a bridge-to-heart transplantation.

The clinical features and short-term outcomes of MCS in patients with advanced heart failure due to therapy-induced cardiomyopathy are distinct. In an analysis of 3812 patients undergoing LVAD implantation in the Interagency Registry for Mechanically Assisted Circulatory Support (INTERMACS) between 2006 and 2011, 75 (2%) of MCS recipients had a history of chemotherapy-induced cardiomyopathy [28]. These recipients were predominantly female (72% as compared to 20% in recipients of MCS for other indications) and a significantly larger proportion underwent LVAD implantation as destination therapy (33% as compared to 17% in recipients of MCS for other indications). Interestingly, pre-MCS markers of right ventricular dysfunction, such as central venous pressure and central venous pressure to pulmonary capillary wedge pressure ratio [29] were significantly higher in the group of patients who underwent LVAD implantation for chemotherapy-induced cardiomyopathy. As such, more patients with chemotherapy-induced cardiomyopathy required right ventricular assist device support devices after LVAD implantation (19% vs. 9.3% in recipients of MCS for other indications). However, survival after MCS implantation for patients with chemotherapy-induced cardiomyopathy was similar to those who received MCS for other indications.

Although recovery of LVEF after LVAD implantation has been observed in approximately 20% of patients [30], only 1% of patients receiving MCS in the INTERMACS registry actually undergo device explantation [24]. Interestingly, there have been three reports of recovery of cardiac function sufficient to permit LVAD explantation in patients with anthracycline-induced cardiomyopathy [31–33]. Although it is unclear if patients with anthracycline-induced cardiomyopathy are more likely to have cardiac recovery in general, these reports suggest that patients with anthracycline-induced cardiomyopathy undergoing LVAD implantation should be monitored closely by serial echocardiograms for potential recovery of cardiac function.

Mechanical Circulatory Support for Primary Cardiac Malignancies

Although rare, primary malignancies of the heart are associated with high morbidity and mortality [34]. The majority of these lesions are sarcomas followed by lymphomas [34,35]. Cardiac angiosarcoma is usually treated by localized resection and chemotherapy [36]. However, for cardiac lymphoma, cardiac explantation with placement of biventricular assist devices followed by heart transplantation has been performed, with survival noted up to 2 years postprocedure [37,38]. Thus, MCS may serve an important role in the management of these malignancies.

HEART TRANSPLANTATION IN CANCER SURVIVORS

The increased risk of malignancy after transplantation was noted by Starzl and Penn almost 50 years ago [39]. The immunosuppression required to maintain the immune system of a transplant recipient in a quiescent state to prevent rejection also leads to an increased risk of cancer recurrence or de novo malignancy after transplant. Indeed, malignancy is one of the major causes of death after heart transplant [40].

Patients with a history of cancer that present for transplant evaluation require a comprehensive assessment of their cancer history and risk of recurrence. Most transplant programs require that transplant candidates with a history of cancer achieve a prespecified cancer-free interval prior to listing. For renal transplant candidates, specific intervals have been proposed for each type of cancer [41,42]. However, the relevance of these intervals to heart transplantation is unclear since heart transplant recipients generally receive greater levels of immunosuppression than renal transplant recipients.

No systematic studies have examined the policies of individual heart transplant programs regarding required cancer-free intervals prior to transplant listing. The International Society of Heart and Lung Transplantation guidelines on listing criteria for heart transplantation do not suggest a firm threshold, and instead suggest that "when tumor recurrence is low based on tumor type, response to therapy and negative metastatic work-up, then cardiac transplantation may be considered" [43].

Many heart transplant programs require a 5-year cancer-free interval prior to heart transplant. The 5-year remission threshold was investigated in a large cohort of heart and lung transplant recipients [44]. Over a 28-year period in a cohort of 3380 heart and lung transplant recipients, 2.9% were diagnosed with malignancy prior to transplant. In this cohort, 42% had a hematologic malignancy, 26% genitourinary malignancy, 13% lung malignancy, and 19% had various other types of malignancy. When divided into three groups by the time between malignancy and transplant (less than 1 year,

1–5 years, and greater than 5 years), malignancy recurrence decreased successively in each group with 63, 26, and 6% recurrence rates, respectively. Overall survival was lower in the first group but was not statistically different in the latter two groups. Thus, a remission threshold of less than 1 year seems imprudent, and a threshold of between 1 year and 5 years can be considered with the caveat that there may be a higher risk of cancer recurrence.

These data support the convention of a 5-year remission threshold policy but should be interpreted with caution. First, the cohort included patients enrolled from between 1983 and 2011 and the treatment and prognosis of cancers has certainly evolved over this time period. Second, a large number of patients in the cohort had lung malignancies, for which there was a 67% recurrence rate which could have skewed the overall results and thus the risk of other cancers might not be as high.

Clinical Considerations Prior to Heart Transplantation in Cancer Survivors

There are sparse guideline-based recommendations for evaluation of cancer survivors prior to heart transplantation but certain general guidelines should be followed. First, cancer survivors should be referred for oncologic assessment at the time of heart transplant evaluation specifically by an oncologist experienced in evaluating potential transplant candidates. The consultation should include an assessment of the transplant candidate's risk of recurrent malignancy and survival from that malignancy. Patients at risk of recurrence within 5 years may not be heart-transplant candidates but may be candidates for left ventricular assist device therapy as a bridge to transplant candidacy.

Epidemiology of Cancer in Patients Undergoing Heart Transplantation

The history of malignancy in heart transplant recipients has been well studied. Using data from the Organ Procurement and Transplantation Network (OPTN) database maintained by the United Network for Organ Sharing, a number of studies have determined that 5.6% of United States heart transplant recipients have a history of prior malignancy [45,46]. The five most common pretransplant malignancies are: breast cancer (14.7%), skin cancer (12.6%), leukemia (12.3%), genitourinary cancer (8.0%), and thyroid cancer (1.9%). Lung cancer composed only 0.8%. Similarly, 4.6% of the patients in the Cardiac Transplant Research Database who underwent heart transplant between 1993 and 2008 had a history of cancer [47] though the types differed somewhat: the three most common malignancies were breast cancer (17.7%), lymphoma (15.2%) and prostate cancer (13.0%). In a cohort of patients undergoing heart transplantation in

Sweden, Norway, and Finland, 2.9% of patients had a pretransplant malignancy [44].

As discussed previously, the two main cardiomyopathies that lead to end-stage heat failure that are caused by cancer therapy are chemotherapy-induced cardiomyopathy frequently with a dilated phenotype and radiation-induced cardiomyopathy with a restrictive phenotype. From the OPTN database, the incidence of chemotherapy-induced cardiomyopathies in heart transplant recipients in the United States between 2000 and 2008 [48] was 2.6%. Chemotherapy-induced cardiomyopathy in this cohort was most common after hematologic malignancies (33%), followed by breast cancer (31%) and sarcomas (7.5%).

We have reviewed the incidence of heart transplantation in the United States for doxorubicin-induced cardiomyopathy using data in the OPTN database (Kransdorf and Kittleson, unpublished). Interestingly, the incidence appears to be increasing, with doxorubicin-induced cardiomyopathy representing 0.7% of all primary heart transplants in 1993 and 1.9% of transplants in 2013 (Fig. 22.2). This trend will likely continue, as the age-adjusted death rate for breast cancer continues to decrease [49].

A small number of patients undergo heart transplantation for restrictive cardiomyopathy, one cause of which is radiation-induced cardiomyopathy. Between 1987 and 2010, only 35 patients in the United States underwent heart transplant for this indication [50]. We have also reviewed the incidence of heart transplantation in the United States for radiation-induced restrictive cardiomyopathy using data in the OPTN database (Kransdorf and Kittleson, unpublished) and found that here too the incidence appears to be increasing (Fig. 22.3).

Survival and Recurrent Malignancy After Heart Transplantation in Cancer Survivors

When assessing heart transplant recipients with pretransplant malignancy in toto, several studies have shown that overall, these patients have posttransplant survival comparable to cancer-free transplant recipients, but patients with hematologic malignancies are at an increased risk [45]. Such patients have twofold increase in mortality at 30 days and 1 year posttransplant, and 1.6-fold increase risk of death at 5 years posttransplant.

From the Cardiac Transplant Research Database, it appears that recurrences of pretransplant malignancy were uncommon, with only 37 of 283 patients (13%) experiencing a recurrence. Freedom from cancer recurrence at 10 years posttransplant was 84% for breast cancer, 58% for lymphoma, 96% for prostate cancer, and 36% for basal or squamous cell skin cancer [47]. Nonetheless, other analyses indicate that any history of pretransplant malignancy was associated with an increased risk of posttransplant malignancy, with

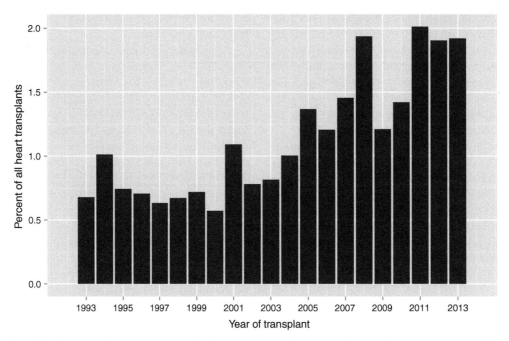

FIGURE 22.2 **Plot of the incidence of heart transplantation for chemotherapy-induced cardiomyopathy, as a percentage of the total number of heart transplants per year, in the United Network for Organ Sharing database.** As can be seen from the plot, the incidence of heart transplantation for chemotherapy-induced cardiomyopathy is increasing.

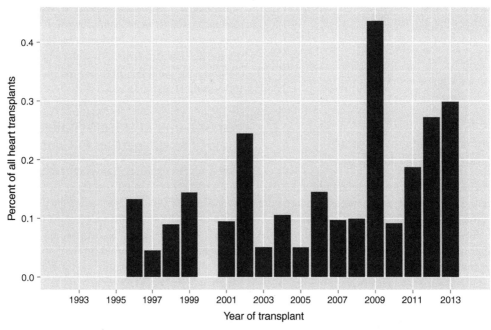

FIGURE 22.3 **Plot of the incidence of heart transplantation for radiation-induced cardiomyopathy, as a percentage of the total number of heart transplants per year, in the United Network for Organ Sharing database.** As can be seen from the plot, the incidence of heart transplantation for radiation-induced cardiomyopathy is increasing.

a hazard ratio of 1.51 [46]. Furthermore, recipients with chemotherapy-induced cardiomyopathy were at a significantly increased risk of malignancy at 1 year posttransplant (5% in the chemotherapy-induced cardiomyopathy group versus 2% in the nonischemic cardiomyopathy group).

Focusing on survival in heart transplant recipients with chemotherapy-induced cardiomyopathies, multiple studies have shown that such patients have comparable posttransplant survival at 1, 3, and 5 years to patients with nonischemic cardiomyopathies [48,51]. In contrast, heart transplant recipients with prior radiation-induced cardiomyopathy have increased mortality [50] with 1-, 5-, and 10-year survival of 71, 47, and 32%, respectively, with an overall hazard ratio of 1.8 compared to patients undergoing heart transplantation for nonrestrictive cardiomyopathies. Two single-center cohorts, from Columbia and Mayo Clinic have confirmed these findings, showing increased perioperative mortality in patients with a history of prior chest radiation [52,53].

DE NOVO MALIGNANCIES AFTER HEART TRANSPLANTATION

The increased incidence of malignancy first recognized in kidney and liver transplant recipients has also been observed in heart transplant recipients. In an early series of heart transplant recipients at Stanford University between 1968 and 1977, 25% of recipients developed cancer by 5 years posttransplant [54]. Subsequently, multiple investigations using large clinical registries have demonstrated this increased incidence of malignancy after heart transplantation.

An analysis of the Scientific Registry of Transplant Recipients linked to 13 state-based cancer registries [55] comprising 175,732 solid organ transplant recipients transplanted between 1987 and 2008 demonstrated that the overall risk of cancer was double that of the general population, with a SIR of 2.10. The four most common malignancies in their analysis were non-Hodgkin lymphoma, lung cancer, liver cancer, and kidney cancer, all of which except liver cancer occurred at an increased incidence after heart transplantation (SIR of 7.8, 2.7, 1.0, and 2.9, respectively).

In a similar analysis of the OPTN database between 1999 and 2008 [56], 11% of heart transplant recipients developed a posttransplant malignancy, with an incidence of 14.3 cases per 1000 person-years. Lung cancer and posttransplant lymphoproliferative disease were most common (3.2 cases and 2.2 cases per 1000-person years, respectively) but comparison to the general population was not performed. In a multivariate regression model including age, sex, race, human leukocyte antigen mismatch, and immunosuppression regimen, increasing age was a strong risk factor for posttransplant malignancy, whereas Hispanic ethnicity

was protective. Of note, skin cancer was not investigated in either study.

An analysis of the Cardiac Transplant Research Database [47] illustrated similar findings. The most common malignancies posttransplant in this cohort were lung (21.2%), lymphoproliferative disease/lymphoma (16.8%), prostate (15.5%), melanoma (6.7%), and colon (4.9%). In a multivariate regression model, older age, African-American ethnicity, history of cigarette use, prior history of invasive malignancy and earlier transplant era were risk factors for development of a posttransplant malignancy.

The risk of malignancy after heart transplantation outside the United States has also been assessed using the Spanish Post-Heart-Transplant Tumor Registry [57]. In this population, 490 recipients (14.4%) experienced 639 malignancies with an overall incidence of 18.7 cases per 1000 person-years at 1 year, 22.7 cases per 1000 person-years at 5 years and 30.4 cases per 1000 person-years at 10 years posttransplant. The most common malignancies were of the skin (50.7%), lymphoma (9.7%), lung (10.1%), and prostate (3.9%).

Beyond the increased incidence of malignancy after transplantation, de novo posttransplant malignancies present at more advanced stages than in the general population. In an analysis of 635 transplant recipients in the Israel Penn International Transplant Tumor Registry compared with over one million adults in the general population [58], cancer of the lung, breast, prostate, and bladder, as well as malignant melanoma all presented at higher cancer stages in transplant recipients as compared to the general population. Furthermore, for most types of cancer, stage-specific survival was worse in transplant recipients.

Role of Specific Immunosuppressive Agents in Malignancies After Heart Transplantation

In the early era of heart transplantation, cyclosporine, an inhibitor of calcineurin, and azathioprine, which inhibits the proliferation of lymphocytes, was the mainstay of chronic immunosuppression. Additional immunosuppression was frequently administered immediately after transplantation, termed "induction" immunosuppression. Pivotal clinical trials have shown that utilization of newer immunosuppressive agents of these same classes, tacrolimus and mycophenolate mofetil, are associated with a reduced incidence of rejection [59]. In the light of these data, clinical utilization of cyclosporine and azathioprine has shifted to predominant use of tacrolimus and mycophenolate mofetil (Fig. 22.4) [40]. More recently another class of immune-modulatory agents, the mammalian target of rapamycin (mTOR) inhibitors have become available and demonstrate antioncogenic activity in renal transplant recipients [60]. Several groups have investigated whether the clinical shift to utilization of these newer immunosuppressive

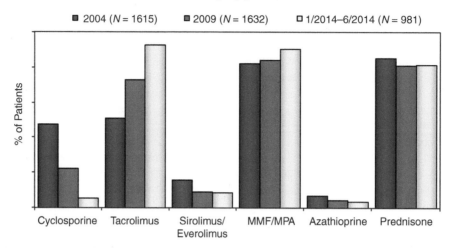

FIGURE 22.4 **Bar plot of the utilization of different immunosuppression agents during 3 successive years (2004, 2009, and 2014) in the International Society for Heart and Lung Transplantation database.** The utilization of cyclosporine has dramatically decreased in favor of tacrolimus, and the utilization of azathioprine has dropped in favor of mycophenolate mofetil.

agents has led to changes in the incidence of cancer after heart transplantation.

In a cohort of patients from the ISHLT registry who received heart transplants between 1995 and 1997, the use of mycophenolate mofetil was associated with a 26% reduced risk of developing malignancy within 5 years of transplant (hazard ratio 0.73). Neither the use of tacrolimus nor induction immunotherapy was associated with an increased risk of malignancy as compared with the use of cyclosporine and no induction, respectively [61]. In contrast, observational studies have demonstrated that the use of tacrolimus over cyclosporine and mycophenolate mofetil over azathioprine was associated with fewer malignancies, though the specific benefit (skin cancer vs. solid organ cancers vs. lymphoma) varied between studies. [57,62].The use of induction immunosuppression increased the risk of both skin cancer and solid organ cancers but the increased risk of lymphoma associated with the use of induction immunosuppression was ameliorated by the use of antiviral agents [63].

Statins are standard of care in heart transplant recipients to reduce the risk of cardiac allograft vasculopathy [64]. However, statin use also appears to protect against malignancy in a small study of 255 heart transplant recipients in Switzerland between 1985 and 2007 [65]. This benefit was independent of age, gender, type of cardiomyopathy, and immunosuppressive therapy with a 67% lower risk of malignancy (hazard ratio 0.33) in a multivariate analysis. The benefit of statin therapy was independent of cholesterol levels, which reflects the known immunomodulatory benefits of statins [66].

Use of mTOR Inhibitors in Kidney Transplantation

While we await that further data on whether more widespread use of mTOR inhibitors will decrease the incidence of malignancy after heart transplantation, there is a substantial body of literature that mTOR inhibitors decrease the incidence of malignancies after kidney transplantation. In an analysis of 33,249 deceased donor kidney transplant recipients between 1996 and 2001 in the OPTN database [67], use of the mTOR inhibitors sirolimus or everolimus as maintenance immunosuppression was associated with a 60% reduced risk of developing any de novo malignancy.

Analysis of clinical trial data has had similar findings. In a post hoc analysis of the Sirolimus CONVERT trial, the overall rate of malignancy was significantly lower in kidney transplant recipients that had been converted to sirolimus (plus azathioprine or mycophenolate) than those that were maintained on tacrolimus or cyclosporine (2.1 vs. 6.0 malignancies per 100 person-years, respectively) [68]. This endpoint was driven by the lower number of skin cancers, which is the most common malignancy after solid organ transplantation. The number of nonskin malignancies was numerically lower in the sirolimus conversion group, but of borderline statistical significance (1.0 vs. 2.1 malignancies per 100 person-years, respectively).

Comparable results were obtained in a meta-analysis of kidney transplant recipients treated with sirolimus [69]. After adjustment for the trial, age, location, and time after transplantation, the use of sirolimus was associated with a 40% reduction in the risk of malignancy. Specifically, the

TABLE 22.2 Recommendations for Management of Heart Transplant Recipients With a History of Cancer

	All Recipients	Recipients With History of Cancer	Recipients With Active Cancer
Risk of malignancy	+	++	+++
Induction immunosuppression	If indicated	–	–
Mammalian target of rapamycin inhibitor	If indicated	+	++
Statin	+	++	++

risk of nonmelanoma skin cancer was reduced by 56% whereas the risk of nonskin cancers was unaffected by sirolimus use.

Clinical Management the Heart Transplant Recipient With Malignancy

Given the increased incidence and severity of malignancies in patients after heart transplantation, specialized management strategies are required to optimize long-term outcomes (Table 22.2). All heart transplant recipients should be regarded as "at risk" for development of malignancy. This is especially true for patients with previously established risk factors for the development of posttransplant malignancy, such as those with history of cancer and older age.

The management of patients after heart transplantation focuses on balance, achieving a state of quiescence whereby the immune system accepts the donor organ as its own (Fig. 22.5). Immunosuppression must be adequate to prevent host immune system activation and rejection of the graft, but not so strong as to increase the risk of infection

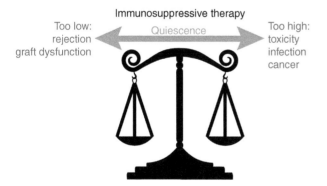

FIGURE 22.5 **General approach to immunosuppression after heart transplantation.** The goal of immunosuppressive therapy is to achieve a state of quiescence whereby the immune system accepts the donor organ as its own. If immunosuppressive intensity is too low, rejection or graft dysfunction due to activation of the recipient's immune system may occur. If immunosuppressive intensity is too high, the recipient may experience toxicities of the immunosuppressive agent (e.g., renal dysfunction), infection, or cancer. *Adapted from Patel J, Kobashigawa JA. Minimization of immunosuppression: transplant immunology. Transpl Immunol 2008;20:48–54.*

and malignancy. After transplantation, a comprehensive immunologic assessment should be performed to determine each recipient's risk of rejection and the immunosuppression regimen should be individualized to this risk. Use of a test of T-cell immune function (ImmunoKnow or Cylex assay) can identify transplant recipients who are overimmunosuppressed [70]. One study of 13 patients with de novo malignancy after solid organ transplantation [71] demonstrated that T-cell immune function levels in transplant recipients who died of their malignancy were significantly lower than that of patients who survived. These results suggest that transplant recipients with malignancy may be profoundly immunosuppressed even at low levels of immunosuppression and as such using biomarkers, such as this T-cell immune function assay may guide appropriate reduction in immunosuppression.

As discussed in this chapter, patients with pretransplant cancer, either incidental to the cause of their cardiomyopathy or with therapy-induced cardiomyopathy, are at substantial risk of recurrence and secondary malignancy after transplant. We recommend immunosuppression be reduced to "as low as reasonably achievable." In these patients, the use of induction immunosuppression should be avoided unless the recipient is at high immunologic risk. An mTOR inhibitor should be initiated within the first year after transplantation. Statin therapy should be prescribed.

For patients who develop malignancies after heart transplantation, further attenuation of the immunosuppression regimen is required. Target levels of calcineurin inhibitors should be reduced to the minimum and mTOR inhibitors should be initiated (usually after surgical procedures are performed as there is some evidence that sirolimus in particular may impair wound healing) [59]. Statin therapy should be continued unless there are other contraindications.

CANCER SURVIVORS AS ORGAN DONORS

Heart transplantation is limited by the supply of donor organs. Thus, every effort should be made to utilize all donor hearts absent of clear contraindications to their use [73]. Organ donors with a history of malignancy constituted 2.2% of 39,455 organ donors in the UNOS database between 2000

TABLE 22.3 Risk Framework for Donor Transmitted Malignancy

Category	Risk of Transmission	Donor Malignancy Examples
0	No significant risk (0%)	Benign tumors
1	Minimal (0–0.1%)	Basal cell carcinoma, skin
2	Low (0.1–1%)	Low-grade CNS tumor (WHO grade I or II)
3	Intermediate (1–10%)	Breast carcinoma (stage 0, i.e., carcinoma in situ)
4	High (>10%)	Malignant melanoma

Source: Adapted from Nalesnik MA, et al. Donor-transmitted malignancies in organ transplantation: assessment of clinical risk. Am J Transplant 2011;11:1140–47.

and 2005 [74]. The four most common types of malignancy were of the skin (30.9%), central nervous system (25.6%), uterine cervix (13.4%), and melanoma (5.6%). In an older study of organ donors in the UNOS database with a history of malignancy between 1994 and 2001, transmission of cancer from cadaveric donors occurred at a rate of 0.04% [76]. The mortality rate in these recipients was 38%, so even though donor transmitted malignancy is a rare occurrence, precautions must be taken to prevent donor transmission of malignancy. In 2011, the Donor Transmission Advisory Committee of the OPTN published a framework to help clinicians assess the risk of donor transmitted malignancy [75]. This framework assigns malignancy types to five categories of increasing risk for donor-to-recipient transmission (Table 22.3). Utilization of donors with malignancies in categories 3 and 4 is not recommended, whereas donors with malignancies in categories 1 and 2 are permissible as long as informed consent is obtained from the potential recipients.

CONCLUSIONS

Cancer survivors constitute a large and important subset of patients with advanced cardiomyopathy. These patients are an approximately equal mix of those that have cardiomyopathy as a result of their cancer therapy in the form of chemotherapy-induced or radiation-induced cardiomyopathy and those that were previously treated for malignancy and have an unrelated cardiomyopathy. Recent data indicate that 10% of patients treated with anthracyclines will experience a drop in LVEF. This drop occurs almost exclusively within the first year after treatment, and in many cases left ventricular function will improve with guideline-directed medical therapy for heart failure. Thus, systematic screening for left ventricular dysfunction in patients treated with anthracyclines may be warranted as a strategy to reduce the incidence of chemotherapy-induced cardiomyopathy.

For patients with advanced heart failure who are at high risk of cancer relapse, mechanical circulatory support as destination therapy with the Thoratec HeartMate II LVAD may be a therapeutic option. An important caveat is that patients with chemotherapy-induced cardiomyopathy undergoing LVAD implantation are at substantially increased risk of perioperative right ventricular failure and the need for a right ventricular assist device, and so appropriate strategies should be undertaken to mitigate this increased risk.

Cancer survivors with advanced heart failure who are at low risk of relapse may be excellent candidates for heart transplantation. Important considerations in the pretransplant assessment include the transplant candidate's risk of recurrent malignancy and survival from that malignancy. Many transplant programs require a 5-year cancer-free interval prior to heart transplant though this interval can be adjusted on the basis of the details of the individual cancer in consultation with an oncologist well-versed in the risks of immunosuppression.

After heart transplantation, both recipients with and without a history of cancer are at an increased risk of malignancies. When malignancies occur posttransplant they frequently present at more advanced stages. Clinical strategies to minimize the posttransplant risk of both recurrent and de novo malignancies include avoidance of induction immunosuppression as well as utilization of mammalian target of rapamycin inhibitors and statin therapy.

REFERENCES

[1] Chabner BA, Roberts TG. Timeline: chemotherapy and the war on cancer. Nat Rev Cancer 2005;5:65–72.

[2] Yeh ETH, Bickford CL. Cardiovascular complications of cancer therapy. J Am Coll Cardiol 2009;53:2231–47.

[3] Shapiro CL, Hardenbergh PH, Gelman R, et al. Cardiac effects of adjuvant doxorubicin and radiation therapy in breast cancer patients. J Clin Oncol 1998;16:3493–501.

[4] Myrehaug S, Pintilie M, Yun L, et al. A population-based study of cardiac morbidity among Hodgkin lymphoma patients with preexisting heart disease. Blood 2010;116:2237–40.

[5] Galper SL, Yu JB, Mauch PM, et al. Clinically significant cardiac disease in patients with Hodgkin lymphoma treated with mediastinal irradiation. Blood 2011;117:412–8.

[6] Cardinale D, Colombo A, Bacchiani G, et al. Early detection of anthracycline cardiotoxicity and improvement with heart failure therapy. Circulation 2015;131:1981–8.

[7] Drafts BC, Twomley KM, D'Agostino R, et al. Low to moderate dose anthracycline-based chemotherapy is associated with early noninvasive imaging evidence of subclinical cardiovascular disease. JACC Cardiovasc Imaging 2013;6:877–85.

[8] Jordan JH, D'Agostino RB, Hamilton CA, et al. Longitudinal assessment of concurrent changes in left ventricular ejection fraction and left ventricular myocardial tissue characteristics after administration of cardiotoxic chemotherapies using T1-weighted and T2-weighted cardiovascular magnetic resonance. Circ Cardiovasc Imaging 2014;7:872–9.

[9] Sawaya H, Sebag IA, Plana JC, et al. Assessment of echocardiography and biomarkers for the extended prediction of cardiotoxicity in patients treated with anthracyclines, taxanes, and trastuzumab. Circ Cardiovasc Imaging 2012;5:596–603.

[10] Ky B, Putt M, Sawaya H, et al. Early increases in multiple biomarkers predict subsequent cardiotoxicity in patients with breast cancer treated with doxorubicin, taxanes, and trastuzumab. J Am Coll Cardiol 2014;63:809–16.

[11] Ewer MS, Ewer SM. Cardiotoxicity of anticancer treatments. Nat Rev Cardiol 2015;12(9):547–1984.

[12] Lotrionte M, Biondi-Zoccai G, Abbate A, et al. Review and meta-analysis of incidence and clinical predictors of anthracycline cardiotoxicity. Am J Cardiol 2013;112:1980–4.

[13] Torti FM, Bristow MM, Lum BL, et al. Cardiotoxicity of epirubicin and doxorubicin: assessment by endomyocardial biopsy. Cancer Res 1986;46:3722–7.

[14] Hoff Von DD, Layard MW, Basa P, et al. Risk factors for doxorubicin-induced congestive heart failure. Ann Intern Med 1979;91:710–7.

[15] Swain SM, Whaley FS, Ewer MS. Congestive heart failure in patients treated with doxorubicin: a retrospective analysis of three trials. Cancer 2003;97:2869–79.

[16] Bosch X, Rovira M, Sitges M, et al. Enalapril and carvedilol for preventing chemotherapy-induced left ventricular systolic dysfunction in patients with malignant hemopathies: the OVERCOME trial (preventiOn of left Ventricular dysfunction with Enalapril and caRvedilol in patients submitted to intensive ChemOtherapy for the treatment of Malignant hEmopathies). J Am Coll Cardiol 2013;61:2355–62.

[17] Kransdorf EP, Kittleson MM. Dissecting the "CHF admission": an evidence-based review of the evaluation and management of acute decompensated heart failure for the hospitalist. J Hosp Med 2012;7:439–45.

[18] Shore S, Grau-Sepulveda MV, Bhatt DL, et al. Characteristics, treatments, and outcomes of hospitalized heart failure patients stratified by etiologies of cardiomyopathy. JACC Heart Fail 2015;3:906–16.

[19] Jaworski C, Mariani JA, Wheeler G, Kaye DM. Cardiac complications of thoracic irradiation. J Am Coll Cardiol 2013;61:2319–28.

[20] Adams MJ. Cardiovascular status in long-term survivors of Hodgkin's disease treated with chest radiotherapy. J Clin Oncol 2004;22:3139–48.

[21] van Nimwegen FA, Schaapveld M, Janus CPM, et al. Cardiovascular disease after Hodgkin lymphoma treatment. JAMA Intern Med 2015;175:1007–11.

[22] Hooning MJ, Botma A, Aleman BMP, et al. Long-term risk of cardiovascular disease in 10-year survivors of breast cancer. J Natl Cancer Inst 2007;99:365–75.

[23] Nativi-Nicolau J, Ryan JJ, Fang JC. Current therapeutic approach in heart failure with preserved ejection fraction. Heart Fail Clin 2014;10:525–38.

[24] Kirklin JK, Naftel DC, Pagani FD, et al. Seventh INTERMACS annual report 15,000 patients and counting. J Heart Lung Transplant 2015;1–10.

[25] Pagani FD, Milano CA, Tatooles AJ, et al. HeartWare HVAD for the treatment of patients with advanced heart failure ineligible for cardiac transplantation_ results of the ENDURANCE destination therapy trial. J Heart Lung Transplant 2015;34:S9.

[26] Heart Failure Society of America, Lindenfeld J, Albert NM, et al. HFSA 2010 Comprehensive Heart Failure Practice Guideline. J Cardiac Failure 2010;16:e1–194.

[27] Feldman D, Pamboukian SV, Teuteberg JJ, et al. The 2013 International Society for Heart and Lung Transplantation Guidelines for mechanical circulatory support: executive summary. J Heart Lung Transplant 2013;32:157–87.

[28] Oliveira GH, Dupont M, Naftel D, et al. Increased need for right ventricular support in patients with chemotherapy-induced cardiomyopathy undergoing mechanical circulatory support: outcomes from the INTERMACS Registry (Interagency Registry for Mechanically Assisted Circulatory Support). J Am Coll Cardiol 2014;63:240–8.

[29] Drazner MH, Velez-Martinez M, Ayers CR, et al. Relationship of right- to left-sided ventricular filling pressures in advanced heart failure: insights from the ESCAPE Trial. Circ Heart Fail 2013;6:264–70.

[30] Drakos SG, Wever Pinzon O, Selzman CH, et al. Magnitude and time course of changes induced by continuous-flow left ventricular assist device unloading in chronic heart failure. J Am Coll Cardiol 2013;61:1985–94.

[31] Castells E, Roca J, Miralles A, et al. Recovery of ventricular function with a left ventricular axial pump in a patient with end-stage toxic cardiomyopathy not a candidate for heart transplantation: first experience in Spain. Transplant Proc 2009;41:2237–9.

[32] Freilich M, Stub D, Esmore D, et al. Recovery from anthracycline cardiomyopathy after long-term support with a continuous flow left ventricular assist device. J Heart Lung Transplant 2009;28:101–3.

[33] Khan N, Husain SA, Husain SI, et al. Remission of chronic anthracycline-induced heart failure with support from a continuous-flow left ventricular assist device. Tex Heart Inst J 2012;39:554–6.

[34] Oliveira GH, Al-Kindi SG, Hoimes C, Park SJ. Characteristics and survival of malignant cardiac tumors: a 40-year analysis of over 500 patients. Circulation 2015;132.

[35] Roberts WC. Primary and secondary neoplasms of the heart. Am J Cardiol 1997;80:671–82.

[36] Bakaeen FG, Jaroszewski DE, Rice DC, et al. Outcomes after surgical resection of cardiac sarcoma in the multimodality treatment era. J Thoracic Cardiovasc Surg 2009;137:1454–60.

[37] Ried M, Rupprecht L, Hirt S, et al. Sequential therapy of primary cardiac lymphoma with cardiectomy, total artificial heart support, and cardiac transplantation. J Heart Lung Transplant 2010;29:707–9.

[38] Ried M, Hirt S, Schmid C. Over 2-year disease-free survival after multimodality therapy of a primary cardiac lymphoma. J Heart Lung Transplant 2012;31:334.

[39] Starzl TE, Penn I, Putnam CW, Groth CG, Halgrimson CG. Iatrogenic alterations of immunologic surveillance in man and their influence on malignancy. Transplantation Rev 1971;7:112–45.

[40] Lund LH, Edwards LB, Kucheryavaya AY, et al. The registry of the International Society for Heart and Lung Transplantation: thirty-first official adult heart transplant report—2014; focus theme: retransplantation. J Heart Lung Transplant 2014;33:996–1008.

[41] Kasiske BL, Cangro CB, Hariharan S, et al. The evaluation of renal transplantation candidates: clinical practice guidelines. Am J Transplant 2001;1(Suppl 2):3–95.

[42] Girndt M, Köhler H. Waiting time for patients with history of malignant disease before listing for organ transplantation. Transplantation 2005;80:S167–70.

[43] Mehra MR, Kobashigawa J, Starling R, et al. Listing criteria for heart transplantation: International Society for Heart and Lung Transplantation guidelines for the care of cardiac transplant candidates—2006. J Heart Lung Transplant 2006;25:1024–42.

[44] Sigurdardottir V, Bjortuft O, Eiskjaer H, et al. Long-term follow-up of lung and heart transplant recipients with pre-transplant malignancies. J Heart Lung Transplant 2012;31:1276–80.

[45] Beaty CA, George TJ, Kilic A, Conte JV, Shah AS. Pre-transplant malignancy: an analysis of outcomes after thoracic organ transplantation. J Heart Lung Transplant 2013;32:202–11.

[46] Yoosabai A, Mehta A, Kang W, et al. Pretransplant malignancy as a risk factor for posttransplant malignancy after heart transplantation. Transplantation 2015;99:345–50.

[47] Higgins RS, Brown RN, Chang PP, et al. A multi-institutional study of malignancies after heart transplantation and a comparison with the general United States population. J Heart Lung Transplant 2014;33:478–85.

[48] Oliveira GH, Hardaway BW, Kucheryavaya AY, Stehlik J, Edwards LB, Taylor DO. Characteristics and survival of patients with chemotherapy-induced cardiomyopathy undergoing heart transplantation. J Heart Lung Transplant 2012;31:805–10.

[49] American Chemical Society. Cancer Facts and Figures 2005. American Chemical Society 2014:1–56.

[50] DePasquale EC, Nasir K, Jacoby DL. Outcomes of adults with restrictive cardiomyopathy after heart transplantation. J Heart Lung Transplant 2012;31:1269–75.

[51] Lenneman AJ, Wang L, Wigger M, et al. Heart transplant survival outcomes for adriamycin-dilated cardiomyopathy. Am J Cardiol 2013;111:609–12.

[52] Uriel N, Vainrib A, Jorde UP, et al. Mediastinal radiation and adverse outcomes after heart transplantation. J Heart Lung Transplant 2010;29:378–81.

[53] Saxena P, Joyce LD, Daly RC, et al. Cardiac transplantation for radiation-induced cardiomyopathy: the Mayo Clinic experience. Ann Thorac Surg 2014;98:2115–21.

[54] Krikorian JG, Anderson JL, Bieber CP, Penn I, Stinson EB. Malignant neoplasms following cardiac transplantation. JAMA 1978;240:639–43.

[55] Engels EA, Pfeiffer RM, Fraumeni JFJ, et al. Spectrum of cancer risk among US solid organ transplant recipients. JAMA 2011;306:1891–901.

[56] Sampaio MS, Cho YW, Qazi Y, Bunnapradist S, Hutchinson IV, Shah T. Posttransplant malignancies in solid organ adult recipients: an analysis of the U.S. National Transplant Database. Transplantation 2012;94:990–8.

[57] Crespo-Leiro MG, Alonso-Pulpon L, Vazquez de Prada JA, et al. Malignancy after heart transplantation: incidence, prognosis and risk factors. Am J Transplant 2008;8:1031–9.

[58] Miao Y, Everly JJ, Gross TG, et al. De novo cancers arising in organ transplant recipients are associated with adverse outcomes compared with the general population. Transplantation 2009;87:1347–59.

[59] Kobashigawa JA, Miller LW, Russell SD, et al. Tacrolimus with mycophenolate mofetil (MMF) or sirolimus vs. cyclosporine with MMF in cardiac transplant patients: 1-year report. Am J Transplant 2006;6:1377–86.

[60] Schena FP, Pascoe MD, Alberu J, et al. Conversion from calcineurin inhibitors to sirolimus maintenance therapy in renal allograft recipients: 24-month efficacy and safety results from the CONVERT trial. Transplantation 2009;87:233–42.

[61] O'Neill JO, Edwards LB, Taylor DO. Mycophenolate mofetil and risk of developing malignancy after orthotopic heart transplantation: analysis of the transplant registry of the International Society for Heart and Lung Transplantation. J Heart Lung Transplant 2006;25:1186–91.

[62] Rivinius R, Helmschrott M, Ruhparwar A, et al. Analysis of malignancies in patients after heart transplantation with subsequent immunosuppressive therapy. Drug Des Devel Ther 2015;9:93–102.

[63] Crespo-Leiro MG, Alonso-Pulpón L, Arizón JM, et al. Influence of induction therapy, immunosuppressive regimen and anti-viral prophylaxis on development of lymphomas after heart transplantation: data from the Spanish Post-Heart Transplant Tumour Registry. J Heart Lung Transplant 2007;26:1105–9.

[64] Kobashigawa JA, Katznelson S, Laks H, et al. Effect of pravastatin on outcomes after cardiac transplantation. N Engl J Med 1995;333:621–7.

[65] Frohlich GM, Rufibach K, Enseleit F, et al. Statins and the risk of cancer after heart transplantation. Circulation 2012;126:440–7.

[66] Fildes JE, Shaw SM, Williams SG, Yonan N. Potential immunologic effects of statins in cancer following transplantation. Cancer Immunol Immunother 2009;58:461–7.

[67] Kauffman HM, Cherikh WS, Cheng Y, Hanto DW, Kahan BD. Maintenance immunosuppression with target-of-rapamycin inhibitors is associated with a reduced incidence of de novo malignancies. Transplantation 2005;80:883–9.

[68] Alberu J, Pascoe MD, Campistol JM, et al. Lower malignancy rates in renal allograft recipients converted to sirolimus-based, calcineurin inhibitor-free immunotherapy: 24-month results from the CONVERT Trial. Transplantation 2011;92:303–10.

[69] Knoll GA, Kokolo MB, Mallick R, et al. Effect of sirolimus on malignancy and survival after kidney transplantation: systematic review and meta-analysis of individual patient data. BMJ 2014;349:g6679.

[70] Kobashigawa JA, Kiyosaki KK, Patel JK, et al. Benefit of immune monitoring in heart transplant patients using ATP production in activated lymphocytes. J Heart Lung Transplant 2010;29:504–8.

[71] Uemura T, Riley TR, Khan A, et al. Immune functional assay for immunosuppressive management in post-transplant malignancy. Clin Transplant 2011;25:E32–7.

[72] Patel J, Kobashigawa JA. Minimization of immunosuppression: transplant immunology. Transpl Immunol 2008;20:48–54.

[73] Kransdorf EP, Stehlik J. Donor evaluation in heart transplantation: the end of the beginning. J Heart Lung Transplant 2014;.

[74] Kauffman HM, Cherikh WS, McBride MA, Cheng Y, Hanto DW. Deceased donors with a past history of malignancy: an organ procurement and transplantation network/united network for organ sharing update. Transplantation 2007;84:272–4.

[75] Nalesnik MA, Woodle ES, DiMaio JM, et al. Donor-transmitted malignancies in organ transplantation: assessment of clinical risk. Am J Transplant 2011;11:1140–7.

[76] Kauffman HM, McBride MA, Cherikh WS, Spain PC, Marks WH, Roza AM. Transplant tumor registry: donor related malignancies. Transplantation 2002;74:358–62.

Chapter 23

Chemotherapy-Associated Arrhythmias

T. Tejada* and M.F. El-Chami**

*Electrophysiology Fellow, Emory University, Atlanta, GA, United States; **Emory University Hospital Midtown, Division of Cardiology-Section of Electrophysiology, Emory University School of Medicine, Atlanta, GA, United States*

INTRODUCTION

The cardiotoxicity of many chemotherapeutic agents is well established. Myocardial damage leading to left ventricular dysfunction, as well as ischemic and pericardial complications are recognized toxic effects of some antineoplastic drugs. Increasingly, however, atrial and ventricular arrhythmias, as well as asymptomatic ECG changes and QT interval prolongation as a risk marker for Torsades des Pointes (TdP), are clinically recognized entities that should be part of patient management and further research (Table 23.1). This chapter will review the current data available on the incidence and associations of atrial and ventricular arrhythmias in cancer patients, with particular attention to the proarrhythmic effects of chemotherapeutic agents.

ATRIAL FIBRILLATION

Atrial fibrillation (AF) is an important arrhythmia to consider in cancer patients not only because it is the most common sustained arrhythmia but also because increasing evidence shows an association between AF and both cancer and chemotherapeutic agents. In addition, treatment of AF represents an important challenge given the cumbersome management of thromboembolic risk in conjunction with an increased bleeding risk in some cancer patients. Finally, the concomitant use of chemotherapy and antiarrhythmic drugs (AAD) may lead to a higher incidence of drug-induced arrhythmia, especially in the common setting of polypharmacy and electrolyte disorders prevalent in cancer patients.

A direct link between AF and cancer has not yet been firmly established, but limited epidemiologic data does suggest a higher incidence of AF in cancer patients. An Italian study in 2008 screened 2339 cancer patients for the presence of AF preoperatively. Nearly half of the group underwent noncancer surgery and the remainder had surgery for a recent diagnosis of colorectal or breast cancer. AF was present in 3.6% of cancer cases and only 1.6% of controls, corresponding to a greater than twofold increased risk of AF

for patients with a cancer diagnosis [1]. Extensive conclusions from this study cannot be reached because patients were only age-matched and multivariate control for cardiovascular risk factors was not included. A larger study with 24,125 patients with newly diagnosed malignant disease, including head and neck, GI, skin, lymphatic, hematopoietic, breast, genitourinary, and other cancers, demonstrated a prevalence of preexisting AF of 2.4%, and a new diagnosis of AF was made in an additional 1.8% of patients. Mortality and incidence of thromboembolism and heart failure was not different between patients with newly diagnosed AF or those with AF at baseline [2]. Yet another large population-based cohort of 28,333 patients, comparing the prevalence of colorectal cancer in patients with and without AF, showed a prevalence of colorectal cancer of 0.59% in AF patients and only 0.05% in those without AF (HR: 11.8; 95% CI 9.3–14.9) [3]. Lastly, an interesting recent Danish cohort study evaluated the incidence of cancer within 3 months of a new diagnosis of AF in 269, 742 patients. There was a low absolute risk (2.5%; 95% confidence interval [CI], 2.4–2.5%) of a cancer diagnosis within those 3 months, but so-called standardized incidence ratios (SIR) calculated by comparing the observed cancer incidence (6656 cancers) with the expected incidence (1302 cancers) on the basis of national cancer rates during the period, yielded an SIR of 5.11 (95% CI, 4.99–5.24) [4]. In juxtaposition, some smaller studies fail to demonstrate cancer as an independent predictor of AF or show any impact of AF on the prognosis of cancer patients [5].

The pathophysiology of any potential causal link between cancer and AF is equally not well established. The coexistence of polypharmacy, comorbid conditions, and cancer-related stressors such as pain, hypoxia, surgery, and chemotherapy obfuscate simple correlations, thus highly controlled studies are required. Currently, some evidence suggests systemic inflammation as an important common operator in the relationship between AF and cancer. More than a decade ago the association between systemic inflammation and AF was first suggested by demonstrating

TABLE 23.1 Risk of SVT, Ventricular Arrhythmia, and Effect on QTc

Drug or Drug Class	Risk of SVT	Risk of VA	QTc Effect
Anthracyclines	Moderate	Small	+
Antimetabolites	Small	Small	+
Cyclophosphamide	Trivial	None	−
Melphalan	High	None	−
Trastuzumab	Trivial	Trivial	−
VEGF TKI	Trivial	High	+++
Antimicrotubules	Trivial	Small	−
Arsenic trioxide	Trivial	Moderate	+++
Thalidomide	Small	Small	−
HDACI	None	High	+++
IL-2	Moderate	Moderate	−
Amsacrine	Moderate	Small	+

Trivial, isolated cases report(s); Small, low incidence in small case series; Moderate, moderate incidence in limited studies; High, moderate to high incidence in several studies and/or box warning for specific risk.

elevated C-reactive protein levels (CRP) in patients with AF, with a noted stepwise CRP elevation with higher AF burden [6]. At a more local level, marked inflammation, myocyte necrosis, and fibrosis have been demonstrated in the atrial biopsies of patients with lone refractory AF compared to an absence of inflammatory changes in control biopsies from Wolff–Parkinson–White patients undergoing surgery [7]. Similarly, evidence exists for a strong inflammatory stimulus following cardiac surgery, with interleukin (IL)-6 levels peaking 6 h after surgery, followed by a second systemic inflammatory response with an increase in CRP that peaks on the second postoperative day, coinciding with the peak incidence of postoperative atrial arrhythmias [8].

Ultimately, the role of inflammation as causal or secondary in AF remains uncertain. This association is nevertheless important in cancer patients given the described existence of systemic inflammation as a function of many particular cancers or related to chemotherapy and comorbid conditions [9]. The common, well-documented, elevated prevalence of postoperative AF in the case of cancer surgery [10] lends itself to speculation on a plausible causative role of inflammation, which may be particularly heightened in these patients. Unfortunately, there has been no direct comparison study evaluating the difference between postoperative AF in cancer patients compared with noncancer patients undergoing similar surgical procedures.

Regardless of the particular relationship between AF and cancer, the prevalence of AF in cancer patients is a clinical reality with unfortunately limited available research regarding optimal management strategies. The current 2014 American Heart Association/American College of Cardiology guidelines make no particular recommendations or discuss the management of AF in the oncology patient [11]. Although there are no studies specifically evaluating the thromboembolic risk in cancer patients with AF, cancer is considered a prothrombotic state. CHADS2 scoring is recommended to help identify those at increased risk of stroke and to guide the use of anticoagulation in the setting of AF. However, a history of cancer is not part of the endorsed $CHADS_2$ [cardiac failure, hypertension, age, diabetes, and stroke (doubled)] and CHA_2DS_2-VASc [congestive heart failure or left ventricular dysfunction, hypertension, age $\geq$ 75 (doubled), diabetes, stroke (doubled)–vascular disease, age 65–74, sex (female)] risk scores used for calculation of thromboembolic risk in AF [11]. Conversely, some malignancies, mostly hematologic and primary or metastatic intracranial tumors are associated with an increased risk of bleeding. Similarly, warfarin (vitamin K antagonist) used for deep venous thrombosis is associated with a sixfold higher risk of hemorrhage in cancer patients [12]. There is no data on the use of novel anticoagulants (dabigatran, rivaroxaban, and apixaban) for stroke prevention in AF as cancer was an exclusion criterion in these trials [13–15]. Interestingly, dalteparin is associated with better survival than vitamin K antagonists in patients with venous thromboembolism and nonmetastatic cancer, and this effect has been speculated to be due to potential antitumor and antimetastatic effects of lower molecular weight heparins (LMWH) that provide a survival benefit in select cancer patients [16–18]. Current American College of Chest Physicians guidelines recommend the use of LMWH over vitamin K antagonists in the first 3 months post venous thromboembolism in cancer patients [19]. The use of LMWH as long-term anticoagulation therapy in cancer patients has not been studied.

Thus, anticoagulation strategies in cancer patients remain a challenge with more questions than answers in the current literature, and an obvious need for a highly individualized approach.

Use of AAD in cancer patients is sometimes necessary due to AF symptom burden and/or to help diminish the thromboembolic risk in patients with contraindications to anticoagulation. Class-III AAD delay ventricular repolarization and place patients at risk for corrected QT (QTc) interval prolongation and ventricular arrhythmias, for example, TdP. Several chemotherapeutic agents, discussed in this chapter, have also been associated with QTc prolongation and risk of drug-induced ventricular arrhythmias. Antibiotics, antifungals, and antiemetics frequently used in cancer patients also increase the risk of TdP. Lastly, commonly occurring electrolyte imbalances, in particular related to potassium and magnesium, further potentiate this risk. For these reasons, use of AAD in this population is quite challenging and limited data exist on the use of these agents in cancer patients. One retrospective analysis of 81 cancer patients who received ibutilide for cardioversion of AF or atrial flutter demonstrated that drug was effective in 75% of cases and no changes in the QTc interval were encountered in patients receiving other QT-prolonging drugs [20].

An additional important consideration when evaluating cancer patients referred for new-onset AF or atrial tachycardia is an assessment of the central venous access location within the heart. At times the PORT catheter is "too deep" in the right atrium (RA) and could be irritating the RA wall. Pulling back the PORT might be necessary to eliminate the problem. In addition, some patients with cancer have preexisting implantable cardiac devices (pacemakers and defibrillators). These patients often require central venous access for chemotherapy infusion and for easier access to the often-required routine blood collection. PORT catheters in these patients should be placed on the contralateral side to the implantable cardiac device to avoid any damage to pacing or defibrillator leads. Also, the subclavian vein is often stenosed or occluded on the ipsilateral side of the pacing/defibrillator system, which might make placement of any catheter technically challenging or not possible.

ANTHRACYCLINES

Anthracyclines are polycyclic aromatic compounds that act as cytostatic antibiotics, exerting their primary antitumor effect by their ability to intercalate into DNA and prevent DNA and RNA synthesis of tumor cells [21]. The specific mechanisms of action elucidated involve inhibition of topoisomerase II [22] and the formation of reactive oxygen species [23]. They are established components in the treatment of many neoplasias, including breast cancer, childhood solid tumors, soft-tissue sarcomata, lymphomas, leukemias, and many others. Danorubicin and doxorubicin were the first isolated compounds in this class and much of the literature regarding cardiac toxicity pertains to these two drugs.

CARDIAC TOXICITY

Anthracyclines have been primarily associated with myocardial damage and a consequent dilated nonischemic cardiomyopathy. First, this is a severe and well-documented late-onset cardiotoxic effect that is closely linked to cumulative dose and which has limited the use of these drugs [24,25]. Second, (*Idarubicin, Epirubicin, Valrubicin*, as well as several others not FDA approved), and third-generation (aclarubicin and others) anthracyclines have been developed, in part, in an effort to improve their therapeutic index relative to adverse cardiac effects [21]. Additionally, molecular modifications by encapsulation (e.g., liposomal doxorubicin) as well as development of new structurally related drugs (e.g., mitoxantrone) [26] have shown some benefit in reducing the incidence of cardiomyopathy. The specific electrophysiological complications reported with certain anthracyclines will be discussed individually as applicable.

The mechanism of anthracycline-induced cardiomyopathy has been attributed to the formation of free radicals and an increase in oxidative stress [25,27]. Initial studies suggested that this increased free radical cascade was a product of: (1) direct intracellular enzymatic reactions with doxorubicin leading to the generation of superoxide and hydrogen peroxide [25,28], and (2) doxorubicin–iron complex formation that served as a catalyst in the conversion of hydrogen peroxide to the hydroxyl radical [29]. Subsequently, doxorubicin inhibition of topoisomerase IIβ in cardiac cells has been shown to be a primary mechanism for the increased formation of free radicals [30] and consequent myocardial toxicity.

Anthracycline-induced cardiac damage manifestations fall into a continuum that extends from asymptomatic elevations of brain natriuretic peptide (BNP), to congestive heart failure symptoms in the setting of a preserved ejection fraction, to advanced dilated cardiomyopathy. Patients with prior cardiovascular disease (hypertension, diabetes, peripheral vascular disease, coronary artery disease) are at higher risk of developing chronic anthracycline cardiotoxicity. Other risk factors include chest irradiation, concomitant use of cardiotoxic agents (e.g., paclitaxel, trastuzumab), and younger age at time of drug exposure. However, the strongest predictor is cumulative anthracycline dose. Ultimately, all patients require long-term monitoring for the development of cardiomyopathy, especially if the ascribed total dose thresholds are reached (e.g., 450–500 mg/m^2 of doxorubicin in adults) [31].

ELECTROPHYSIOLOGIC TOXICITY

ECG changes, dysrhythmias, and other conduction system alterations, as well as a pericarditis–myocarditis syndrome [32], are anthracycline-triggered toxic effects that are less common and have been mostly documented to occur acutely (during infusion, during the first 24 h of drug administration, or in the initial week following completion of therapy). Data on close long-term electrocardiographic monitoring of patients that have received anthracyclines are lacking.

Decreased limb lead QRS voltage by 15–30% may occur in patients treated with first-generation anthracyclines and may be an early sign of myocardial damage [33,34]. There are limited experimental models evaluating the proarrhythmic effects of anthracyclines. One study administrating doxorubicin to mice led to PVCs and ventricular tachycardia (VT) in the presence of ether anesthesia. Noted effects were dose-dependent and fatal arrhythmias occurred at very high doses not comparable to standard doses in humans [35]. Doxorubicin has also been shown to prolong the action potential in a dose-dependent manner in canine Purkinje fibers [36]. Limited data in humans shows primarily nonspecific ST changes and premature atrial contractions (PACs) in patients treated with doxorubicin, with very variable incidence reported (6 and 40%) [37–39]. Incidence of PVCs of up to 24% during the first 24 h of doxorubicin infusion has been reported, but the prevalence may vary depending on the specific anthracycline [39,40]. A single prospective study used Holter monitors to evaluate only 29 patients treated with doxorubicin and demonstrated primarily PACs and premature ventricular contraction (PVCs), but there was also a reported AF incidence of 10% [41].

Rare case reports have also documented development of both Mobitz type-II and complete atrioventricular blocks in patients that have received doxorubicin. Two cases were more clearly associated with acute doxorubicin administration and were treated with pacemaker implantation [41,42]. Two other reported cases from a retrospective series actually developed complete heart block during treatment with cyclophosphamide, although they had previously received doxorubicin. Notably, these patients were treated with isoproterenol, completed the chemotherapy regimen, and did not require pacemaker implantation [43].

QT prolongation has been documented with anthracycline therapy but its clinical significance remains incompletely understood. An early study documented corrected QT (QTc) intervals >480 ms in 14% of children treated with doxorubicin but no clear association with higher incidence of VT [44]. More recent studies comparing QT dispersion between anthracycline-treated and control patients showed no significant difference [45]. TdP has been reported in patients treated with anthracyclines and hypokalemia. However, we are aware of only one case report clearly identifying QT prolongation followed by TdP development in two patients treated with aclarubicin in the absence of a concomitant QT prolonging drug or hypokalemia. Rare cases of monomorphic VT have also been reported without apparent relationship to dose and in the absence of other contributing factors [46,47]. Unfortunately, the paucity of cases does not allow for the identification of risk factors for the development of ventricular arrhythmias in anthracycline-treated patients.

In summary, anthracyclines are a major risk factor for the development of myocardial damage and cardiomyopathy. Myocardial injury is dose dependent and ventricular surveillance with echocardiography or other modalities should be employed for most patients. Approaches to curtail the cardiotoxicity of these agents should be considered when clinically applicable. AF, on the basis of limited data, has a modest but significant incidence in these patients and use of AAD and anticoagulation strategy should be highly individualized. Strict avoidance of hypokalemia and careful ECG monitoring may be considered, especially when QT prolonging drugs are used concomitantly. Aclarubicin may be associated with a higher incidence of QT prolongation and TdP.

ANTIMETABOLITES

Like anthracyclines, antimetabolites interfere with DNA synthesis. These include 5-fluorouracil, capecitabine, gemcitabine, and cytarabine. After anthracyclines, 5-fluorouracil is the antineoplastic agent with the highest incidence of symptomatic cardiotoxicity.

5-Fluorouracil and Capecitabine

The antimetabolite 5-flourouracil (5-FU) is a fluoropyrimidine nucleoside analog widely used in the treatment of gastrointestinal, breast, and head and neck tumors. Capecitabine is an oral prodrug of 5-FU with a very similar cardiotoxicity profile; it is approved for the treatment of colorectal and metastatic breast cancer.

Symptomatic cardiotoxicity is highly variable in both drugs with reports ranging from 0% to 35%. Larger studies show a cardiac symptom burden of 1.2–4.3% and a risk of sudden cardiac death of up to 0.5% [48]. Chest pain is the most frequently reported symptom and is commonly accompanied by ST changes suggestive of ischemia or injury on ECG. However, biomarker evidence of acute myocardial infarction is rare, with an incidence of 14% in only one of three studies measuring troponin and CK-MB in 5-FU-treated patients [48]. Troponin values were not elevated in the remaining studies. Furthermore, a study of patients with angina after 5-FU administration showed no obstructive disease on coronary angiography [49]. Generally, coronary vasospasm has been attributed as the cause of the ischemic clinical picture observed. This is in part supported by two studies measuring brachial artery diameter with high-resolution ultrasound, which demonstrated reproducible, transient contractions of the brachial artery after 5-FU-infusion while no vasoconstriction was observed in controls [50,51]. Glyceryltrinitrate prevented the vascular contractions. Myocarditis [52], endothelial cytotoxicity leading to a thrombogenic effect [53], and Takotsubo cardiomyopathy [54] have also been implicated in the pathogenesis of 5-FU cardiotoxicity.

AF in one series of 76 patients was reported to have an incidence of 6% in 5-FU-treated patients [55]. Most studies show palpitations as a common complaint but supraventricular arrhythmias have mostly been primarily a subclinical phenomenon [48]. 5-FU has been associated with QTc prolongation in two studies [49,56], without documentation of TdP. A small study of continuous Holter monitoring during 5-FU therapy also demonstrated an increase in premature ventricular complexes (PVCs) but no episodes of ventricular tachycardia or ventricular fibrillation (VT or VF) [57].

Overall the incidence of atrial and ventricular arrhythmias or sudden cardiac death with 5-FU or capecitabine is low and clinical surveillance of cardiotoxicity should be focused on ECG monitoring in patients that develop angina. Prompt drug discontinuation and nitrate therapy should be instituted in cases of presumed cardiotoxicity.

The remaining antimetabolites, gemcitabine, and cytarabine, have been rarely associated with arrhythmias. Cases of gemcitabine-associated AF, atrial flutter, and VT with cardiac arrest have been documented. Cytarabine has only been associated with atropine-responsive bradycardia.

ALKYLATING AGENTS

Alkylating agents are cytotoxic agents that act by transferring alkyl groups to DNA, thus interfering with DNA transcription and cell division. Agents in this class include melphalan, cisplatin, cyclophosphamide, chlorambucil, and busulfan.

Cyclophosphamide

High-dose cyclophosphamide (HDC) is arguably the most well established cause of *acute* cardiac toxicity following chemotherapy [58]. An acute cardiomyopathy with left ventricular dysfunction and congestive heart-failure symptoms is typical, but other presentations including hemorrhagic myopericarditis with pericardial effusions, tamponade, and death have also been reported shortly after treatment [59,60]. Unlike anthracyclines, cyclophosphamide-associated cardiotoxicity is not related to cumulative

dose [60]. Previous heart failure, older age, type of cancer (e.g., lymphoma), dose administration regimen, and simultaneous use of other cytotoxic drugs, have all emerged as risk factors [58]. Currently, clinically significant cardiac complications now occur in less than 5% of patients treated with HDC. There is scant data on the association of cyclophosphamide and arrhythmic complications. AF has only once been documented without associated cardiomyopathy [61]. QT prolongation, TdP or VT/VF have not been reported in direct association with cyclophosphamide use.

Ifosfamide is structurally similar to cyclophosphamide and has also been associated with acute cardiomyopathy. Fatal ventricular arrhythmias have been reported in context of acute cardiac damage [62], but otherwise a proarrhythmic effect per se has not been reported. Atrial arrhythmia has only been documented once in a pediatric patient [63].

Melphalan

High dose melphalan (as low as $140 \, \text{mg/m}^2$ in one study, ≥ 200 in mg/m^2 in others) has been associated with the development of AF in several studies in patients ≥ 40 years of age [64–66]. One study with patients age 65 and older treated with melphalan at a dose of $200 \, \text{mg/m}^2$ had an AF incidence of 33% [64]. Patients that developed AF in all studies were treated effectively with propafenone or amiodarone; a minority had spontaneous conversion to normal sinus rhythm. Importantly, all patients in these series had structurally normal hearts. Probably the most compelling evidence of melphalan's association with AF comes from a retrospective study that compared supraventricular tachycardia (SVT) incidence in bone-marrow transplant recipients treated with melphalan or other alkylating or antimicrotubule agents. From a total of 1221 patients, 5.1% developed SVT. The incidence of atrial arrhythmias was higher in the melphalan-treatment groups than all others, with an incidence of 11%. Of these atrial arrhythmias, 70% were AF. As expected, older individuals, those with pre-existing cardiac disease and/or larger left atriums had a higher incidence of AF, as did patients with chronic kidney disease [67].

In short, alkylating agents have been associated in small numbers with atrial arrhythmias, but the data is most compelling for an association of AF with melphalan. Patient's treated with melphalan should be monitored for the development of AF, especially in older patients with predisposing factors such as hypertension, diabetes, and structural heart disease. Cyclophosphamide and isofosfamide cardiotoxicity involves primarily acute myocardial or pericardial disease, and this should be the focus of clinical surveillance. Severe acute cardiomyopathy may be complicated by ventricular arrhythmias that would necessitate standard treatment.

HER2-TARGETING AGENTS AND TYROSINE KINASE INHIBITORS

Trastuzumab is a monoclonal antibody that acts upon the human epidermal growth factor receptor-2 (HER2) and has become an important adjuvant treatment of breast cancer with HER2 overexpression [21]. Trastuzumab has been associated primarily with asymptomatic left ventricular dysfunction, although a cohort of patients does develop symptomatic cardiomyopathy. Unlike anthracycline toxicity, trastuzumab-mediated ventricular damage is not dependent on cumulative dose and is largely reversible [68–70]. Lapatinib, a tyrosine kinase inhibitor (TKI) that also targets HER2, is similarly associated with myocardial toxicity, but limited data suggests a safer cardiotoxic profile than that of trastuzumab [71,72]. The myocardial toxicity of trastuzumab and other HER2-targeted therapies will not be discussed in detail in this chapter.

Trastuzumab has not been found to be proarrhythmic. Exceptions are represented by an isolated case report of VT that resolved after discontinuation of therapy [73] and another of atrial tachycardias following the development of myocardial dysfunction [74].

TKIs broadly include agents that target the human epidermal growth factor receptor-2 (HER2) (e.g., lapatinib) and vascular endothelial growth factor (VEGF) receptor TKIs (vandetanib, sunitinib, sorafenib, lenvatinib, ponatinib). The cardiotoxicity of VEGF-TKIs is primarily related to QT prolongation and a consequent potential for life-threatening ventricular arrhythmias, not cardiomyopathy. A trial-level meta-analysis of 6548 patients compared patients from 18 randomized controlled trials in which one of the arms was a VEGFR TKI [75]. A 4.4 and 0.83% increase in all-grade (>0.45 s) and high-grade (>0.50 s) QTc prolongation, respectively, were observed in VEGR TKI-treated patients. A subgroup analysis showed that only sunitinib and vandetanib were both associated with a statistically significant risk of QTc prolongation; the increased relative risk seen with pazopanib and axitinib was not statistically significant. The effect with vandetanib was dose dependent, but not dependent on duration of therapy. In this particular meta-analysis, the incidence of ventricular arrhythmias including TdP was not higher in patients who developed high-grade QTc prolongation. However, in individual trials, vandetanib has been associated with TdP and sudden death [76,77]. FDA recommends that vandetanib should not be initiated in a patient with a QTc interval greater than 450 ms. Further, routine electrolyte monitoring should be employed prior to drug administration in order to correct any hypocalcemia, hypokalemia, and/or hypomagnesemia. Vandetanib has a 19-day half-life, thus ECGs are recommended to monitor the QT interval at baseline, at 2–4 weeks, and 8–12 weeks after treatment initiation, as well as every 3 months thereafter. Electrolyte and TSH monitoring is recommended on the same schedule. Concurrent administration of drugs known to prolong the QTc interval should be avoided. Therapy should be discontinued in patients who develop a QTc interval greater than 500 ms, and can be resumed at a lower dose when QTc returns to less than 450 ms. Due to this proarrhythmic risk, vandetanib is only available through a restricted distribution program (the Vandetanib Risk Evaluation and Mitigation Strategy [REMS] Program).

Several other TKIs have also been associated with QTc prolongation. Sunitinib has a dose-dependent effect on the QTc interval [77–80]. Conversely, sorafenib affects the QTc interval only in modest degree and is unlikely to be of clinical significance [77,81]. Guidelines for ECG monitoring during sunitinib therapy have not been established. At a minimum, a baseline ECG should be obtained in these patients, as well as avoiding QTc prolonging drugs or conditions. Recurring ECG monitoring during therapy may be considered. Ponatinib is associated with symptomatic bradyarrhythmias in 1% of patients and AF in 5% of patients, according to the US Food and Drug Administration (FDA)-approved manufacturer's package insert. QTc prolongation has not been reported.

Since April 2015, nine more TKIs have been introduced for clinical use (afatinib, cabozantinib, ceritinib, dabrafenib, ibrutinib, lenvatinib, nintedanib, ponatinib, and trametinib). Of these, cabozantinib and ceritinib have been shown to induce a moderate degree of QTc interval prolongation, but primarily cardiac dysfunction has been reported with the use of afatinib, dabrafenib, lenvatinib, ponatinib, and trametinib [82].

In conclusion, trastuzumab and other HER2-targeting agents are associated primarily with left ventricular dysfunction and do not require specific monitoring for arrhythmia development. Patients with baseline QTc prolongation may benefit from a repeat ECG after initiation of therapy to establish a "new baseline," but based on current evidence, would not require more rigorous monitoring. VEFG TKIs on the other hand are clearly associated with QTc prolongation and consequent risk of life-threatening ventricular arrhythmias. These agents require close electrocardiographic monitoring. Further, these drugs should be avoided in patients with conditions that further prolong the QTc interval, namely: patients on AAD or other QTc-prolonging agents; patients with prolonged QTc intervals at baseline, especially ≥500 ms; patients with hypokalemia, hypocalcemia, or hypomagnesemia; and bradycardic patients. Furthermore, concomitant treatment with strong CYP3A4 inhibitors, which may increase plasma concentrations of antiangiogenic TKIs, may require a dose reduction of the TKI.

ANTIMICROTUBULE AGENTS

Antimicrotubule agents act by stabilizing microtubules, thus blocking cell division. Clinically used agents include vinca alkaloids and taxanes (e.g., paclitaxel and docetaxel).

Paclitaxel cardiotoxicity primarily relates to asymptomatic sinus bradycardia (29%) [83] and first-degree atrioventricular block (25%) [84,85]. The National Cancer Institute database demonstrated an almost complete absence of significant conduction or arrhythmia complications, with minimal cases of atrial and ventricular arrhythmias and only four patients of approximately 3400 with second or third degree atrioventricular heart block. VT and VF occurred in only 0.26% patients [84]. Additionally, cardiomyopathy has only been observed in conjunction with anthracyclines [86], albeit it seems lower doses of doxorubicin are required for cardiotoxicity when paclitaxel is used concomitantly [87,88]. Other taxanes have a similarly benign cardiac profile.

ARSENIC TRIOXIDE

Arsenic trioxide is used alone or in combination for the treatment of acute promyelocytic leukemia. It is reserved for patients that do not respond to (or relapse with) first line therapy with retinoid and anthracycline chemotherapy [21]. Arsenic trioxide is an established cardiac toxin. Chronic exposure in drinking water has been linked to prenatal cardiac anomalies, and increased cardiovascular disease in adults. The pathophysiology of arsenic cardiotoxicity is believed to be a function of several mechanisms, including increased intracellular reactive oxygen species formation which in turn leads to increased apoptosis via mitochondrial disruption, MAP kinase activation and caspase activation [21]. Importantly, arsenic trioxide inhibits the rapid component of the delayed rectifier potassium current (IKr) or the slow component of the potassium current (IKs) and activation of the adenosine triphosphate-sensitive potassium current (IKATP) [89]. This may lead to prolonged ventricular repolarization with consequent QTc interval prolongation and risk of TdP.

ECG evidence of arsenic poisoning includes prolongation of the QTc interval, QRS widening, ST depression, and T-wave flattening. Approximately 38.4% of patients on arsenic develop QTc prolongation, with 27% developing QTc duration $\geq$ 500 ms. In this series of 100 patients, one individual with concomitant hypokalemia developed asymptomatic TdP that resolved spontaneously and did not recur after electrolyte repletion [90]. Other studies have also demonstrated QTc prolongation and development of TdP, but nearly all cases have been in association with either hypokalemia, baseline cardiomyopathy, or simply arsenic poisoning not as a result of chemotherapy [90–93]. In one series of 10 patients with acute promyelocytic leukemia, three had sudden deaths. Two of these patients were off the monitor and no definitive cause of death was identified on autopsy, and one developed asystole [94].

Thus, although a mechanism by which arsenic trioxide can lead to QTc prolongation and TdP (cardiac potassium channel modulation) has been established, and documented clinically, the overall incidence of TdP and sudden cardiac death is low and likely associated with other QTc-prolonging conditions. Ultimately, patients treated with arsenic trioxide need ECG monitoring during therapy and require proactive clinical attention to avoiding factors that may contribute to ventricular arrhythmias.

THALIDOMIDE

The mechanism of action of thalidomide is incompletely understood but it is used in multiple myeloma regimens. Thalidomide is primarily associated with venous thromboembolism but case reports of third-degree atrioventricular block [95] and sustained VT [96] have been documented. Of note, baseline ECG changes in these cases were not noted. The data related to electrocardiographic monitoring for arrhythmia-risk in thalidomide-treated patients is limited, and currently there are no specific recommendations for arrhythmia monitoring in these patients. Prospective Holter monitoring during thalidomide therapy may be a relevant approach in future studies to determine arrhythmic risk.

HISTONE DEACETYLASE INHIBITORS

Histone deacetylase inhibitors (HDACI) alter gene expression and modulate apoptosis by reactivating transcription of dormant tumor-suppressor genes. Three HDACIs are available: vorinostat and romidepsin (depsipeptide), used for the treatment of cutaneous T-cell lymphoma, and panobinostat that is approved for treatment of refractory multiple myeloma.

All of these agents have been associated with ECG changes (QTc interval prolongation and ST and T wave changes) [97–99]. A study of 15 patients receiving depsipeptide was terminated prematurely due to significant cases of arrhythmic complications (one had sudden death, two episodes of asymptomatic VT, and three occurrences of QTc prolongation were recorded) [100]. Risk of arrhythmias may be related to rate of drug infusion [101]. Although the available data of cardiotoxicity with panobinostat is limited, the US prescribing information includes a boxed warning about severe or fatal cardiac ischemic events, severe arrhythmias, and ECG changes. The drug is contraindicated in patients with unstable angina or a history of a recent myocardial infarction, and in those with a QTc interval greater than 450 ms, or significant baseline ST-segment or T-wave abnormalities.

INTERLEUKIN-2

Interleukin-2 (IL-2) is produced by activated lymphocytes and induces T-cell proliferation. It is effective in the treatment of metastatic renal cell carcinoma and malignant melanoma. IL-2 has been associated with virtually all arrhythmias (AF, SVT, VT, and bradycardia) [102–104]. In patients with underlying CAD, ischemic events and death have also been reported [104]. A mechanistic link has not been identified but most patients treated with high doses of IL-2 develop a capillary leak syndrome with associated hypotension and tachycardia, which may conceivably contribute to tachyarrhythmias in susceptible patients. One of the larger studies analyzed over 300 patients treated with 423 courses of IL-2. AF was associated with 8% of drug courses administered, and 1.7% were associated with prolonged atrial arrhythmias and hypotension [105]. Given these association, patients with underlying CAD and those with increased hemodynamic susceptibility require closer hemodynamic and ECG monitoring with IL-2 administration.

AMSACRINE

Amsacrine is used in the treatment of leukemia and acts at least in part by topoisomerase II inhibition, similar to anthracyclines. Not surprisingly, QTc prolongation, atrial and ventricular arrhythmias, heart failure, and sudden death have all been reported. However, the overall incidence of amsacrine-related arrhythmia may be low. A study of 5340 patients treated with amsacrine had only a 0.7% occurrence of arrhythmia. Other authors report higher incidence of arrhythmias with this chemotherapeutic agent [101].

CONCLUSIONS

The proarrhythmic cardiotoxicity of chemotherapeutic agents is an increasingly recognized phenomenon. Although the data on prevalence and risk factors for the development of chemotherapy-induced arrhythmias is limited, there is an evident association with many agents. Cardiologists and oncologists alike must maintain a high index of suspicion in patients that develop palpitations, presyncope, or syncope in the course of their cancer treatment and pursue more aggressive electrocardiographic monitoring in such cases. More importantly, the clinician needs to proactively minimize the proarrhythmic risk of patients with or without underlying cardiovascular disease that in the course of their chemotherapy are exposed to multiple QTc-prolonging agents and to substantial electrolyte disturbances. A common theme with most of the agents discussed is that despite their inherent proarrhythmic risk as evidenced by ECG changes, actual incidence of serious ventricular arrhythmias is low and highly associated with other predisposing conditions. Further research will be necessary regarding optimal surveillance strategies and more controlled studies for the identification of individuals at high-risk of chemotherapy-induced arrhythmias.

REFERENCES

[1] Guzzetti S, et al. First diagnosis of colorectal or breast cancer and prevalence of atrial fibrillation. Intern Emerg Med 2008;3(3): p227–31.

[2] Hu YF, et al. Incident thromboembolism and heart failure associated with new-onset atrial fibrillation in cancer patients. Int J Cardiol 2013;165(2):355–7.

[3] Erichsen R, et al. Colorectal cancer and risk of atrial fibrillation and flutter: a population-based case-control study. Intern Emerg Med 2012;7(5):431–8.

[4] Ostenfeld EB, et al. Atrial fibrillation as a marker of occult cancer. PLoS One 2014;9(8):pe102861.

[5] Velagapudi P, Turagam MK, Kocheril AG. Atrial fibrillation in cancer patients: an underrecognized condition. South Med J 2011;104(9):667–8.

[6] Chung MK, et al. C-reactive protein elevation in patients with atrial arrhythmias: inflammatory mechanisms and persistence of atrial fibrillation. Circulation 2001;104(24):2886–91.

[7] Frustaci A, et al. Histological substrate of atrial biopsies in patients with lone atrial fibrillation. Circulation 1997;96(4):1180–4.

[8] Bruins P, et al. Activation of the complement system during and after cardiopulmonary bypass surgery: postsurgery activation involves C-reactive protein and is associated with postoperative arrhythmia. Circulation 1997;96(10):3542–8.

[9] Roxburgh CS, McMillan DC. Cancer and systemic inflammation: treat the tumour and treat the host. Br J Cancer 2014;110(6): 1409–12.

[10] Farmakis D, Parissis J, Filippatos G. Insights into onco-cardiology: atrial fibrillation in cancer. J Am Coll Cardiol 2014;63(10):945–53.

[11] January CT, et al. 2014 AHA/ACC/HRS guideline for the management of patients with atrial fibrillation: a report of the American College of Cardiology/American Heart Association Task Force on Practice Guidelines and the Heart Rhythm Society. J Am Coll Cardiol 2014;64(21):pe1–pe76.

[12] Hutten BA, et al. Incidence of recurrent thromboembolic and bleeding complications among patients with venous thromboembolism in relation to both malignancy and achieved international normalized ratio: a retrospective analysis. J Clin Oncol 2000;18(17):3078–83.

[13] Connolly SJ, et al. Dabigatran versus warfarin in patients with atrial fibrillation. N Engl J Med 2009;361(12):1139–51.

[14] Patel MR, et al. Rivaroxaban versus warfarin in nonvalvular atrial fibrillation. N Engl J Med 2011;365(10):883–91.

[15] Granger CB, et al. Apixaban versus warfarin in patients with atrial fibrillation. N Engl J Med 2011;365(11):981–92.

[16] Lee AY, et al. Randomized comparison of low molecular weight heparin and coumarin derivatives on the survival of patients with cancer and venous thromboembolism. J Clin Oncol 2005;23(10):2123–9.

[17] Klerk CP, et al. The effect of low molecular weight heparin on survival in patients with advanced malignancy. J Clin Oncol 2005;23(10):2130–5.

[18] Niers TM, et al. Mechanisms of heparin induced anti-cancer activity in experimental cancer models. Crit Rev Oncol Hematol 2007;61(3):195–207.

[19] Kearon C, et al. Antithrombotic therapy for venous thromboembolic disease: American College of Chest Physicians Evidence-Based Clinical Practice Guidelines (8th Edition). Chest 2008;133 (6 Suppl):454S–545S.

[20] Bickford CL, et al. Efficacy and safety of ibutilide for chemical cardioversion of atrial fibrillation and atrial flutter in cancer patients. Am J Med Sci 2014;347(4):277–81.

[21] Weber GF. Molecular therapies of cancer. Springer International Publishing; Switzerland.

[22] Liu LF. DNA topoisomerase poisons as antitumor drugs. Annu Rev Biochem 1989;58:351–75.

[23] Taatjes DJ, et al. Redox pathway leading to the alkylation of DNA by the anthracycline, antitumor drugs adriamycin and daunomycin. J Med Chem 1997;40(8):1276–86.

[24] Lefrak EA, et al. A clinicopathologic analysis of adriamycin cardiotoxicity. Cancer 1973;32(2):302–14.

[25] Singal PK, Iliskovic N. Doxorubicin-induced cardiomyopathy. N Engl J Med 1998;339(13):900–5.

[26] Smith LA, et al. Cardiotoxicity of anthracycline agents for the treatment of cancer: systematic review and meta-analysis of randomised controlled trials. BMC Cancer 2010;10:337.

[27] Doroshow JH. Doxorubicin-induced cardiac toxicity. N Engl J Med 1991;324(12):843–5.

[28] Sinha BK, et al. Adriamycin-stimulated hydroxyl radical formation in human breast tumor cells. Biochem Pharmacol 1987;36(6):793–6.

[29] Myers C. The role of iron in doxorubicin-induced cardiomyopathy. Semin Oncol 1998;25(4 Suppl 10):10–4.

[30] Zhang S, et al. Identification of the molecular basis of doxorubicin-induced cardiotoxicity. Nat Med 2012;18(11):1639–42.

[31] Hensley ML, et al. American Society of Clinical Oncology 2008 clinical practice guideline update: use of chemotherapy and radiation therapy protectants. J Clin Oncol 2009;27(1):127–45.

[32] Harrison DT, Sanders LA, Letter:. Pericarditis in a case of early daunorubicin cardiomyopathy. Ann Intern Med 1976;85(3):339–41.

[33] Ali MK, et al. Noninvasive cardiac evaluation of patients receiving adriamycin-containing adjuvant chemotherapy (FAC) for stage II or III breast cancer. J Surg Oncol 1983;23(3):212–6.

[34] Shapira J, et al. Reduced cardiotoxicity of doxorubicin by a 6-hour infusion regimen. A prospective randomized evaluation. Cancer 1990;65(4):870–3.

[35] Aversano RC, Boor PJ. Acute doxorubicin-induced cardiac arrhythmias during ether anesthesia. Res Commun Chem Pathol Pharmacol 1983;41(2):345–8.

[36] Binah O, Cohen IS, Rosen MR. The effects of adriamycin on normal and ouabain-toxic canine Purkinje and ventricular muscle fibers. Circ Res 1983;53(5):655–62.

[37] Middleman E, Luce J, Frei E 3rd. Clinical trials with adriamycin. Cancer 1971;28(4):844–50.

[38] Dindogru A, et al. Electrocardiographic changes following adriamycin treatment. Med Pediatr Oncol 1978;5(1):65–71.

[39] Friess GG, et al. Effects of first-dose doxorubicin on cardiac rhythm as evaluated by continuous 24-hour monitoring. Cancer 1985;56(12):2762–4.

[40] Salminen E, et al. Docetaxel with epirubicin—investigations on cardiac safety. Anticancer Drugs 2003;14(1):73–7.

[41] Kilickap S, et al. Early and late arrhythmogenic effects of doxorubicin. South Med J 2007;100(3):262–5.

[42] Kilickap S, et al. Doxorubicin-induced second degree and complete atrioventricular block. Europace 2005;7(3):227–30.

[43] Ando M, et al. Cardiac conduction abnormalities in patients with breast cancer undergoing high-dose chemotherapy and stem cell transplantation. Bone Marrow Transplant 2000;25(2):185–9.

[44] Larsen RL, et al. Electrocardiographic changes and arrhythmias after cancer therapy in children and young adults. Am J Cardiol 1992;70(1):73–7.

[45] Amoozgar H, et al. Heart repolarization changes after anthracycline therapy in the children with cancer. Iran J Ped Hematol Oncol 2014;4(3):103–8.

[46] Wortman JE, et al. Sudden death during doxorubicin administration. Cancer 1979;44(5):1588–91.

[47] Rudzinski T, et al. Doxorubicin-induced ventricular arrhythmia treated by implantation of an automatic cardioverter-defibrillator. Europace 2007;9(5):278–80.

[48] Polk A, et al. Cardiotoxicity in cancer patients treated with 5-fluorouracil or capecitabine: a systematic review of incidence, manifestations and predisposing factors. Cancer Treat Rev 2013;39(8):974–84.

[49] Wacker A, et al. High incidence of angina pectoris in patients treated with 5-fluorouracil. A planned surveillance study with 102 patients. Oncology 2003;65(2):108–12.

[50] Salepci T, et al. 5-Fluorouracil induces arterial vasoconstrictions but does not increase angiotensin II levels. Med Oncol 2010;27(2):416–20.

[51] Sudhoff T, et al. 5-Fluorouracil induces arterial vasocontractions. Ann Oncol 2004;15(4):661–4.

[52] Sasson Z, et al. 5-Fluorouracil related toxic myocarditis: case reports and pathological confirmation. Can J Cardiol 1994;10(8):861–4.

[53] Cwikiel M, et al. The appearance of endothelium in small arteries after treatment with 5-fluorouracil. An electron microscopic study of late effects in rabbits. Scanning Microsc 1996;10(3):805–18. discussion 819.

[54] Grunwald MR, Howie L, Diaz LA Jr. Takotsubo cardiomyopathy and Fluorouracil: case report and review of the literature. J Clin Oncol 2012;30(2):e11–4.

[55] Eskilsson J, Albertsson M, Mercke C. Adverse cardiac effects during induction chemotherapy treatment with cis-platin and 5-fluorouracil. Radiother Oncol 1988;13(1):41–6.

[56] Oztop I, et al. Evaluation of cardiotoxicity of a combined bolus plus infusional 5-fluorouracil/folinic acid treatment by echocardiography, plasma troponin I level, QT interval and dispersion in patients with gastrointestinal system cancers. Jpn J Clin Oncol 2004;34(5):262–8.

[57] Yilmaz U, et al. 5-fluorouracil increases the number and complexity of premature complexes in the heart: a prospective study using ambulatory ECG monitoring. Int J Clin Pract 2007;61(5):795–801.

[58] Morandi P, et al. Cardiac toxicity of high-dose chemotherapy. Bone Marrow Transplant 2005;35(4):323–34.

[59] Appelbaum F, et al. Acute lethal carditis caused by high-dose combination chemotherapy. A unique clinical and pathological entity. Lancet 1976;1(7950):58–62.

[60] Gottdiener JS, et al. Cardiotoxicity associated with high-dose cyclophosphamide therapy. Arch Intern Med 1981;141(6):758–63.

[61] Ifran A, Kaptan K, Beyan C. High-dose cyclophosphamide and MESNA infusion can cause acute atrial fibrillation. Am J Hematol 2005;80(3):247.

[62] Quezado ZM, et al. High-dose ifosfamide is associated with severe, reversible cardiac dysfunction. Ann Intern Med 1993;118(1):31–6.

[63] Muller L, et al. Recurrent atrial ectopic tachycardia following chemotherapy with ifosfamide. Pediatr Hematol Oncol 2004;21(4):307–11.

[64] Olivieri A, et al. Paroxysmal atrial fibrillation after high-dose melphalan in five patients autotransplanted with blood progenitor cells. Bone Marrow Transplant 1998;21(10):1049–53.

[65] Moreau P, et al. Melphalan 220 mg/m2 followed by peripheral blood stem cell transplantation in 27 patients with advanced multiple myeloma. Bone Marrow Transplant 1999;23(10):1003–6.

[66] Phillips GL, et al. Amifostine and autologous hematopoietic stem cell support of escalating-dose melphalan: a phase I study. Biol Blood Marrow Transplant 2004;10(7):473–83.

[67] Feliz V, et al. Melphalan-induced supraventricular tachycardia: incidence and risk factors. Clin Cardiol 2011;34(6):356–9.

[68] Romond EH, et al. Trastuzumab plus adjuvant chemotherapy for operable HER2-positive breast cancer. N Engl J Med 2005;353(16):1673–84.

[69] Smith I, et al. 2-year follow-up of trastuzumab after adjuvant chemotherapy in HER2-positive breast cancer: a randomised controlled trial. Lancet 2007;369(9555):29–36.

[70] Slamon D, et al. Adjuvant trastuzumab in HER2-positive breast cancer. N Engl J Med 2011;365(14):1273–83.

[71] Geyer CE, et al. Lapatinib plus capecitabine for HER2-positive advanced breast cancer. N Engl J Med 2006;355(26):2733–43.

[72] Perez EA, et al. Cardiac safety of lapatinib: pooled analysis of 3689 patients enrolled in clinical trials. Mayo Clin Proc 2008;83(6):679–86.

[73] Ferguson C, Clarke J, Herity NA. Ventricular tachycardia associated with trastuzumab. N Engl J Med 2006;354(6):648–9.

[74] Olin RL, et al. Non-myopathic cardiac events in two patients treated with trastuzumab. Breast J 2007;13(2):211–2.

[75] Ghatalia P, et al. QTc interval prolongation with vascular endothelial growth factor receptor tyrosine kinase inhibitors. Br J Cancer 2015;112(2):296–305.

[76] Zang J, et al. Incidence and risk of QTc interval prolongation among cancer patients treated with vandetanib: a systematic review and meta-analysis. PLoS One 2012;7(2):pe30353.

[77] Shah RR, Morganroth J, Shah DR. Cardiovascular safety of tyrosine kinase inhibitors: with a special focus on cardiac repolarisation (QT interval). Drug Saf 2013;36(5):295–316.

[78] Bello CL, et al. Electrocardiographic characterization of the QTc interval in patients with advanced solid tumors: pharmacokinetic–pharmacodynamic evaluation of sunitinib. Clin Cancer Res 2009;15(22):7045–52.

[79] Strevel EL, Ing DJ, Siu LL. Molecularly targeted oncology therapeutics and prolongation of the QT interval. J Clin Oncol 2007;25(22):3362–71.

[80] Schmidinger M, et al. Cardiac toxicity of sunitinib and sorafenib in patients with metastatic renal cell carcinoma. J Clin Oncol 2008;26(32):5204–12.

[81] Tolcher AW, et al. A phase I open-label study evaluating the cardiovascular safety of sorafenib in patients with advanced cancer. Cancer Chemother Pharmacol 2011;67(4):751–64.

[82] Shah RR, Morganroth J. Update on cardiovascular safety of tyrosine kinase inhibitors: with a special focus on QT interval, left ventricular dysfunction and overall risk/benefit. Drug Saf 2015;38(8):693–710.

[83] Rowinsky EK, et al. Clinical toxicities encountered with paclitaxel (Taxol). Semin Oncol 1993;20(4 Suppl 3):1–15.

[84] Arbuck SG, et al. A reassessment of cardiac toxicity associated with Taxol. J Natl Cancer Inst Monogr 1993;(15):117–30.

[85] McGuire WP, et al. Taxol: a unique antineoplastic agent with significant activity in advanced ovarian epithelial neoplasms. Ann Intern Med 1989;111(4):273–9.

[86] Gehl J, et al. Combined doxorubicin and paclitaxel in advanced breast cancer: effective and cardiotoxic. Ann Oncol 1996;7(7):687–93.

[87] Giordano SH, et al. A detailed evaluation of cardiac toxicity: a phase II study of doxorubicin and one- or three-hour-infusion paclitaxel in patients with metastatic breast cancer. Clin Cancer Res 2002;8(11):3360–8.

[88] Biganzoli L, et al. Doxorubicin-paclitaxel: a safe regimen in terms of cardiac toxicity in metastatic breast carcinoma patients. Results from a European Organization for Research and Treatment of Cancer multicenter trial. Cancer 2003;97(1):40–5.

[89] Alamolhodaei NS, Shirani K, Karimi G. Arsenic cardiotoxicity: an overview. Environ Toxicol Pharmacol 2015;40(3):1005–14.

[90] Barbey JT, Pezzullo JC, Soignet SL. Effect of arsenic trioxide on QT interval in patients with advanced malignancies. J Clin Oncol 2003;21(19):3609–15.

[91] Naito K, et al. Two cases of acute promyelocytic leukemia complicated by torsade de pointes during arsenic trioxide therapy. Int J Hematol 2006;83(4):318–23.

[92] Goldsmith S, From AH. Arsenic-induced atypical ventricular tachycardia. N Engl J Med 1980;303(19):1096–8.

[93] Beer TM, et al. Southwest Oncology Group phase II study of arsenic trioxide in patients with refractory germ cell malignancies. Cancer 2006;106(12):2624–9.

[94] Westervelt P, et al. Sudden death among patients with acute promyelocytic leukemia treated with arsenic trioxide. Blood 2001;98(2):266–71.

[95] Hinterseer M, et al. Thalidomide-induced symptomatic third-degree atrioventricular block. Clin Res Cardiol 2006;95(9):474–6.

[96] Ballanti S, et al. Sustained ventricular tachycardia in a thalidomide-treated patient with primary plasma-cell leukemia. Nat Clin Pract Oncol 2007;4(12):722–5.

[97] Richardson PG, et al. Bortezomib or high-dose dexamethasone for relapsed multiple myeloma. N Engl J Med 2005;352(24):2487–98.

[98] Berenson JR, et al. Safety of prolonged therapy with bortezomib in relapsed or refractory multiple myeloma. Cancer 2005;104(10):2141–8.

[99] Siegel DS, et al. A phase 2 study of single-agent carfilzomib (PX-171-003-A1) in patients with relapsed and refractory multiple myeloma. Blood 2012;120(14):2817–25.

[100] Shah MH, et al. Cardiotoxicity of histone deacetylase inhibitor depsipeptide in patients with metastatic neuroendocrine tumors. Clin Cancer Res 2006;12(13):3997–4003.

[101] Guglin M, et al. Introducing a new entity: chemotherapy-induced arrhythmia. Europace 2009;11(12):1579–86.

[102] White RL Jr, et al. Cardiopulmonary toxicity of treatment with high dose interleukin-2 in 199 consecutive patients with metastatic melanoma or renal cell carcinoma. Cancer 1994;74(12):3212–22.

[103] Oleksowicz L, et al. Sustained ventricular tachycardia and its successful prophylaxis during high-dose bolus interleukin-2 therapy for metastatic renal cell carcinoma. Am J Clin Oncol 2000;23(1):34–6.

[104] Margolin KA, et al. Interleukin-2 and lymphokine-activated killer cell therapy of solid tumors: analysis of toxicity and management guidelines. J Clin Oncol 1989;7(4):486–98.

[105] Lee RE, et al. Cardiorespiratory effects of immunotherapy with interleukin-2. J Clin Oncol 1989;7(1):7–20.

Index